A CONSUMER'S GUIDE TO PRESCRIPTION MEDICINES

Dr Barrington Cooper and Dr Laurence Gerlis
Consultant Pharmacist: Dawn Hurrell

With a Foreword by
TP Astill LLB, BPharmS, FRPharmS, FBIM
Director, National Pharmaceutical Association

- All commonly prescribed medicines,
vaccines and contraceptives included •
- All known side effects listed •
- Key medical terms explained •
- Easy-to-follow table of drug interactions •

NEW EDITION
Fully revised in line with new prescribing practices

TED SMART

Edited by Neil Curtis
Designed by Richard Garratt

This edition first published 1996 for The Book People
Guardian House, Borough Road, Godalming, Surrey GU7 2AE
by Hamlyn, an imprint of Reed International Books
Michelin House, 81 Fulham Road, London SW3 6RB
and Auckland, Melbourne, Singapore and Toronto

A catalogue record for this book is available from the British Library

ISBN 1 85613 332 X

Printed in Great Britain

In the introductory sections of this book, it has been emphasized that
A Consumer's Guide to Prescription Medicines must not be used for
self-prescription. Nor is it intended to be a substitute for the advice of
a prescribing physician or the instructions on the medicine's package.

Every effort has been made to ensure that the information contained
in the book is as accurate and up-to-date as possible at the time of
going to press but medical and pharmaceutical knowledge continues
to progress, and the use of a particular medicine may be different for
every patient. **Always** consult your medical practitioner or other
qualified medical specialist for advice.

The authors, editors, consultants, and publishers of this book can
not be held liable for any errors or omissions, nor for any consequences
of using it.

Preface to the Third Edition

The continued demand for more and better information has led to people turning to this book. It provides information on their treatment, not only on which condition is being treated but also on the dose, interactions, and side effects, as well as the availability of treatment. Barely thirty years ago, patients were denied access to this type of information and were not even told which treatment they were receiving.

The need for information and openness in medicine is to be encouraged, not suppressed. Recent changes in providing patient information leaflets have underlined the trend. Other changes in the practise of medicine include full patient access to their own notes, and more products switching to over-the-counter status. These form part of the overall revolution in medical care.

This third edition has been expanded to include more products, such as common injectables, vaccines, medicated dressings, fluoride supplements, contraceptives, and so on. It also reflects changes in medical practice such as the trend towards prescribing generic, as opposed to branded, products, as well as the opportunity for nurses to prescribe some preparations (on a trial basis at the moment) without reference to a doctor. We are grateful to our consulting pharmacist Dawn Hurrell for all her hard work, advice, and energy, without which this work would not have been completed. In addition, Charles Fowkes, Neil Curtis, and Richard Garratt have been essential to the development of the Guide.

We have also incorporated many readers' suggestions, and we continue to invite comment.

Dr Barrington Cooper and Dr Laurence Gerlis
21 Devonshire Place, London W1
1996

Preface to the Second Edition

The acceptance this Guide has received since it was first published in 1990 has been gratifying. We offered information to patients that was previously not available to them and, as consumers, they have responded warmly to the book. Providing patients with information about their treatment has proved to be part of the new wave in medical care in which the person participates actively rather than passively accepting authority.

This fully revised second edition incorporates the hundreds of changes to prescription medicines which have occurred over the past three years. Many new products are included and many amendments have been made. The work of Dawn Hurrell has been invaluable in the preparation of this edition and, as a practising pharmacist, she underlines our belief in the team concept of medical treatment and in the importance of the pharmacist's role.

A Consumer's Guide to Prescription Medicines has been used by pharmacists to offer information to patients at the time the prescription is collected. In addition to the doctor/patient relationship, the pharmacist/patient interaction provides an opportunity to involve patients in the pharmaceutical aspects of their medical care.

It is our intention to continue to improve and update this book. Reader's enquiries have always been helpful, and they contribute to the interaction between patient and doctor. We see this book as an integral part of that relationship.

Dr Barrington Cooper and Dr Laurence Gerlis
21 Devonshire Place, London W1
1992

Preface to the First Edition

We have always felt that patient education is a vital part of the healing process in preventive and therapeutic medicine. Those patients who are best informed are also those for whom treatment is most likely to be successful.

The main purpose of this book is only to reinforce advice which a prescribing doctor has given already to a patient receiving that prescription. It confirms information about drug names and type, as well as the condition which is being treated.

As prescribing physicians, we have made a conscious effort to provide information without, in any way, undermining the vitally important doctor-patient relationship. Thus, we have excluded inject-able preparations and a small number of other sensitive areas of information. Our decision to use brand and generic names is not a statement of medical politics, but it is designed to help people who may have medication prescribed in either way. New European laws on product liability require a physician to explain possible side effects to patients, and this book will, to some extent, fulfil this role. Thus, *A Consumer's Guide to Prescription Medicines* should also be a valu-able aid to doctors who are prescribing the medications listed.

Dr Barrington Cooper and Dr Laurence Gerlis
21 Devonshire Place, London W1
1989

Foreword

It is no exaggeration to say that the last fifty years have seen a revolution in pharmacy and medicine. In the 'good old days', the family doctor would write a prescription which was usually in the form of a recipe and, quite deliberately, in semi-legible handwriting so that the patient could not read it — just in case the patient was able to decipher the writing, the names of the ingredients were in abbreviated Latin! The pharmacist would look at the prescription, nod sagely, and disappear out of sight behind his dispensary screen to make the pills or to mix the ingredients of the ointment or medicine. The name of the product never appeared on the label because everyone, including most patients, felt that it was undesirable for ordinary people to know what had been prescribed. It can now be revealed that what was in the bottle was probably innocuous and pharmacologically ineffective. The curative power of medicine in those days derived in large measure from the mystery and mystique which surrounded its preparation, coupled always with the doctor's bedside manner and confident reassurance.

Since then, there has been an enormous increase in scientific knowledge, especially of the way in which chemical substances affect the organs of the human body and of the way in which the body itself works. Antibiotics and other anti-infective agents have also been discovered, with the result that many hitherto fatal diseases have either disappeared altogether or can now be cured easily. Those who criticize the pharmaceutical industry forget too readily the former ravages of tuberculosis, polio, meningitis, septicaemia, typhoid fever, endocarditis, and other killing and crippling diseases. Many people suffering from asthma, epilepsy, hormone deficiency, or allergy can now lead a normal life whereas they would previously have been severely handicapped, confined to a wheelchair, or dead at an early age. Modern advances in surgery, such as organ transplants, have also been made possible by the drugs which control the body's natural tendency to reject 'invaders'.

Alongside this pharmaceutical revolution, there has also been a consumer revolution. Nowadays, you want to **know** what kind of drugs you are taking, and rightly so. While some people may regret the passing of the age of medicinal mystique, most of us prefer to be told precisely what is wrong with us and what is being provided to put us right. We want to know what effect the medicine is likely to have, what side effects might occur, and what precautions we need to take to ensure that the medicine behaves as it should. The modern medicine is certainly a powerful weapon for good, but it is also often complex in its chemistry and formulation. It is important, therefore, that patients are properly informed about their medicines, not only for their own peace of mind, but also so that the product gives them the maximum possible benefit with the minimum risk of harm.

For these reasons, I welcome warmly this new book by Dr Cooper and Dr Gerlis. In simple language it tells us what we need to know about our prescribed medicines. It reinforces and supplements what we have been told by our doctor and pharmacist, it will help us to understand why a particular medicine has been selected; and it tells us how it should be used. As the authors emphasize in their introduction, the book is not intended to be a substitute for professional advice. You should not hesitate to talk to your doctor or pharmacist if you are in serious doubt about any aspect of your treatment. But this book is a very usable source of reference and will fill reassuringly many gaps in our knowledge. It will help to remove those little apprehensions which many of us feel when we leave the surgery with the prescription and the pharmacy with our medicine.

T P Astill LLB, BPharmS, FRPharmS, FBIM
Director, National Pharmaceutical Association

How the book works

Apart from some injectables and a small number of other medicines and appliances, all medicines which may be commonly prescribed through the National Health Service or private practice in the United Kingdom should be found in this book. They are arranged in strict alphabetical order throughout with brand names, generic names, and any commonly used medical terms contained within the same sequence. There is also a chart to be found on page 713 which explains the way in which various drugs may interact with one another or with other substances such as alcohol. Some drugs are required to be prescribed by its generic, or scientific, name only and it is then up to the dispensing pharmacist to select a particular manufacturer's product. Other drugs are prescribed by a brand name. In this book, the main description of any preparation is to be found under its most commonly prescribed name, which may be either a brand name or a generic, and then the alternative generic or brand name, also found within the alphabetic sequence, will cross refer to the main entry.

Similarly, one particular medicine may be manufactured by more than one drug company under a variety of brand names. In such cases the authors have selected one preparation to be given the complete description, and then other preparations are, once again, cross-referred to the main entry. And, of course, the main entry also refers in its 'Other preparations' to any other manufacturer's version of the medicine. Thus, no matter what name has been used on the container of a medicine dispensed to a patient, it is a simple matter quickly to find a full description of the preparation.

The name of the medicine is given in bold type at the beginning of each entry, with the name of the manufacturing company in brackets on the next line. A short paragraph then follows describing the medicine in terms of its appearance, strength where this is relevant, what kind of drug it is — eg antacid, and what it is used to treat — eg dyspepsia. The usual dose or dose range is given for the particular uses of the medicine, including any variations that may be required to treat children, the elderly, or in any other special circumstances. The next section indicates whether the drug is available through the NHS, by private prescription, or over the counter without any prescription being needed. Any possible side effects that the medicine might produce are explained as well as any cautionary advice in its use. It is clearly stated If a medicine is not to be used for particular groups of patients, such as pregnant women, or to treat certain conditions or states. And any known interactions with other medicines or substances such as alcohol are also indicated. The components of the preparation are given in terms of their scientific names, and any other preparations of these components are also included at the end of the entry.

How to use this book (including how *not* to use it)

When a doctor prescribes a medicine for a patient, then he or she will always explain carefully to the patient how it is to be used. Similarly, the pharmacist will always write instructions for the drug's dose on the container, and the name of the drug will also be clearly visible. If you look up the name in *A Consumer's Guide to Prescription Medicines*, you will be able to confirm that you have understood the doctor's instructions fully so that you can be confident you are making the best possible use of the medicine. It will also help you to anticipate and prepare for any possible side effects, and ensure that you are not taking anything else which perhaps the doctor was not made aware of and which might interact with the prescription. More importantly perhaps, the book will enable you to become better informed generally about the medicine(s) which has been prescribed to treat or prevent a particular condition.

A Consumer's Guide to Prescription Medicines is **not** a guide to self-prescription. Nor is it a 'home doctor'. The authors recognize clearly that it is the advice of the prescribing doctor, given after a careful investigation of the patient and his or her symptoms, that should always be followed by patients. If the information given in this book differs in any particular from the doctor's recommendations about a medicine, this must only be a basis for discussing such differences with the prescribing doctor or perhaps with the dispensing pharmacist.

The information contained in this book should not be followed in preference to the recommendations of the prescription even though it has been compiled by highly qualified physicians and a pharmacist using the most up-to-date sources. There are few doctors or pharmacists who do not welcome well-informed questioning by their patients, and it is the purpose of this book to add to the information already given by the prescribing physician in the surgery and on the product's labelling. On the other hand, the authors have chosen not to include the names and addresses of the manufacturers of the drugs described because it is the policy of most drug companies not to respond directly to enquiries concerning their medicines from individual patients; generally, they will refer such enquiries back to the general practitioner.

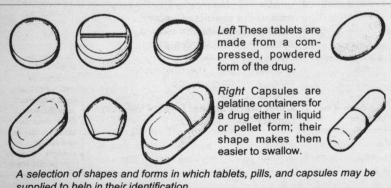

Left These tablets are made from a compressed, powdered form of the drug.

Right Capsules are gelatine containers for a drug either in liquid or pellet form; their shape makes them easier to swallow.

A selection of shapes and forms in which tablets, pills, and capsules may be supplied to help in their identification.

An annotated guide to understanding the entries

manufacturer's brand name or scientific name

Depixol
(Lundbeck)

manufacturer

dose range, including any variations for children or the elderly (note: this is for guidance only and you should always follow the physician's advice)

A yellow tablet supplied at a strength of 3 mg and used as a sedative to treat schizophrenia and other mental disorders, especially withdrawal or apathy.

general description including physical appearance, strength where appropriate, the type of drug, and the conditions it is used to treat

Dose: usually 1-3 tablets a day, up to a maximum of 6 tablets a day.
Availability: NHS and private prescription.

these are the most commonly noted side effects. In many cases, however, no side effects or only some will be experienced

Side effects: muscle spasms, restlessness, hands shaking, dry mouth, blocked nose, constipation, blurred vision, urine retention, palpitations, low blood pressure, weight gain, changes in sexual function, low body temperature, breast swelling, menstrual changes, jaundice, blood and skin changes, drowsiness, tiredness, rarely fits.

not all medicines are available through the National Health Service, while some are available over the counter without prescription

circumstances where care should be exercised by certain groups of patients or those taking other medicines

Caution: in the elderly, and in patients suffering from kidney, liver, heart, or lung disease, Parkinson's disease, or anyone who is intolerant of those drugs taken by mouth.
Not to be used for: children, pregnant women, nursing mothers, or for very excitable or overactive patients.

any groups of patients who should **not** take this medicine

these are substances, such as alcohol or foods, or other drugs with which this medicine should not usually be taken

Caution needed with: alcohol, sedatives, tranquillizers, pain killers, blood-pressure lowering drugs, antidepressants, anticonvulsants, antidiabetic drugs, LEVODOPA.
Contains: FLUPENTHIXOL dihydrochloride.

the active ingredients of the medicine

Other preparations: Depixol Injection, Depixol-Conc, FLUANXOL.

this lists other forms of the same medicine, or equivalent drugs from a different manufacturer (note: since the medicine may be of a different strength, the doses may be different)

(note: CAPITALS indicate a separate entry in the book)

Abidec
(Warner Wellcome Consumer)

Drops used as a multivitamin preparation to treat vitamin deficiencies.

Dose: children aged 1-12 years 0.6 ml a day; infants under 1 year 0.3 ml a day.
Availability: NHS, private prescription, over the counter.
Side effects:
Caution: in pregnant women. Not recommended for use in adults
Not to be used for:
Caution needed with: LEVODOPA, some DIURETICS.
Contains: VITAMINS A, D, B_1, B_2, B_3 B_6, C.
Other preparations: DALIVIT.

AC Vax
(Smith Kline & French)

A vaccination used to provide active immunization against meningitis A and meningitis C.

Dose: adults and children over 2 months old, 1 injection of 0.5 ml.
Availability: NHS, private prescription.
Side effects: mild fever, discomfort at the site of the injection.
Caution: in pregnant women and nursing mothers.
Not to be used for: children under 2 months, or for patients suffering from acute infections or feverish illness.
Caution needed with: drugs that suppress the body's immune system.
Contains: meningococcal polysaccharide vaccine.
Other preparations: MENGIVAC (A and C).

---

acarbose *see* Glucobay

Accupro
(Parke-Davis)

A brown, elliptical, triangular, or round tablet according to strengths 5 mg, 10 mg, and 20 mg, and used as an ACE INHIBITOR in addition to DIURETICS and DIGOXIN in the treatment of congestive heart failure and high blood pressure.

Dose: To treat high blood pressure, 10 mg once a day at first (or 2.5 mg if diuretics also given); adjust according to response (maximum 40 mg a day). To treat congestive heart failure, 2.5 mg once a day at first, adjusted according to response (maximum 20 mg a day). Elderly patients may require lower doses.

Availability: NHS and private prescription.
Side effects: headache, dizziness, inflammation of the nose, cough, upper respiratory tract infection, tiredness, nausea, stomach, abdominal, chest, or muscle pain, low blood pressure, severe allergy.
Caution: in the elderly, and in patients suffering from kidney disease, some vascular diseases, and in those undergoing anaesthesia. Your doctor may advise blood and urine checks.
Not to be used for: children, pregnant women, nursing mothers, or for patients suffering from some heart valve diseases, some kidney disorders.
Caution needed with: some diuretics, some potassium supplements, NON-STEROIDAL ANTI-INFLAMMATORY DRUGS, TETRACYCLINE ANTIBIOTICS, LITHIUM.
Contains: QUINAPRIL.
Other preparations:

Accuretic
(Parke-Davis)

A pink, scored, film-coated tablet used as an ACE INHIBITOR and DIURETIC to treat raised blood pressure.

Dose: usually 1 tablet a day, and a maximum of 2 tablets a day.
Availability: NHS, private prescription.
Side effects: headache, dizziness, coughing, tiredness, stomach upset, chest pain and infections, sleeplessness, rhinitis, allergy, muscle pain, severe allergic swelling of the blood vessels, skin disorder.
Caution: in patients suffering from kidney or liver damage, severe congestive heart failure, narrowing of the arteries supplying the kidneys, collagen vascular disease, diabetes, or who are undergoing anaesthesia or haemodialysis. Your doctor may advise regular blood, kidney, and urine tests before and during treatment.
Not to be used for: children, pregnant women, nursing mothers, or for patients suffering from a failure to produce urine.
Caution needed with: potassium supplements, LITHIUM, some antibiotics, CORTICOSTEROIDS, NON-STEROIDAL ANTI-INFLAMMATORY DRUGS, some DIURETICS.
Contains: QUINAPRIL, HYDROCHLOROTHIAZIDE.
Other preparations:

ACE inhibitor (angiotension converting enzyme inhibitor)
a drug which blocks the production of water-retaining hormones and thus functions as a DIURETIC. Example captopril *see* CAPOTEN.

---

acebutolol *see* **Secadrex, Sectral**

acemetacin *see* **Emflex**

Acepril *see* **Capoten**
(Squibb)

acetazolamide *see* **acetazolamide tablets, Diamox**

acetazolamide tablets

A tablet supplied at a strength of 250 mg used as a weak DIURETIC and fluid balance drug to treat congestive heart failure, fluid retention, premenstrual swelling, epilepsy, glaucoma, and to help prevent mountain sickness.

Dose: 250-375 mg a day or every other day in the morning at first. For premenstrual swelling 125-375 mg a day as a single dose. For epilepsy adults 250-1000 mg a day in divided doses; children 8-30 mg a day in divided doses. For glaucoma 250-1000 mg a day in divided doses.
Availability: NHS and private prescription.
Side effects: flushing, thirst, headache, drowsiness, increased urination, pins and needles, blood changes, excitement, rash.
Caution: in nursing mothers and in patients suffering from emphysema, lung blockages, gout or diabetes. Not generally recommended for prolonged treatment. Your doctor may advise that potassium supplements may be needed, and that blood, fluids, and electrolytes should be checked regularly.
Not to be used for: children except for epilepsy, pregnant women, or for patients suffering from chronic closed angle glaucoma, some kidney conditions, liver failure, adrenal insufficiency, low sodium or potassium levels, sensitivity to sulphonamides.
Caution needed with: ASPIRIN, anti-arrhythmic drugs, drugs used to treat ulcers, other diuretics, CORTICOSTEROIDS, PHENYTOIN, antidiabetics, ANTICOAGULANTS taken by mouth, alcohol, sedatives, NON-STEROIDAL ANTI-INFLAMMATORY DRUGS, LITHIUM, METHOTREXATE.
Contains: ACETAZOLAMIDE.
Other preparations: Diamox tablets, Diamox SR.

Acetest
(Bayer Diagnostics)

A tablet used as a reagent to test for the presence of ketones in the blood or urine. Raised ketone levels indicate an imbalance in the metabolism of fat in the body, such as occurs when a patient is suffering from diabetes.

---

acetic acid *see* **Aci-Jel, Otomize, Phytex**

---

acetomenaphthone *see* **Ketovite**

Acetoxyl
(Stiefel)

A gel, available in two strengths (2.5% and 5%), used as an antibacterial and skin softener to treat acne.

Dose: wash and dry the affected area and apply the gel once a day.
Availability: NHS, private prescription, over the counter.
Side effects: irritation, peeling.
Caution: keep out of the eyes, nose, and mouth; children should use the weaker gel; may bleach fabrics.
Not to be used for:
Caution needed with:
Contains: BENZOYL PEROXIDE.
Other preparations: ACNECIDE, ACNEGEL, BENOXYL, NERICUR, PANOXYL, QUINODERM. (Other brands available over the counter.)

---

acetylcysteine *see* **Fabrol, Ilube, Parvolex**

Acezide *see* **Capozide**
(Squibb)

Achromycin capsules *see* **tetracycline tablets**
(Lederle)

Achromycin ointment
(Lederle)

An ointment used as an antibiotic to treat skin infections.

Dose: apply once a day or as needed.
Availability: NHS and private prescription.

A

Side effects: additional infection.
Caution:
Not to be used for: children, pregnant women, or nursing mothers.
Caution needed with:
Contains: TETRACYCLINE HYDROCHLORIDE.
Other preparations:

---

aciclovir *see* aciclovir tablets, Zovirax Cream, Zovirax Eye Ointment, Zovirax Tablets

---

aciclovir tablets

A tablet supplied at strengths of 200 mg, 400 mg, 800 mg, and used as an antiviral treatment for chicken pox, shingles, cold sores and other skin herpes infections.

Dose: adults shingles and chicken pox, 800 mg 5 times a day every 4 hours for 7 days; other herpes infections 200 mg 5 times a day for 5 days; reduced doses for prevention or in children.
Availability: NHS and private prescription.
Side effects: rash, stomach upset, liver changes, blood changes, headache, dizziness and other brain reactions, tiredness, convulsions.
Caution: in pregnant women, nursing mothers, and in patients suffering from kidney damage; drink plenty of fluids.
Not to be used for:
Caution needed with: PROBENECID.
Contains: ACICLOVIR.
Other preparations: ZOVIRAX Tablets and Suspension, ZOVIRAX CREAM, Zovirax Cold Sore Cream (available without prescription only to treat cold sores), Zovirax Infusion, ZOVIRAX EYE OINTMENT (for herpes eye infections).

Aci-Jel
(Cilag)

A jelly with applicator used as an antiseptic to treat non-specific vaginal infection.

Dose: 1 application into the vagina twice a day.
Availability: NHS, private prescription, over the counter.
Side effects: irritation and inflammation.
Caution: in pregnant women
Not to be used for: children.
Caution needed with:
Contains: ACETIC ACID.

Other preparations:

acipimox *see* **Olbetam**

Acitak *see* **cimetidine**
(Opus)

acitretin *see* **Neotigason**

Acnecide *see* **Acnegel**
(Galderma)

Acnegel
(Stiefel)

A gel, available in two strengths (5% and 10%), used as an antibacterial and skin softener to treat acne.

Dose: wash and dry the affected area and apply the gel once a day. (Start with the weaker strength.)
Availability: NHS, private prescription, over the counter.
Side effects: irritation, peeling.
Caution: keep out of the eyes, nose, mouth; may bleach fabrics.
Not to be used for:
Caution needed with:
Contains: BENZOYL PEROXIDE.
Other preparations: Acnegel Forte (10%), ACETOXYL, ACNECIDE, BENOXYL, NERICUR, PANOXYL, QUINODERM. (Other brands also available over the counter.)

Acnisal
(Euroderma)

A solution used as an antibacterial skin softener to treat acne.

Dose: lather with warm water, rub into the skin, and then rinse off, 2-3 times a day.
Availability: NHS, private prescription, over the counter.
Side effects: local irritation, and, with excessive use, symptoms of ASPIRIN poisoning including headache, dizziness, tinnitus, disturbed vision, vomiting.

A

Caution: avoid contact with eyes, mucous membranes.
Not to be used for: children.
Caution needed with:
Contains: SALICYLIC ACID.
Other preparations:

---

acrivastine *see* **Semprex**

---

acrosoxacin *see* **Eradacin**

ACT-HIB
(Pasteur Merieux MSD)

A vaccination used to provide active immunization against infections giving rise to such diseases as meningitis and epiglottitis.

Dose: children 2-12 months old, 3 injections at 4-weekly intervals of 0.5 ml (children over 13 months require only 1 single dose).
Availability: NHS, private prescription.
Side effects: local reddening of the skin.
Caution: in children over 4 years, if immunization is begun with this vaccine, the course should be completed with it.
Not to be used for: adults, children under 2 months, or for patients suffering from acute infections.
Caution needed with:
Contains: Haemophilus influenza type B polysaccharide vaccine.
Other preparations:

Actinac
(Hoechst Roussel)

A lotion used as an antibacterial, STEROID, and skin softener to treat acne and associated disorders.

Dose: apply to the affected area night and morning for 4 days, then at night only until 3 nights after the spots have gone.
Availability: NHS and private prescription.
Side effects: severe reddening of the skin.
Caution: in pregnant women. Remove jewellery before applying.
Not to be used for:
Caution needed with:
Contains: CHLORAMPHENICOL, HYDROCORTISONE acetate, BUTOXYETHYL NICOTINATE, ALLANTOIN, precipitated SULPHUR.

Other preparations:

Actraphane *see* Insulin
(Novo Nordisk)

Actrapid *see* Insulin
(Novo Nordisk)

Acupan
(3M Healthcare)

A white tablet supplied at a strength of 30 mg and used as an ANALGESIC to relieve pain.

Dose: 1-3 tablets 3 times a day.
Availability: NHS and private prescription.
Side effects: nausea, nervousness, dry mouth, dizziness.
Caution: in the elderly and in patients suffering from kidney or liver disease, pregnant women.
Not to be used for: children or for patients with a history of convulsions or suffering from heart attack.
Caution needed with: MAOIS, ANTICHOLINERGICS, SYMPATHOMIMETICS, TRICYCLIC ANTIDEPRESSANTS.
Contains: NEFOPAM HYDROCHLORIDE.
Other preparations: Acupan Injection.

Adalat *see* nifedipine capsules
(Bayer)

Adalat Retard *see* nifedipine modified release tablets
(Bayer)

Adcortyl Cream
(Squibb)

A cream used as a strong STEROID treatment for dermatitis, psoriasis, eczema, and external ear infections.

Dose: apply to the affected area 2-4 times a day.
Availability: NHS and private prescription.
Side effects: fluid retention, suppression of adrenal glands, thinning of the

skin may occur.
Caution: use for short periods of time only.
Not to be used for: patients suffering from acne or any other skin infections caused by tuberculosis, ringworm, viruses, or fungi, or continuously especially in pregnant women.
Caution needed with:
Contains: TRIAMCINOLONE ACETONIDE.
Other preparations: Adcortyl with Graneodin (with added antibacterial – additionally suitable for treating infected skin conditions, but not psoriasis).

Adcortyl in Orabase
(Squibb)

A paste used as a STEROID treatment for mouth ulcers, mouth infections, gingivitis, and damage in the mouth.

Dose: apply the paste to the affected area 2-4 times a day without rubbing in.
Availability: NHS and private prescription. (May be purchased from pharmacies for use on mouth ulcers only.)
Side effects:
Caution: in pregnant women, nursing mothers, and patients suffering from chicken pox or diabetes, or with a history of stomach ulcers. Do not use for infants over extended periods.
Not to be used for: patients suffering from untreated mouth infections.
Caution needed with:
Contains: TRIAMCINOLONE ACETONIDE.
Other preparations:

Adcortyl intra-articular injection
(Squibb)

An injection supplied in 1 ml ampoules and 5 ml vials at a strength of 10 mg/ml, and used as a STEROID treatment for the pain, stiffness, and swelling of the joints associated with rheumatoid arthritis and other inflammatory joint conditions.

Dose: adults 2.5-15 mg; children over 6 years according to age, weight, joint size, and severity of condition.
Availability: NHS, private prescription.
Side effects: raised blood sugars, osteoporosis, euphoria, depression, stomach ulcer, weight gain, raised blood pressure, mental disturbances, low potassium levels, fluid retention.
Caution: in pregnant women and in patients suffering from stress, underactive thyroid, cirrhosis of the liver, diabetes, epilepsy, glaucoma,

raised blood pressure, kidney disorders, chickenpox, tuberculosis, stomach ulcer, osteoporosis, measle-like illnesses, mental disorders, thrombophlebitis, or who have undergone recent stomach surgery.
Not to be used for: children under 6 years, for intravenous injection, or where there is infection near the proposed injection site.
Caution needed with: PHENYTOIN, PHENOBARBITONE, EPHEDRINE, RIFAMPICIN, DIURETICS, ANTICHOLINESTERASES, some heart and antidiabetic drugs, ANTICOAGULANTS taken by mouth, NON-STEROIDAL ANTI-INFLAMMATORY DRUGS.
Contains: TRIAMCINOLONE ACETONIDE.
Other preparations: KENALOG, LEDERSPAN, LEDERCORT (tablet form).

Adifax
(Servier)

A white capsule supplied at a strength of 15 mg and used in addition to dietary measures in the treatment of severe obesity.

Dose: 1 capsule in the morning and 1 capsule in the evening at meal times.
Availability: NHS and private prescription.
Side effects: dry mouth, nausea, constipation, diarrhoea, drowsiness, dizziness, headache, frequency of urination.
Caution: treatment limited to 3 months, and withdrawn gradually.
Not to be used for: children, the elderly, pregnant women, nursing mothers, or for patients suffering from glaucoma, history of anorexia, mental illness, kidney or liver disease, drug or alcohol abuse.
Caution needed with: MAOIS, blood-pressure lowering drugs, antidiabetics, antidepressants, alcohol, sedatives, other drugs used to reduce appetite.
Contains: DEXFENFLURAMINE
Other preparations:

Adizem *see* diltiazem tablets
(Napp)

Adizem SR *see* diltiazem modified release
(Napp)

Adizem XL *see* diltiazem modified release
(Napp)

---

adrenal glands

the adrenal glands are organs situated above the kidneys which produce hormones, including STEROIDS.

---

adrenaline *see* Eppy, Ganda, Medihaler-EPI, Min-i-jet Adrenaline, Simplene

---

Aerobec *see* beclomethasone inhaler
(3M Healthcare)

Aerocrom Inhaler
(Fisons)

A metered-dose aerosol containing 200 doses, and used as an anti-inflammatory treatment for asthma sufferers.

Dose: 2 puffs 4 times a day continuously.
Availability: NHS, private prescription.
Side effects: low potassium levels, hands shaking, headache, dilation of the blood vessels in hands and feet, coughing, sore throat, rarely bronchial spasm.
Caution: in pregnant women, nursing mothers, and in patients suffering from overactive thyroid, weak heart, angina, raised blood pressure, heart rhythm disturbances.
Not to be used for: children, or for patients suffering from acute asthma.
Caution needed with: SYMPATHOMIMETICS, ß-BLOCKERS.
Contains: SODIUM CROMOGLYCATE, SALBUTAMOL.
Other preparations: Aerocrom Syncroner (with spacer device).

Aerocrom Syncroner *see* Aerocrom Inhaler
(Fisons)

Aerolin Auto *see* salbutamol inhaler
(3M Healthcare)

Ailax *see* co-danthramer suspension
(Galen)

Airomir *see* salbutamol inhaler

Akineton
(Knoll)

A white, scored tablet supplied at a strength of 2 mg and used as an ANTICHOLINERGIC to treat Parkinson's disease.

Dose: ½ tablet twice a day at first, then increasing to 1 tablet 3 times a day, increasing again and then reducing.
Availability: NHS and private prescription.
Side effects: drowsiness, dry mouth, blurred vision.
Caution: in patients suffering from abnormal heart rhythm or recent heart attack, convulsions, urinary obstruction.
Not to be used for: children, pregnant women, nursing mothers, or patients suffering from gastro-intestinal obstruction, untreated narrow-angle glaucoma, other types of involuntary movements.
Caution needed with: other anti-parkinson drugs, sedatives, alcohol.
Contains: BIPERIDEN HYDROCHLORIDE.
Other preparations:

Aknemin *see* minocycline capsules

---

albendazole *see* Eskazole

Albustix
(Bayer Diagnostics)

A plastic strip used as an indicator for the detection of protein in the urine. Protein in the urine may indicate damage to, or disease of, the kidneys.

Albym Test
(Boehringer Mannheim Diagnostics)

A plastic strip used as an indicator for the detection of protein in the urine. Protein in the urine may indicate damage to, or disease of, the kidneys.

---

alclometasone diproprionate *see* Modrasone

Alcoderm
(Galderma)

A cream or lotion used as an emollient to treat dry skin conditions.

Dose: apply to the affected area as needed.
Availability: NHS, private prescription, over the counter.
Side effects:
Caution:
Not to be used for:
Caution needed with:
Contains: LIQUID PARAFFIN, moisturizer.
Other preparations: KERI lotion.

Aldactide 50
(Searle)

A buff coated tablet supplied at a strength of 50 mg and used as a DIURETIC to treat congestive heart failure.

Dose: adults 2 tablets a day at first with food, increasing to 4 tablets a day; children 1.5-3 mg per kg bodyweight a day in divided doses.
Availability: NHS and private prescription.
Side effects: breast enlargement, stomach upset, drowsiness, rash, confusion, shaky movements, sensitivity to light, blood changes, irregular periods, deepening of voice.
Caution: in pregnant women, young patients, the elderly, and in patients suffering from liver or kidney disease, gout, or diabetes. Your doctor may advise regular blood tests.
Not to be used for: nursing mothers or for patients suffering from severe kidney or liver failure, progressive kidney failure, raised potassium levels, raised calcium levels, Addison's disease, or with allergy to sulphonamide.
Caution needed with: potassium supplements, other diuretics, LITHIUM, DIGOXIN, CARBENOXOLONE, blood-pressure lowering drugs, ACE INHIBITORS, alcohol, sedatives, NON-STEROIDAL ANTI-INFLAMMATORY DRUGS, some other heart drugs.
Contains: SPIRONOLACTONE, HYDROFLUMETHIAZIDE, (CO-FLUMACTANE).
Other preparations: Aldactide 25.

Aldactone *see* spironolactone tablets
(Searle)

Aldomet see methyldopa tablets
(M.S.D.)

alendronate sodium *see* Fosamax

Alfa D
(Du Pont)

A pink capsule or orange capsule according to strengths of 0.25 mcg and 1 mcg, and used as a VITAMIN D treatment for bone changes due to kidney failure, low blood calcium due to underactive parathyroid glands, rickets, softening of the bones, and other vitamin D deficiencies.

Dose: adults, 1 mcg a day at first, then adjusted as needed; elderly half adult dose; children over 20 kg bodyweight, 1 mcg a day at first, then adjusted as needed.
Availability: NHS, private prescription.
Side effects:
Caution: in pregnant women, nursing mothers, and in patients suffering from kidney failure. Your doctor may advise regular blood tests.
Not to be used for: children under 20 kg bodyweight.
Caution needed with: BARBITURATES, anticonvulsants, DANAZOL, DIGOXIN, ANTACIDS, some DIURETICS, mineral oils, SUCRALFATE, COLESTIPOL, CHOLESTYRAMINE.
Contains: ALFACALCIDOL.
Other preparations: ONE ALPHA.

---

alfacalcidol *see* Alfa D, One-Alpha

---

alfuzosin *see* Xatral

Algesal
(Solvay Healthcare)

A cream used as an ANALGESIC rub to treat rheumatic conditions.

Dose: massage into the affected area 3 times a day.
Availability: NHS, private prescription, over the counter.
Side effects:
Caution: in pregnant women.
Not to be used for: children under 6 years.
Caution needed with:
Contains: DIETHYLAMINE SALICYLATE.
Other preparations:

Algicon
(Rhône-Poulenc Rorer)

A white tablet used as an ANTACID to treat heartburn, hiatus hernia, indigestion.

Dose: adults 1-2 tablets 4 times a day after meals and at night.
Availability: NHS, private prescription, over the counter.
Side effects: few; constipation or diarrhoea.
Caution: patients suffering from diabetes owing to sucrose content.
Not to be used for: children, or in kidney failure or severe debilitation.
Caution needed with: tablets coated to protect the stomach, some antibiotics, iron.
Contains: MAGNESIUM ALGINATE, ALUMINIUM HYDROXIDE/MAGNESIUM CARBONATE, MAGNESIUM CARBONATE, POTASSIUM BICARBONATE.
Other preparations: Algicon Suspension.

---

alginic acid *see* **Gastrocote, Gastron, Gaviscon, Pyrogastrone, Topal**

Algitec
(SmithKline Beecham)

A tablet and suspension used as an H$_2$-BLOCKER and reflux suppressant to treat reflux from the stomach.

Dose: 1-2 tablets (chewed) or 10-20 ml 4 times a day after meals and at bedtime.
Availability: NHS and private prescription.
Side effects: stomach upset, rash, tiredness, breast changes, occasionally liver damage, confusion, kidney disorder, inflamed pancreas, blood changes, headache, joint and muscle pain.
Caution: in pregnant women, nursing mothers, and in patients with kidney disorders.
Not to be used for: children.
Caution needed with: ANTICOAGULANTS, PHENYTOIN, THEOPHYLLINE.
Contains: CIMETIDINE, SODIUM ALGINATE.
Other preparations: Tagamet Dual Action (available over the counter).

Alimix *see* Prepulsid
(Janssen)

---

allantoin *see* **Actinac, Alphosyl, Alphosyl HC, Anodesyn, Dermalex**

Allegron
(Dista)

A white tablet or an orange, scored tablet according to strengths of 10 mg, 25 mg and used as a TRICYCLIC ANTIDEPRESSANT to treat depression, bedwetting in children.

Dose: adults 25 mg 3-4 times a day, to a maximum of 150 mg a day; elderly 10 mg 3 times a day at first; children over 6 years 10-35 mg half an hour before bed time. Reduced doses in the elderly.
Availability: NHS and private prescription.
Side effects: dry mouth, constipation, urine retention, blurred vision, palpitations, breast changes, drowsiness, sleeplessness, dizziness, hands shaking, low blood presure, weight change, skin reactions, jaundice or blood changes, and convulsions at high doses. Loss of sexual desire may occur.
Caution: in nursing mothers or in patients suffering from heart disease, thyroid disease, epilepsy, diabetes, glaucoma, urinary retention, adrenal tumour, some other psychiatric conditions. Your doctor may advise regular blood tests.
Not to be used for: children under 6 years, pregnant women, or for patients suffering from heart attacks, liver disease, heart block, mania.
Caution needed with: alcohol, sedatives, ANTICHOLINERGICS, ADRENALINE, MAOIS, BARBITURATES, other antidepressants, blood-pressure lowering drugs, drugs that affect heart rhythm, anticonvulsants, ASTEMIZOLE, TERFENADINE, SOTALOL, CIMETIDINE, local anaesthetics.
Contains: NORTRIPTYLINE hydrochloride.
Other preparations:

allopurinol tablets
(Wellcome)

A tablet supplied at strengths of 100 mg, 300 mg and used as an enzyme blocker to prevent gout.

Dose: 100 mg a day at first increasing to 300 mg if required. (Usual maintenance 200-900 mg a day in divided doses.) At the beginning of treatment and for 1 month thereafter, colchicine or an anti-inflammatory drug should be prescribed.
Availability: NHS and private prescription.
Side effects: skin reactions, rash, nausea, acute gout. Rarely headache, vertigo, drowsiness, hair loss, liver disorder, pins and needles, general

feeling of being unwell.
Caution: in pregnant women, the elderly, and in patients suffering from kidney or liver disease. Be sure to drink plenty of fluids.
Not to be used for: children or for patients suffering from acute gout.
Caution needed with: NICOUMALONE, WARFARIN, CAPTOPRIL, CHLORPROPAMIDE, mercaptopurine, AZATHIOPRINE, CYCLOSPORIN.
Contains: ALLOPURINOL.
Other preparations: CAPLENAL, COSURIC, RIMAPURINOL, XANTHOMAX, ZYLORIC.

Almevax *see* rubella vaccine
(Evans)

Almodan *see* amoxycillin capsules

Alomide
(Galen)

A solution used as an anti-allergy eye drop to treat allergic conjunctivitis.

Dose: adults and children over 4 years, 1-2 drops in each eye 4 times a day.
Availability: NHS, private prescription.
Side effects: irritation.
Caution: in pregnant women and nursing mothers.
Not to be used for: children under 4 years, or for patients who wear soft contact lenses.
Caution needed with:
Contains: LODOXAMIDE.
Other preparations:

Alpha Keri
(Westwood)

A liquid used to treat dry, itchy skin conditions.

Dose: adults and children add 1-2 capsful to the bath, or rub a small amount on to wet skin; infants use half a capful per bath.
Availability: NHS, private prescription, over the counter.
Side effects:
Caution:
Not to be used for:
Caution needed with:
Contains: MINERAL OIL, LANOLIN OIL.

Alphaderm
(Procter & Gamble Pharmaceuticals)

A cream used as a STEROID and wetting agent to treat eczema, dermatitis.

Dose: wash and dry the affected area, and apply twice a day.
Availability: NHS and private prescription.
Side effects: fluid retention, suppression of adrenal glands. Thinning of the skin may occur.
Caution: use for short periods of time only.
Not to be used for: patients suffering from acne or any other skin infections caused by tuberculosis, ringworm, viruses, or fungi, or continuously especially in pregnant women.
Caution needed with:
Contains: HYDROCORTISONE, UREA.
Other preparations: CALMURID HC.

Alphavase *see* prazosin tablets
(Ashbourne)

Alphosyl
(Stafford-Miller)

A cream and lotion used as an anti-psoriatic to treat psoriasis.

Dose: massage thoroughly into the affected area 2-4 times a day. (On scalp, use lotion and wash off after 12 hours.)
Availability: NHS, private prescription, over the counter.
Side effects: irritation, sensitivity to light.
Caution: keep out of the eyes.
Not to be used for: patients suffering from acute psoriasis.
Caution needed with:
Contains: COAL TAR EXTRACT, ALLANTOIN.
Other preparations: Alphosyl 2-in-1 Shampoo. CLINITAR, GELCOTAR, POLYTAR, PSORIDERM, PSORIGEL, T-GEL.

Alphosyl HC
(Stafford-Miller)

A cream used as an anti-psoriatic and STEROID treatment for psoriasis.

Dose: apply to the affected area twice a day.
Availability: NHS and private prescription.
Side effects: thinning of the skin, fluid retention, suppression of adrenal glands.
Caution: in pregnant women, and in patients on extended treatment – withdraw gradually.
Not to be used for: children under 5 years, or for patients suffering from acne or other skin infections unless otherwise directed, or continuously especially in pregnancy.
Caution needed with:
Contains: COAL TAR EXTRACT, ALLANTOIN, HYDROCORTISONE.
Other preparations: TARCORTIN.

---

alprazolam *see* **Xanax**

---

alprostadil *see* **Caverject, Prostin**

Alrheumat *see* **ketoprofen capsules**
(Bayer)

Altacite Plus
(Hoechst Roussel)

A white liquid used as an ANTACID and anti-wind preparation to treat wind, excess stomach acid, gastritis, indigestion, wind, and stomach ulcers.

Dose: adults 10 ml between meals and at bedtime; children 8-12 years half adult dose.
Availability: NHS, private prescription, over the counter.
Side effects: few; occasional diarrhoea and constipation.
Caution:
Not to be used for: children under 8 years.
Caution needed with: tablets coated to protect the stomach, some antibiotics, iron.
Contains: HYDROTALCITE, activated DIMETHICONE (CO-SIMALCITE).
Other preparations: Altacite Plus tablets (not available on NHS), Altacite suspension and tablets (antacids only – available on NHS prescription only if prescribed generically).

Alu-Cap
(3M Health Care)

A green/red capsule supplied at a strength of 475 mg and used as an ANTACID to treat excess stomach acid and to regulate blood phosphate levels in patients with kidney failure.

Dose: adults 1 tablet 4 times a day and at bedtime (higher doses for phosphate regulation).
Availability: NHS, private prescription, over the counter.
Side effects: few; occasional bowel disorders such as constipation.
Caution:
Not to be used for: children, or for patients suffering from low blood phosphate levels.
Caution needed with: tablets coated to protect the stomach, some antibiotics, iron.
Contains: ALUMINIUM HYDROXIDE GEL.
Other preparations: ALUDROX (not available on NHS), ALUMINIUM HYDROXIDE TABLETS AND MIXTURE.

Aludrox *see* **aluminium hydroxide mixture**
(Charwell)

---

aluminium acetate *see* **aluminium acetate ear drops, aluminium acetate lotion, Xyloproct**

---

aluminium acetate ear drops

Drops supplied at strengths of 8% and 13%, and used as an astringent to treat inflammation of the outer ear.

Dose: insert directly into the ear or saturate a gauze wick and apply into the ear.
Availability: NHS, private prescription, over the counter.
Side effects:
Caution:
Not to be used for:
Caution needed with:
Contains: ALUMINIUM ACETATE.
Other preparations:

---

aluminium acetate lotion

A lotion used as an astringent to treat weeping eczema and wounds.

Dose: to be used undiluted as a wet dressing.

Availability: NHS, private prescription, over the counter.
Side effects:
Caution:
Not to be used for:
Caution needed with:
Contains: ALUMINIUM ACETATE.
Other preparations:

---

aluminium chloride *see* Anhydrol Forte, Driclor, Odaban

---

aluminium dihydroxyallantoinate *see* Zeasorb

---

aluminium hydroxide *see* Algicon, Alu-Cap, Aludrox, Asilone, Caved-S, Diovol, Gastrocote, Gastron, Gaviscon, Kolanticon, Maalox, Mucaine, Pyrogastrone, Topal

---

aluminium hydroxide tablets

A tablet supplied at a strength of 500 mg and used as an ANTACID to treat excess stomach acid, indigestion.

Dose: 1-2 tablets chewed 4 times a day and at bedtime, or as required.
Availability: NHS, private prescription, and over the counter.
Side effects: occasionally constipation.
Caution: in patients suffering from PORPHYRIA.
Not to be used for: children, or for patients with low blood phosphate levels.
Caution needed with: tablets coated to protect the stomach, some antibiotics, iron.
Contains: ALUMINIUM HYDROXIDE.
Other preparations: ALUMINIUM HYDROXIDE MIXTURE. ALU-CAP, Aludrox (not available on NHS.)

---

aluminium hydroxide mixture

A sugar-free mixture/gel used as an ANTACID to treat excess stomach acid, indigestion, stomach ulcer, and excess blood phosphate.

Dose: adults 5-10 ml 4 times a day between meals and at bedtime, up to a maximum of 100 ml per day; children aged 6-12 years up to 5 ml 3 times a day.
Availability: NHS, private prescription, and over the counter.

Side effects: occasionally constipation.
Caution: in patients suffering from PORPHYRIA.
Not to be used for: children under 6 years, or for patients with low blood phosphate levels.
Caution needed with: tablets coated to protect the stomach, some antibiotics, iron.
Contains: ALUMINIUM HYDROXIDE.
Other preparations: ALUMINIUM HYDROXIDE TABLETS. ALU-CAP, Aludrox (not available on NHS).

A

---

aluminium oxide *see* Brasivol

Alupent
(Boehringer Ingelheim)

An off-white, scored tablet supplied at a strength of 20 mg and used as an anti-asthma drug to treat bronchial spasm brought on by chronic bronchitis, asthma, emphysema.

Dose: adults 1 tablet 4 times a day; children use syrup.
Availability: NHS and private prescription.
Side effects: abnormal heart rhythm, tremor, nervous tension, headache, dilation of the veins, rapid heart rate.
Caution: in diabetics and patients suffering from high blood pressure.
Not to be used for: patients suffering from cardiac asthma, acute heart disease, overactive thyroid gland.
Caution needed with: MAOIS, TRICYCLIC ANTIDEPRESSANTS, SYMPATHOMIMETICS.
Contains: ORCIPRENALINE SULPHATE.
Other preparations: Alupent Syrup, Alupent Aerosol.

Alvedon
(Novex)

A suppository used to treat pain and fever in children.

Dose: children aged 1-5 years, 1-2 suppositories up to 4 times a day.
Availability: NHS, private prescription, over the counter.
Side effects:
Caution: in patients suffering from kidney or liver damage.
Not to be used for: children under 1 year or over 5 years, adults.
Caution needed with: other preparations containing PARACETAMOL.
Contains: paracetamol
Other preparations: CALPOL INFANT, DISPROL PAEDIATRIC, PALDESIC, PARACETAMOL PAEDIATRIC ELIXIR.

31

Alvercol
(Norgine)

Beige, coated granules used as an antispasm and bulking agent to treat irritable bowel syndrome and other spasm disorders of the colon.

Dose: adults 1-2 heaped 5 ml spoonsful once or twice a day after meals; children over 6 years half adult dose.
Availability: NHS, private prescription, over the counter.
Side effects: occasionally mild bloating
Caution: in women in the first 3 months of pregnancy. Do not chew or crush the granules. Swallow with plenty of fluids.
Not to be used for: children under 6 years, or for patients with obstructed bowel, or absence of bowel movements.
Caution needed with:
Contains: STERCULIA, ALVERINE CITRATE.
Other preparations:

---

alverine citrate *see* **Alvercol, Relaxyl, Spasmonal**

---

amantadine *see* **Symmetrel**

Ambaxin
(Upjohn)

An off-white, oblong, scored tablet supplied at a strength of 400 mg and used as a broad-spectrum penicillin to treat respiratory, ear, nose, and throat, skin, soft tissue, urinary tract, and venereal infections, paratyphoid fever.

Dose: adults 1-2 tablets 2-3 times a day (higher doses in venereal infections); children over 5 years ½ tablet 3 times a day.
Availability: NHS and private prescription.
Side effects: allergy, stomach disturbances.
Caution: in patients suffering from kidney disease, severe liver disease, glandular fever.
Not to be used for: children under 5 years.
Caution needed with:
Contains: BACAMPICILLIN hydrochloride.
Other preparations:

Ames Lancet
(Bayer Diagnostics)

A device (lancet) for obtaining blood samples from the finger, compatible with Autolet, Autolet Lite, and Glucolet finger-pricking devices. Blood-glucose monitoring enables individual patients suffering from diabetes accurately to control blood glucose and manage their condition.

amethocaine *see* Eludril

Amfipen *see* ampicillin capsules
(Yamanouchi)

Amidose Saline *see* sterile saline
(Abatron)

Amilco *see* co-amilozide tablets
(Baker Norton)

Amilmaxco 5/50 *see* co-amilozide tablets
(Ashbourne)

amiloride *see* Amilco, Amilmaxco, Amilospare, amiloride tablets, Berkamil, Burinex A, Delvas, Fru-Co, Frumil, Kalten, Lasoride, Midamor, Moducren, Moduret-25, Moduretic, Navispare, Synuretic

amiloride tablets

A yellow, diamond-shaped tablet supplied at a strength of 5 mg and used as a potassium-sparing DIURETIC to maintain potassium level when used with other diuretics.

Dose: 1-2 tablets a day at first, then up to 4 tablets a day if needed.
Availability: NHS and private prescription.
Side effects: stomach upset, rash.
Caution: in pregnant women or nursing mothers and in patients suffering from diabetes with a predisposition to high potassium levels, gout, liver or kidney disease. Your doctor may advise blood tests for potassium levels.
Not to be used for: children or for patients suffering from high potassium levels or progressive kidney failure.
Caution needed with: potassium supplements, potassium-sparing diuretics, ACE INHIBITORS.

A

Contains: AMILORIDE hydrochloride.
Other preparations: AMILOSPARE, BERKAMIL, MIDAMOR.

Amilospare *see* amiloride tablets
(Ashbourne)

aminophylline tablets

A tablet supplied at a strength of 100 mg and used as a bronchodilator to treat bronchial spasm associated with severe acute asthma, chronic bronchitis, emphysema. (The slow-release preparations are also used to treat heart failure.)

Dose: 100-300 mg 3-4 times a day after food.
Availability: NHS, private prescription, over the counter.
Side effects: nausea, stomach upset, headache, brain stimulation, abnormal heart rhythm.
Caution: in pregnant women, nursing mothers, the elderly, and in patients suffering from other forms of heart disease, liver disease, stomach ulcer, PORPHYRIA.
Not to be used for: children.
Caution needed with: CIMETIDINE, some antibiotics, STEROIDS, DIURETICS, some other bronchodilators, STEROIDS, FLUVOXAMINE, DILTIAZEM, VERAPAMIL, LITHIUM, some contraceptive pills, INFLUENZA VACCINE.
Contains: AMINOPHYLLINE.
Other preparations: aminophylline SR tablets. AMNIVENT, PECRAM, PHYLLOCONTIN (all slow-release products).

amiodarone tablets

A tablet supplied at strength of 100 mg and used as an anti-arrhythmic drug to treat heart rhythm disturbances.

Dose: adults 200 mg 3 times a day for 7 days, then 200 mg twice a day for 7 days, and 200 mg a day thereafter; children as advised by the physician.
Availability: NHS and private prescription.
Side effects: corneal deposits, sensitivity to light, lung disorders, tremor, sleeplessness, tiredness, rash, nervous system, liver, heart, eye, and thyroid effects.
Caution: in pregnant women, the elderly, and in patients suffering from heart or kidney failure, or PORPHYRIA. Your doctor may advise thyroid, eyes, heart, and liver tests. Treatment to be started only under specialist supervision or in hospital.
Not to be used for: nursing mothers or for patients suffering from cardiac

shock, some types of heart block or failure, thyroid disease, very low blood
pressure, or who are allergic to iodine.
Caution needed with: ANTICOAGULANTS taken by mouth, ß-BLOCKERS, DIGOXIN,
PHENYTOIN, DIURETICS, anaesthetics, drugs to treat abnormal heart rhythm,
antidepressants, ASTEMIZOLE, TERFENADINE, CIMETIDINE, CYCLOSPORIN, some
drugs used to treat angina and high blood pressure.
Contains: AMIODARONE hydrochloride.
Other preparations: CORDARONE X.

---

amitriptyline *see* amitriptyline tablets, Domical, Elavil, Lentizol-SR, Triptafen-M, Tryptizol

---

amitriptyline tablets

A coated tablet supplied at strengths of 10 mg, 25 mg, 50 mg and used as
a TRICYCLIC ANTIDEPRESSANT to treat depression with anxiety especially where
sedation is valuable, and bedwetting in children.

Dose: adults 75 mg a day in divided doses at first increasing to up to 150
mg a day if needed, then usually 50-100 mg at night; elderly 25-75 mg a
day at first. To treat bedwetting in children: 7-10 years, 10-20 mg at night;
10-16 years 25-50 mg (maximum treatment period 3 months withdrawing
gradually).
Availability: NHS and private prescription.
Side effects: dry mouth, tinnitus, tiredness, constipation, urine retention,
blurred vision, nausea, palpitations, drowsiness, sleeplessness, dizziness,
hands shaking, low blood pressure, weight change, sweating, fever,
behavioural changes in children, confusion in the elderly, skin reactions,
jaundice or blood changes, loss of sexual function may occur.
Caution: in pregnant women, nursing mothers or in patients suffering from
heart disease, liver and kidney disorders, thyroid disease, adrenal
tumours, epilepsy, diabetes, glaucoma, urine retention, constipation, some
other psychiatric conditions. Your doctor may advise regular blood tests.
Not to be used for: children under 7 years, children under 16 years to
treat depression, or for patients suffering from recent heart attacks, heart
block, severe liver disease.
Caution needed with: alcohol, sedatives, ANTICHOLINERGICS, ASTEMIZOLE,
ADRENALINE, MAOIS, BARBITURATES, other antidepressants, TERFENADINE, blood-
pressure lowering drugs, CIMETIDINE, anticonvulsants, the contraceptive pill.
Contains: AMITRIPTYLINE hydrochloride.
Other preparations: amitriptyline syrup. DOMICAL, ELAVIL, LENTIZOL SR (a
slow-release product), TRYPTIZOL.

Amix *see* **amoxycillin capsules**
(Ashbourne)

---

amlodipine *see* **Istin**

Amnivent *see* **aminophylline tablets**
(Ashbourne)

Amopen *see* **amoxycillin capsules**
(Yorkshire)

Amoram *see* **amoxycillin capsules**
(Eastern)

---

amorolfine *see* **Loceryl**

---

amoxapine *see* **Asendis**

Amoxil *see* **amoxycillin capsules**
(Bencard)

---

amoxycillin *see* **Almodan, Amix, Amoram, Amoxil, amoxycillin capsules, Amrit, Augmentin, Galenmox, Rimoxallin**

---

amoxycillin capsules

A capsule supplied at strengths of 250 mg and 500 mg and used as a broad-spectrum penicillin antibiotic to treat respiratory, ear, nose, and throat, urinary, venereal, and soft tissue infections. Also for dental abscess, and to prevent infection of the heart during dental procedures

Dose: adults 250-500 mg 3 times a day; children up to 10 years half adult dose. (Infants use paediatric suspension.) Doses may be increased in severe infections. To prevent heart infection during dental treatment: adults, 3 g, children 750-1500 mg, 1 hour before procedure.
Availability: NHS and private prescription.
Side effects: stomach upset, allergy.

Caution: in patients suffering from glandular fever, kidney disorder, leukaemia, HIV infection.
Not to be used for: patients suffering from penicillin allergy.
Caution needed with: the contraceptive pill.
Contains: AMOXYCILLIN trihydrate.
Other preparations: amoxycillin oral suspension, amoxycillin sachets. AMOXIL (including Paediatric Suspension), ALMODAN, AMIX, AMORAM, AMRIT, GALENAMOX, RIMOXALLIN.

---

amphotericin *see* Fungilin, Fungilin Lozenges

---

ampicillin *see* ampicillin capsules, Magnapen, Penbritin, Rimacillin, Vidopen

---

ampicillin capsules

A capsule supplied at strengths of 250 mg, 500 mg and used as a broad-spectrum penicillin to treat respiratory, ear, nose, and throat, and soft tissue infections. Also for urinary tract and venereal infections.

Dose: adults 250 mg-1 g 4 times a day; children half adult dose.
Availability: NHS and private prescription.
Side effects: stomach upset, allergy.
Caution: in patients suffering kidney disease, glandular fever, leukaemia, HIV infection.
Not to be used for: patients suffering from penicillin allergy.
Caution needed with: the contraceptive pill.
Contains: AMPICILLIN.
Other preparations: Ampicillin Syrup, Ampicillin Injection, AMFIPEN, PENBRITIN, RIMACILLIN, VIDOPEN.

Ampiclox
(SmithKline Beecham)

A black/purple capsule or a syrup used as a penicillin antibiotic for the emergency treatment of serious infections or for the prevention of infections during surgery.

Dose: adults, 1-2 capsules or 10-20 ml of syrup every 4-6 hours; children 1 month-2 years 2.5-5 ml syrup, 2-12 years 5-10 ml syrup, both every 4-6 hours. (Children under 1 month use neonatal suspension.)
Availability: NHS, private prescription.
Side effects: allergy, stomach upset.

A

Caution: in patients suffering from glandular fever.
Not to be used for:
Caution needed with: the contraceptive pill.
Contains: AMPICILLIN, CLOXACILLIN.
Other preparations: Ampiclox Neonatal Suspension, Ampiclox Injection, Ampiclox Neonatal Injection.

Amrit *see* **amoxycillin capsules**
(BHR)

---

amylobarbitone *see* **Amytal, Sodium Amytal, Tuinal**

Amytal
(Distriphar)

A white tablet supplied at a strength of 50 mg and used as a BARBITURATE for the short-term treatment of severe sleeplessness.

Dose: 100-200 mg before going to bed.
Availability: controlled drug; NHS and private prescription.
Side effects: drowsiness, hangover, dizziness, allergies, headache, shaky movements, breathing difficulties, confusion, excitement.
Caution: in patients suffering from liver, kidney, or lung disease. Dependence (addiction) may develop.
Not to be used for: children, young adults, pregnant women, nursing mothers, the elderly, patients with a history of drug or alcohol abuse, or suffering from PORPHYRIA, or in the management of pain.
Caution needed with: ANTICOAGULANTS, alcohol, other tranquillizers, sedatives, STEROIDS, the contraceptive pill, GRISEOFULVIN, RIFAMPICIN, PHENYTOIN, METRONIDAZOLE, CHLORAMPHENICOL.
Contains: AMYLOBARBITONE.
Other preparations: SODIUM AMYTAL.

Anacal
(Panpharma)

An ointment used as a soothing, anti-inflammatory treatment for haemorrhoids, anal fissure, anal itch, inflammation of the rectum.

Dose: apply one or more times a day as required.
Availability: NHS, private prescription, over the counter.
Side effects:
Caution:

Not to be used for: children.
Caution needed with:
Contains: HEPARINOID, LAUROMACROGOL.
Other preparations: Anacal Suppositories.

Anaflex Cream
(Geistlich)

A cream used as an antibacterial and antifungal treatment for skin infections.

Dose: apply the cream to the affected area 1-2 times a day.
Availability: NHS, private prescription, over the counter.
Side effects:
Caution:
Not to be used for:
Caution needed with:
Contains: POLYNOXYLIN.
Other preparations:

Anafranil *see* clomipramine capsules
(Ciba)

---

analgesic
A preparation used to relieve pain. Example PARACETAMOL tablets.

Androcur
(Schering Health Care)

A white, scored tablet supplied at a strength of 50 mg and used as an anti-androgen to treat severe hypersexuality and sexual deviation in men.

Dose: 1 tablet in the morning and 1 tablet in the evening.
Availability: NHS and private prescription.
Side effects: tiredness, depression, weight gain, breast enlargement, changes in hair pattern, osteoporosis, liver disorder.
Caution: in patients suffering from diabetes or liver disease. Patients must give consent to treatment. Your doctor may advise regular blood and sperm tests.
Not to be used for: men under 18 years or where bones and testes have not reached full development, or for patients suffering from acute liver disease, malignant or wasting disease, severe chronic depression, history of blood clots.

Caution needed with: alcohol.
Contains: CYPROTERONE ACETATE.
Other preparations: CYPROSTAT.

---

anethol *see* **Rowatinex**

Angeze *see* **isosorbide mononitrate tablets**
(Opus)

Angilol *see* **propranolol tablets**
(DDSA)

Angiopine *see* **nifedipine capsules/nifedipine modified release**
(Ashbourne)

Angiozem *see* **diltiazem tablets**
(Ashbourne)

Angitate *see* **isosorbide mononitrate**
(Berk)

Angitil SR *see* **diltiazem tablets**
(Trinity)

Anhydrol Forte
(Dermal)

A roll-on solution used to treat excessive sweating of the armpits, hands, or feet.

Dose: apply if necessary at night. Wash off in the morning. Children only to be treated on the feet.
Availability: NHS, private prescription, over the counter.
Side effects:
Caution: in children. Avoid contact with clothes or jewellery. Ensure that area is dry and not shaved for 12 hours before or after use.
Not to be used for: inflamed and broken skin areas.
Caution needed with:

Contains: ALUMINIUM CHLORIDE.
Other preparations:

---

anise *see* **simple linctus**

Anodesyn
(Seton Healthcare)

An ointment or suppository used as an anaesthetic, soothing, and astringent treatment for the symptoms of haemorrhoids (piles).

Dose: to be used twice a day and after each bowel movement.
Availability: NHS, private prescription, over the counter.
Side effects:
Caution:
Not to be used for: children under 12 years.
Caution needed with:
Contains: LIGNOCAINE hydrochloride, ALLANTOIN.
Other preparations:

Anquil
(Janssen-Cilag)

A white tablet supplied at a strength of 0.25 mg and used as a sedative to control unacceptable sexual behaviour.

Dose: 1-6 tablets a day in divided doses.
Availability: NHS and private prescription.
Side effects: muscle spasms, restlessness, hands shaking, changes in sexual function, dry mouth, urine retention, blurred vision, palpitations, low blood pressure, weight gain, low body temperature, breast swelling, menstrual changes, jaundice, blood and skin changes, stomach upset, drowsiness, constipation, rarely fits.
Caution: in pregnant women, nursing mothers. Your doctor may advise regular blood and liver tests.
Not to be used for: children or for patients with parkinson-like disorders or movement disorders.
Caution needed with: alcohol, sedatives, tranquillizers, pain killers, blood-pressure lowering drugs, antidepressants, anticonvulsants, antidiabetic drugs, LEVODOPA.
Contains: BENPERIDOL.
Other preparations:

Antabuse
(Dumex)

A white, scored tablet supplied at a strength of 200 mg and used as an enzyme inhibitor for additional treatment for alcoholism.

Dose: initially as advised by doctor.
Availability: NHS and private prescription.
Side effects: drowsiness, tiredness, nausea, bad breath, reduced sex drive, skin allergy, liver damage, weakness or numbness of hands and feet, rarely mental disturbances.
Caution: in patients suffering from liver, kidney, or breathing diseases, diabetes, epilepsy, drug addiction.
Not to be used for: children, pregnant women, or patients suffering from heart failure, coronary artery disease, raised blood pressure, mental disorders.
Caution needed with: alcohol, BARBITURATES, WARFARIN, sedatives.
Contains: DISULFIRAM.
Other preparations:

---

antacid
A preparation which reduces the acid content of the stomach, used to relieve indigestion. Example MAGNESIUM TRISILICATE mixture.

Antepsin
(Wyeth)

A white, oblong tablet supplied at a strength of 1 g and used as a cell-surface protector in the treatment of gastritis and ulcers, and for the prevention of haemorrhage from stomach ulcers.

Dose: 2 tablets twice a day or 1 tablet 4 times a day an hour before meals, up to a maximum of 8 tablets a day; treatment period usually 4-6 weeks but up to 12 weeks if necessary. For prevention of haemorrhage, 1 tablet 6 times a day, up to a maximum of 8 tablets a day.
Availability: NHS and private prescription.
Side effects: stomach upset, dry mouth, rash, constipation or diarrhoea.
Caution: in kidney function impairment.
Not to be used for: children.
Caution needed with: TETRACYCLINE antibiotics, PHENYTOIN, DIGOXIN, CIMETIDINE.
Contains: SUCRALFATE.
Other preparations: Antepsin suspension.

Anthisan
(Rhône-Poulenc Rorer Family Health)

An antihistamine cream used to relieve allergic skin reactions, including insect bites, stings, and nettle rash.

Dose: apply to the affected area 2-3 times a day for up to 3 days.
Availability: NHS, private prescription, over the counter.
Side effects: rarely allergy.
Caution:
Not to be used for: areas or broken skin or eczema.
Caution needed with:
Contains: MEPYRAMINE maleate.
Other preparations:

---

anthraquinone glycosides *see* Pyralvex

---

anticholinergic
a drug which blocks the action of acetyl choline, a nerve transmitter. Anticholinergics are used to reduce muscle spasm. The effects include dry mouth, difficulty passing urine, and possibly confusion. Example, HYOSCINE *see* Buscopan.

---

anticholinesterase
A drug which enhances the action of acetyl choline, a nerve transmitter. Example NEOSTIGMINE *see* Prostigmin.

---

anticoagulant
A substance used to prevent the blood from clotting. Example WARFARIN.

---

antihistamine
A preparation which blocks the histamine response in the body which occurs during an allergic reaction. Antihistamines are used to treat all types of allergy (skin rashes, hay fever, etc). Example CHLORPHENIRAMINE *see* Piriton.

---

antihypertensive
A preparation used to lower blood pressure. Example ß-BLOCKERS *see* Inderal.

Antipressan *see* **atenolol tablets**
(Berk)

Anturan
(Ciba)

A yellow tablet supplied at strengths of 100 mg, 200 mg and used as a uric acid-lowering drug to treat gout, gouty arthritis, high uric acid levels.

Dose: 100-200 mg a day with food at first increasing to 600 mg a day over 2-3 weeks and then reduce to the minimum effective dose.
Availability: NHS and private prescription.
Side effects: acute gout, stones in the urinary tract, kidney colic, stomach upset, gastro-intestinal bleeding or ulcers, kidney or liver disease, rash, blood changes.
Caution: in pregnant women, nursing mothers, and in patients suffering from kidney disease, heart failure. Drink plenty of fluids. Your doctor may advise blood and kidney tests.
Not to be used for: children, patients with a history of peptic ulcer, severe liver or kidney disease, acute gout, blood disorders, PORPHYRIA, allergies induced by anti-inflammatory drugs.
Caution needed with: ASPIRIN, ANTICOAGULANTS, some antidiabetics, THEOPHYLLINE, PHENYTOIN, some antibiotics.
Contains: SULPHINPYRAZONE.
Other preparations:

Anugesic-HC
(Parke-Davis)

A cream used as a soothing, antiseptic, STEROID treatment for haemorrhoids, anal itch, and other rectal disorders.

Dose: apply night and morning, and after passing motions.
Availability: NHS and private prescription.
Side effects: systemic CORTICOSTEROID effects (*see* prednisolone tablets).
Caution: do not use for prolonged periods; special care is required for pregnant women.
Not to be used for: children or for patients suffering from tuberculous, fungal, and viral infections.
Caution needed with:
Contains: PRAMOXINE hydrochloride, HYDROCORTISONE acetate, ZINC OXIDE, PERU BALSAM, BENZYL BENZOATE, BISMUTH OXIDE.
Other preparations: Anugesic-HC suppositories.

Anusol
(Warner Wellcome Consumer)

A suppository used as a soothing, antiseptic, astringent treatment for haemorrhoids, anal itch, and other rectal and anal disorders.

Dose: 1 suppository night and morning, and after passing motions.
Availability: NHS, private prescription, over the counter.
Side effects:
Caution:
Not to be used for: children.
Caution needed with:
Contains: BISMUTH SUBGALLATE, BISMUTH OXIDE, PERU BALSAM, ZINC OXIDE.
Other preparations: Anusol cream, Anusol ointment.

Anusol HC
(Warner Wellcome Consumer)

A suppository used as a STEROID, antiseptic, astringent treatment for haemorrhoids and inflammation of the anus and rectum.

Dose: 1 suppository night and morning after passing motions.
Availability: NHS and private prescription.
Side effects: systemic CORTICOSTEROID effects (see prednisolone tablets).
Caution: in pregnant women; do not use for prolonged periods.
Not to be used for: children or for patients suffering from tuberculous, fungal, and viral infections.
Caution needed with:
Contains: HYDROCORTISONE acetate, BENZYL BENZOATE, BISMUTH SUBGALLATE, BISMUTH OXIDE, RESORCINOL, PERU BALSAM, ZINC OXIDE.
Other preparations: Anusol HC ointment, ANUSOL PLUS HC (available over the counter only to treat haemorrhoids and anal itching).

Anusol Plus HC *see* Anusol HC

---

apraclonidine *see* Iopidine

Apresoline *see* hydralazine tablets
(Ciba)

Aprinox *see* **bendrofluazide tablets**
(Knoll Pharma)

Apsifen *see* **ibuprofen tablets**

Apsin *see* **penicillin V tablets**
(APS)

Apsolol *see* **propranolol tablets**
(APS)

Aquadrate
(Procter & Gamble Pharmaceuticals)

A cream used as an emollient to treat chronic dry skin conditions, scaly and thickening skin.

Dose: apply to clean dry skin twice a day.
Availability: NHS, private prescription, over the counter.
Side effects:
Caution:
Not to be used for:
Caution needed with:
Contains: UREA.
Other preparations: NUTRAPLUS.

Aquasept
(Hough, Hoseason)

A solution used as a disinfectant for skin and body cleansing and disinfecting.

Dose: use as a soap.
Availability: NHS, private prescription, over the counter.
Side effects:
Caution: keep out of the eyes.
Not to be used for:
Caution needed with:
Contains: TRICLOSAN.
Other preparations: MANUSEPT, STER-ZAC BATH CONCENTRATE.

---

aqueous cream BP

A cream used as an emollient to treat dry skin conditions.

Dose: apply as required.
Availability: NHS, private prescription, over the counter.
Side effects:
Caution:
Not to be used for:
Caution needed with:
Contains: aqueous cream BP.
Other preparations:

---

arachis oil *see* Cerumol, Fletchers' Arachis Oil, Oilatum Cream, Polytar AF, Polytar Emollient, Polytar Liquid

---

Arbralene *see* metoprolol tablets
(Berk)

Arelix
(Hoechst-Roussel)

A green/orange capsule supplied at a strength of 6 mg and used as a DIURETIC to treat high blood pressure.

Dose: 1-2 a day as a single morning dose.
Availability: NHS and private prescription.
Side effects: electrolyte imbalance.
Caution: in pregnant women, nursing mothers, or in patients suffering from liver or kidney disease, gout, diabetes, enlarged prostate, or impaired urination. Your doctor may advise regular blood tests. Potassium supplements may also be needed.
Not to be used for: children or for patients suffering from cirrhosis of the liver.
Caution needed with: DIGOXIN, LITHIUM, some antibiotics, blood pressure-lowering drugs, NON-STEROIDAL ANTI-INFLAMMATORY DRUGS.
Contains: PIRETANIDE.
Other preparations:

Arpicolin *see* procyclidine tablets
(Rosemont)

Artane *see* **benzhexol tablets**
(Lederle)

Arthrofen *see* **ibuprofen tablets**
(Ashbourne)

Arthrosin *see* **naproxen tablets**
(Ashbourne)

Arthrotec
(Searle Pharmaceuticals)

A white tablet used as a PROSTAGLANDIN and NON-STEROIDAL ANTI-INFLAMMATORY DRUG to treat rheumatoid arthritis, osteoarthritis.

Dose: 1 tablet twice a day with food, up to 1 tablet 3 times a day if required.
Availability: NHS, private prescription.
Side effects: stomach upset, heavy periods, bleeding from the vagina, headache, dizziness, nausea, swelling, skin reactions.
Caution: in patients suffering from stomach ulcer, heart, kidney, or liver failure, blood vessel disorders. Patients on long-term treatments should have regular blood tests and women of child-bearing age should use effective contraception.
Not to be used for: pregnant women, women planning pregnancy, nursing mothers, or patients suffering from stomach bleeding or allergy to ASPIRIN or anti-inflammatory drugs.
Caution needed with: antidiabetic drugs taken by mouth, DIURETICS, STEROIDS, other non-steroidal anti-inflammatory drugs, LITHIUM, DIGOXIN, ANTICOAGULANTS, METHOTREXATE, some antibiotics.
Contains: DICLOFENAC SODIUM, MISOPROSTOL.
Other preparations:

Arthroxen *see* **naproxen tablets**
(Ashbourne)

Artificial Tears Minims
(Chauvin Pharmaceuticals)

Single-dose eye drops used to treat tear deficiencies.

Dose: as needed.

Availability: NHS, private prescription, over the counter.
Side effects:
Caution:
Not to be used for:
Caution needed with:
Contains: HYDROXYETHYLCELLULOSE, SODIUM CHLORIDE.
Other preparations:

Artracin SR *see* indomethacin tablets
(Trinity)

Arythmol
(Knoll)

A white coated tablet supplied in strengths of 150 mg, 300 mg and used as an anti-arrhythmic drug to treat heart rhythm disturbances

Dose: 150-300 mg 3 times a day.
Availability: NHS and private prescription.
Side effects: nausea, vomiting, dizziness, diarrhoea or constipation, headache, tiredness, skin rash, bitter taste in the mouth, slow heart rate.
Caution: in the elderly, patients with pace makers, and in patients suffering from heart failure, liver and kidney disorders. Treatment with this drug should be started under hospital supervision.
Not to be used for: children, pregnant women, nursing mothers, or for patients suffering from uncontrolled heart failure, obstructive lung disease, electrolyte disturbances, some heart rhythm disturbances, very low blood pressure, MYASTHENIA GRAVIS.
Caution needed with: other anti-arrhythmics, DIGOXIN, WARFARIN, CIMETIDINE, PROPRANOLOL, METOPROLOL, RIFAMPICIN, TRICYCLIC ANTIDEPRESSANTS, tranquillizers, CYCLOSPORIN, THEOPHYLLINE, TERFENADINE, ASTEMIZOLE, NICOUMALONE.
Contains: PROPAFENONE.
Other preparations:

Asacol
(Smith Kline & French)

A red, coated, oblong tablet supplied at a strength of 400 mg and used as a salicylate to treat ulcerative colitis.

Dose: 3-6 tablets a day in divided doses.
Availability: NHS and private prescription.
Side effects: stomach disturbances, headache, blood changes, kidney

failure.

Caution: in pregnant women, nursing mothers, the elderly, and in patients suffering from kidney disease, raised blood urea, protein in the urine. You should tell your doctor if there is any bleeding, bruising, sore throat, or general feeling of illness. Your doctor may advise blood tests.

Not to be used for: children or for patients suffering from severe kidney damage.

Caution needed with: LACTULOSE or any preparations that increase the acidity of the motions.

Contains: MESALAZINE.

Other preparations: Asacol suppositories, Asacol foam enema, PENTASA (a long-acting product), SALOFALK.

Ascabiol
(Rhône-Poulenc Rorer)

An emulsion used as an insect-destroying drug to treat scabies, lice.

Dose: as advised by doctor. (Infants and children use diluted preparation).

Availability: NHS, private prescription, over the counter.

Side effects: irritation.

Caution: in pregnant women, nursing mothers. Keep out of the eyes.

Not to be used for:

Caution needed with:

Contains: BENZYL BENZOATE.

Other preparations: BENZYL BENZOATE APPLICATION BP.

---

ascorbic acid *see* ascorbic acid tablets, vitamin C

---

ascorbic acid tablets

A tablet supplied at strengths of 25 mg, 50 mg, 100 mg, 200 mg, 500 mg, and used to prevent and treat scurvy.

Dose: prevention 25-75 mg a day; treatment at least 250 mg a day.

Availability: NHS and private prescription.

Side effects:

Caution:

Not to be used for:

Caution needed with:

Contains: VITAMIN C.

Other preparations: Redoxon (not available on NHS).

Asendis
(Wyeth)

A white, orange, or blue, seven-sided tablet according to strengths of 25 mg, 50 mg, 100 mg, and used as a TRICYCLIC ANTIDEPRESSANT to treat depression.

Dose: 100-150 mg a day increasing to 150-250 mg a day. for maintenance and up to a maximum of 300 mg a day; elderly reduced doses
Availability: NHS and private prescription.
Side effects: dry mouth, constipation, retention of urine, changes in eyesight, heart rhythm changes, tinnitus, drowsiness, nervousness, sleeplessness, shaking, low blood pressure on standing, dizziness, sweating, weakness, tiredness, shaky movements, stomach upset, weight changes, blood changes, allergy, jaundice, changes in sexual function, inappropriate production of breast milk, impotence, breast enlargement, convulsions at high doses.
Caution: in the elderly, nursing mothers, and in patients who are a suicide risk, or who are suffering from epilepsy, glaucoma, urine retention, constipation, kidney disease, confusion, agitation, blood circulation disease, liver disorders, overactive thyroid gland, diabetes, .
Not to be used for: children, pregnant women, or for patients suffering from recent heart attack, heart block, heart rhythm disturbances, severe liver disease, mania.
Caution needed with: MAOIS, BARBITURATES, anticonvulsants, tranquillizers, alcohol, ANTICHOLINERGICS, other antidepressants, sedatives, blood-pressure lowering drugs, local anaesthetics, ADRENALINE.
Contains: AMOXAPINE.
Other preparations:

Aserbine
(Forley)

A cream and solution used as a wound cleanser to treat varicose ulcers, burns, bed sores, and for cleansing of wounds.

Dose: wash the wound with the solution and apply cream twice a day.
Availability: NHS, private prescription, over the counter.
Side effects:
Caution: avoid the eyes.
Not to be used for:
Caution needed with:
Contains: MALIC ACID, BENZOIC ACID, SALICYLIC ACID, PROPYLENE GLYCOL.
Other preparations:

Ashbourne *see* Oilatum Emollient
(Ashbourne)

Asilone Suspension
(Seton Healthcare)

A white liquid used as an ANTACID, anti-wind preparation to treat gastritis, stomach ulcers, indigestion, heartburn, wind.

Dose: adults 5-10 ml after meals and at bedtime
Availability: NHS, private prescription, over the counter.
Side effects: occasionally constipation.
Caution:
Not to be used for: infants and children.
Caution needed with: tablets coated to protect the stomach, some antibiotics, iron.
Contains: activated DIMETHICONE, ALUMINIUM HYDROXIDE GEL, MAGNESIUM OXIDE.
Other preparations: Asilone liquid and tablets (not available on NHS), MAALOX PLUS (tablets not available on NHS), INFACOL – for infants.

Asmaven *see* salbutamol tablets/inhaler
(Berk)

Aspav
(Hoechst-Roussel)

A white, dispersible tablet used as ANALGESIC to relieve pain after operations and other chronic pain.

Dose: 1-2 tablets dispersed in water every 4-6 hours up to a maximum of 8 tablets in 24 hours.
Availability: NHS and private prescription.
Side effects: allergies, asthma, stomach bleeding, constipation, nausea, confusion.
Caution: in pregnant women, women in labour, nursing mothers, the elderly, and in patients suffering from head injury, underactive thyroid gland, a history of bronchospasm or anti-inflammatory induced allergies, kidney or liver disease, stomach disorders.
Not to be used for: children, unconscious patients, or patients suffering from haemophilia, breathing disorders.
Caution needed with: MAOIS, sedatives, ANTICOAGULANTS, antidiabetic drugs, NON-STEROIDAL ANTI-INFLAMMATORY DRUGS, uric acid-lowering drugs, METHOTREXATE, sulphonamide antibiotics.
Contains: ASPIRIN, PAPAVERETUM.

Other preparations:

aspirin *see* **Aspav, aspirin tablets, aspirin 75 mg tablets, Caprin, Co-Codaprin Dispersible, Disprin CV, Doloxene Co., Equagesic, Migravess, Nu-Seals Aspirin, postMI, Robaxisal Forte**

aspirin 75 mg tablets

A white tablet supplied at a strength of 75 mg and used to prevent heart attack or stroke, in patients known to be at risk.

Dose: 1-4 tablets a day (dissolved in water).
Availability: NHS, private prescription, over the counter.
Side effects: stomach upsets, allergy, asthma.
Caution: in pregnant women and in patients suffering from uncontrolled high blood pressure or asthma.
Not to be used for: children under 12 years, nursing mothers, or for patients suffering from haemophilia or stomach ulcer.
Caution needed with: ANTICOAGULANTS, some antidiabetic drugs, anti-inflammatory agents, METHOTREXATE, SPIRONOLACTONE, STEROIDS, some uric-acid lowering drugs.
Contains: ASPIRIN.
Other preparations: BEECHAM ASPIRIN 75 MG, NU-SEALS ASPIRIN 75 MG, POST-MI 75. (Some available as a non-dissolving form or with a coating to protect the stomach – do not take the latter with ANTACIDS.)

aspirin tablets

A white tablet supplied at a strength of 300 mg and used as an ANALGESIC to relieve pain and reduce fever.

Dose: 1-3 tablets every 4-6 hours as needed to a maximum of 12 tablets a day.
Availability: NHS, private prescription, over the counter.
Side effects: stomach upsets, allergy, asthma.
Caution: in pregnant women, the elderly, or in patients with a history of allergy to aspirin, asthma, impaired kidney or liver function, indigestion.
Not to be used for: children, nursing mothers, or patients suffering from haemophilia, or stomach ulcers.
Caution needed with: ANTICOAGULANTS, some antidiabetic drugs, anti-inflammatory agents, METHOTREXATE, SPIRONOLACTONE, STEROIDS, some ANTACIDS, some uric acid-lowering drugs.
Contains: ASPIRIN.

Other preparations: Dispersible Aspirin, NU-SEALS ASPIRIN (with coating to protect the stomach – do not take with ANTACIDS).

---

astemizole *see* **Hismanal**

AT 10
(Sanofi Winthrop)

A solution used as a source of VITAMIN D to treat a nerve disorder due to low calcium levels in patients with underactive parathyroid glands.

Dose: 1-7 ml taken by mouth each week, or as directed by a doctor.
Availability: NHS, private prescription, over the counter.
Side effects: loss of appetite, raised blood calcium levels, listlessness, vertigo, stupor, nausea, urgent need to urinate, passing large volumes of pale-coloured urine, paralysis, headache, thirst.
Caution: in pregnant women, nursing mothers.Your doctor may advise that your calcium levels should be checked regularly.
Not to be used for: children.
Caution needed with: CHOLESTYRAMINE, some DIURETICS, DIGOXIN and similar drugs.
Contains: DIHYDROTACHYSTEROL.
Other preparations:

Atarax
(Pfizer)

An orange tablet or a green tablet according to strengths of 10 mg, 25 mg and used as an ANTIHISTAMINE to treat anxiety and itching.

Dose: adults: anxiety 50-100 mg 4 times a day; itching 25 mg 1-4 times a day. (Children use syrup.)
Availability: NHS and private prescription.
Side effects: drowsiness, ANTICHOLINERGIC effects, involuntary movements if a high dosage is taken.
Caution: in patients suffering from kidney disease. Patients should be warned of reduced judgement and abilities. Only to be used in children for itching (reduced doses).
Not to be used for: pregnant women, infants under 6 months.
Caution needed with: alcohol and sedatives.
Contains: HYDROXYZINE HYDROCHLORIDE.
Other preparations: Atarax Syrup, UCERAX.

Atenix *see* **atenolol tablets**
(Ashbourne)

Atenixco *see* **co-tenidone tablets**
(Ashbourne)

---

atenolol *see* **Antipressan, Atenix, Atenixco, atenolol tablets, Beta-Adalat, Kalten, Tenchlor, Tenif, Tenoret 50, Tenoretic, Tenormin, Totamol**

---

atenolol tablets

A tablet supplied at strengths of 25 mg, 50 mg, and 100 mg, and used as a ß-BLOCKER to treat angina, abnormal heart rhythm, high blood pressure.

Dose: 50-100 mg a day.
Availability: NHS and private prescription.
Side effects: cold hands and feet, sleep disturbance, slow heart rate, tiredness, wheezing, heart failure, low blood pressure, stomach upset, dry eyes, rash.
Caution: in pregnant women, nursing mothers, the elderly, and in patients suffering from diabetes, kidney or liver disorders, MYASTHENIA GRAVIS. May need to be withdrawn before surgery. Withdraw gradually. Your doctor may advise additional treatment with DIURETICS or DIGOXIN.
Not to be used for: children or for patients suffering from heart block or failure, asthma, or a history of blocked airways disease.
Caution needed with: VERAPAMIL, CLONIDINE withdrawal, some anti-arrhythmic drugs and anaesthetics, some blood-pressure lowering drugs, ERGOTAMINE, CIMETIDINE, sedatives, antidiabetics, SYMPATHOMIMETICS, CORTICOSTEROIDS, INDOMETHACIN, NON-STEROIDAL ANTI-INFLAMMATORY DRUGS, oestrogens, the contraceptive pill.
Contains: ATENOLOL.
Other preparations: ANTIPRESSAN, ATENIX, TOTAMOL, TENORMIN.

Ativan *see* **lorazepam tablets**
(Wyeth)

---

atovaquone *see* **Wellvone**

Atromid-S
(Zeneca)

A red capsule supplied at a strength of 500 mg and used as a lipid-lowering agent to treat elevated cholesterol.

Dose: 20-30 mg per kg body weight a day in 2-3 divided doses after meals.
Availability: NHS and private prescription.
Side effects: stomach upset, gallstones, muscle aches.
Caution: in patients with low blood proteins. Your doctor may advise diet and other changes in lifestyle as well as regular blood tests.
Not to be used for: children, pregnant women, or for patients with a history of gall bladder problems or kidney or liver disease.
Caution needed with: ANTICOAGULANTS, antidiabetic drugs, PHENYTOIN.
Contains: CLOFIBRATE.
Other preparations:

Atropine Minims *see* atropine sulphate eye drops
(Chauvin)

---

atropine sulphate *see* Atropine Minims, atropine sulphate eye drops, Isopto Atropine, Lomotil, Lotharin, Tropergen

---

atropine sulphate eye drops

Drops used as an ANTICHOLINERGIC preparation for pupil dilation.

Dose: 1 drop into the eye as needed.
Availability: NHS and private prescription.
Side effects: stinging in the eye, dry mouth, blurred vision, intolerance of light, rapid heart rate, rarely psychological changes.
Caution: effects may be long lasting.
Not to be used for: patients suffering from narrow angle glaucoma.
Caution needed with:
Contains: atropine sulphate.
Other preparations: atropine sulphate eye ointment. ISOPTO ATROPINE, ATROPINE MINIMS (single-use containers).

Atrovent
(Boehringer Ingelheim)

An inhaler used as an ANTICHOLINERGIC preparation to relieve blocked airways especially as a result of bronchitis.

Dose: adults 1-2 metered doses 3-4 times a day; children under 6 years 1 dose 3 times a day; 6-12 years 1-2 doses 3 times a day.
Availability: NHS and private prescription.
Side effects: dry mouth, constipation, retention of urine.
Caution: in patients suffering from enlarged prostate, glaucoma.
Not to be used for:
Caution needed with:
Contains: IPRATROPIUM bromide.
Other preparations: Atrovent aerocaps, Atrovent aerohaler, Atrovent autohaler, Atrovent Forte inhaler, Atrovent nebules (unit dose vials for use in a nebulizer), IPRATROPIUM (solution for use in a nebulizer), STERI-NEB.

Audax
(Napp Consumer)

Drops used as an ANALGESIC and wax softener to relieve pain associated with acute inflammation of the outer or middle ear.

Dose: every four hours fill the ear with the liquid and plug it.
Availability: NHS, private prescription, over the counter.
Side effects:
Caution:
Not to be used for: patients suffering from perforated ear drum.
Caution needed with:
Contains: CHOLINE SALICYLATE, GLYCEROL.
Other preparations:

Audicort
(Lederle)

Drops used as an antibiotic and STEROID treatment for inflammation and infection of the outer ear.

Dose: 2-5 drops into the ear 3-4 times a day.
Availability: NHS and private prescription.
Side effects: additional infection, irritation.
Caution: in pregnant women and nursing mothers.
Not to be used for: children or for patients suffering from perforated ear drum.
Caution needed with:
Contains: TRIAMCINOLONE ACETONIDE, NEOMYCIN.
Other preparations:

Augmentin
(Beecham)

A white, oval tablet available at strengths of 375 mg, 625 mg, and used as a broad-spectrum penicillin to treat respiratory, ear, nose, and throat, urinary tract, skin, and soft tissue infections, bone, joint, and dental infections.

Dose: 375-625 mg 3 times a day for up to 14 days (children use suspension). For dental infections treat only for 5 days.
Availability: NHS and private prescription.
Side effects: allergy and stomach disturbances. Rarely liver, kidney, blood or skin changes.
Caution: in pregnant women, nursing mothers, and in patients suffering from kidney or liver disease, glandular fever.
Not to be used for: patients suffering from penicillin allergy.
Caution needed with:
Contains: CLAVULANIC ACID, AMOXYCILLIN (CO-AMOXICLAV).
Other preparations: Augmentin Dispersible, Augmentin Intravenous, Augmentin Suspension, Augmentin Duo.

---

auranofin *see* Ridaura Tiltab

Aureocort
(Lederle)

A cream used as a strong STEROID, antibacterial treatment for skin disorders where there is inflammation and infection.

Dose: apply a small quantity of the cream to the affected area 2-3 times a day.
Availability: NHS and private prescription.
Side effects: fluid retention, suppression of adrenal glands. Thinning, spotting, or streaking of the skin may occur.
Caution: use for short periods of time only.
Not to be used for: children, or for patients suffering from acne or any other skin infections caused by tuberculosis, ringworm, viruses, or fungi, scabies, leg ulcers, or continuously especially in pregnant women.
Caution needed with:
Contains: TRIAMCINOLONE ACETONIDE, CHLORTETRACYCLINE HYDROCHLORIDE.
Other preparations: Aureocort Ointment.

Aureomycin Ointment/Eye Ointment
(Lederle)

An ointment and eye ointment used as an antibiotic to treat eye and skin infections.

Dose: apply eye ointment into the eye every 2 hours, or skin ointment on gauze to the affected area once a day or as needed.
Availability: NHS and private prescription.
Side effects: additional infection.
Caution:
Not to be used for: children, women in the latter half of pregnancy, nursing mothers.
Caution needed with:
Contains: CHLORTETRACYCLINE HYDROCHLORIDE.
Other preparations: Aureomycin Cream.

Aveeno
(Bioglan)

A bath oil, cream, or powder in sachets (with or without added mineral oil) used as an emollient to treat eczema and itchy and infective skin conditions.

Dose: 20-30 ml of bath oil added to bath or applied to skin before bathing or showering; cream used as required; 1 sachet of powder (children half sachet) added to bath and soak for 10-15 minutes.
Availability: NHS, private prescription, over the counter.
Side effects:
Caution: take care not to slip in the bath/shower.
Not to be used for:
Caution needed with:
Contains: colloidal OATMEAL.
Other preparations:

Avloclor
(Zeneca)

A white, scored tablet supplied at a strength of 250 mg and used as an antimalarial, amoebicide preparation for the prevention and treatment of malaria, and the treatment of some forms of hepatitis.

Dose: prevention of malaria adults 2 tablets on the same day once a week, children reduced doses (start 1 week before entering endemic area, and continue for 4 weeks after leaving); treatment of hepatitis adults only 4 tablets a day for 2 days then 1 tablet twice a day for 2-3 weeks.
Availability: NHS, private prescription, over the counter (for prevention of malaria).

A

Side effects: headache, stomach upset, skin eruptions, hair loss or loss of hair colour, blurred vision, eye damage, blood disorders, loss of pigments.
Caution: in pregnant women, nursing mothers, and in patients suffering from PORPHYRIA, kidney or liver disease, or psoriasis. Your doctor may advise regular eye tests before and during treatment.
Not to be used for:
Caution needed with:
Contains: CHLOROQUINE phosphate.
Other preparations: NIVAQUINE.

Avomine
(Rhône-Poulenc Rorer)

A white, scored tablet supplied at a strength of 25 mg and used as an ANTIHISTAMINE treatment for travel sickness, nausea, vomiting, vertigo.

Dose: adults travel sickness 1 at bedtime before long journeys or 1-2 hours before short journeys, nausea 1 tablet 1-4 times a day; children 5-10 years half adults dose.
Availability: NHS, private prescription, over the counter (for travel sickness).
Side effects: drowsiness (do not drive or operate machinery if affected), reduced reactions, rarely skin eruptions and blood disorders.
Caution: in pregnant women, nursing mothers, and in patients suffering from liver or kidney disease, epilepsy, enlarged prostate, galucoma.
Not to be used for: children under 5 years.
Caution needed with: alcohol, sedatives, and some antidepressants (MAOIS), ANTICHOLINERGICS.
Contains: PROMETHAZINE theoclate.
Other preparations: PHENERGAN, SOMINEX.

Axid
(Eli Lilly)

A pale-yellow/ dark-yellow capsule supplied at a strength of 150 mg and 300 mg and used as a HISTAMINE H_2-ANTAGONIST for treatment and prevention of ulcers and to treat reflux from the stomach.

Dose: ulcers: 300 mg in the evening or 150 mg twice a day for 4-8 weeks; prevention: 150 mg in the evening for up to a year. Reflux: 150-300 mg twice a day for up to 12 weeks.
Availability: NHS and private prescription.
Side effects: headache, chest pain, muscle ache, fatigue, dreams, runny nose, sore throat, cough, itch, sweating, changes in liver enzymes, anaemia.

Caution: in pregnant women and nursing mothers, and in patients suffering from impaired kidney and liver functions.
Not to be used for: children.
Caution needed with:
Contains: NIZATIDINE.
Other preparations: Axid Injection.

Axsain
(Euroderma)

A cream used as a topical ANALGESIC to treat pain following shingles.

Dose: apply to the painful area 3-4 times a day.
Availability: NHS, private prescription.
Side effects: irritation.
Caution:
Not to be used for: children or on broken or irritated skin.
Caution needed with:
Contains: CAPSAICIN.
Other preparations:

Azamune *see* azathioprine tablets
(Penn)

---

azapropazone *see* Rheumox

---

azatadine *see* Optimine

---

azathioprine tablets

A tablet supplied at strengths of 25 mg, 50 mg and used to suppress the rejection of newly transplanted organs by the body's immune system. It is also used to treat MYASTHENIA GRAVIS, ulcerative colitis, and rheumatoid arthritis.

Dose: up to 5 mg per kilogram of body weight at first, but generally 1-4 mg/kg per day in divided doses according to condition.
Availability: NHS and private prescription.
Side effects: general debility, rash, dizziness, nausea and vomiting, fever, joint and muscle pain, liver damage, heart rhythm disturbance, low blood pressure, bone marrow effects such as bruising or bleeding (must be reported to the physician immediately), hair loss, infections.

Caution: in the elderly, pregnant women, and in patients suffering from liver or kidney disorder, infection, or where there is excessive exposure to the sun. Your doctor will insist on regular check-ups and blood tests.
Not to be used for: patients suffering from stagnation of the biliary system or toxic inflammation of the liver.
Caution needed with: ALLOPURINOL, RIFAMPICIN, muscle relaxants.
Contains: AZATHIOPRINE.
Other preparations: AZAMUNE, IMMUNOPRIN, IMURAN.

---

azelaic acid *see* **Skinoren**

---

azelastine *see* **Rhinolast**

---

azithromycin *see* **Zithromax**

---

azlocillin *see* **Securopen**

---

bacampicillin hydrochloride *see* **Ambaxin**

---

bacitracin *see* **Cicatrin, Polyfax**

---

baclofen tablets

A tablet supplied at a strength of 10 mg and used as a muscle relaxant to treat voluntary muscle spasticity caused by cerebrovascular accidents, cerebral palsy, meningitis, multiple sclerosis, spinal lesions.

Dose: adults ½ tablet 3 times a day after food at first increasing as needed by ½ tablet 3 times a day every 3 days to a maximum of 10 tablets a day; children as advised by doctor.
Availability: NHS and private prescription.
Side effects: nausea, sedation, drowsiness, confusion, dizziness, muscle tiredness, reduced alertness, low blood pressure, heart, lung, and circulation disorder, sleeplessness, headache, problems with urination. Rarely visual disturbance, rash, convulsions, taste disturbance, sweating, or liver disorder.
Caution: in the elderly, pregnant women, nursing mothers, and in patients suffering from epilepsy, stroke, liver/kidney disorder, diabetes, or mental disorders, respiratory problems, or with a history of stomach ulcer. Withdraw treatment gradually.

Not to be used for: patients suffering from stomach ulcer.
Caution needed with: blood-pressure lowering drugs, LITHIUM, TRICYCLIC ANTIDEPRESSANTS, IBUPROFEN, LEVODOPA, CARBIDOPA, ACE INHIBITORS, sedatives, alcohol.
Contains: BACLOFEN.
Other preparations: BACLOSPAS, BALGIFEN, LIORESAL.

B

Baclospas *see* baclofen tablets
(Ashbourne)

Bactigras
(Smith & Nephew Healthcare)

A sterile gauze dressing impregnated with antiseptic, supplied in sizes of 5 cm square or 10 cm square, and used as a dressing for wounds where there may be bacterial infection.

Availability: NHS, private prescription, over the counter.
Contains: CHLORHEXIDINE acetate, WHITE SOFT PARAFFIN.

Bactrim *see* co-trimoxazole tablets
(Roche)

Bactroban
(Beecham)

A nasal ointment or an ointment used as an antibiotic to treat infections of the nose or skin.

Dose: apply to the openings of the nose 2-3 times a day for 5-7 days, or up to 10 days for skin infections.
Availability: NHS and private prescription.
Side effects:
Caution: in patients suffering from kidney disease. Keep out of the eyes.
Not to be used for:
Caution needed with:
Contains: MUPIROCIN.
Other preparations:

Balgifen *see* baclofen tablets
(Berk)

Balmosa
(Pharmax)

A cream used as an ANALGESIC rub to treat muscular rheumatism, fibrositis, lumbago, sciatica, unbroken chilblains.

Dose: massage into the affected area as needed.
Availability: NHS, private prescription, over the counter.
Side effects: may be irritant.
Caution:
Not to be used for: areas near the eyes, on broken or inflamed skin, or on membranes (such as the mouth).
Caution needed with:
Contains: MENTHOL, CAMPHOR, METHYL SALICYLATE, CAPSICUM OLEORESIN.
Other preparations:

Balneum
(Merck)

A liquid used as a bath emollient to treat dry skin conditions.

Dose: adults, 1-3 measures added to bath; infants, ½-¾ measure, other children, ½-1½ measure.
Availability: NHS, private prescription, over the counter.
Side effects:
Caution: take care not to slip in the bath.
Not to be used for:
Caution needed with:
Contains: SOYA OIL.
Other preparations: BALNEUM PLUS (with added LAUROMACROGOLS for itchy conditions).

Balneum Plus
(Merck)

A liquid used as a bath oil to treat itching and dry skin conditions.

Dose: 1-3 measures added to the bath; children use ¼-¾ measures.
Availability: NHS, private prescription, over the counter.
Side effects:
Caution:
Not to be used for:
Caution needed with:
Contains: SOYA OIL, LAUROMACROGOLS.
Other preparations:

Balneum with Tar
(Merck)

A bath oil used as an emollient and antipsoriatic to treat eczema, itchy or thickening skin disorders, psoriasis, dandruff.

Dose: adults add 20 ml to the bath water; children add 10 ml and use for a maximum of 6 weeks.
Availability: NHS, private prescription, over the counter.
Side effects:
Caution: avoid exposing skin to bright sunlight for long periods.
Not to be used for: patients suffering from wet or weeping skin problems or where the skin is badly broken.
Caution needed with:
Contains: COAL TAR, SOYA OIL.
Other preparations: POLYTAR EMOLLIENT.

Baltar
(Merck)

A liquid used as an antipsoriatic treatment for psoriasis, dandruff, eczema, itchy and scaly conditions of the scalp.

Dose: shampoo the hair with the liquid 1-3 times a week.
Availability: NHS, private prescription, over the counter.
Side effects:
Caution: keep out of the eyes.
Not to be used for: children under 2 years or for patients suffering from wet or weeping dermatoses, or where the skin is badly broken.
Caution needed with:
Contains: COAL TAR.
Other preparations: POLYTAR.

Bambec
(Novex Pharma)

A white, oval, scored tablet supplied at strengths of 10 mg and 20 mg, and used as a BRONCHODILATOR to treat reversible airways disease, bronchial spasm in asthma.

Dose: 10-20 mg once a day at night
Availability: NHS, private prescription.
Side effects: low potassium levels, hands shaking, headache, cramps, palpitations.
Caution: in pregnant women, nursing mothers, and in patients suffering

from kidney damage, weak heart, overactive thyroid, diabetes. In asthmatics blood potassium levels should be checked regularly.

Not to be used for: children or for patients suffering from severe liver failure.

Caution needed with: ß-BLOCKERS.

Contains: BAMBUTEROL hydrochloride.

Other preparations:

---

bambuterol *see* Bambec

Baratol
(Monmouth)

A blue tablet or a green, scored tablet according to strengths of 25 mg, 50 mg and used as an ANTIHYPERTENSIVE to treat high blood pressure.

Dose: 25 mg twice a day at first increasing by 25-50 mg a day at two-weekly intervals to a maximum of 200 mg a day if needed in 2-3 divided doses.

Availability: NHS and private prescription.

Side effects: drowsiness, dry mouth, blocked nose, increase in bodyweight, inability to ejaculate.

Caution: in patients suffering from kidney or liver weakness, Parkinson's disease, epilepsy, depression; patients with weak hearts should be treated with DIGOXIN and DIURETICS.

Not to be used for: children or patients suffering from heart failure.

Caution needed with: alcohol, sedatives, MAOIS, blood-pressure lowering drugs.

Contains: INDORAMIN hydrochloride.

Other preparations: DORALESE.

---

barbiturate
A sedative drug used to treat the most severe cases of sleeplessness and epilepsy. Examples AMYLOBARBITONE *see* Amytal, and PHENOBARBITONE.

Baxan
(Bristol-Myers Squibb)

A white capsule supplied at a strength of 500 mg and used as a cephalosporin antibiotic to treat respiratory, skin, and soft tissue infections, ear infections, urine infections.

Dose: adults 1-2 capsules twice a day; children use suspension.

Availability: NHS and private prescription.
Side effects: allergy, stomach disturbances.
Caution: in pregnant women, nursing mothers, and in patients suffering from kidney disease or who are sensitive to penicillins.
Not to be used for:
Caution needed with:
Contains: CEFADROXIL.
Other preparations: Baxan Suspension.

Baycaron
(Bayer)

A white, scored tablet supplied at a strength of 25 mg and used as a DIURETIC to treat high blood pressure, fluid retention.

Dose: 1-2 a day as a single dose in the morning for 10-14 days, then 1 a day or 1 every other day. (Up to 4 a day for fluid retention.)
Availability: NHS and private prescription.
Side effects: stomach upset, blood and other metabolic changes, rash, sensitivity to light, dizziness, pancreatitis, anorexia, impotence.
Caution: in pregnant women, nursing mothers, the elderly, and in patients suffering from kidney or liver disease, diabetes, gout, LUPUS.
Not to be used for: children or for patients suffering from severe kidney failure, Addison's disease, sensitivity to sulphonamides, or severely raised calcium levels.
Caution needed with: DIGOXIN, LITHIUM, blood-pressure lowering drugs, some ANALGESICS, BARBITURATES, alcohol, antidiabetics, NON-STEROIDAL ANTI-INFLAMMATORY DRUGS, CARBENOXOLONE, CORTICOSTEROIDS.
Contains: MEFRUSIDE.
Other preparations:

BCG *see* tuberculosis vaccine

Beclazone *see* beclomethasone inhaler
(Baker Norton)

Beclazone Easi-Breathe *see* beclomethasone inhaler
(Baker Norton)

Becloforte *see* beclomethasone inhaler
(A & H)

Becloforte integra *see* beclomethasone inhaler
(A & H)

Becloforte VM *see* beclomethasone inhaler
(A & H)

beclomethasone *see* Aerobec, Beclazone, Beclofortebeclomethasone inhaler, Beconase, Becotide, Filair, Propaderm, Ventide

beclomethasone inhaler

An aerosol supplied at a strength of 50 mcg, 100 mcg, and 250 mcg per inhalation, and used as a STEROID to prevent asthma.

Dose: adults 400-800 mcg daily; children 200-400 mcg daily. (Adult dose may be increased to 2000 mcg daily in severe cases.) Total daily intake is usually divided into 2-4 equal doses, spaced throughout the day.
Availability: NHS and private prescription.
Side effects: hoarseness, thrush in the mouth and throat. High doses may give rise to general CORTICOSTEROID side effects (see PREDNISOLONE TABLETS).
Caution: in pregnant women, in patients transferring from steroids taken by mouth, and in patients suffering from tubercular lungs.
Not to be used for: (250 mcg strength inhalers not recommended for children.)
Caution needed with:
Contains: BECLOMETHASONE dipropionate.
Other preparations: AEROBEC, BECLAZONE, BECLOFORTE, BECODISKS, BECOTIDE INHALER, BECOTIDE ROTACAPS, FILAIR.

Becodisks *see* beclomethasone inhaler
(A & H)

Beconase
(A & H)

A powder in an aerosol or a suspension in an atomizer supplied at a strength of 50 micrograms and used as a STEROID to treat rhinitis, hay fever.

Dose: 2 sprays into each nostril twice a day regularly.
Availability: NHS and private prescription.
Side effects: irritation of the nose, nose bleeds, disturbance of taste and

smell.

Caution: in pregnant women, nursing mothers, in patients with nasal infections, and in patients transferring from steroids taken by mouth.

Not to be used for: children under 6 years.

Caution needed with:

Contains: BECLOMETHASONE dipropionate.

Other preparations: Beconase Aqueous, Beconase Hayfever (available without prescription to treat hay fever only).

Becotide *see* beclomethasone inhaler
(A & H)

Bedranol SR *see* propranolol tablets
(Lagap)

Beecham Aspirin 75 mg *see* aspirin 75 mg tablets
(SmithKline Beecham Consumer)

---

belladonna *see* Bellocarb

Bellocarb
(Sinclair)

A beige scored tablet used as an ANTACID and anti-spasm treatment for bowel spasm, ulcers, indigestion, gastritis.

Dose: 1-2 tablets, crushed and chewed, 4 times a day.

Availability: over the counter and private presecription.

Side effects: occasionally constipation.

Caution: in patients with enlarged prostate, heart, kidney, or liver problems.

Not to be used for: children or for patients suffering from glaucoma.

Caution needed with: tablets coated to protect the stomach, some antibiotics, iron.

Contains: BELLADONNA, MAGNESIUM TRISILICATE, MAGNESIUM CARBONATE.

Other preparations:

Bendogen *see* bethanidine tablets
(Lagap)

---

bendrofluazide *see* **Aprinox, bendrofluazide tablets, Berkozide, Corgaretic 40, Inderetic, Neo-Bendramax, Neo-Naclex, Neo-Naclex-K, Prestim**

B

bendrofluazide tablets

A white tablet or a white, scored tablet according to strengths of 2.5 mg, 5 mg used as a DIURETIC to treat fluid retention and high blood pressure.

Dose: fluid retention 5-10 mg a day or every other day; high blood pressure usually 2.5 mg a day in the morning.
Availability: NHS and private prescription.
Side effects: low blood presure on standing, mild stomach upset, reversible impotence, pancreatitis, low potassium levels, allergy, rash, sensitivity to light, blood changes, gout, tiredness
Caution: in pregnant women, nursing mothers, the elderly, and in patients suffering from liver or kidney disease, diabetes, gout, LUPUS.
Not to be used for: children or for patients suffering from kidney failure or severe kidney failure, Addison's disease, raised blood sodium, potassium, or calcium levels, or PORPHYRIA.
Caution needed with: DIGOXIN, LITHIUM, blood-pressure lowering drugs, some diuretics, calcium salts, CORTICOSTEROIDS, SYMPATHOMIMETICS, CARBENOXOLONE
Contains: BENDROFLUAZIDE.
Other preparations: APRINOX, BERKOZIDE, NEO-BENDRAMAX, NEO-NACLEX.

Benemid
(M.S.D.)

A white, scored tablet supplied at a strength of 500 mg and used as a uric acid-lowering agent to to treat gout, high uric acid levels in the blood. Also used to prolong the action of certain antibiotics.

Dose: ½ tablet twice a day for the first 7 days then 1 tablet twice a day. (To prolong antibiotics 4 tablets a day; children as advised by a doctor.)
Availability: NHS and private prescription.
Side effects: headache, stomach upset, frequent urination, allergy, sore gums, flushes, acute gout, kidney stones, kidney colic.
Caution: in pregnant women, the elderly, and in patients with kidney disease or a history of stomach ulcer. Drink plenty of fluids.
Not to be used for: children (except to prolong antibiotics), patients suffering from blood disorders, kidney uric acid stones, or to start treatment during an acute attack.
Caution needed with: salicylates, PYRAZINAMIDE, some antibiotics, INDOMETHACIN, METHOTREXATE, some antidiabetic drugs, ASPIRIN.

Contains: PROBENECID.
Other preparations:

Benoral *see* benorylate tablets
(Sanofi Winthrop)

---

benorylate tablets

A tablet used as an ANALGESIC for the relief of pain and inflammation, fever, rheumatoid arthritis, osteoarthritis, pain in bones or muscles.

Dose: for mild to moderate pain 2 g twice a day; for rheumatic disease up to 8 g per day in divided doses (reduced doses for the elderly).
Availability: NHS, private prescription, over the counter.
Side effects: stomach upsets, allergy, asthma.
Caution: in the elderly, in pregnant women, and in patients with a history of allergy to ASPIRIN or asthma, or who are suffering from impaired kidney or liver function, indigestion, uncontrolled high blood pressure.
Not to be used for: children, nursing mothers, haemophiliacs, or patients suffering from stomach ulcers.
Caution needed with: ANTICOAGULANTS, some antidiabetic drugs, NON-STEROIDAL ANTI-INFLAMMATORY DRUGS, METHOTREXATE, SPIRONOLACTONE, CORTICOSTEROIDS, some ANTACIDS, some uric acid-lowering drugs, MIFEPRISTONE, METOCLOPRAMIDE. Do not take with any other medicine containing ASPIRIN or PARACETAMOL.
Contains: BENORYLATE.
Other preparations: benorylate suspension. BENORAL.

Benoxyl 5
(Stiefel)

A cream used as an antibacterial and skin softener to treat acne.

Dose: wash and dry the affected area, then apply once a day. (Progress to stronger product, Benoxyl 10, if necessary.)
Availability: NHS, private prescription, over the counter.
Side effects: irritation, peeling.
Caution: keep out of the eyes, nose, and mouth. May bleach fabrics.
Not to be used for:
Caution needed with:
Contains: BENZOYL PEROXIDE.
Other preparations: Benoxyl 10 Lotion, ACETOXYL, ACNEGEL, ACNECIDE, NERICUR, PANOXYL, QUINODERM. (Other brands available over the counter.)

---

benperidol *see* **Anquil**

---

benserazide hydrochloride *see* **Madopar**

---

benzalkonium chloride *see* **Capitol, Conotrane, Drapolene, Ionax, Ionil T, Oilatum Plus, Timodine**

Benzamycin
(Bioglan)

A gel used as an antibiotic and skin softener to treat acne.

Dose: wash and dry the skin, then apply gel twice a day.
Availability: NHS, private prescription.
Side effects: irritation.
Caution: in pregnant women, nursing mothers, and on mucous membranes.
Not to be used for:
Caution needed with: CLINDAMYCIN and other acne treatments applied to the skin.
Contains: ERYTHROMYCIN, BENZOYL PEROXIDE.
Other preparations:

---

benzhexol tablets

A tablet used as an ANTICHOLINERGIC preparation to treat parkinsonism and tremor.

Dose: 1 mg a day at first gradually increasing if necessary to 5-15 mg a day in divided doses.
Availability: NHS and private prescription.
Side effects: dry mouth, stomach upset, dizziness, blurred vision, occasionally retention of urine, allergy, confusion, excitement, mental disturbances, rapid heart rate.
Caution: in patients suffering from heart disease, liver or kidney failure. Withdraw slowly.
Not to be used for: undiagnosed retention of urine, stomach block, closed angle glaucoma.
Caution needed with: NEFOPAM, DISOPYRAMIDE, TRICYCLIC ANTIDEPRESSANTS, MAOIS, ANTIHISTAMINES, some sedatives, CISAPRIDE, DOMPERIDONE, METOCLOPRAMIDE, AMANTADINE, some SYMPATHOMIMETICS.
Contains: benzhexol hydrochloride

Other preparations: ARTANE, BROFLEX.

---

benzocaine *see* **Intralgin, Merocaine**

---

benzoic acid *see* **Aserbine**

---

benzoic acid compound ointment BP

An ointment used as an antifungal preparation to treat infections such as ringworm.

Dose: apply twice a day.
Availability: NHS, private prescription, over the counter.
Side effects:
Caution:
Not to be used for:
Caution needed with:
Contains: BENZOIC ACID, SALICYLIC ACID, EMULSIFYING OINTMENT.
Other preparations:

---

benzoyl peroxide *see* **Acetoxyl, Acnecide, Acnegel, Benoxyl 5, Benzamycin, Nericur, Panoxyl, Quinoderm Cream, Quinoped**

---

benzthiazide *see* **Dytide**

---

benztropine *see* **Cogentin**

---

benzydamine *see* **Difflam, Difflam Oral Rinse**

---

benzyl alcohol *see* **Sudocrem**

---

benzyl benzoate *see* **Anugesic-HC, Anusol HC, Ascabiol, benzyl benzoate application BP, Sudocrem**

---

benzyl benzoate application BP

An emulsion used as an insect-destroying drug to treat scabies.

Dose: adults: apply the emulsion to the whole body, repeat treatment the next day without bathing, and then wash off 24 hours later. Or as advised by doctor. (Infants and children use diluted preparation.)
Availability: NHS, private prescription, over the counter.
Side effects: irritation, burning sensation, rarely, rash.
Caution: in children. Keep out of the eyes and avoid mucous membranes.
Not to be used for: nursing mothers, pregnant women, or on broken or infected skin.
Caution needed with:
Contains: BENZYL BENZOATE.
Other preparations: ASCABIOL.

---

benzyl cinnamate *see* Sudocrem

---

benzyl nicotinate *see* Salonair

Berkamil *see* amiloride tablets
(Berk)

Berkatens *see* verapamil tablets
(Berk)

Berkmycen *see* oxytetracycline tablets
(Berk)

Berkolol *see* propranolol tablets
(Berk)

Berkozide *see* bendrofluazide tablets
(Berk)

Berotec
(Boehringer Ingelheim)

An aerosol supplied at a strength of 0.1 mg and 0.2 mg and used as a BRONCHODILATOR to treat bronchial asthma, emphysema, bronchitis.

Dose: adults 1-2 sprays 3 times a day up to a maximum of 2 sprays every 6 hours; children over 6 years1 spray 3 times a day up to a maximum of 2 spray every 6 hours (using lower strength only).
Availability: NHS and private prescription.
Side effects: headache, dilation of the blood vessels, nervous tension.
Caution: in pregnant women and in patients suffering from heart disease, angina, abnormal heart rhythms, high blood pressure, overactive thyroid gland.
Not to be used for: children under 6 years.
Caution needed with: SYMPATHOMIMETICS.
Contains: FENOTEROL hydrobromide.
Other preparations:

Beta-Adalat
(Bayer)

A reddish-brown capsule used as a ß-BLOCKER and calcium antagonist to treat high blood pressure, angina.

Dose: adults 1 capsule a day increasing to 2 capsules a day if necessary; elderly no more than 1 capsule a day.
Availability: NHS and private prescription.
Side effects: flushing, headache, dizziness, tiredness, dry eyes, skin rash, fluid retention, jaundice, gum swelling.
Caution: in patients under anaesthesia or those with weak heart, lung, kidney or liver disease, diabetes.
Not to be used for: children, pregnant women, nursing mothers, or for patients suffering from heart block, failure, or shock.
Caution needed with: CIMETIDINE, QUINIDINE, other heart drugs.
Contains: ATENOLOL, NIFEDIPINE.
Other preparations: TENIF.

---

beta-blocker (ß-blocker)
a drug which blocks some of the effects of ADRENALINE in the body. Beta-blockers are used to treat angina, high blood pressure, and other conditions. Example PROPANOLOL *see* propranolol tablets.

Beta-Cardone
(Evans)

A green tablet, pink tablet, or white tablet according to strengths of 40 mg,

80 mg, 200 mg and used as a ß-BLOCKER to treat angina, high blood pressure, heart rhythm disturbance, and as an additional treatment for overactive thyroid.

Dose: heart rhythm disturbance 40 mg 3 times a day for 7 days, then 120-240 mg a day in single or divided doses. For angina 80 mg twice a day for 7-10 days, then 200-600 mg a day in single or divided doses. High blood pressure 80 mg twice a day for 7-10 days, then 200-600 mg a day. Overactive thyroid 120-240 mg a day.
Availability: NHS and private prescription.
Side effects: cold hands and feet, sleep disturbances, slow heart rate, tiredness, wheezing, heart failure, low blood pressure, stomach upset, dry eyes, rash.
Caution: in pregnant women, nursing mothers, and in patients suffering from diabetes, kidney or liver disorders, asthma. May need to be withdrawn before surgery. Withdraw gradually. Your doctor may advise additional treatment with DIURETICS or DIGOXIN.
Not to be used for: children or for patients suffering from heart block or failure, low blood pressure, untreated PHAEOCHROMOCYTOMA, asthma.
Caution needed with: VERAPAMIL, CLONIDINE withdrawal, some anti-arrhythmic drugs and anaesthetics, some blood-pressure lowering drugs, CIMETIDINE, sedatives, SYMPATHOMIMETICS, INDOMETHACIN, antidiabetics, ERGOTAMINE.
Contains: SOTALOL hydrochloride.
Other preparations: SOTACOR.

Beta-Prograne *see* propranolol tablets
(Tillomed)

Betacap *see* Betnovate
(Dermal)

Betadine Gargle and Mouthwash
(Seton Healthcare)

A solution used as an antiseptic to treat inflammation of the mouth and pharynx brought on by thrush and other bacterial infections.

Dose: Wash out the mouth or gargle with the diluted or undiluted solution up to 4 times a day.
Availability: NHS, private prescription, over the counter.
Side effects: rarely local irritation and sensitivity.
Caution:
Not to be used for: children under 6 years.

Caution needed with:
Contains: POVIDONE-IODINE.
Other preparations:

Betadine Ointment
(Seton Healthcare)

An ointment used as an antiseptic to treat skin ulcers.

Dose: apply to the affected area and cover once or twice a day for up to 14 days.
Availability: NHS, private prescription, over the counter.
Side effects: rarely irritation.
Caution: in patients sensitive to iodine.
Not to be used for: children under 2 years.
Caution needed with:
Contains: POVIDONE-IODINE.
Other preparations: BETADINE SPRAY.

Betadine Pessaries
(Seton Healthcare)

A pessary and applicator supplied at a strength of 200 mg and used as an antiseptic to treat inflammation of the vagina.

Dose: 1 pessary to be inserted into the vagina night and morning for at least 14 days.
Availability: NHS, private prescription, over the counter.
Side effects: irritation and sensitivity.
Caution:
Not to be used for: children.
Caution needed with:
Contains: POVIDONE-IODINE.
Other preparations: Betadine Vaginal Gel, Betadine VC Kit.

Betadine Scalp Cleanser
(Seton Healthcare)

A solution used as an antiseptic and detergent to treat scaly scalp disorders.

Dose: use as a shampoo twice a week at first and then once a week as condition improves.
Availability: NHS, private prescription, over the counter.

Side effects: rarely irritation or sensitivity.
Caution:
Not to be used for: children under 2 years.
Caution needed with:
Contains: POVIDONE-IODINE.
Other preparations: Betadine Skin Cleanser, Betadine Shampoo.

Betadine Spray
(Seton Healthcare)

A dry powder spray used as an antiseptic to treat skin infections.

Dose: spray on to the affected area once a day or as needed until the area is covered with powder.
Availability: NHS, private prescription, over the counter.
Side effects:
Caution: keep out of the eyes.
Not to be used for: patients suffering from non-toxic colloid goitre.
Caution needed with:
Contains: POVIDONE-IODINE.
Other preparations: Betadine Antiseptic Paint, Betadine Antiseptic Solution, Betadine Alcoholic Solution, Betadine Surgical Scrub.

Betagan
(Allergan)

Drops used as a ß-BLOCKER to treat glaucoma and high blood pressure in the eye.

Dose: 1 drop once or twice a day.
Availability: NHS and private prescription.
Side effects: eye irritation, headache, dizziness, systemic ß-blocker effects (*see* propranolol tablets).
Caution: in nursing mothers, and in patients suffering from diabetes or breathing problems.
Not to be used for: children, pregnant women, and in patients suffering from asthma or some heart disorders, heart failure, or with a history of blocked lung disease.
Caution needed with: RESERPINE, ß-BLOCKERS taken by mouth.
Contains: LEVOBUNOLOL
Other preparations:

---

betahistine dihydrochloride *see* **betahistine tablets, Serc**

---

betahistine tablets

A tablet used as a histamine-type drug to treat vertigo, tinnitus, and hearing loss caused by Ménière's disease.

Dose: 16 mg 3 times a day at first then 24-48 mg a day.
Availability: NHS and private prescription.
Side effects: stomach upset, headache, itching, rash.
Caution: in pregnant women and nursing mothers, and in patients suffering from bronchial asthma, or with a history of stomach ulcer.
Not to be used for: children or for patients suffering from PHAEOCHROMOCYTOMA (a disease of the adrenal glands).
Caution needed with: ANTIHISTAMINES.
Contains: BETAHISTINE dihydrochloride.
Other preparations: SERC.

---

betaine hydrochloride *see* Kloref

Betaloc *see* metoprolol tablets
(Astra)

---

betamethasone *see* Betacap, Betnelan, Betnesol, Betnesol Drops, Betnovate, Betnovate Rectal, Diprosalic, Diprosone, Fucibet, Vista-Methasone

---

betaxolol *see* Betoptic, Kerlone

---

bethanechol *see* Myotonine

---

bethanidine sulphate *see* Bendogen, bethanidine tablets

---

bethanidine tablets

A tablet supplied at a strength of 10 mg and used to treat high blood pressure when the condition has not responded to other blood-pressure lowering drugs.

Dose: 10 mg 3 times a day after meals at first, increasing to a maximum of 200 mg a day if required; elderly half dose at first.

Availability: NHS and private prescription.
Side effects: low blood pressure on standing, fluid retention, blocked nose, headache, drowsiness, failure to ejaculate.
Caution: in the elderly, in pregnant women, and in patients suffering from reduced blood flow to the heart or brain, asthma, or a history of stomach ulcer. Your doctor may advise the use of DIURETICS or other blood-pressure lowering drugs.
Not to be used for: children or for patients suffering from PHAEOCHROMOCYTOMA (a disease of the adrenal glands), heart or kidney failure.
Caution needed with: SYMPATHOMIMETICS, TRICYCLIC ANTIDEPRESSANTS, MAOIS, alcohol, anaesthetics, other blood-pressure lowering drugs, NON-STEROIDAL ANTI-INFLAMMATORY DRUGS, ß-BLOCKERS, some angina treatments, CARBENOXOLONE, CORTICOSTEROIDS, DIURETICS, LEVODOPA, nitrates, oestrogens, some contraceptive pills, PIZOTIFEN, some sedatives and tranquillizers (e.g. CHLORPROMAZINE).
Contains: BETHANIDINE SULPHATE.
Other preparations: BENDOGEN.

Betim *see* Blocadren
(Leo)

Betnelan
(Evans)

A white, scored tablet supplied at a strength of 0.5 mg and used as a STEROID to treat severe asthma, allergies, rheumatoid arthritis, collagen diseases.

Dose: adults 1-10 tablets a day, then reduce as needed; children 1-7 years quarter to half adult dose, 7-12 years half to three-quarters adult dose.
Availability: NHS and private prescription.
Side effects: high blood sugar, thin bones, mood changes, ulcers, high blood pressure, water retention, weak muscles.
Caution: in pregnant women, in patients who have had recent bowel surgery, or who are suffering from inflamed veins, psychiatric disorders, virus infections, some cancers, some kidney diseases, thinning of the bones, ulcers, tuberculosis, other infections, high blood pressure, glaucoma, epilepsy, diabetes, underactive thyroid, liver disease, stress. Withdraw gradually. Avoid contact with chicken pox and shingles.
Not to be used for: children under 1 year.
Caution needed with: PHENYTOIN, PHENOBARBITONE, EPHEDRINE, RIFAMPICIN, DIURETICS, ANTICHOLINESTERASES, DIGOXIN, antidiabetic agents, ANTICOAGULANTS, NON-STEROIDAL ANTI-INFLAMMATORY DRUGS.

Contains: BETAMETHASONE.
Other preparations: BETNESOL TABLETS.

Betnesol Tablets
(Evans)

A pink, scored tablet supplied at a strength of 0.5 mg and used as a STEROID to treat severe asthma, allergies, rheumatoid arthritis, collagen diseases.

Dose: adults 1-10 tablets a day, then reduce as needed; children 1-7 years quarter to half adult dose, 7-12 years half to three-quarters adult dose.
Availability: NHS and private prescription.
Side effects: high blood sugar, thin bones, mood changes, ulcers, high blood pressure, water retention, weak muscles.
Caution: in pregnant women, in patients who have had recent bowel surgery, or who are suffering from inflamed veins, psychiatric disorders, virus infections, some cancers, some kidney diseases, thinning of the bones, ulcers, tuberculosis, other infections, high blood pressure, glaucoma, epilepsy, diabetes, underactive thyroid, liver disease, stress. Withdraw gradually. Avoid contact with chicken pox and shingles.
Not to be used for: children under 1 year.
Caution needed with: PHENYTOIN, PHENOBARBITONE, EPHEDRINE, RIFAMPICIN, DIURETICS, ANTICHOLINESTERASES, DIGOXIN, antidiabetic agents, ANTICOAGULANTS, NON-STEROIDAL ANTI-INFLAMMATORY DRUGS.
Contains: BETAMETHASONE sodium phosphate.
Other preparations: Betnesol Injection.

Betnesol Drops
(Evans)

Drops used as a STEROID to treat inflammation of the ear, nasal passages, or eyes where infection is not present. (Use Betnesol-N for infected conditions.)

Dose: 2-3 drops into each nostril or ear every 2-3 hours, or 1-2 drops into the eye every 1-2 hours.
Availability: NHS and private prescription.
Side effects: sensitivity, resistance to NEOMYCIN (with Betnesol-N), thinning of the cornea, cataract, rise in the eye pressure.
Caution: do not use for longer than is necessary especially in pregnancy.
Not to be used for: patients suffering from viral, tubercular, or fungal conditions of the nose, ear, or eye, dendritic ulcer, glaucoma, or where soft contact lenses are worn. Betnesol-N not to be used on perforated ear

drum.
Caution needed with:
Contains: BETAMETHASONE sodium phosphate.
Other preparations: Betnesol-N, Betnesol Ointment, Betnesol-N Ointment, BETNESOL TABLETS.

___

Betnovate
(Glaxo)

A cream or ointment used as a strong STEROID to treat psoriasis, eczema, external ear and other skin disorders, dermatitis. (Use Betnovate-N and Betnovate-C for infected conditions.)

Dose: apply a small quantity of the cream to the affected area 2-3 times a day.
Availability: NHS and private prescription.
Side effects: fluid retention, suppression of adrenal glands, thinning, spotting, or streaking of the skin may occur.
Caution: use for short periods of time only.
Not to be used for: children under 1 year, or for patients suffering from acne or any other skin infections caused by tuberculosis, ringworm, viruses, or fungi, or continuously especially in pregnant women.
Caution needed with:
Contains: BETAMETHASONE valerate.
Other preparations: Betnovate RD, Betnovate Scalp Application, Betnovate-N, Betnovate-C. BETACAP scalp application, DIPROSONE. Also LOTRIDERM – with CLOTRIMAZOLE for infected conditions.

___

Betnovate Rectal
(Glaxo)

An ointment with applicator used as a STEROID, local anaesthetic treatment for haemorrhoids and mild proctitis.

Dose: apply 2 or 3 times a day at first and then reduce.
Availability: NHS and private prescription.
Side effects: systemic CORTICOSTEROID effects (*see* prednisolone tablets).
Caution: do not use for prolonged periods; caution in pregnant women.
Not to be used for: children or for patients suffering from tuberculous, bacterial, fungal, or viral infections.
Caution needed with:
Contains: BETAMETHASONE valerate, PHENYLEPHRINE hydrochloride, LIGNOCAINE hydrochloride.
Other preparations:

___

Betoptic
(Alcon)

Drops used as a ß-BLOCKER to treat hypertension of the eyes, glaucoma.

Dose: 1 drop into the eye twice a day.
Availability: NHS and private prescription.
Side effects: temporary discomfort, rarely reduction in the sensitivity of the cornea, reddening, staining, or inflammation of the cornea.
Caution: in patients with a history of blocked airways disease, diabetes, overactive thyroid, or who are under general anaesthetic.
Not to be used for: children, or for patients using soft contact lenses or suffering from some heart diseases.
Caution needed with:
Contains: BETAXOLOL hydrochloride.
Other preparations:

bezafibrate *see* **Bezalip-Mono**

Bezalip-Mono
(Boehringer-Mannheim)

A white tablet supplied at a strength of 400 mg and used as a lipid-lowering drug to treat high blood lipids.

Dose: 1 tablet a day after food at night or in the morning.
Availability: NHS and private prescription.
Side effects: stomach upset, muscle aches, rash.
Caution: in patients with kidney disease. Your doctor may advise change in diet or lifestyle.
Not to be used for: children, pregnant women, nursing mothers, or for patients suffering from severe kidney or liver disease.
Caution needed with: ANTICOAGULANTS, antidiabetics, MAOIS.
Contains: BEZAFIBRATE.
Other preparations: Bezalip.

BiNovum
(Janssen-Cilag)

A white tablet and a peach tablet used as an oestrogen, progestogen contraceptive.

Dose: 1 tablet a day for 21 days starting on day 1 of the period.

Availability: NHS and private prescription.

Side effects: enlarged breasts, bloating and fluid retention, cramps, leg pains, mood change, reduction in sexual desire, headaches, nausea, vaginal erosion, discharge, and bleeding, weight gain, skin changes, rarely thrombosis, raised blood pressure, jaundice.

Caution: in patients suffering from high blood pressure, diabetes, Raynaud's disease, vascular disorders, asthma, depression, kidney disease, multiple sclerosis, womb diseases. Your doctor may advise you not to smoke, to have regular examinations. You should stop treatment at the first sign of serious symptoms such as severe headache or jaundice. Treatment should be stopped before surgery.

Not to be used for: pregnant women, or for patients suffering from sickle-cell anaemia, history of heart disease or thrombosis, raised blood pressure supplying the lungs, liver disorders, some cancers, undiagnosed vaginal bleeding, some ear, skin, and kidney disorders, PORPHYRIA.

Caution needed with: RIFAMPICIN, TETRACYCLINE ANTIBIOTICS, GRISEOFULVIN, BARBITURATES, PHENYTOIN, PRIMIDONE, CARBAMAZEPINE, ETHOSUXIMIDE, CHLORAL HYDRATE, DICHLORALPHENAZONE, GLUTETHIMIDE.

Contains: ETHINYLOESTRADIOL, NORETHISTERONE.

Other preparations:

Bioplex
(Thames)

Granules supplied in sachets and used as a protective mouthwash to treat mouth ulcers.

Dose: dissolve contents of sachet in 30-50 ml of warm water and rinse mouth 3 times a day and at night.

Availability: NHS, private prescription.

Side effects:

Caution: do not swallow mouthwash.

Not to be used for:

Caution needed with:

Contains: CARBENOXOLONE sodium.

Other preparations:

Bioral
(SmithKline Beecham)

A gel used as a cell-surface protector to treat mouth ulcers.

Dose: apply after meals and at bed time.

Availability: NHS, private prescription, over the counter.

Side effects:

Caution:
Not to be used for:
Caution needed with:
Contains: CARBENOXOLONE sodium.
Other preparations:

Biorphen
(Bioglan)

A solution to be taken by mouth, supplied at a concentration of 25 mg/5 ml and used as an ANTICHOLINERGIC preparation to treat Parkinson's disease.

Dose: 30 ml a day at first in divided doses increasing every 2-3 days by 5-10 ml to up to 60 ml a day.
Availability: NHS and private prescription.
Side effects: euphoria, anticholinergic effects, confusion, agitation, rash.
Caution: in patients with heart disorders or gastro-intestinal blockage. Dose should be reduced slowly.
Not to be used for: patients suffering from glaucoma, enlarged prostate, some movement disorders.
Caution needed with: some sedative drugs, ANTIHISTAMINES, antidepressants.
Contains: ORPHENADRINE.
Other preparations: DISIPAL.

---

biotin *see* vitamin H

---

biperiden hydrochloride *see* Akineton

---

bisacodyl *see* bisacodyl tablets, Dulcolax

---

bisacodyl tablets

A tablet (coated to protect the stomach) supplied at a strength of 5 mg and used as a stimulant to treat constipation.

Dose: children under 10 years 1 tablet at night, adults and children over 10 years 2 tablets at night (increased to 4 tablets if necessary).
Availability: NHS, private prescription, over the counter.
Side effects: abdominal cramp.
Caution: avoid prolonged use.

85

Not to be used for: patients suffering from intestinal blockage.
Caution needed with: no ANTACIDS should be taken within 1 hour.
Contains: bisacodyl.
Other preparations: Bisacodyl Suppositories. DULCO-LAX (available on NHS only if prescribed as a generic).

---

bismuth oxide *see* **Anugesic-HC, Anusol, Anusol HC**

---

bismuth subgallate *see* **Anusol, Anusol HC**

---

bismuth subnitrate *see* **Caved S**

---

bisoprolol fumarate *see* **Emcor, Monocor, Monozide 10**

Blemix *see* **minocycline tablets**
(Ashbourne)

Blocadren
(MSD)

A blue, scored tablet supplied at a strength of 10 mg and used as a ß-BLOCKER to treat angina, high blood pressure, migraine, and as a treatment following heart attack.

Dose: following heart attack ½ tablet twice a day for 2 days, then 1 tablet twice a day. For angina ½ tablet 2-3 times a day at first increasing if required by 1-1½ tablets a day every 3 days. For high blood pressure 1 tablet a day at first increasing to a maximum of 6 tablets a day if needed. For migraine 1-2 tablets once a day.
Availability: NHS and private prescription.
Side effects: cold hands and feet, sleep disturbances, slow heart rate, tiredness, wheezing, heart failure, stomach upset, dry eyes, rash.
Caution: in pregnant women, nursing mothers, and in patients suffering from diabetes, kidney or liver disorders. May need to be withdrawn before surgery. Withdraw gradually. Your doctor may advise additional treatment with DIGOXIN and DIURETICS.
Not to be used for: children, or for patients suffering from heart block or failure, asthma, low blood pressure, untreated PHAEOCHROMOCYTOMA.
Caution needed with: VERAPAMIL, CLONIDINE withdrawal, some anti-arrhythmic drugs and anaesthetics, some blood-pressure lowering drugs, ERGOTAMINE, antidiabetics, CIMETIDINE, sedatives, SYMPATHOMIMETICS,

INDOMETHACIN.
Contains: TIMOLOL maleate.
Other preparations: BETIM.

BM-Accutest
(Boehringer Mannheim Diagnostics)

A plastic reagent strip used in conjunction with Accutrend, Accutrend Alpha, or Accutrend Mini meters, to detect blood glucose levels. Blood-glucose monitoring enables individual patients suffering from diabetes accurately to control blood glucose and manage their condition.

BM-Test 1–44
(Boehringer Mannheim Diagnostics)

A plastic reagent strip used, either visually or – more accurately – in conjunction with a Reflolux S meter, to detect blood glucose levels. Blood-glucose monitoring enables individual patients suffering from diabetes accurately to control blood glucose and manage their condition.

Bocasan
(Oral-B)

A sachet of white granules used as a disinfectant to treat gingivitis, mouth infections.

Dose: dissolve a sachet of granules in warm water and rinse out the mouth 3 times a day after meals.
Availability: NHS, private prescription, over the counter.
Side effects:
Caution:
Not to be used for: children under 5 years, or for patients suffering from kidney disease.
Caution needed with:
Contains: SODIUM PERBORATE monohydrate, SODIUM HYDROGEN TARTRATE.
Other preparations:

Bolvidon *see* mianserin tablets
(Organon)

---

boric acid *see* Phytex

---

borneol *see* **Rowachol, Rowatinex**

B

Brasivol
(Stiefel)

A paste used as an abrasive to treat acne. (Available in two grades.)

Dose: wet the area then rub in vigorously for 15-20 seconds, rinse and repeat 1-3 times a day. (Start with Grade 1 and progress if necessary to Grade 2.)
Availability: NHS, private prescription, over the counter.
Side effects:
Caution:
Not to be used for: patients suffering from visible superficial arteries or veins on the skin.
Caution needed with:
Contains: ALUMINIUM OXIDE.
Other preparations:

Brevinor
(Roche)

A white tablet used as an oestrogen, progestogen contraceptive.

Dose: 1 tablet a day for 21 days starting on day 5 of the period.
Availability: NHS and private prescription.
Side effects: enlarged breasts, bloating and fluid retention, cramps, leg pains, mood change, reduction in sexual desire, headaches, nausea, vaginal erosion, discharge, and bleeding, weight gain, skin changes, rarely thrombosis, raised blood pressure, jaundice.
Caution: in patients suffering from high blood pressure, Raynaud's disease, diabetes, vascular disorders, asthma, depression, kidney disease, multiple sclerosis, womb diseases. Your doctor may advise you not to smoke, to have regular examinations. You should stop treatment at the first sign of serious symptoms such as severe headache or jaundice. Treatment should be stopped before surgery.
Not to be used for: pregnant women, or for patients suffering from sickle-cell anaemia, history of heart disease or thrombosis, angina, raised blood pressure supplying the lungs, liver disorders, some cancers, undiagnosed vaginal bleeding, some ear, skin, and kidney disorders, PORPHYRIA.
Caution needed with: RIFAMPICIN, TETRACYCLINE ANTIBIOTICS, GRISEOFULVIN, BARBITURATES, PHENYTOIN, PRIMIDONE, CARBAMAZEPINE, ETHOSUXIMIDE, CHLORAL HYDRATE, DICHLORALPHENAZONE, GLUTETHIMIDE.
Contains: ETHINYLOESTRADIOL, NORETHISTERONE.

Other preparations: OVYSMEN.

Bricanyl Tablets
(Astra)

A white, scored tablet supplied at a strength of 5 mg and used as a BRONCHODILATOR to treat bronchial spasm brought on by asthma or other breathing disorders.

Dose: adults ½-1 tablet 3 times a day; children under 7 years use syrup, 7-15 years ½ tablet 2-3 times a day. Leave an interval of at least 7 hours between doses.
Availability: NHS and private prescription.
Side effects: shaking of the hands, tension, headache, palpitations. low potassium levels, rash, muscle spasm, sleep or behaviour changes in children.
Caution: in pregnant women and in diabetics, or in patients suffering from some heart disorders, overactive thyroid gland.
Not to be used for: children under 2 years.
Caution needed with: SYMPATHOMIMETICS, ß-BLOCKERS, drugs that lower potassium levels.
Contains: TERBUTALINE sulphate.
Other preparations: Bricanyl SA, Bricanyl Syrup, Bricanyl Inhaler, Bricanyl Spacer Inhaler, Bricanyl Refill Canister, Bricanyl Turbohaler, Bricanyl Respirator Solution, Bricanyl Respules, Bricanyl Injection. MONOVENT (syrup form).

Britiazim *see* diltiazem tablets
(Thames)

BritLofex
(Britannia)

A peach-coloured, film-coated tablet supplied at a strength of 0.2 mg and used to control the symptoms of withdrawal from opioid drugs.

Dose: 1 tablet twice a day at first, increasing if necessary by 1-2 tablets a day up to a maximum of 12 tablets a day. Treatment should be maintained for 7-10 days then withdrawn over the next 2-4 days
Availability: NHS, private prescription.
Side effects: drowsiness, dry nose and mouth
Caution: in pregnant women, nursing mothers, and in patients suffering from very weak heart, slow heart rate, chronic kidney failure, brain disease, recent heart attack, or with a history of depression.

Not to be used for: children.
Caution needed with: alcohol, sedatives.
Contains: LOFEXIDINE.
Other preparations:

Brocadopa see Larodopa
(Yamanouchi)

Broflex see benzhexol tablets
(Bioglan)

---

bromazepam see Lexotan

---

bromocriptine mesylate see bromocriptine tablets, Parlodel

---

bromocriptine tablets

A tablet supplied at a strength of 2.5 mg and used as a hormone blocker to treat Parkinson's disease, infertility, cyclical benign breast disease, and other disorders due to raised hormone levels. Also used to dry up breast milk

Dose: 1-30 mg a day, depending on condition. (Low doses used initially, increasing gradually if necessary.)
Availability: NHS and private prescription.
Side effects: low blood pressure on standing, brain and stomach disturbances, nausea, vomiting, constipation, headache, drowsiness, poor circulation, movement disorders, dry mouth, leg cramps, lung changes, dizziness.
Caution: in women, patients suffering from a history of mental disorder, severe cardiovascular disease, kidney or liver damage, Raynaud's syndrome, or PORPHYRIA. Your doctor may advise regular examinations.
Not to be used for: children, nursing mothers, women with complications of pregnancy, or for patients suffering from allergy to ERGOTAMINE.
Caution needed with: alcohol, sedatives, ERYTHROMYCIN, drugs affecting blood pressure, some tranquillizers, METOCLOPRAMIDE, DOMPERIDONE.
Contains: BROMOCRIPTINE MESYLATE.
Other preparations: PARLODEL.

---

brompheniramine see Dimotane Expectorant, Dimotane Plus,

Dimotapp LA

Bronchodil
(ASTA Medica)

An aerosol supplied at a strength of 0.5 mg and used as a BRONCHODILATOR to treat and prevent bronchial asthma, bronchitis, emphysema.

Dose: treatment, adults1-2 sprays every 3-6 hours; children over 6 years 1 spray every 3-6 hours. Prevention, adults 2 puffs 3 times a day; children over 6 years half adult dose.
Availability: NHS and private prescription.
Side effects: shaking of hands, nervous tension, headache, dilation of the blood vessels.
Caution: in pregnant women and in patients suffering from heart muscle disorders, angina, high blood pressure, abnormal heart rhythms, overactive thyroid gland.
Not to be used for: children under 6 years.
Caution needed with: SYMPATHOMIMETICS.
Contains: REPROTEROL hydrochloride.
Other preparations:

---

bronchodilator
a substance that enlarges the airways bringing relief in conditions such as asthma and bronchitis. Example, SALBUTAMOL.

Brufen *see* ibuprofen tablets
(Knoll Pharma)

Buccastem
(Reckitt & Colman)

A pale-yellow tablet supplied at a strength of 3 mg and used as an ANTIHISTAMINE treatment for vertigo as a result of Ménière's disease or labyrinthitis, nausea, vomiting, migraine.

Dose: 1-2 tablets twice a day allowed to dissolve between the upper lip and gum.
Availability: NHS and private prescription.
Side effects: low blood pressure especially in elderly or dehydrated patients, drowsiness, ANTICHOLINERGIC effects, sleeplessness, skin reactions.

Caution: in pregnant women or nursing mothers.
Not to be used for: children or for patients suffering from kidney or liver disease, blood disorders, epilepsy, Parkinson's disease, prostate enlargement, glaucoma.
Caution needed with: alcohol, sedatives, some drugs used to lower blood pressure or treat prostate disorders.
Contains: PROCHLORPERAZINE maleate.
Other preparations: STEMETIL.

---

buclizine hydrochloride *see* Migraleve

---

budesonide *see* Preferid, Pulmicort, Rhinocort

---

bumetanide *see* Burinex, Burinex A, Burinex K

---

buprenorphine *see* Temgesic

Burinex
(Leo)

A white, scored tablet supplied at strengths of 1 mg, 5 mg and used as a DIURETIC to treat fluid retention associated with congestive heart failure, liver and kidney disease, including the nephrotic syndrome.

Dose: 1 mg a day according to patient's response.
Availability: NHS and private prescription.
Side effects: low blood potassium, stomach discomfort, rash, cramps, blood changes, breast enlargement.
Caution: in pregnant women, nursing mothers, and in patients suffering from kidney or liver damage, diabetes, gout, enlarged prostate, or impaired urination. Your doctor may advise that potassium supplements may be needed.
Not to be used for: children or patients suffering from cirrhosis of the liver.
Caution needed with: LITHIUM, DIGOXIN, blood-pressure lowering drugs, some antibiotics.
Contains: BUMETANIDE.
Other preparations: Burinex Liquid, Burinex Injection. BURINEX A, BURINEX K.

Burinex A
(Leo)

A cream, oval, scored tablet used as a DIURETIC.

Dose: 1-2 tablets a day.
Availability: NHS and private prescription.
Side effects: stomach upset, cramp, rash, blood changes.
Caution: in pregnant women, nursing mothers, and in patients suffering from diabetes, gout, enlarged prostate, problems in passing urine. Your doctor may advise regular blood tests.
Not to be used for: children, or for patients suffering from liver or kidney disease, adrenal gland disorder, high potassium levels or other body fluid imbalance.
Caution needed with: some diuretics, potassium supplements, ACE INHIBITORS, LITHIUM, some antibiotics, DIGOXIN, blood-pressure lowering drugs.
Contains: BUMETANIDE, AMILORIDE.
Other preparations:

Burinex K
(Leo)

A white, egg-shaped tablet used as a DIURETIC/potassium supplement to treat fluid retention associated with congestive heart failure, liver disease, and kidney disease where potassium supplement is required.

Dose: 1-4 tablets a day.
Availability: NHS and private prescription.
Side effects: rash, cramps, stomach discomfort, blood changes, breast enlargement.
Caution: in pregnant women, nursing mothers, and in patients suffering from enlarged prostate, or impaired urination, kidney or liver disease, gout, diabetes.
Not to be used for: children, or for patients suffering from raised potassium levels, Addison's disease, liver cirrhosis.
Caution needed with: LITHIUM, DIGOXIN, blood-pressure lowering drugs, some diuretics, some antibiotics.
Contains: BUMETANIDE, POTASSIUM CHLORIDE.
Other preparations:

Buscopan
(Boehringer Ingelheim)

A white tablet supplied at a strength of 10 mg and used as an anti-spasm treatment for bowel spasm, painful periods.

Dose: adults painful periods 2 tablets 4 times a day for 5 days starting 2 days before the period begins; bowel spasm children 6-12 years 1 tablet 3 times a day, adults 2 tablets 4 times a day.
Availability: NHS, private prescription, over the counter.
Side effects: blurred vision, confusion, dry mouth.
Caution: in patients with intestinal obstruction or inflammation, enlarged prostate.
Not to be used for: patients with glaucoma.
Caution needed with:
Contains: HYOSCINE butylbromide.
Other preparations:

---

buserelin *see* **Suprecur, Suprefact**

Buspar
(Bristol-Myers Squibb)

A white, oval tablet supplied at a strengths of 5 mg, 10 mg, and used as a tranquillizer for the short-term treatment of anxiety.

Dose: 5 mg 2-3 times a day at first increasing every 2-3 days to a maximum of 45 mg a day; usual maintenance 15-30 mg a day in divided doses.
Availability: NHS and private prescription.
Side effects: dizziness, headache, nervousness, excitement, nausea; rarely rapid heart rate, chest pain, confusion, dry mouth, sweating, tiredness.
Caution: in patients with a history of kidney or liver disease.
Not to be used for: children, pregnant women, nursing mothers, or for patients suffering from severe kidney or liver disease, epilepsy.
Caution needed with: MAOIS.
Contains: BUSPIRONE hydrochloride.
Other preparations:

---

buspirone *see* **Buspar**

---

butobarbitone *see* **Soneryl**

---

butoxyethyl nicotinate *see* **Actinac**

---

cabergoline *see* **Dostinex**

Cacit
(Proctor & Gamble)

A pink effervescent tablet used as a calcium supplement to treat calcium deficiency and thinning of the bones.

Dose: 1-6 tablets a day (depending on condition), dissolved in water.
Availability: NHS, private prescription, over the counter.
Side effects: stomach upset.
Caution: in patients suffering from kidney disorder, intestinal disorder, or with a history of kidney stones.
Not to be used for: patients suffering from high calcium levels in the blood or urine.
Caution needed with: TETRACYCLINE ANTIBIOTICS, VITAMIN D.
Contains: CALCIUM CARBONATE.
Other preparations: CALCICHEW, CALCIDRINK (granular form), CITRICAL.

---

cade oil *see* **Polytar AF, Polytar Emollient, Polytar Liquid, Pixol**

---

cadexomer iodine *see* **Iodoflex, Iodosorb**

Cafergot
(Sandoz)

A white tablet used as an ergot preparation to treat migraine.

Dose: 1-2 tablets at the beginning of a migraine attack to a maximum of 4 tablets in a day. Do not repeat within 4 days; maximum of 8 tablets in a week.
Availability: NHS and private prescription.
Side effects: nausea, vomiting, muscular pain, abdominal pain, reduced circulation, weak legs.
Caution:
Not to be used for: children, pregnant women, nursing mothers, or in patients suffering from coronary, peripheral, or occlusive vascular disease, Raynaud's syndrome, severe high blood pressure, kidney or liver disease, sepsis.
Caution needed with: ERYTHROMYCIN, ß-BLOCKERS.
Contains: ERGOTAMINE TARTRATE, CAFFEINE.

Other preparations: Cafergot Suppositories. LINGRAINE, MEDIHALER-ERGOTAMINE, MIGRIL.

caffeine *see* Cafergot, Doloxene Co.

Calaband
(Seton Healthcare)

A medicated bandage supplied at a size of 7.5 cm x 6 m, and used in conjunction with a compression bandage to treat varicose and gravitational ulcers.

Availability: NHS, private prescription, over the counter. (Also available on a trial basis from nurses.)
Contains: zinc paste, calamine.

Calabren *see* glibenclamide tablets
(Berk)

Caladryl
(Warner Wellcome Consumer)

A cream or lotion used as an antihistamine, anti-itching treatment for sunburn, insect bites and stings, and other forms of skin irritation.

Dose: apply cream or lotion to the affected area 3-4 times a day.
Availability: NHS, private prescription, over the counter.
Side effects:
Caution:
Not to be used for: mucous membranes, broken skin, or for the rash associated with measles, chickenpox, eczema, or other weeping skin conditions.
Caution needed with:
Contains: ZINC OXIDE, CAMPHOR, DIPHENHYDRAMINE HYDROCHLORIDE.
Other preparations:

calamine *see* calamine and coal tar ointment, calamine lotion, Quinaband

calamine and coal tar ointment BP

An ointment used to treat chronic eczema and psoriasis.

Dose: apply 1-3 times a day.
Availability: NHS, private prescription, over the counter.
Side effects: irritation, acne-like skin eruptions, sensitivity to light.
Caution: avoid broken or inflamed skin. Stains hair, skin, and fabrics.
Not to be used for:
Caution needed with:
Contains: CALAMINE, strong COAL TAR solution, ZINC OXIDE, WHITE SOFT PARAFFIN, hydrous WOOL FAT.
Other preparations:

calamine lotion BP

A lotion used to treat itchy skin conditions.

Dose: apply when required.
Availability: NHS, private prescription, over the counter.
Side effects:
Caution:
Not to be used for:
Caution needed with:
Contains: CALAMINE.
Other preparations: aqueous calamine cream BP, oily calamine lotion BP 1980, calamine ointment BP.

Calanif *see* nifedipine capsules
(Berk)

Calcicard CR *see* diltiazem long-acting tablets
(Norton)

Calcichew
(Shire)

A white, chewable tablet supplied at a strength of 500 mg and used as a calcium supplement to treat calcium deficiency, osteoporosis, and regulate blood phosphate levels in patients with kidney failure.

Dose: 1 tablet chewed 2-3 times a day.
Availability: NHS, private prescription, over the counter.

Side effects: constipation, wind.
Caution:
Not to be used for: patients suffering from overactive parathyroid glands, severe kidney disease, some tumours.
Caution needed with: TETRACYCLINE ANTIBIOTICS.
Contains: CALCIUM CARBONATE.
Other preparations: Calcichew D3, Calcichew Forte, CALCIDRINK. CACIT, CALCIUM-500 (non-chewable form), CITRICAL.

Calcidrink *see* Cacit
(Shire)

calciferol tablets

Tablets used as a vitamin D$_2$ supplement to prevent VITAMIN D deficiency.

Dose: 0.01-2.5 mg (400-100 000 units) a day, depending on condition.
Availability: NHS, private prescription, over the counter.
Side effects: loss of appetite, nausea, vomiting, diarrhoea, weight loss, excessive urine output, sweating, headache, thirst, vertigo, raised calcium and phosphate levels, lack of energy.
Caution: in infants. Patients receiving high doses may need regular blood tests.
Not to be used for: patients suffering from high calcium levels in the blood.
Caution needed with: some DIURETICS.
Contains: calciferol (vitamin D).
Other preparations: calciferol injection. (Many compound vitamin preparations available over the counter contain small quantities of calciferol.)

Calcilat *see* nifedipine capsules
(Eastern)

calcipotriol *see* Dovonex

Calcisorb
(3M Health Care)

A powder in a sachet of 4.7 g and used as an ion-exchange compound to treat raised calcium levels in the urine, recurring kidney stones, osteopetrosis.

Dose: adults 1 sachet dispersed in water with meals or sprinkled on to food 3 times a day; children 2 sachets a day in 3 divided doses with food.
Availability: NHS, private prescription, over the counter.
Side effects: diarrhoea.
Caution: treatment of children should be monitored, and the treatment should be accompanied by a low-calcium diet with foods rich in oxalates restricted.
Not to be used for: pregnant women, nursing mothers, or for patients suffering from kidney disease, congestive heart disease, or any other conditions in which a low-sodium diet is needed.
Caution needed with:
Contains: SODIUM CELLULOSE phosphate.
Other preparations:

---

calcitriol *see* **Rocaltrol**

Calcium-500 *see* **Calcichew**

---

calcium and ergocalciferol tablets

A tablet used as a calcium and VITAMIN D supplement to treat vitamin D deficiency.

Dose: as advised by your physician or in accordance with the manufacturer's instructions. The tablets should be crushed or chewed before swallowing.
Availability: NHS, private prescription, and over the counter.
Side effects: excessive intake may give rise to anorexia, tiredness, nausea and vomiting, diarrhoea, weight loss, excessive urinations, sweating, headache, thirst, vertigo, high calcium and phosphate levels in blood and urine.
Caution: in nursing mothers, infants, and in patients suffering from kidney failure, stomach ulcer or block. Your doctor may advise regular check-ups.
Not to be used for: patients suffering from raised calcium levels, or who are suffering from overactive parathyroid glands, severe kidney disease, decalcifying tumours.
Caution needed with: some DIURETICS, some antibiotics.
Contains: CALCIUM LACTATE, CALCIUM PHOSPHATE, ERGOCALCIFEROL (vitamin D).
Other preparations: various brands of calcium and vitamin D are available for purchase without prescription, but strengths may vary.

---

calcium carbonate *see* **Cacit, Calcium-500, Citrical, Calcichew, Gaviscon, Sandocal, Titralac**

---

calcium chloride *see* **Glandosane, Salivace**

---

calcium folinate *see* **Refolinon**

C

calcium gluconate *see* **calcium gluconate tablets**

---

calcium gluconate tablets

A tablet or effervescent tablet used as a calcium supplement to treat calcium deficiency, osteoporosis, and bones which have been softened by VITAMIN D deficiency.

Dose: as advised by your physician.
Availability: NHS, private prescription, over the counter.
Side effects: stomach upset, heart rhythm disturbances, slow pulse.
Caution: in patients suffering from kidney failure, sarcoidosis.
Not to be used for: patients suffering from raised calcium levels.
Caution needed with: some DIURETICS, some antibiotics.
Contains: calcium gluconate.
Other preparations:

---

calcium glycine hydrochloride *see* **Calcimax**

---

calcium lactate *see* **calcium and ergocalciferol tablets, calcium lactate tablets**

---

calcium lactate gluconate *see* **Sandocal**

---

calcium lactate tablets

A tablet used as a calcium supplement to treat calcium deficiency, osteoporosis, and bones which have been softened by VITAMIN D deficiency.

Dose: as advised by your physician.
Availability: NHS, private prescription, over the counter.
Side effects: stomach upset, heart rhythm disturbances, slow pulse.

100

Caution: in patients suffering from kidney failure, sarcoidosis.
Not to be used for: patients suffering from raised calcium levels.
Caution needed with: some DIURETICS, some antibiotics.
Contains: calcium lactate.
Other preparations:

---

calcium pantothenate *see* Calcimax, Ketovite

---

calcium phosphate *see* calcium and erogocalciferol tablets

---

calcium polystyrene *see* Calcium Resonium

Calcium Resonium
(Sanofi Winthrop)

A powder used as an ion-exchange resin to treat raised potassium levels.

Dose: adults 15 g 3-4 times a day; children 0.5-1 g per kg body weight a day in divided doses.
Availability: NHS, private prescription, over the counter.
Side effects: raised calcium levels, low potassium levels, impaction of resin.
Caution: in new-born infants. Potassium and calcium levels should be checked.
Not to be used for: for patients suffering from overactive parathyroid glands, multiple myeloma (a bone marrow tumour), sarcoidosis (a disease causing raised calcium levels), certain forms of cancer with kidney failure and hypercalcaemia (raised calcium levels), obstructive bowel disease, or for newborn infants with low gut activity.
Caution needed with:
Contains: CALCIUM POLYSTYRENE sulphonate.
Other preparations:

Calcium Sandoz *see* Sandocal
(Sandoz)

Calmurid
(Novex Pharma)

A cream used as a moisturizer and skin softener to treat chronic dry skin conditions.

Dose: wash and dry skin, then apply twice a day; leave on skin for 3-5 minutes, then rub in and remove any excess cream.
Availability: NHS, private prescription, over the counter.
Side effects:
Caution:
Not to be used for:
Caution needed with:
Contains: UREA, LACTIC ACID.
Other preparations:

Calmurid HC
(Galderma)

A cream used as a STEROID, wetting agent and skin softener to treat dry eczemas and other skin disorders.

Dose: wash and dry the affected area, and apply twice a day.
Availability: NHS and private prescription.
Side effects: fluid retention, suppression of adrenal glands, thinning, streaking, or spotting of the skin may occur.
Caution: use for short periods of time only.
Not to be used for: patients suffering from acne or any other skin infections caused by tuberculosis, ringworm, viruses, or fungi, leg ulcers, scabies, or continuously especially in pregnant women.
Caution needed with:
Contains: HYDROCORTISONE, UREA, LACTIC ACID.
Other preparations: ALPHADERM.

Calpol Paediatric
(Warner Wellcome Consumer)

A suspension or sugar-free suspension supplied at a strength of 120 mg/5 ml and used as an ANALGESIC to relieve pain and reduce fever.

Dose: under 3 months 2.5 ml 4 times a day; 3 months-1 year 2.5-5 ml 4 times a day; 1-6 years 5-10 ml 4 times a day.
Availability: NHS, private prescription, over the counter.
Side effects:
Caution: in patients suffering from kidney or liver disease.
Not to be used for:
Caution needed with: other medicines containing PARACETAMOL.
Contains: paracetamol.
Other preparations: Calpol Infant, Calpol Six Plus. DISPROL PAEDIATRIC, PARACETAMOL PAEDIATRIC ELIXIR. Many other brands are available over the counter (most available on NHS only if prescribed as a generic).

CAM
(Shire)

A sugar-free syrup used as a BRONCHODILATOR to treat bronchial spasm.

Dose: adults 20 ml 3-4 times a day; children 6 months-2 years 2.5 ml 3-4 times a day, 2-4 years 5 ml 3-4 times a day, over 4 years 10 ml 3-4 times a day.
Availability: NHS, private prescription, over the counter.
Side effects: nervousness, sleeplessness, restlessness, abnormal heart rhythms, shaking.
Caution: in patients suffering from diabetes.
Not to be used for: infants under 6 months or for patients suffering from heart disease, high blood pressure, overactive thyroid gland, enlarged prostate, excitability, closed-angle glaucoma.
Caution needed with: MAOIS, TRICYCLIC ANTIDEPRESSANTS, anaesthetics.
Contains: EPHEDRINE hydrochloride.
Other preparations:

Camcolit
(Norgine)

A white, scored tablet supplied at strengths of 250 mg, 400 mg and used as a LITHIUM salt to treat mania, manic depression, aggressive and self-injuring behaviour.

Dose: your doctor may advise a blood test to check correct dose.
Availability: NHS and private prescription.
Side effects: nausea, diarrhoea, shaking hands, muscular weakness, brain and heart disturbances, weight gain, fluid retention, overactive or underactive thyroid gland, thirst, frequent urination, skin reactions.
Caution: in pregnant women. Patients should be treated in hospital at first and then monitored. Maintain an adequate salt and liquid intake.
Not to be used for: children, nursing mothers, or for patients suffering from kidney or heart disease, Addison's disease, underactive thyroid gland, disturbed sodium balance.
Caution needed with: DIURETICS, NON-STEROIDAL ANTI-INFLAMMATORY DRUGS, CARBAMAZEPINE, FLUPENTHIXOL, METHYLDOPA, PHENYTOIN, HALOPERIDOL, METOCLOPRAMIDE, antidepressants, TETRACYCLINE ANTIBIOTICS.
Contains: LITHIUM CARBONATE.
Other preparations: LISKONUM, LITHONATE, PRIADEL.

---

camomile *see* **Kamillosan**

---

camphene *see* **Rowachol, Rowatinex**

---

camphor *see* **Balmosa, Caladryl, Salonair**

Canesten
(Bayer)

A solution used as an antifungal treatment for fungal inflammation and infection of the outer ear, skin, and nails.

Dose: 2-3 applications a day until 14 days after the symptoms have gone.
Availability: NHS, private prescription, over the counter.
Side effects: local irritation, allergy.
Caution:
Not to be used for:
Caution needed with:
Contains: CLOTRIMAZOLE, POLYETHYLENE GLYCOL solution.
Other preparations: Canesten Cream, Canesten Powder, Canesten Spray. CLOTRIMAZOLE CREAM, MASNODERM.

Canesten 1
(Bayer)

A white, vaginal tablet plus applicator supplied at a strength of 500 mg and used as an antifungal, antibacterial treatment for vaginal infections. (This product may be purchased without prescription only for the treatment of vaginal thrush.)

Dose: 1 tablet inserted into the vagina at night.
Availability: NHS, private prescription, over the counter (*see* above).
Side effects: mild burning or irritation, allergy.
Caution:
Not to be used for: children.
Caution needed with:
Contains: CLOTRIMAZOLE.
Other preparations: Canesten 10% VC, Canesten Vaginal Tablets, Canesten Cream, Canesten Duopak, Canesten Vaginal Cream, Canesten Combi.

Canesten-HC
(Bayer)

A cream used as a STEROID, antifungal, antibacterial treatment for fungal skin infections where there is also inflammation.

Dose: apply to the affected area twice a day.
Availability: NHS and private prescription.
Side effects: burning or irritation, allergy.
Caution: use for short periods of time only.
Not to be used for: patients suffering from acne or any other skin infections caused by tuberculosis, ringworm, viruses, or fungi, leg ulcers, scabies, or continuously especially in pregnant women.
Caution needed with:
Contains: CLOTRIMAZOLE, HYDROCORTISONE.
Other preparations:

Capasal
(Dermal)

A shampoo used as an emollient and skin softener to treat psoriasis or seborrhoeic dermatitis of the scalp, cradle cap.

Dose: use as a shampoo, daily if necessary.
Availability: NHS, private prescription, over the counter.
Side effects:
Caution:
Not to be used for:
Caution needed with:
Contains: SALICYCLIC ACID, COCONUT OIL, distilled COAL TAR.
Other preparations:

Capitol
(Dermal)

A gel used as an antibacterial treatment for dandruff and other similar scalp disorders.

Dose: use as a shampoo.
Availability: NHS, private prescription, over the counter.
Side effects:
Caution:
Not to be used for:
Caution needed with:
Contains: BENZALKONIUM CHLORIDE.
Other preparations:

Caplenal *see* **allopurinol tablets**
(Berk)

Capoten
(Squibb)

A mottled white, capsule-shaped scored tablet, a mottled white, quarter-scored, square tablet, or a mottled white, oval tablet according to strengths of 12.5 mg, 25 mg, 50 mg and used as an ACE INHIBITOR in addition to DIURETICS and DIGOXIN in the treatment of severe congestive heart failure, high blood pressure, diabetic kidney disease in patients dependent on insulin.

Dose: adults, heart failure 6.25 mg or 12.5 mg at first then 25 mg 2-3 times a day up to a maximum of 150 mg a day. For moderate to mild high blood pressure 12.5 mg twice a day then 25 mg twice a day increasing to 50 mg twice a day at 2-4 week intervals if needed. Severe high blood pressure 12.5 mg twice a day at first, then 50 mg 3 times a day if needed. For diabetic kidney disease, 75-100 mg a day in divided doses. Children as advised by the physician.
Availability: NHS and private prescription.
Side effects: rash, loss of taste, rarely a cough, blood changes, protein in the urine, low blood pressure, swelling, pancreatitis.
Caution: in the elderly and in patients suffering from kidney disease, auto-immune diseases, severe congestive heart failure, or patients undergoing anaesthesia, dialysis. Your doctor may advise regular blood tests.
Not to be used for: pregnant women, nursing mothers, or for patients suffering from some heart valve diseases.
Caution needed with: some diuretics, potassium supplements, NON-STEROIDAL ANTI-INFLAMMATORY DRUGS, CLONIDINE, ALLOPURINOL, PROCAINAMIDE, PROBENECID, immunosuppressants, LITHIUM drugs that affect the circulation or immune system.
Contains: CAPTOPRIL.
Other preparations: ACEPRIL.

Capozide
(Squibb)

A white, scored tablet used as a DIURETIC/ACE INHIBITOR combination to treat high blood pressure.

Dose: 1-2 tablets a day.
Availability: NHS and private prescription.
Side effects: protein in the urine, low blood pressure, rash, loss of taste, blood changes, sensitivity to light, tiredness, rarely a cough, rapid heart

rate, stomach upset, pancreatitis.

Caution: in patients undergoing anaesthesia or dialysis, and those suffering from kidney disease, auto-immune diseases, diabetes, gout, liver disease.

Not to be used for: children, pregnant women, nursing mothers or for patients suffering from some heart valve diseases.

Caution needed with: LITHIUM, NON-STEROIDAL ANTI-INFLAMMATORY DRUGS, ALLOPURINOL, PROCAINAMIDE, PROBENECID, CLONIDINE, some diuretics, potassium supplements, blood-pressure lowering drugs, and drugs that affect the circulation or immune system. Your doctor may advise regular blood tests.

Contains: CAPTOPRIL, HYDROCHLOROTHIAZIDE.

Other preparations: Capozide LS. ACEZIDE.

Caprin
(Sinclair)

A pink tablet, coated to protect the stomach, supplied at a strength of 300 mg and used as an ANALGESIC to treat rheumatic and associated conditions, and to reduce risk of heart attack.

Dose: for pain 3 tablets 3-4 times a day; to reduce risk of heart attack 1 tablet a day.

Availability: NHS, private prescription, over the counter.

Side effects: stomach upsets, allergy, asthma.

Caution: in the elderly, pregnant women, patients with a history of allergy to ASPIRIN or asthma, or who are suffering from impaired liver or kidney function.

Not to be used for: children, nursing mothers, or patients suffering from haemophilia or ulcers.

Caution needed with: ANTICOAGULANTS, some antidiabetic drugs, NON-STEROIDAL ANTI-INFLAMMATORY DRUGS, METHOTREXATE, SPIRONOLACTONE, STEROIDS, ANTACIDS, some uric acid-lowering drugs.

Contains: ASPIRIN.

Other preparations: ASPIRIN TABLETS, NU-SEALS ASPIRIN.

---

capsaicin *see* Axsain

---

capsicum oleoresin *see* Balmosa, Cremalgin

Capsuvac *see* co-danthrusate capsules
(Galen)

---

captopril *see* **Acepril, Acezide, Capoten, Capozide**

Carace
(Du Pont)

A blue, oval tablet, a white, oval, scored tablet, a yellow, oval, scored tablet, or an orange, oval, scored tablet according to strengths of 2.5 mg, 5 mg, 10 mg, 20 mg and used as an ACE INHIBITOR to treat congestive heart failure in addition to DIURETICS and/or DIGOXIN; high blood pressure, and following acute heart attack in some patients.

Dose: for heart failure 2.5 mg once a day at first, increasing to 5-20 mg a day over 2-4 weeks. After heart attack 5 mg at first, then another 5 mg after 24 hours, 10 mg after 48 hours, then 10 mg a day. For high blood pressure 2.5 mg once a day at first, increasing to 10-20 mg once a day and a maximum of 40 mg a day.
Availability: NHS and private prescription.
Side effects: low blood pressure, kidney failure, swelling, rash, dizziness, headache, diarrhoea, nausea, cough, tiredness, palpitations, chest pains, weakness.
Caution: in nursing mothers and in patients suffering from kidney disease, severe congestive heart failure, or undergoing anaesthesia or dialysis.
Not to be used for: children, pregnant women, or for patients suffering from some heart valve or lung diseases, or some types of fluid retention.
Caution needed with: some diuretics, potassium supplements, INDOMETHACIN, LITHIUM, blood-pressure lowering drugs.
Contains: LISINOPRIL.
Other preparations: ZESTRIL.

Carace Plus
(Du Pont)

A blue hexagonal tablet (Carace 10 Plus) or a yellow hexagonal, tablet (Carace 20 Plus) used as an ACE INHIBITOR and DIURETIC to treat high blood pressure.

Dose: 1-2 tablets a day.
Availability: NHS and private prescription.
Side effects: dizziness, headache, cough, tiredness, low blood pressure, severe allergy, nausea, diarrhoea, swelling, impotence.
Caution: in patients undergoing surgery, anaesthesia, or dialysis, or suffering from body fluid imbalance, heart or circulatory disorder, liver or kidney disease, gout, high uric acid levels, diabetes.
Not to be used for: pregnant women, nursing mothers, children, or for patients suffering from reduced urine output, swelling, or who have

previously suffered severe allergic reaction to ACE inhibitors.
Caution needed with: potassium supplements, LITHIUM, NON-STEROIDAL INFLAMMATORY DRUGS, antidiabetics.
Contains: LISINOPRIL, HYDROCHLOROTHIAZIDE.
Other preparations: ZESTORETIC.

---

carbachol *see* carbachol tablets, Isopto Carbachol

C

---

carbachol tablets

Tablets supplied at a strength of 2 mg and used to treat urine retention after surgical procedures.

Dose: 1 tablet 3 times a day, half an hour before food.
Availability: NHS and private prescription.
Side effects: nausea, vomiting, sweating, blurred vision, heartbeat irregularities, colic.
Caution:
Not to be used for: pregnant women, or patients suffering from blockage in the intestine or urinary tract, asthma, irregular heartbeat, overactive thyroid, recent heart attack, epilepsy, low blood pressure, Parkinson's disease, stomach ulcer, or where increased muscle activity in the urinary tracts could be harmful.
Caution needed with:
Contains: CARBACHOL.
Other preparations: carbachol injection.

Carbalax
(Pharmax)

A suppository used to treat constipation, local anal conditions.

Dose: 1 suppository 30 minutes before evacuation required.
Availability: NHS, private prescription, over the counter.
Side effects:
Caution:
Not to be used for: children.
Caution needed with:
Contains: SODIUM BICARBONATE, anyhdrous SODIUM ACID PHOSPHATE.
Other preparations:

C

...engths of 100 mg, 200 mg, 400 mg and used as an ...ent for manic depression, hypermania, epilepsy, and ...at trigeminal neuralgia, migraine.

Dose: ...epression 400 mg a day in divided doses at first increasing ...ally until symptoms are controlled and up to a maximum of 1.6 g a day. ...or epilepsy and neuralgia adults 100-200 mg 1-2 times a day at first increasing usually to 800 mg-1.2 g a day up to a maximum of 2 g; children up to 1 year 100-200 mg a day, 1-5 years 200-400 mg a day, 5-10 years 400-600 mg a day, 10-15 years 600 mg-1 g a day.

Availability: NHS and private prescription.

Side effects: nausea, vomiting, stomach upset, double vision, dry mouth, drowsiness, dizziness, confusion and agitation (in the elderly), fluid retention, low blood sodium, blood changes, rash, acute kidney failure, jaundice, hair loss, hepatitis, fever, sensitivity to light, heart disturbances, depression, hypersensitivity.

Caution: in the elderly, pregnant women, nursing mothers, and in patients suffering from severe cardiovascular disease, liver or kidney disease, glaucoma. Your doctor may advise that blood tests should be made regularly.

Not to be used for: patients suffering from heart conduction block, PORPHYRIA, or a history of bone marrow depression.

Caution needed with: ANTICOAGULANTS taken by mouth, alcohol, sedatives, MAOIS, CYCLOSPORIN, contraceptive pill, ERYTHROMYCIN, ISONIAZID, CIMETIDINE, antidepressants, DEXTROPROPOXYPHENE, DILTIAZEM, VERAPAMIL, VILOXAZINE, STEROIDS, DANAZOL, PHENYTOIN, LITHIUM, DOXYCYCLINE, TERFENADINE, antimalarial drugs, DIURETICS.

Contains: CARBAMAZEPINE.

Other preparations: TEGRETOL (available as tablets, long-acting tablets, liquid, or suppositories).

---

carbaryl *see* **Carylderm, Clinicide, Derbac-C, Suleo-C**

---

carbenoxolone *see* **Bioplex, Bioral, Pyrogastrone**

---

carbldopa monohydrate *see* **Sinemet**

---

carbimazole *see* **Neo-Mercazole**

Carbo-Cort
(Lagap)

A cream used as a STEROID, anti-psoriatic treatment for eczema, lichen planus (a rare skin disorder).

Dose: apply to the affected area 2-3 times a day.
Availability: NHS and private prescription.
Side effects: fluid retention, suppression of adrenal glands, thinning, streaking, or spotting of the skin may occur.
Caution: use for short periods of time only, especially in children or on the face. Withdraw gradually.
Not to be used for: patients suffering from acne or any other skin infections caused by tuberculosis, ringworm, viruses, or fungi, scabies, leg ulcers, or continuously especially in pregnant women.
Caution needed with:
Contains: HYDROCORTISONE, COAL TAR solution.
Other preparations: ALPHOSYL HC, TARCORTIN.

Carbo-Dome
(Lagap)

A cream used as an anti-psoriatic treatment for psoriasis.

Dose: apply to the affected area 2-3 times a day.
Availability: NHS, private prescription, over the counter.
Side effects: irritation, sensitivity to light.
Caution:
Not to be used for: patients suffering from acute psoriasis.
Caution needed with:
Contains: COAL TAR.
Other preparations: CLINITAR, GELCOTAR, PSORIDERM, PSORIGEL.

---

carbocisteine *see* Mucodyne

Carbomix
(Penn)

Granules used as an adsorbent to treat acute poisoning, overdose of drugs.

Dose: adults dissolve 50 g in water and take by mouth as soon as possible after poisoning; children usually 25-50 mg. Repeat dose up to 200 g over 4-8 hours if required.

Availability: NHS, private prescription, over the counter.
Side effects:
Caution: your doctor may advise additional treatment for certain overdoses.
Not to be used for:
Caution needed with: antidotes, emetics, or any drugs taken by mouth.
Contains: activated CHARCOAL.
Other preparations: MEDICOAL.

---

carboxymethylcellulose *see* **Glandosane, Luborant, Salivace**

Cardene
(Roche)

A blue/white or blue/pale-blue capsule according to strengths of 20 mg, 30 mg and used as an anti-anginal, ANTIHYPERTENSIVE drug to treat chronic stable angina, high blood pressure.

Dose: for angina, 20 mg 3 times a day increasing after not less than 3-day intervals to 30 mg 3 times a day or as required. Not more than 120 mg a day. For high blood pressure (use Cardene SR), 20 mg 3 times a day at first, up to 60 mg twice a day if needed.
Availability: NHS and private prescription.
Side effects: chest pain, dizziness, headache, swelling of lower limbs, flushing, feeling warm, palpitations and nausea.
Caution: in patients suffering from weak heart, congestive heart failure, or liver or kidney disease.
Not to be used for: children, pregnant women, nursing mothers, or for patients suffering from some heart valve diseases.
Caution needed with: DIGOXIN, CIMETIDINE.
Contains: NICARDIPINE hydrochloride.
Other preparations: Cardene SR.

Cardilate MR *see* nifedipine modified-release tablets
(Norton)

Cardinol *see* propranolol tablets
(CP Pharmaceuticals)

Cardura
(Invicta)

A white five-sided tablet, a white egg-shaped tablet, or a white square tablet according to strengths of 1 mg, 2 mg, 4 mg and used as a selective alpha-blocker to treat high blood pressure and symptoms associated with enlarged prostate.

Dose: high blood pressure,1 mg once a day at first increasing after 1-2 weeks if needed to 2 mg once a day and then 4 mg once a day, up to a maximum of of 16 mg a day; prostate disorder, 8 mg a day.
Availability: NHS, private prescription.
Side effects: low blood pressure on standing, vertigo, dizziness, headache, tiredness, weakness, fluid retention, sleepiness, rhinitis, nausea.
Caution: in pregnant women.
Not to be used for: children or nursing mothers.
Caution needed with:
Contains: DOXAZOSIN.
Other preparations:

Carisoma
(Pharmax)

A white tablet supplied at strengths of 125 mg, 350 mg and used as a sedative to treat muscle and bone problems associated with muscle spasm.

Dose: elderly 125 mg 3 times a day; adults 350 mg 3 times a day.
Availability: NHS and private prescription.
Side effects: drowsiness, dizziness, nausea, lassitude, flushes, headache, constipation, rash.
Caution: in patients suffering from kidney or liver disease, or a history of alcoholism or drug addiction. Avoid long-term treatment and withdraw gradually.
Not to be used for: children, pregnant women, nursing mothers, or for patients suffering from acute intermittent PORPHYRIA.
Caution needed with: alcohol, sedatives, ANTICOAGULANTS, STEROIDS, the contraceptive pill, PHENYTOIN, GRISEOFULVIN, RIFAMPICIN, TRICYCLIC ANTIDEPRESSANTS.
Contains: CARISOPRODOL.
Other preparations:

---

carisoprodol *see* **Carisoma**

---

carmellose sodium *see* **Orabase**

---

carteolol hydrochloride *see* **Teoptic**

---

carvedilol *see* **Eucardic**

Carylderm
(Seton Healthcare)

A lotion used as a pediculicide to treat lice in the head and pubic areas.

Dose: rub into the hair and allow to dry. Leave it for at least 2 hours before shampooing. Repeat after 7-9 days if needed.
Availability: NHS, private prescription.
Side effects:
Caution: in infants under 6 months, and in patients suffering from asthma or eczema. Keep out of the eyes. Flammable liquid – do not dry hair with hair dryer.
Not to be used for:
Caution needed with:
Contains: CARBARYL.
Other preparations: Carylderm Shampoo. CLINICIDE, DERBAC-C, SULEO-C.

Catapres
(Boehringer Ingelheim)

A white tablet scored on one side supplied at strengths of 0.1 mg, 0.3 mg and used to treat high blood pressure.

Dose: 0.05-0.1 mg 3 times a day increasing every second or third day.
Availability: NHS and private prescription.
Side effects: drowsiness, dry mouth, dizziness, fluid retention.
Caution: in nursing mothers, in patients suffering from depression or peripheral vascular disease, and where ß-BLOCKERS are being withdrawn.
Not to be used for: children.
Caution needed with: TRICYCLIC ANTIDEPRESSANTS, other blood-pressure lowering drugs, alcohol, sedatives, some drugs used to treat enlarged prostate.
Contains: CLONIDINE hydrochloride.
Other preparations: Catapres Perlongets (long-acting preparation), Catapres Injection.

Caved-S
(Pharmacia)

A brown tablet used as a cell-surface protector and ANTACID to treat peptic ulcer.

Dose: adults 2 tablets chewed 3-6 times a day between meals.
Availability: NHS, private prescription, over the counter.
Side effects: few; occasionally constipation.
Caution:
Not to be used for: children.
Caution needed with: tablets coated to protect the stomach, some antibiotics, iron.
Contains: LIQUORICE extract, ALUMINIUM HYDROXIDE, MAGNESIUM CARBONATE, SODIUM BICARBONATE, BISMUTH SUBNITRATE.
Other preparations:

Caverject
(Upjohn)

A powder in a vial with prefilled syringe and needles, and used as a PROSTAGLANDIN to treat erectile impotence in men.

Dose: 2.5 mcg by intracavernosal injection, increasing in steps of 5-10 mcg to obtain a dose that produces an erection lasting not more than 1 hour; (maximum dose 60 mcg, maximum frequency once a day and 3 times in any 1 week). Injections may be self administered after proper training.
Availability: NHS, private prescription.
Side effects: burning or pain in the penis during erection, thickening of the tissue, flushing, pain around the anus or in the testicles, iron and protein deposits in the penis, persistent painful erection, blood pressure changes, abnormal heart rhythm, dizziness, headache, collapse, shock.
Caution: in patients suffering from tightness of the foreskin, angulation, thickening of the tissue of the penis, Peyronie's disease. If erection persists for more than 4 hours medical advice should be sought.
Not to be used for: children or for patients suffering from sickle cell anaemia, leukaemia, some forms of cancer.
Caution needed with: WARFARIN, HEPARIN.
Contains: ALPROSTADIL.
Other preparations:

Ceanel Concentrate
(Quinoderm)

A liquid used as an antibacterial, antifungal treatment for psoriasis, seborrhoeic inflammation of the scalp.

Dose: use as a shampoo 3 times a week at first and then twice a week or

apply directly to other areas of skin as needed.
Availability: NHS, private prescription, over the counter.
Side effects:
Caution: keep out of the eyes.
Not to be used for:
Caution needed with:
Contains: PHENYLETHYL ALCOHOL, CETRIMIDE, UNDECANOIC ACID.
Other preparations:

Cedax
(Schering-Plough)

A white capsule supplied at a strength of 400 mg and used as an antibiotic to treat pharyngitis, tonsillitis, bronchitis in adults, middle ear infection in children, urinary tract infections.

Dose: adults, 1 capsule once a day for 5-14 days; children use suspension.
Availability: NHS, private prescription.
Side effects: stomach upset, headache, rash; rarely dizziness, blood changes, colitis, convulsions.
Caution: in pregnant women, and in patients suffering from kidney damage, allergy to penicillin, or with a history of gastro-intestinal disease.
Not to be used for: children under 6 months.
Caution needed with:
Contains: CEFTIBUTEN dihydrate.
Other preparations: Cedax Suspension.

Cedocard *see* isosorbide dinitrate tablets
(Pharmacia)

Cedocard Retard *see* isosorbide dinitrate tablets
(Pharmacia)

cefaclor *see* cefaclor capsules, Distaclor

cefaclor capsules

A capsule supplied at strengths of 250 mg, 500 mg, and used as a cephalosprin antibiotic to treat infections.

Dose: adults and children over 5 years 250-500 mg every 8 hours,

children 1 month-1 year 62.5-125 mg (as syrup) every 8 hours, children 1-5 years 125-250 mg (as syrup) every 8 hours.
Availability: NHS and private prescription.
Side effects: allergy, headache, stomach disturbances.
Caution: in pregnant women, nursing mothers, and in patients suffering from kidney disease or who are allergic to penicillin.
Not to be used for: patients suffering from PORPHYRIA or extreme allergy to cephalosporin antibiotics.
Caution needed with: ANTICOAGULANTS.
Contains: CEFACLOR monohydrate.
Other preparations: DISTACLOR capsules and syrup, Distaclor MR (long-acting) tablets.

---

cefadroxil *see* **Baxan**

---

cefixime *see* **Suprax**

---

cefpodoxime *see* **Orelox**

---

ceftibufen *see* **Cedax**

---

cefuroxime axetil *see* **Zinnat**

Celance
(Lilly)

An ivory, green, or pink, rectangular, scored tablet according to strengths of 0.05 mg, 0.25 mg, 1 mg, and used as an antiparkinsonian drug as an additional treatment for Parkinson's disease.

Dose: Initially 0.05 mg a day for 2 days, then gradually increasing to a maximum of 5 mg a day.
Availability: NHS and private prescription.
Side effects: hallucinations, confusion, movement disorder, drowsiness, low blood pressure, heartbeat abnormalities, nausea, indigestion, inflammation of the nose, breathing difficulty, double vision.
Caution: in pregnant women, nursing mothers, and in patients suffering from heart disease, abnormal heart rhythm, or with a history of hallucinations. Treatment should be withdrawn gradually.
Not to be used for: children.

Caution needed with: other similar antiparkinsonian drugs, alcohol, sedatives, blood-pressure lowering drugs, ANTICOAGULANTS.
Contains: PERGOLIDE MESYLATE.
Other preparations:

Celectol
(Rhône-Poulenc Rorer)

A yellow, heart-shaped, scored tablet or a white, heart-shaped, scored tablet according to strengths of 200 mg, 400 mg, and used as a ß-BLOCKER to treat high blood pressure.

Dose: 200 mg a day in the morning 30 minutes before food, up to a maximum of 400 mg a day.
Availability: NHS and private prescription.
Side effects: cold hands and feet, sleep disturbance, slow heart rate, tiredness, wheezing, heart failure, stomach upset, dry eyes, skin rash.
Caution: in pregnant women, nursing mothers, and in patients suffering from diabetes, kidney or liver disorders, asthma. May need to be withdrawn before surgery. Withdraw gradually. Your doctor may advise additional treatment with DIURETICS or DIGOXIN.
Not to be used for: children or for patients suffering from heart block or failure.
Caution needed with: VERAPAMIL, CLONIDINE withdrawal, some anti-arrhythmic drugs, some anaesthetics, RESERPINE, some blood-pressure lowering drugs, ERGOTAMINE, CIMETIDINE, sedatives, SYMPATHOMIMETICS, INDOMETHACIN, antidiabetics.
Contains: CELIPROLOL.
Other preparations:

Celevac
(Monmouth)

A pink tablet supplied at a strength of 500 mg and used as an adsorbent and bulking agent to treat constipation, colostomy control, diarrhoea, ulcerative colitis, diverticular disease, obesity.

Dose: to treat constipation adults 3-6 tablets night and morning with at least 300 ml liquid; to treat diarrhoea adults 3-6 tablets night and morning with little liquid; to treat obesity 3 tablets with liquid 30 minutes before a meal or when hungry; children in proportion to the dosage for a 70 kg adult.
Availability: NHS, private prescription, over the counter.
Side effects:
Caution: if treating diarrhoea, do not drink for 30 minutes before and after each dose.

Not to be used for: treating obesity in children or for patients suffering from blocked intestine.
Caution needed with:
Contains: METHYLCELLULOSE.
Other preparations:

---

celiprolol *see* Celectol

---

cephalexin capsules

A capsule supplied at strengths of 250 mg and 500 mg, and used as a cephalosporin antibiotic to treat respiratory, skin, and soft tissue infections, ear infections, urinary infections, gonorrhoea.

Dose: adults and children over 7 years 1-2 g a day in 2-4 divided doses (up to 4.5 g a day may be needed for severe infections); children under 1 year 125 mg twice a day, 1-5 years 125 mg every 8 hours, 6-12 years 250 mg every 8 hours.
Availability: NHS and private prescription.
Side effects: allergy, headache, stomach disturbances.
Caution: in pregnant women, nursing mothers, and in patients suffering from kidney disease or who are sensitive to penicillins.
Not to be used for: patients suffering from PORPHYRIA or extreme sensitivity to cephalosporin antibiotics.
Caution needed with: some DIURETICS, ANTICOAGULANTS.
Contains: CEPHALEXIN
Other preparations: cephalexin tablets, cephalexin oral suspension and syrup. CEPOREX, KEFLEX.

---

cephradine *see* Velosef

Ceporex *see* cephalexin capsules
(Glaxo)

Cerebrovase *see* dipyridamole tablets
(Ashbourne)

Cerumol
(LAB)

Drops used as a wax softener to remove wax from the ears.

Dose: 5 drops into the ear twice a day for 3 days may enable syringing to be avoided.
Availability: NHS, private prescription, over the counter.
Side effects:
Caution:
Not to be used for: inflammation of the outer ear, dermatitis, eczema, perforated ear drum.
Caution needed with:
Contains: PARADICHLOROBENZENE, CHLORBUTOL, ARACHIS OIL.
Other preparations:

C

Cetavlex
(Zeneca)

A cream used as an antiseptic to treat minor cuts and wounds, nappy rash.

Dose: apply as needed.
Availability: NHS, private prescription, over the counter.
Side effects:
Caution:
Not to be used for:
Caution needed with:
Contains: CETRIMIDE.
Other preparations:

---

cetirizine dihydrochloride *see* **Zirtek**

---

cetomacrogol *see* **Diprobase, Lipobase**

---

cetostearyl alcohol *see* **Diprobase, Lipobase, Unguentum Merck**

---

cetrimide *see* **Ceanel, Cetavlex, Drapolene, Tisept, Torbetol**

---

cetyl alcohol/coal tar distillate *see* **Pragmatar**

---

cetylpyridinium *see* **Merocaine, Merocet**

---

charcoal *see* **Carbellon, Carbomix, Medicoal**

Chemotrim Paediatric *see* **co-trimoxazole tablets**
(Rosemont)

Chendol
(CP Pharmaceuticals)

An orange/ivory capsule supplied at a strength of 125 mg and used as a bile acid to dissolve non-calcified gallstones.

Dose: 10-15 mg per kilogram bodyweight a day. Maintain treatment for 3 months after stones have dissolved.
Availability: NHS and private prescription.
Side effects: diarrhoea, itching.
Caution: your doctor may advise liver-function tests.
Not to be used for: children, pregnant women, nursing mothers, or for patients suffering from chronic liver disease or inflammatory intestinal disease.
Caution needed with: the contraceptive pill.
Contains: CHENODEOXYCHOLIC ACID.
Other preparations: CHENOFALK.

---

chenodeoxycholic acid *see* **Chendol, Combidol**

Chenofalk *see* **Chendol**
(Thames)

Chloractil *see* **chlorpromazine tablets**
(DDSA)

---

choral hydrate *see* **chloral mixture BP, Noctec, Welldorm**

---

chloral mixture BP

An oral solution used as a sedative for the short-term treatment of sleeplessness.

Dose: adults 5-20 ml well diluted in water taken before going to bed; children 1-5 years 2.5-5 ml diluted in water; 6-12 years 5-10 ml.

Availability: NHS and private prescription.
Side effects: stomach upset, wind, rash, ketones in the urine, headache, excitement, dependence, confusion in the elderly.
Caution: in pregnant women, nursing mothers, the elderly or those with general debility, and in patients suffering from respiratory disease, PORPHYRIA, a history of drug addiction or alcoholism, some psychiatric disorders. Withdraw slowly and avoid contact with the skin. Patients should be warned of reduced judgement and abilities.
Not to be used for: patients suffering from severe heart disease, gastritis, or kidney or liver disorder.
Caution needed with: alcohol, other sedatives, ANTICOAGULANTS.
Contains: CHLORAL HYDRATE.
Other preparations: chloral elixir paediatric BP (suitable for children under 1 year, chloral syrup BPC 1968 (double-strength preparation). NOCTEC, WELLDORM.

---

chloramphenicol *see* Actinac, chloramphenicol capsules, chloramphenicol ear drops, chloramphenicol eye drops, Chloramphenicol Minims, Chloromycetin Hydrocortisone, Chloromycetin Eye Ointment, Sno Phenicol

---

chloramphenicol capsules

A capsule supplied at a strength of 250 mg and used as an antibiotic to treat typhoid and other life-threatening infections.

Dose: adults and children over 2 weeks 50 mg per kg body weight a day in divided doses every 6 hours; children under 2 weeks half adult dose.
Availability: NHS and private prescription.
Side effects: blood changes, stomach disturbances, nerve inflammation.
Caution: in patients with kidney or liver disorders. Not for repeated or prolonged use. Your doctor may advise regular blood tests.
Not to be used for: pregnant women, nursing mothers, or for patients suffering from PORPHYRIA.
Caution needed with: ANTICOAGULANTS, anticonvulsants, PARACETAMOL.
Contains: CHLORAMPHENICOL.
Other preparations:

---

chloramphenicol ear drops

Drops used as an antibiotic to treat bacterial infection of the outer ear.

Dose: apply 2-3 times a day.
Availability: NHS and private prescription.

Side effects: allergy.
Caution: avoid prolonged use.
Not to be used for:
Caution needed with:
Contains: CHLORAMPHENICOL.
Other preparations:

---

chloramphenicol eye drops

Drops used as an antibiotic to treat bacterial infections of the eye.

Dose: adults 1 or more drops into the eye as needed or at least every 2 hours, reducing as infection subsides; children 1 drop into the eye as needed. Continue for 48 hours after infection subsides.
Availability: NHS and private prescription.
Side effects: stinging, rarely anaemia.
Caution: remove contact lenses before using.
Not to be used for:
Caution needed with:
Contains: CHLORAMPHENICOL.
Other preparations: chloramphenicol eye ointment. CHLOROMYCETIN EYE OINTMENT, CHLORAMPHENICOL MINIMS (in single-use containers), SNO PHENICOL.

Chloramphenicol Minims *see* chloramphenicol eye drops
(Chauvin)

Chlorasol
(Seton Healthcare)

A solution in a sachet used as a disinfectant for cleaning and removing dead skin from ulcers.

Dose: apply to the affected areas as needed.
Availability: NHS, private prescription, over the counter.
Side effects: irritation.
Caution: keep away from the eyes and the clothes; throw away any remaining solution immediately.
Not to be used for: internal use.
Caution needed with:
Contains: SODIUM HYPOCHLORITE.
Other preparations:

---

chlorbutol *see* **Cerumol, Eludril, Monphytol**

---

chlordiazepoxide *see* **chlordiazepoxide capsules, Librium, Tropium**

---

chlordiazepoxide capsules

A capsule supplied at strengths of 5 mg and 10 mg, and used as a tranquillizer for the short-term treatment of severe anxiety, and symptoms of acute alcohol withdrawal.

Dose: anxiety: elderly 15 mg a day at first then half adult dose; adults up to 30 mg a day in divided doses at first to a maximum of 100 mg a day in severe cases; other conditions as advised by a doctor.
Availability: NHS and private prescription.
Side effects: drowsiness, confusion, forgetfulness, vertigo, stomach upset, unsteadiness, low blood pressure, rash, changes in vision, changes in sexual function, retention of urine. Risk of addiction increases with dose and length of treatment. May impair judgement.
Caution: in the elderly, pregnant women, nursing mothers, and in patients suffering from lung disorders, kidney or liver disorders, PORPHYRIA, or with a history of drug or alcohol abuse. Avoid long-term use and withdraw gradually.
Not to be used for: children or for patients suffering from acute breathing disorder, some chronic lung diseases, some mental disorders.
Caution needed with: alcohol, sedatives, and other tranquillizers and anticonvulsants, CIMETIDINE, RIFAMPICIN.
Contains: CHLORDIAZEPOXIDE.
Other preparations: chlordiazepoxide hydrochloride tablets. LIBRIUM, TROPIUM (neither available on NHS).

---

chlorhexidine *see* **Bactigras, Chlorhexitulle, Corsodyl, CX Powder, Eludril, Hibiscrub, Hibisol, Naseptin, Nystaform, Nystaform-HC, pHiso-Med, Rotersept, Serotulle, Sterexidine, Tisept, Unisept**

---

chlormethiazole edisylate *see* **Heminevrin**

Chloromycetin Eye Ointment
(Parke-Davis)

An ointment used as an antibiotic to treat bacterial conjunctivitis.

Dose: apply the ointment into the eye every 3 hours or more often if needed and continue until 2 days after the symptoms have gone.
Availability: NHS and private prescription.
Side effects: rarely bone marrow suppression.
Caution:
Not to be used for:
Caution needed with:
Contains: CHLORAMPHENICOL.
Other preparations: Chloromycetin Redidrops. Chloramphenicol eye ointment, CHLORAMPHENICOL MINIMS.

Chloromycetin Hydrocortisone
(Parke-Davis)

An ointment used as an antibiotic, STEROID to treat eye infections.

Dose: apply into the eye up to once an hour depending on the severity of the infection.
Availability: NHS and private prescription.
Side effects: rise in eye pressure, thinning cornea, cataract, rarely bone marrow suppression.
Caution: in infants and pregnant women; do not use for extended periods; do not stop treatment abruptly.
Not to be used for: patients suffering from glaucoma, viral, fungal, tuberculous, or weeping infections.
Caution needed with:
Contains: CHLORAMPHENICOL, HYDROCORTISONE.
Other preparations:

---

chloroquine *see* **Avloclor, Nivaquine**

---

chlorothiazide *see* **Saluric**

---

chloroxylenol *see* **Zeasorb**

---

chlorpheniramine maleate *see* **chlorpheniramine tablets, Galpseud Plus, Haymine, Piriton, Rimarin**

---

chlorpheniramine tablets

A tablet supplied at a strength of 4 mg and used as an ANTIHISTAMINE treatment for allergies such as hay fever and nettle rash.

Dose: adults 1 tablet every 4-6 hours up to 6 tablets a day; children 6-12 years ½ tablet every 4-6 hours up to 3 tablets a day (children aged 1-6 years use syrup).
Availability: NHS, private prescription, over the counter.
Side effects: drowsiness, reduced reactions, dizziness, excitation.
Caution: in pregnant women and nursing mothers.
Not to be used for: infants under 1 year.
Caution needed with: sedatives, MAOIS, alcohol.
Contains: CHLORPHENIRAMINE MALEATE.
Other preparations: CALIMAL, PIRITON (also available as syrup), RIMARIN.

---

chlorpromazine *see* chlorpromazine tablets, Largactil

---

chlorpromazine tablets

A coated tablet supplied at strengths of 10 mg, 25 mg, 50 mg, 100 mg and used as a sedative to treat brain disturbances needing sedation, nausea, vomiting, schizophrenia, mood change, hiccups, anxiety.

Dose: adults 25 mg 3 times a day at first increasing if needed by 25 mg a day to 75-300 mg a day; children as advised by physician.
Availability: NHS and private prescription.
Side effects: muscle spasms, restlessness, hands shaking, dry mouth, palpitations, heart rhythm disturbance, low blood pressure, weight gain, blurred vision, changes in sexual function, low body temperature, breast swelling, menstrual changes, blood, liver, eye, and skin changes, drowsiness, apathy, nightmares, sleeplessness, depression, blocked nose, difficulty passing water, rarely fits.
Caution: in pregnant women, nursing mothers, the elderly, and in patients suffering from heart, lung, or circulation disorders, epilepsy, Parkinson's disease, thyroid disorder, infections, MYASTHENIA GRAVIS, kidney or liver disease, glaucoma, prostate disorder, some blood disorders.
Not to be used for: unconscious patients, or for patients suffering from bone marrow depression, PHAEOCHROMOCYTOMA.
Caution needed with: alcohol, sedatives, tranquillizers, pain killers, ASTEMIZOLE, TERFENADINE, CIMETIDINE, blood-pressure lowering drugs, some ß-BLOCKERS, LITHIUM, antidepressants, anticonvulsants, antidiabetic drugs, LEVODOPA, ANTACIDS, anaesthetics, drugs affecting heart rhythm.
Contains: CHLORPROMAZINE HYDROCHLORIDE.
Other preparations: chlorpromazine elixir, injection, suppositories. CHLORACTIL, LARGACTIL.

---

chlorpropamide *see* chlorpropamide tablets, Diabinese

chlorpropamide tablets

A tablet supplied at strengths of 100 mg, 250 mg and used as an antidiabetic drug to treat diabetes.

Dose: 100-250 mg a day with breakfast, to a maximum of 500 mg a day.
Availability: NHS and private prescription.
Side effects: allergy, including skin rash, stomach upset, low blood sodium levels, sensitivity to light, blood disorders, headache.
Caution: in the elderly and in patients suffering from kidney failure.
Not to be used for: children, pregnant women, nursing mothers, during surgery, or for patients suffering from juvenile diabetes, liver or kidney disorders, stress, infections, or PORPHYRIA.
Caution needed with: ß-BLOCKERS, MAOIS, STEROIDS, DIURETICS, alcohol, CIMETIDINE, RANITIDINE, ANTICOAGULANTS, lipid-lowering agents, ASPIRIN, some antibiotics, some antifungals, GLUCAGON, cyclophosphamide, the contraceptive pill, ACE INHIBITORS, NON-STEROIDAL ANTI-INFLAMMATORY DRUGS, KETOTIFEN, SULPHINPYRAZONE.
Contains: CHLORPROPAMIDE.
Other preparations: DIABINESE, GLYMESE.

---

chlorquinaldol *see* Locoid C

---

chlortetracycline *see* Aureocort, Aureomycin Ointment, Deteclo

---

chlorthalidone *see* Atenixco, co-tenidone tablets, Hygroton, Kalspare, Tenchlor, Tenoret 50, Tenoretic

---

Choledyl
(Parke Davis)

A syrup supplied at a strength of 62.5 mg/5 ml, and used as a BRONCHODILATOR to treat bronchial spasm brought on by chronic bronchitis or asthma.

Dose: adults 100-400 mg 4 times a day; children 3-6 years 5-10 ml 3 times a day, 6-12 years 100 mg 3-4 times a day.
Availability: NHS, private prescription , over the counter.
Side effects: rapid heart rate, sleeplessness, nausea, change in heart

rhythms, stomach upset.

Caution: in pregnant women, nursing mothers, and in patients suffering from heart or liver disease, peptic ulcer, diabetes.

Not to be used for: children under 3 years.

Caution needed with: CIMETIDINE, ERYTHROMYCIN, CIPROFLOXACIN, STEROIDS, DIURETICS, some other bronchodilators.

Contains: CHOLINE THEOPHYLLINATE.

Other preparations:

C

cholera vaccine
(Evans)

Cholera vaccine is not very effective and is no longer a legal requirement anywhere in the world. For travellers going to and from areas where cholera is known to exist, border controls may still require evidence of vaccination so that it may be better to be vaccinated before going to such countries rather than risk vaccination abroad.

Dose: 1 injection is sufficient to enable travellers to be provided with a certificate of vaccination but 2 injections 1-4 weeks apart provides improved protection.

---

cholestyramine *see* **Questran**

---

choline bitartrate *see* **Lipoflavonoid, Lipotriad**

---

choline chloride *see* **Ketovite**

---

choline salicylate *see* **Audax**

---

choline theophyllinate *see* **Choledyl**

---

chorionic gonadotrophin *see* **Gonadotrophon LH, Pregnyl, Profasi**

Cicatrin
(Wellcome)

A cream used as an aminoglycoside antibiotic to treat skin infections.

Dose: apply to the affected area up to 3 times a day.
Availability: NHS and private prescription.
Side effects: hearing damage, sensitization.
Caution: where there are large areas of damaged skin.
Not to be used for:
Caution needed with:
Contains: NEOMYCIN sulphate, BACITRACIN zinc, L-CYSTEINE, GLYCINE, DL-THREONINE.
Other preparations: Cicatrin Powder.

Cidomycin Cream
(Hoechst Roussel)

A cream used as an aminoglycoside antibiotic to treat skin infections.

Dose: apply to the affected area 3-4 times a day.
Availability: NHS and private prescription.
Side effects: hearing damage, sensitization.
Caution: where there are large areas of damaged skin.
Not to be used for:
Caution needed with:
Contains: GENTAMICIN sulphate.
Other preparations: Cidomycin Ointment.

Cidomycin Drops
(Hoechst Roussel)

Drops used as an antibiotic to treat infections of the outer ear or eye.

Dose: 2-4 drops into the ear 3-4 times a day and at night, or 1-3 drops into the eye 3-4 times a day.
Availability: NHS and private prescription.
Side effects: additional infection.
Caution:
Not to be used for: patients suffering from perforated ear drum.
Caution needed with:
Contains: GENTAMICIN sulphate.
Other preparations: Cidomycin Eye Ointment. GARAMYCIN, GENTICIN.

cilazapril *see* Vascace

Cilest
(Janssen-Cilag)

A blue tablet used as an oestrogen, progestogen contraceptive.

Dose: 1 tablet a day for 21 days, starting on day 1 of period.
Availability: NHS and private prescription.
Side effects: enlarged breasts, bloating and fluid retention, cramps, leg pains, mood change, reduction in sexual desire, headaches, nausea, vaginal erosion, discharge and bleeding, weight gain, skin changes, rarely thrombosis, raised blood pressure, jaundice.
Caution: in patients on dialysis or who are suffering from high blood pressure, Raynaud's disease, diabetes, vascular disorders, asthma, depression, kidney disease, multiple sclerosis, womb diseases. Your doctor may advise you not to smoke, and to have regular examinations. You should stop treatment at the first sign of serious symptoms such as severe headache or jaundice. Treatment should be stopped before surgery.
Not to be used for: pregnant women, or for patients suffering from sickle-cell anaemia, history of heart disease or thrombosis, liver disorders, some cancers, undiagnosed vaginal bleeding, PORPHYRIA, some ear, skin and kidney disorders.
Caution needed with: RIFAMPICIN, TETRACYCLINE ANTIBIOTICS, GRISEOFULVIN, BARBITURATES, PHENYTOIN, PRIMIDONE, CARBAMAZEPINE, ETHOSUXIMIDE, CHLORAL HYDRATE, DICHLORAL PHENAZONE, GLUTETHIMIDE.
Contains: ETHINYLOESTRADIOL, NORGESTIMATE.
Other preparations:

Ciloxan
(Alcon)

Drops used as an antibiotic to treat superficial infections of the eye and surrounding areas, ulcerated cornea.

Dose: ulcerated cornea, first day 2 drops into the eye every 15 minutes for 6 hours, then every 30 minutes for the remainder of the day, second day 2 drops every hour, days 3-14 (and up to a maximum of 21 days) 2 drops every 4 hours; conjunctivitis, 1-2 drops 4 times a day; severe infection, 1-2 drops every 2 waking hours for 2 days, then 1-2 drops 4 times a day.
Availability: NHS, private prescription.
Side effects: irritation, skin rash (stop treatment), bitter taste in the mouth.
Caution: in pregnant women, nursing mothers.
Not to be used for: children, for patients who wear soft contact lenses, or for longer than 21 days.
Caution needed with:
Contains: CIPROFLOXACIN.

Other preparations:

---

cimetidine *see* **Acitak, Algitec, cimetidine tablets, Dyspamet, Galenamet, Peptimax, Phimetin, Tagamet, Ultec, Zita**

---

cimetidine tablets

A tablet supplied at strengths of 200 mg, 400 mg, and 800 mg and used as a HISTAMINE H$_2$ BLOCKER to treat duodenal and gastric ulcers, hiatus hernia, indigestion, oesophageal reflux.

Dose: children over 1 year 25-30 mg per 1 kg body weight a day in divided doses; adults 400 mg–2.4 g a day, depending on condition.
Availability: NHS, private prescription, and over the counter to adults only for the short-term treatment of heartburn, dyspepsia, and excess stomach acid.
Side effects: rash, tiredness, dizziness, liver changes, confusion, breast swelling; rarely kidney, pancreas, bone marrow, joint, and muscle problems; headache, altered bowel habit.
Caution: in pregnant women, nursing mothers and in patients suffering from impaired liver or kidney function. Monitor patients on long-term therapy.
Not to be used for:
Caution needed with: ANTICOAGULANTS taken by mouth, ANALGESICS, MEBENDAZOLE, some heart rhythm drugs, some antibacterials, TRICYCLIC ANTIDEPRESSANTS, antidiabetics, CARBAMAZEPINE, tranquillizers, ß-BLOCKERS, CYCLOSPORIN, PHENYTOIN, some antifungals, THEOPHYLLINE, CHLORPROMAZINE, CLOZAPINE, CHLORAQUINE, QUININE, some drugs used to treat angina, high blood pressure.
Contains: CIMETIDINE.
Other preparations: ACITAK, DYSPAMET, GALENMET, PEPTIMAX, PHIMETIN, TAGAMET, ULTEC, ZITA. Tagamet-100 (a 100 mg tablet available over the counter only to treat heartburn, excess acid, and indigestion). Tagamet Dual Action (a liquid combination of cimetidine and sodium alginate, available over the counter only to treat heartburn associated with acid reflux).

Cinazière 15 *see* **cinnarizine tablets**
(Ashbourne)

---

cinchocaine *see* **Nupercainal, Proctosedyl, Scheriproct, Ultraproct, Uniroid-HC**

---

cineole *see* **Rowachol, Rowatinex**

---

cinnarizine *see* **Cinazière, cinnarizine tablets, Stugeron, Stugeron Forte**

---

cinnarizine tablets

A tablet supplied at a strength of 15 mg and used as an ANTIHISTAMINE treatment for vestibular disorders such as vertigo, tinnitus, Ménière's disease, travel sickness, and for vascular disorders such as Raynaud's syndrome.

Dose: vestibular disorders adults, 2 tablets 3 times a day; travel sickness 2 tablets 2 hours before journey, then 1 every 8 hours during the journey. Children 5-12 years half adult dose. For vascular disorders adults 75 mg 2-3 times a day.
Availability: NHS, private prescription, over the counter.
Side effects: drowsiness, reduced reactions, rarely skin eruptions and tiredness, dry mouth, blurred vision.
Caution: in pregnant women, nursing mothers, and in patients suffering from liver or kidney disease, glaucoma, PORPHYRIA, epilepsy, low blood pressure, or enlarged prostate.
Not to be used for: children under 5 years.
Caution needed with: alcohol, sedatives, some antidepressants (MAOIS), ANTICHOLINERGICS.
Contains: CINNARIZINE.
Other preparations: CINAZIERE, STUGERON.

Cinobac
(Eli Lilly)

A green/orange capsule supplied at a strength of 500 mg and used as a quinolone antibiotic to treat infections of the urinary tract.

Dose: 1 capsule twice a day for 7-14 days; for prevention 1 at night.
Availability: NHS and private prescription.
Side effects: allergy, brain and stomach disturbances.
Caution: in patients suffering from kidney disease, or with a history of liver disease.
Not to be used for: children, pregnant women, nursing mothers or for patients suffering from severe kidney disease.
Caution needed with: ANTICOAGULANTS, THEOPHYLLINE, NON-STEROIDAL ANTI-INFLAMMATORY DRUGS.

Contains: CINOXACIN.
Other preparations:

---

cinoxacin *see* Cinobac

Cipramil
(Lundbeck)

A white, oval, scored, film-coated tablet supplied at a strength of 20 mg, and used as an antidepressant to treat and prevent depression.

Dose: adults, 1 tablet a day at first, increasing if necessary to 3 tablets a day; elderly, 1 tablet a day at first increasing to 2 tablets a day if needed.
Availability: NHS, private prescription.
Side effects: nausea, sweating, shaking, drowsiness, dry mouth.
Caution: in pregnant women, nursing mothers, and in patients suffering from liver or severe kidney failure.
Not to be used for: children.
Caution needed with: MAOIS, LITHIUM, TRYPTOPHAN, tranquillizers, antidepressants.
Contains: CITALOPRAM hydrobromide.
Other preparations:

---

ciprofibrate *see* Modalim

---

ciprofloxacin *see* Ciloxan, Ciproxin

Ciproxin
(Bayer)

Tablets supplied at strengths of 250 mg, 500 mg, 750 mg, and used as an antibiotic to treat infections of the ear, nose, throat, urinary system, respiratory system, skin, soft tissues, bone, joints, stomach, and gonorrhoea (a venereal disease), and major infections.

Dose: adults, 250-750 mg twice a day; gonorrhoea, 1 dose of 250 mg. Children as advised by a doctor.
Availability: NHS and private prescription.
Side effects: stomach and intestinal disturbances, dizziness, headache, tiredness, confusion, convulsions, rash, pain in the joints, changes in blood, liver, or kidneys, blurred vision, rapid heart rate, changes in taste and smell, sleep disturbance, sensitivity to light, hearing disorder.

C

Caution: in patients suffering from severe kidney disease, epilepsy, or with a history of convulsions. Plenty of liquid should be drunk. If pain, inflammation, and creaking in a limb occurs, treatment should be stopped and limb rested. If judgement or dexterity are affected, patients should not drive or operate machinery. Children are treated only in extreme circumstances.

Not to be used for: growing youngsters unless absolutely necessary, and pregnant women or nursing mothers.

Caution needed with: THEOPHYLLINE, ANTACIDS, alcohol, opiate ANALGESICS, GLIBENCLAMIDE, PROBENECID, magnesium, aluminium, or iron salts, ANTICOAGULANTS, NON-STEROIDAL ANTI-INFLAMMATORY DRUGS, CYCLOSPORIN.

Contains: CIPROFLOXACIN.

Other preparations: Ciproxin Infusion.

---

cisapride *see* **Alimix, Prepulsid**

---

citalopram *see* **Cipramil**

Citramag
(Bioglan)

An effervescent powder in a sachet used as a laxative to induce the total emptying of the bowels before X-ray or bowel surgery.

Dose: 1 sachet in 200 ml of water taken by mouth the day before the procedure.

Availability: NHS, private prescription, over the counter.

Side effects:

Caution: in the elderly and in patients suffering from kidney failure. Patients should be advised to have a high-fluid, low-residue diet.

Not to be used for: children.

Caution needed with:

Contains: MAGNESIUM CITRATE.

Other preparations:

---

citric acid *see* **Effercitrate, Mictral, Rehidrat, Sandocal, simple linctus**

Citrical
(Shire)

Orange-flavoured granules supplied in sachets of 500 mg and used as a calcium supplement to treat calcium deficiency.

Dose: 1 sachet dissolved in water up to 3 times a day.
Availability: NHS, private prescription, over the counter.
Side effects: constipation, wind.
Caution:
Not to be used for: for patients suffering from overactive parathyroid
gland, decalcifying tumours, severe kidney failure.
Caution needed with: TETRACYCLINE ANTIBIOTICS.
Contains: CALCIUM CARBONATE.
Other preparations: CACIT, CALCICHEW, CALCIDRINK, CALCIUM-500.

---

clarithromycin *see* Klaricid

Clarityn
(Schering-Plough)

A white, oval, scored tablet supplied at a strength of 10 mg and used as an
ANTIHISTAMINE treatment for allergic rhinitis and other allergies.

Dose: 1 tablet a day (children use syrup).
Availability: NHS, private prescription, over the counter.
Side effects: tiredness, headache, nausea, heart rhythm changes,
fainting, hair loss, severe allergy, liver changes.
Caution:
Not to be used for: children under 2 years, pregnant women, or nursing
mothers.
Caution needed with: CIMETIDINE, ERYTHROMYCIN, KETOCONAZOLE, QUINIDINE,
FLUCONAZOLE, FLUOXETINE.
Contains: LORATADINE.
Other preparations: Clarityn Syrup (available only on prescription).

---

clavulanic acid *see* Augmentin

Cleanlet 25
(Gainor Medical Europe)

A device (lancet) for obtaining blood samples from the finger, compatible
with Autoclix, Autolet, Glucolet, Monojector, Penlett II, Softouch finger-
pricking devices. Blood-glucose monitoring enables individual patients
suffering from diabetes accurately to control blood glucose and manage
their condition.

Cleanlet 25XL
(Gainor Medical Europe)

A device (lancet) for obtaining blood samples from the finger, compatible with Autolet, Glucolet finger-pricking devices. Blood-glucose monitoring enables individual patients suffering from diabetes accurately to control blood glucose and manage their condition.

---

clemastine *see* Tavegil

Climagest 1 mg
(Sandoz)

16 grey/blue tablets and 12 white tablets used as an oestrogen and progestogen treatment for menopausal symptoms.

Dose: 1 grey/blue tablet for 16 days followed by 1 white tablet for the next 12 days. Begin on day 1 of period if present.
Availability: NHS and private prescription.
Side effects: enlarged breasts, fluid retention, nausea, vaginal bleeding, weight gain, headache, dizziness. Rarely jaundice, raised blood pressure, thrombosis.
Caution: in patients suffering from high blood pressure, diabetes, epilepsy, womb diseases, gall bladder disorder, migraine, multiple sclerosis, PORPHYRIA, liver disorders, some ear disorders, or a history or increased risk of breast disorders (including cancer) and thrombosis. Your doctor may advise you to have regular examinations.
Not to be used for: children, pregnant women, nursing mothers, or for patients suffering from thombosis, severe liver, kidney, or heart disorders, some cancers, undiagnosed vaginal bleeding, endometriosis.
Caution needed with: ACE INHIBITORS, ANTICOAGULANTS, BARBITURATES, ß-BLOCKERS, CARBAMAZEPINE, PHENYTOIN, RIFAMPICIN.
Contains: OESTRADIOL valerate, NORETHISTERONE.
Other preparations: Climagest 2 mg.

Climaval
(Sandoz)

A grey-blue or blue tablet supplied at a strength of 1 mg, 2 mg and used as an oestrogen to treat menopausal symptoms in women who have had a hysterectomy.

Dose: 1-2 mg a day. May be taken continuously for up to 24 months.
Availability: NHS and private prescription.

Side effects: enlarged breasts, fluid retention, nausea, vaginal bleeding, weight gain, headache, dizziness. Rarely jaundice, raised blood pressure, thrombosis.

Caution: in patients suffering from high blood pressure, diabetes, epilepsy, womb diseases, gall bladder disorder, migraine, multiple sclerosis, PORPHYRIA, liver disorders, some ear disorders, or a history or increased risk of breast disorders (including cancer) and thrombosis. Your doctor may advise you to have regular examinations.

Not to be used for: children, pregnant women, nursing mothers, or for patients suffering from thombosis, severe liver, kidney, or heart disorders, some cancers, undiagnosed vaginal bleeding, endometriosis.

Caution needed with: ACE INHIBITORS, ANTICOAGULANTS, BARBITURATES, ß-BLOCKERS, CARBAMAZEPINE, PHENYTOIN, RIFAMPICIN.

Contains: OESTRADIOL valerate.

Other preparations: PROGYNOVA, ZUMENON.

---

clindamycin *see* Dalacin C, Dalacin Cream, Dalacin T

Clinicide
(De Witt)

A liquid used as a pediculicide to treat lice of the head and pubic areas.

Dose: apply to the hair and allow to dry, then shampoo the following day.
Availability: NHS, private prescription.
Side effects:
Caution: keep out of the eyes.
Not to be used for:
Caution needed with:
Contains: CARBARYL.
Other preparations: CARYLDERM, DERBAC-C, SULEO-C.

Clinistix
(Bayer Diagnostics)

A plastic strip used for the detection of glucose in the urine and suitable only for screening purposes.

Clinitar Cream
(Shire)

A cream used as an antipsoriatic treatment for psoriasis, eczema.

Dose: apply to the affected area 1-2 times a day.
Availability: NHS, private prescription, over the counter.
Side effects: sensitivity to light.
Caution:
Not to be used for: patients suffering from pustular psoriasis.
Caution needed with:
Contains: COAL TAR EXTRACT.
Other preparations: Clinitar Shampoo. ALPHOSYL, GELCOTAR, PSORIDERM, PSORIGEL, T-GEL.

Clinitest
(Bayer Diagnostics)

A reagent tablet used by some patients suffering from diabetes for the detection of glucose and other reducing substances in the urine. This gives an approximate estimate of blood glucose levels which may be adequate for the management of Type II diabetes.

Clinoril
(MSD)

A hexagonal, yellow, scored tablet supplied at strengths of 100 mg, 200 mg and used as a NON-STEROIDAL ANTI-INFLAMMATORY DRUG to treat rheumatoid arthritis, osteoarthritis, ankylosing spondylitis, acute gouty arthritis, other joint disorders.

Dose: 200 mg twice a day with drink or food.
Availability: NHS and private prescription.
Side effects: stomach pain or bleeding, indigestion, inflammation of the tongue, fluid retention, muscle weakness, rash, dizziness, buzzing in the ears, breathing difficulties, changes in the blood, urine, eyesight, heart rhythm disturbance, high blood sugar, kidney stones, pancreatitis. Withdraw if fever or liver disorders occur.
Caution: in the elderly, and in patients with a history of stomach haemorrhage, ulcer or kidney or gall stones, kidney or liver disease, or heart failure. Drink plenty of fluids.
Not to be used for: children, pregnant women, nursing mothers, or for patients suffering from anti-inflammatory or ASPIRIN-induced allergy, peptic ulcer, or stomach bleeding.
Caution needed with: DIMETHYL SULPHOXIDE, METHOTREXATE, CYCLOSPORIN, ASPIRIN, ANTICOAGULANTS, DIFLUSINAL, antidiabetics.
Contains: SULINDAC.
Other preparations:

clioquinol *see* **Betnovate-C, Haelan-C, Locorten-Vioform, Oralcer, Quinaband, Synalar-C, Vioform-Hydrocortisone**

---

clobazam *see* **Frisium**

---

clobetasol propionate *see* **Dermovate**

---

clobetasone butyrate *see* **Cloburate, Eumovate Cream, Trimovate**

Cloburate
(Cusi)

Drops used as a CORTICOSTEROID to treat eye inflammations where there is no infection present.

Dose: 1-2 drops into the eye, usually 4 times a day but 1-2 hourly in severe conditions.
Availability: NHS, private prescription.
Side effects: rise in eye pressure, thinning of the cornea, cataract, fungal infection, sensitization
Caution: avoid prolonged use in pregnant women and in infants.
Not to be used for: patients suffering from fungal, viral, tuberculous, or weeping infections, corneal ulcer, glaucoma, or who wear soft contact lenses.
Caution needed with:
Contains: CLOBETASONE BUTYRATE.
Other preparations: Cloburate-N (for infected conditions).

---

clofazimine *see* **Lamprene**

---

clofibrate *see* **Atromid-S, Modalim**

Clomid
(Marion Merrell Dow)

A beige, scored tablet supplied at a strength of 50 mg and used as an anti-oestrogen treatment for sterility caused by failure of ovulation.

Dose: 1 tablet a day for five days starting on the fifth day of the period. Do

not use for more than 3 cycles.
Availability: NHS and private prescription.
Side effects: enlargement of the ovaries, hot flushes, uncomfortable abdomen, rash, thinning hair, blurred vision.
Caution:
Not to be used for: children, pregnant women, or for patients suffering from liver disease, large ovarian cyst, womb cancer, undiagnosed bleeding.
Caution needed with:
Contains: CLOMIPHENE CITRATE.
Other preparations: SEROPHENE.

---

clomiphene citrate *see* Clomid, Serophene

---

clomipramine hydrochloride *see* Anafranil, clomipramine capsules, Tranquax

---

clomipramine capsules

A capsule supplied at strengths of 10 mg, 25 mg, 50 mg and used as a TRICYCLIC ANTIDEPRESSANT to treat depression, obsessions, phobias.

Dose: adults 10 mg at first increasing to 30-250 mg a day; elderly 10 mg a day at first up to a maximum of 75 mg a day.
Availability: NHS and private prescription.
Side effects: dry mouth, constipation, urine retention, blurred vision, palpitations, drowsiness, sleeplessness, dizziness, low blood pressure, weight change, skin reactions, jaundice or blood changes, loss of sexual function, sweating, confusion, convulsions.
Caution: in pregnant women, nursing mothers, the elderly, and in patients suffering from heart disease, liver disease, thyroid disease, adrenal tumour, glaucoma, urine retention, epilepsy, diabetes, some other psychiatric conditions. Your doctor may advise regular blood tests.
Not to be used for: children, or for patients suffering from recent heart attack, liver disease, heart rhythm disturbances, or some mental disorders.
Caution needed with: alcohol, sedatives, ANTICHOLINERGICS, ADRENALINE, ASTEMIZOLE, TERFENADINE, BARBITURATES, MAOIS, other antidepressants, blood-pressure lowering drugs, anticonvulsants, DIURETICS, CIMETIDINE, some local anaesthetics, anti-arrhythmic drugs, RIFAMPICIN, NITRATES, the contraceptive pill.
Contains: CLOMIPRAMINE hydrochloride.
Other preparations: ANAFRANIL, TRANQUAX.

---

clonazepam *see* **Rivotril**

---

clonidine *see* **Catapres, Dixarit**

---

clopamide *see* **Viskaldix**

Clopixol
(Lundbeck)

A pink tablet, light-brown tablet, or brown tablet according to strengths of 2 mg, 10 mg, 25 mg and used as a tranquillizer to treat mental disorders especially schizophrenia.

Dose: 20-30 mg a day at first, then usually 20-50 mg a day up to a maximum of 150 mg a day.
Availability: NHS and private prescription.
Side effects: muscle spasms, restlessness, hands shaking, dry mouth, blocked nose, urine retention, constipation, palpitations, low blood pressure, blurred vision, weight gain, changes in sexual function, low body temperature, breast swelling, menstrual changes, jaundice, blood and skin changes, drowsiness, tiredness, rarely fits.
Caution: in pregnant women, nursing mothers, in the elderly who should take smaller dosage, and in patients suffering from Parkinson's disease, kidney, liver, or heart disease, or breathing disorders.
Not to be used for: children, unconscious patients, or for patients suffering from some mental disorders.
Caution needed with: alcohol, sedatives, ANALGESICS, blood-pressure lowering drugs, anticonvulsants, antidepressants, antidiabetics, LEVODOPA.
Contains: ZUCLOPENTHIXOL hydrochloride.
Other preparations: Clopixol Injection, Clopixol-Conc, Clopixol Acuphase.

Clorhexitulle
(Hoechst Roussel)

A sterile gauze tulle dressing, impregnated with antiseptic, supplied at a size of 10 cm square, and used as a dressing for wounds where there may be bacterial infection.

Availability: NHS, private prescription, over the counter.
Contains: CHLORHEXIDINE acetate, WHITE SOFT PARAFFIN.

Clostet *see* **tetanus vaccine**
(Evans)

---

clotrimazole *see* **Canesten, Canesten 1, Canesten-HC, clotrimazole cream, Lotriderm, Masnoderm**

---

clotrimazole cream

A cream used as an antifungal preparation to treat fungal skin infections such as ringworm.

Dose: apply cream 2-3 times a day until 14 days after the symptoms have gone.
Availability: NHS, private prescription, over the counter.
Side effects: irritation or allergy.
Caution:
Not to be used for:
Caution needed with:
Contains: CLOTRIMAZOLE.
Other preparations: CANESTEN (available as cream, powder, solution, and spray), MASNODERM.

---

cloxacillin *see* **Ampiclox, Ampiclox Neonatal Suspension, cloxacillin capsules, Orbenin**

---

cloxacillin capsules

An capsule supplied at strengths of 250 mg, 500 mg and used as a penicillin antibiotic to treat infections.

Dose: adults 500 mg every 6 hours at least half an hour before food; children over 2 years half adult dose; children under 2 years quarter adult dose.
Availability: NHS and private prescription.
Side effects: allergy, stomach disturbances, rash, blood changes.
Caution: in patients with a history of allergies or kidney disorders.
Not to be used for: patients suffering from penicillin allergy.
Caution needed with: METHOTREXATE, ANTICOAGULANTS, the contraceptive pill.
Contains: CLOXACILLIN.
Other preparations: cloxacillin injection. ORBENIN.

---

clozapine *see* **Clozaril**

Clozaril
(Sandoz)

A yellow, scored tablet supplied at strengths of 25 mg, 100 mg, and used as a sedative to treat schizophrenia.

Dose: 12.5-25 mg on first day, increasing to a maximum of 900 mg a day. Usual maintenance dose 150-300 mg a day in divided doses.
Availability: NHS and private prescription.
Side effects: blood changes, skin changes, drowsiness, watering of the mouth, rapid heart beat, tiredness, dizziness, headache, difficulty in passing urine, incontinence, stomach upset, change in electrical activity of the brain and heart, temporary upset of automatic body functions, low blood pressure on standing, persistent painful erection, weight gain, increased blood sugar levels.
Caution: in pregnant women, the elderly, and in patients with a history of epilepsy or suffering from enlarged prostate, glaucoma, liver disease, or intestinal abnormality. Patients should report any symptoms of infection. Your doctor may advise regular blood tests.
Not to be used for: children, nursing mothers, or for patients suffering from severe kidney or liver disease, alcoholism, drug intoxication, drowsiness or reduced reactions, heart failure, or for those in a coma or having a history of drug-induced blood disorder.
Caution needed with: other drugs that cause blood disorder, some sedatives, alcohol, MAOIS, ANTICHOLINERGICS, drugs that lower blood pressure, LITHIUM, ANTIHISTAMINES, CIMETIDINE, PHENYTOIN.
Contains: CLOZAPINE.
Other preparations:

co-amilofruse *see* co-amilofruse tablets, Fru-Co, Frumil, Lasoride

co-amilofruse tablets

A tablet available in 3 strengths and used as a DIURETIC to treat swelling and fluid retention associated with heart failure, liver and kidney disease.

Dose: 1 tablet in the morning. (2 tablets of the medium strength may be used if necessary.)
Availability: NHS and private prescription.
Side effects: stomach upset, rash, general feeling of being unwell, dry mouth, confusion, blood changes.

Caution: in pregnant women, nursing mothers, the elderly and in patients suffering from liver or kidney impairment, diabetes, excess acid in the body, enlarged prostate, gout, difficulty in passing water, or PORPHYRIA.
Not to be used for: children, or for patients suffering from progressive kidney failure, high blood potassium levels, cirrhosis of the liver.
Caution needed with: potassium supplements, some other diuretics, ASTEMIZOLE, TERFENADINE, LITHIUM, blood-pressure lowering drugs, CARBAMAZEPINE, NON-STEROIDAL ANTI-INFLAMMATORY DRUGS, ACE INHIBITORS, CYCLOSPORIN, DIGOXIN, some antibiotics, antidiabetic drugs, STEROIDS.
Contains: AMILORIDE hydrochloride, FRUSEMIDE.
Other preparations: FRU-CO, FRUMIL, FRUMIL LS, LASORIDE (some available in capsule form).

---

co-amilozide *see* co-amilozide tablets, Moduretic

---

co-amilozide tablets

A tablet available in 2 strengths and used as a DIURETIC to treat high blood pressure, congestive heart failure, liver cirrhosis with fluid retention.

Dose: usually 1-4 tablets a day. (Up to 8 of the weaker-strength tablets may be used daily.)
Availability: NHS and private prescription.
Side effects: rash, sensitivity to light, blood changes, gout.
Caution: in pregnant women, nursing mothers, the elderly, and in patients suffering from diabetes, electrolyte changes, gout, kidney or liver damage, PORPHYRIA.
Not to be used for: children, or for patients suffering from raised potassium levels, progressive or severe kidney failure.
Caution needed with: potassium supplements, other diuretics, DIGOXIN, LITHIUM, blood-pressure lowering drugs, ACE INHIBITORS, NON-STEROIDAL ANTI-INFLAMMATORY DRUGS, CARBAMAZEPINE, calcium supplements, STEROIDS, CYCLOSPORIN, antidiabetics.
Contains: AMILORIDE hydrochloride, HYDROCHLOROTHIAZIDE (CO-AMILOZIDE).
Other preparations: co-amilozide oral solution. Moduretic Solution. AMIL-CO, AMILMAXCO, CO-AMILOZIDE, DELVAS, MODURETIC, MODURET-25.

---

co-amoxiclav *see* Augmentin

---

co-beneldopa *see* Madopar

Co-Betaloc
(Astra)

A white, scored tablet used as a ß-BLOCKER and DIURETIC combination to treat high blood pressure.

Dose: 1-3 tablets a day in single or divided doses.
Availability: NHS and private prescription.
Side effects: cold hands and feet, sleep disturbances, slow heart rate, tiredness, wheezing, heart failure, stomach upset, dry eyes, rash, blood changes, gout, sensitivity to light.
Caution: in pregnant women, nursing mothers, or patients suffering from asthma, diabetes, gout, kidney or liver disorders. May need to be withdrawn before surgery. Withdraw gradually. Your doctor may advise addititional treatment with DIURETICS and DIGOXIN.
Not to be used for: children or patients suffering from heart block or failure, or severe kidney disorder.
Caution needed with: VERAPAMIL, CLONIDINE withdrawal, some anti-arrhythmic drugs and anaesthetics, RESERPINE, some blood-pressure lowering drugs, ERGOTAMINE, CIMETIDINE, antidiabetics, sedatives, SYMPATHOMIMETICS, INDOMETHACIN, LITHIUM, NON-STEROIDAL ANTI-INFLAMMATORY DRUGS, DIGOXIN, ALLOPURINOL, AMANTADINE.
Contains: METOPROLOL tartrate, HYDROCHLOROTHIAZIDE.
Other preparations: Co-Betaloc SA.

Co-careldopa *see* Sinemet

Co-Codamol

A tablet used as an ANALGESIC to relieve pain.

Dose: adults 1-2 tablets every 4-6 hours to a maximum of 8 tablets a day; children 6-12 years ½-1 tablet every 4-6 hours to a maximum of 4 tablets a day.
Availability: NHS, private prescription, over the counter
Side effects:
Caution: in patients suffering from kidney or liver disease.
Not to be used for: children under 6 years.
Caution needed with: other medicines containing PARACETAMOL.
Contains: CODEINE PHOSPHATE, paracetamol.
Other preparations: Co-Codamol Dispersible. PARAKE. (Various other branded products are available but not on NHS prescription.)

Co-Codaprin Dispersible

A dispersible tablet used as an ANALGESIC to relieve pain.

Dose: 1-2 tablets in water every 4-6 hours as needed.
Availability: NHS, private prescription, over the counter.
Side effects: stomach upsets, allergy, asthma.
Caution: in the elderly, pregnant women, in patients with a history of allergy to ASPIRIN or asthma, or who are suffering from impaired kidney or liver function.
Not to be used for: children, nursing mothers, or for patients suffering from haemophilia, ulcers.
Caution needed with: ANTICOAGULANTS, some antidiabetic drugs, anti-inflammatory agents, METHOTREXATE, SPIRONOLACTONE, STEROIDS, some uric acid-lowering drugs.
Contains: ASPIRIN, CODEINE PHOSPHATE.
Other preparations: Co-Codaprin – available on NHS only when prescribed as generic.

---

co-danthramer *see* co-danthramer suspension and capsules, Codalax

---

co-danthramer suspension and capsules

A liquid or capsule used as a laxative to treat constipation in the elderly, and in patients with heart failure or coronary thrombosis, or caused by ANALGESICS.

Dose: adults 5-10 ml or 1-2 capsules at night; children 2.5-5 ml or 1 capsule at night.
Availability: NHS and private prescription.
Side effects: colouring of urine and skin around the anus, skin irritation in incontinent patients.
Caution: in incontinent patients.
Not to be used for: pregnant women, nursing mothers, infants in nappies or patients suffering from intestinal blockage or pain in the abdomen.
Caution needed with:
Contains: poloxamer 188, DANTHRON.
Other preparations: co-danthramer strong suspension and capsules. AILAX, CODALAX, Codalax Forte (all available on NHS only if prescribed as a generic).

---

co-danthrusate capsules

Capsules used as a stimulant laxative and faecal softener to treat constipation in the elderly and in patients with heart failure or coronary thrombosis, or caused by ANALGESICS.

Dose: adults 1-3 capsules at night; children over 6 years 1 capsule at night.
Availability: NHS and private prescription.
Side effects: red colour in urine, skin irritation and discoloration.
Caution: in incontinent patients.
Not to be used for: children under 6 years, pregnant women, or for patients with blocked intestine.
Caution needed with:
Contains: DANTHRON, DOCUSATE sodium.
Other preparations: Co-Danthrusate Suspension. CAPSUVAC, NORMAX (available on NHS only when prescribed as a generic).

co-dydramol *see* co-dydramol tablets, Galake

co-dydramol

A tablet used as an opiate ANALGESIC to control pain.

Dose: 1-2 tablets every 4-6 hours up to a maximum of 8 tablets a day.
Availability: NHS, private prescription.
Side effects: constipation, nausea, headache.
Caution: in pregnant women, the elderly, and in patients suffering from allergies, kidney or liver disease, or underactive thyroid.
Not to be used for: children or patients suffering from respiratory depression or blocked airways.
Caution needed with: alcohol, sedatives, other medicines containing PARACETAMOL.
Contains: DIHYDROCODEINE tartrate, paracetamol.
Other preparations: GALAKE (available on NHS only if prescribed as a generic), Paramol (a weaker-strength tablet available over the counter).

co-fluampicil *see* co-fluampicil capsules, Magnapen

co-fluampicil capsules

A capsule used as a penicillin antibiotic to treat infections.

Dose: adults 1-2 capsules 4 times a day; children under 10 years use

syrup form
Availability: NHS and private prescription.
Side effects: allergies, stomach disturbances; rarely blood changes, jaundice.
Caution: in patients suffering from glandular fever, kidney disorders, PORPHYRIA, leukaemia, or HIV infection.
Not to be used for: for patients suffering from penicillin allergy.
Caution needed with: ANTICOAGULANTS, the contraceptive pill, METHOTREXATE
Contains: AMPICILLIN, FLUCLOXACILLIN.
Other preparations: MAGNAPEN (available as capsules and syrup).

---

co-flumactane *see* Aldactide

---

co-phenotrope *see* Lomotil, Lotharin

---

co-prenozide *see* Trasidrex

---

co-proxamol *see* co-proxamol tablets, Cosalgesic, Distalgesic

---

co-proxamol tablets

A tablet used as an opiate ANALGESIC to control pain.

Dose: 2 tablets 3-4 times a day.
Availability: NHS and private prescription.
Side effects: tolerance, dependence, drowsiness, constipation, dizziness, nausea, rash.
Caution: in pregnant women, the elderly, and in patients suffering from liver or kidney disease.
Not to be used for: children.
Caution needed with: alcohol, sedatives, anticonvulsant drugs, ANTICOAGULANTS, other medicines containing PARACETAMOL.
Contains: DEXTROPROPOXYPHENE hydrochloride, PARACETAMOL.
Other preparations: COSALGESIC, DISTALGESIC – available on NHS only when prescribed as generics.

---

co-simalcite *see* Altacite Plus

---

co-tenidone *see* co-tenidone tablets, Tenoret-50, Tenoretic

---

co-tenidone tablets

A tablet available in 2 strengths, and used as a ß-BLOCKER/thiazide DIURETIC to treat high blood pressure.

Dose: 1 tablet a day (of either strength).
Availability: NHS and private prescription.
Side effects: cold hands and feet, sleep disturbance, slow heart rate, tiredness, wheezing, heart failure, stomach upset, gout, sensitivity to light, blood changes, weakness, dry eyes, rash, impotence.
Caution: in pregnant women, nursing mothers, and in patients suffering from diabetes, gout, myasthenia gravis, LUPUS, PORPHYRIA, kidney or liver disorders. May need to be withdrawn before surgery. Withdraw gradually. Your doctor may advise additional treatment with diuretics or DIGOXIN.
Not to be used for: children or for patients suffering from asthma, heart block or failure, kidney failure, Addison's disease.
Caution needed with: VERAPAMIL, CLONIDINE withdrawal, some anti-arrhythmic drugs and anaesthetics, RESERPINE, some blood-pressure lowering drugs, CYCLOSPORIN, ERGOTAMINE, sedatives, antidiabetics, LITHIUM, DIGOXIN, STEROIDS, SYMPATHOMIMETICS, INDOMETHACIN, STEROIDS, NON-STEROIDAL ANTI-INFLAMMATORY DRUGS, MEFLOQUINE, CARBAMAZEPINE, calcium supplements, VITAMIN D, DILTIAZEM.
Contains: ATENOLOL, CHLORTHALIDONE.
Other preparations: ATENIXCO, KALTEN, TENCHLOR, TENORET 50, TENORETIC.

---

co-triamterzide *see* co-triamterzide tablets, Diazide, Triamaxco, Triam-co

---

co-triamterzide

A tablet used as a DIURETIC to treat high blood pressure, fluid retention.

Dose: high blood pressure 1 tablet a day at first; fluid retention 1 tablet twice a day at first after meals and then 1 tablet a day or every other day for maintenance. No more than 4 tablets a day.
Availability: NHS and private prescription.
Side effects: nausea, diarrhoea, cramps, weakness, headache, dry mouth, rash, blood changes, blue colour in urine, sensitivity to light, gout, impotence.
Caution: in pregnant women, nursing mothers, and in patients suffering from liver or kidney disease, diabetes, electrolyte changes, gout, pancreatitis, LUPUS, PORPHYRIA.
Not to be used for: children or for patients suffering from severe or progressive kidney failure, raised potassium levels, Addison's disease (a disease of the adrenal glands).

Caution needed with: potassium supplements, potassium-sparing diuretics, LITHIUM, ASTEMIZOLE, TERFENADINE, DIGOXIN, blood-pressure lowering drugs, INDOMETHACIN, ACE INHIBITORS, NON-STEROIDAL ANTI-INFLAMMATORY DRUGS, STEROIDS, antidiabetics, CARBAMAZEPINE, calcium supplements, CYCLOSPORIN, VITAMIND D.
Contains: TRIAMTERENE, HYDROCHLOROTHIAZIDE.
Other preparations: DYAZIDE, TRIAMAXCO, TRIAM-CO.

C

co-trimoxazole *see* co-trimoxazole tablets, Septrin

---

co-trimoxazole tablets

A tablet supplied at strengths of 480 mg and 960 mg and used as an antibiotic to treat respiratory, ear, urinary tract, and other specific infections where there is good reason to prefer the combination to another antibiotic.

Dose: adults 960 mg every 12 hours, increased to 1.44 g in severe infections; infants 6 weeks to 5 months 120 mg every 12 hours, 6 months to 5 years 240 mg, 6-12 years 480 mg.
Availability: NHS and private prescription.
Side effects: nausea, vomiting, diarrhoea, tongue inflammation, rash, blood changes, folate (vitamin) deficiency, rarely skin changes, jaundice.
Caution: in the elderly, nursing mothers, and in patients suffering from kidney disease or sensitivity to light. Drink plenty of non-alcoholic fluids. Your doctor may advise that patients undergoing prolonged treatment should have regular blood tests.
Not to be used for: pregnant women, new-born infants, or for patients suffering from severe kidney or liver disease, PORPHYRIA, or blood disorders.
Caution needed with: ANTICOAGULANTS, anticonvulsants, some antidiabetics, CYCLOSPORIN, METHOTREXATE.
Contains: TRIMETHOPRIM, SULPHAMETHOXAZOLE.
Other preparations: co-trimoxazole dispersible tablets, paediatric oral suspension, oral suspension. BACTRIM, CHEMOTRIM PAEDIATRIC SUSPENSION, COMIXCO, FECTRIM, LARATRIM, SEPTRIN.

---

coal tar *see* **Alphosyl, Alphosyl HC, Balneum with Tar, Baltar, calamine and coal tar ointment, Capasal, Carbo-Cort, Carbo-Dome, Clinitar Cream, coal tar paste, coal tar and salicylic acid ointment, Cocois, Gelcosal, Gelcotar, Genisol, Ionil T, Pentrax, Pixol, Polytar, Polytar Emollient, Psoriderm, Psorigel, Psorin, T Gel, Tarband, Tarcortin**

---

coal tar paste BP

A paste used to treat chronic eczema and psoriasis.

Dose: apply 1-3 times a day.
Availability: NHS, private prescription, over the counter.
Side effects: irritation, acne-like skin eruptions, sensitivity to light.
Caution: avoid broken or inflamed skin.
Not to be used for:
Caution needed with:
Contains: strong COAL TAR solution, compound zinc paste,
Other preparations: ZINC AND COAL TAR PASTE BP.

---

coal tar and salicylic acid ointment BP

An ointment used to treat chronic eczema and psoriasis.

Dose: apply 1-3 times a day.
Availability: NHS, private prescription, over the counter.
Side effects: irritation, acne-like skin eruptions, sensitivity to light.
Caution: avoid broken or inflamed skin. Stains skin, hair, and fabrics.
Not to be used for:
Caution needed with:
Contains: COAL TAR, SALICYLIC ACID, emulsifying wax, WHITE SOFT PARAFFIN, COCONUT OIL, POLYSORBATE 80, LIQUID PARAFFIN.
Other preparations:

Cobadex
(Cox)

A cream used as a STEROID treatment for skin disorders, itch of the anus and vulva.

Dose: apply a small quantity to the affected area 2-3 times a day.
Availability: NHS and private prescription.
Side effects: fluid retention, suppression of adrenal glands, thinning, spotting, or streaking of the skin may occur.
Caution: use for short periods of time only, especially in children or on the face.
Not to be used for: patients suffering from acne or any other skin infections caused by tuberculosis, ringworm, viruses, or fungi, leg ulcers, scabies, or continuously especially in pregnant women.
Caution needed with:
Contains: HYDROCORTISONE, DIMETHICONE.
Other preparations:

Cobalin-H *see* Neo-Cytamen
(Link)

Cocois
(Bioglan)

An ointment used for dry and scaly scalp conditions, including eczema and psoriasis.

Dose: apply and then remove after 1 hour by shampooing. Use once a day for 3-7 days, then occasionally.
Availability: NHS, private prescription, over the counter.
Side effects: irritation, sensitivity to light.
Caution:
Not to be used for: children under 6 years, or for patients suffering from acute infections or pustular psoriasis.
Caution needed with:
Contains: COAL TAR solution, SALICYLIC ACID, SULPHUR, COCONUT OIL.
Other preparations: compound coconut oil ointment.

---

coconut oil *see* Capasal, coal tar and salicylic acid ointment, Cocois, Dermamist

---

Codafen Continus
(Napp)

A pink/white, capsule-shaped tablet used as an ANALGESIC and NON-STEROIDAL ANTI-INFLAMMATORY DRUG to treat pain associated with arthritis, rheumatism, and other joint conditions, periods, and surgical and dental procedures, and to treat soft tissue injuries and musculo-skeletal disorders.

Dose: 1-3 tablets every 12 hours.
Availability: NHS and private prescription.
Side effects: stomach upset and bleeding, stomach ulcer, headache, constipation, dizziness, drowsiness, blurred vision, liver or kidney disorder, blood changes.
Caution: in pregnant women, nursing mothers, and in patients suffering from kidney, liver, or heart disorder, underactive thyroid gland, low blood pressure, head injury, raised pressure in the brain, or with a history of asthma or allergy to ASPIRIN or anti-inflammatory drugs.
Not to be used for: children, or patients suffering from breathing difficulty, chronic constipation, or stomach ulcer (including those with a history of stomach ulcer).

Caution needed with: MAOIS, alcohol, sedatives, some antibiotics, some DIURETICS, ANTICOAGULANTS.
Contains: CODEINE PHOSPHATE, IBUPROFEN.
Other preparations: Nurofen Plus (a weaker-strength product available over the counter).

Codalax *see* co-danthramer suspension
(Napp)

---

codeine linctus BP

A linctus supplied at a strength of 15 mg in 5 ml and used as an opiate cough suppressant to treat dry cough.

Dose: adults 5-10 ml 3-4 times a day; children 1-5 years use paediatric formula, 5-12 years 2.5-5 ml 3-4 times a day.
Availability: NHS, private prescription, and over the counter provided a maximum single dose does not exceed 15 ml.
Side effects: constipation, breathing difficulty.
Caution: in patients suffering from asthma, liver or kidney impairment, history of drug addiction.
Not to be used for: infants under 1 year, or for patients suffering from liver disease or breathing difficulties.
Caution needed with: MAOIS.
Contains: CODEINE PHOSPHATE.
Other preparations: codeine linctus paediatric. GALCODINE. Sugar-free products are available for diabetics.

---

codeine phosphate *see* Aspav, Co-Codamol, Co-Codaprin Dispersible, codeine linctus BP, codeine tablets, Codafen, Diarrest, Galcodine, Kapake, Migraleve, Solpadol, Tylex

---

codeine tablets

A tablet supplied at strengths of 15 mg, 30 mg, 60 mg and used as an opiate ANALGESIC to treat pain.

Dose: adults 30-60 mg every 4 hours as needed to a maximum of 240 mg a day; children 1-12 years 3 mg per kg body weight a day in divided doses.
Availability: NHS and private prescription.
Side effects: tolerance, dependence, drowsiness, dry mouth, blurred vision, constipation, difficulty passing urine, low blood pressure, mood

changes, allergy.

Caution: in pregnant women, women in labour, nursing mothers, the elderly, and in patients suffering from underactive thyroid gland, liver disease, low blood pressure, asthma, kidney disease.

Not to be used for: infants under 1 year or for patients suffering from head injury or breathing difficulty.

Caution needed with: MAOIS, sedatives, alcohol.

Contains: CODEINE PHOSPHATE.

Other preparations: CODEINE PHOSPHATE syrup.

---

codergocrine mesylate *see* Hydergine

Cogentin
(MSD)

A white, quarter-scored tablet supplied at a strength of 2 mg and used as an ANTICHOLINERGIC treatment for Parkinson's disease.

Dose: adults ¼ tablet a day at first increasing by ¼ tablet a day every 5-6 days to a maximum of 3 tablets a day; children 3-12 years as advised by physician.

Availability: NHS and private prescription.

Side effects: anticholinergic effects, confusion, agitation, and rash at high doses.

Caution: in patients suffering from rapid heart rate, enlarged prostate, glaucoma, stomach blockage. Dose should be reduced gradually.

Not to be used for: infants under 3 years or for patients suffering from certain movement disorders.

Caution needed with: ANTIHISTAMINES, antidepressants, some tranquillizers.

Contains: BENZTROPINE mesylate.

Other preparations: Cogentin Injection.

---

colchicine tablets

Tablets supplied at a strength of 500 micrograms and used to treat gout, or to prevent attacks while other therapy is initiated.

Dose: treatment, 2 tablets initially, then 1 every 2-3 hours until relief is obtained or until vomiting/diarrhoea occurs, or until a total of 20 tablets has been taken. The course should not be repeated within 3 days. Preventive dose, 1 tablet 2-3 times a day.

Availability: NHS and private prescription.

Side effects: nausea, vomiting, abdominal pain, diarrhoea, bleeding in the

stomach or intestine, rash, kidney damage, hair loss, blood disorders, nerve inflammation.
Caution: in pregnant women, nursing mothers, and in patients suffering from stomach, intestinal, or kidney disorder.
Not to be used for: children.
Caution needed with: CYCLOSPORIN.
Contains: colchicine.
Other preparations:

Colestid
(Upjohn)

Granules in sachets containing 5 g used as a lipid-lowering agent to reduce lipids.

Dose: adults, 5-30 g a day in 1-2 divided doses in fluid; children, as advised by your physician.
Availability: NHS and private prescription.
Side effects: constipation.
Caution: in pregnant women, nursing mothers. VITAMINS A, D, E, and K supplements may be required.
Not to be used for:
Caution needed with: DIGOXIN, antibiotics, DIURETICS. Take any other drugs 1 hour before or 4 hours after Colestid.
Contains: COLESTIPOL.
Other preparations: Colestid Orange.

---

colestipol *see* Colestid

Colifoam
(Stafford-Miller)

Foam supplied in an aerosol and used as a STEROID treatment for ulcerative colitis and other bowel inflammations.

Dose: 1 application once or twice a day for 2 or 3 weeks followed by reduced applications.
Availability: NHS and private prescription.
Side effects: high blood sugar, thin bones, mood changes, ulcers.
Caution: in pregnant women and in patients suffering from severe ulcerative disease. Do not use for prolonged periods.
Not to be used for: children or for patients suffering from obstruction, abscess, fresh intestinal surgery, tuberculous, fungal or viral infections.
Caution needed with:

Contains: HYDROCORTISONE acetate.
Other preparations:

---

colistin sulphomethate sodium *see* Colomycin

Colofac *see* mebeverine tablets
(Solvay Healthcare)

Colomycin
(Pharmax)

A white, quarter-scored tablet used as an antibiotic to treat some stomach infections and to prepare the bowel before surgery.

Dose: adults, 1-2 tablets every 8 hours; children under 30 kg bodyweight use syrup, over 30 kg as adult. (Injection may be nebulized and used for inhalation.)
Availability: NHS, private prescription.
Side effects: pins and needles, vertigo, breathing difficulty, kidney damage. Rarely changes in blood vessels, slurred speech, visual disturbances, mental disturbances.
Caution: in patients suffering from kidney disorder or PORPHYRIA.
Not to be used for: pregnant women, nursing mothers, or for patients suffering from myasthenia gravis.
Caution needed with: ANTICOAGULANTS, CYCLOSPORIN, some DIURETICS, cisplatin, NEOSTIGMINE, PYRIDOSTIGMINE.
Contains: COLISTIN SULPHOMETHATE SODIUM.
Other preparations: Colomycin injection, Colomycin Syrup, Colomycin Powder.

Colpermin
(Pharmacia)

A light blue/dark blue capsule, designed to resist stomach acid, and used as an antispasm treatment for irritable bowel syndrome.

Dose: adults 1-2 capsules 3 times a day, 30 minutes before meals for up to 3 months.
Availability: NHS, private prescription, over the counter.
Side effects: heartburn, allergy, rash, headache, irregular heartbeat, tremor, loss of co-ordination.
Caution: must not be broken or chewed.
Not to be used for: children.

Caution needed with: ANTACIDS.
Contains: PEPPERMINT OIL.
Other preparations: MINTEC.

Colven *see* Fybogel Mebeverine
(Reckitt & Colman)

Combantrin
(Pfizer)

An orange tablet supplied at a strength of 125 mg and used as an anti-worm agent to treat worms.

Dose: adults and children over 6 months 10 mg per kg body weight in one dose.
Availability: NHS and private prescription.
Side effects: rash, stomach and brain disturbances.
Caution: in patients suffering from liver disease.
Not to be used for:
Caution needed with:
Contains: PYRANTEL embonate.
Other preparations:

Combidol
(CP Pharmaceuticals)

A white film-coated tablet used as a bile acid to disperse gallstones.

Dose: 5 mg per kilogram bodyweight per day as a single dose before retiring or in divided doses after meals with last dose before going to bed (patients one-fifth over ideal bodyweight, 7.5 mg/kg/day).
Availability: NHS, private prescription.
Side effects: diarrhoea, rise in certain blood enzymes, calcification of gallstones
Caution: women should use non-hormonal contraception.
Not to be used for: children, pregnant women, nursing mothers, or for patients suffering from poor gall bladder function, chronic liver disease, chronic inflammatory intestinal disorder, stomach ulcer.
Caution needed with: the contraceptive pill, oestrogens, other drugs that alter levels of cholesterol, ANTACIDS, drugs that remove bile acids.
Contains: CHENODEOXYCHOLIC ACID, URSODEOXYCHOLIC ACID.
Other preparations:

Combivent
(Boehringer Ingelheim)

A metered dose aerosol or nebulizer solution (UDVs) used as a BRONCHODILATOR and ANTICHOLINERGIC to treat bronchial spasm associated with chronic obstructive lung disease.

Dose: 2 puffs 4 times a day or 1 vial of solution nebulized 3-4 times a day.
Availability: NHS, private prescription.
Side effects: shaking, nervousness, rapid heart rate, dizziness, headache, low potassium levels, dry mouth, irritated throat, retention of urine.
Caution: in pregnant women, nursing mothers, and in patients suffering from overactive thyroid, severe heart or circulatory disorders, recent heart attack, diabetes, rapid irregular heart rhythm, heart muscle disorder.
Not to be used for: children.
Caution needed with: CORTICOSTEROIDS, DIURETICS, SYMPATHOMIMETICS, ANTICHOLINERGICS, ß-BLOCKERS, THEOPHYLLINE, AMINOPHYLLINE, CHOLINE THEOPHYLLINE.
Contains: SALBUTAMOL, IPRATROPIUM bromide.
Other preparations:

Comixco *see* co-trimoxazole tablets
(Ashbourne)

Concordin
(M.S.D.)

A pink tablet or a white tablet according to strengths of 5 mg, 10 mg and used as a TRICYCLIC ANTIDEPRESSANT to treat depression.

Dose: adults 15-60 mg a day in divided doses at first; elderly 5 mg 3 times a day at first.
Availability: NHS and private prescription.
Side effects: dry mouth, constipation, urine retention, blurred vision, palpitations, drowsiness, sleeplessness, dizziness, hands shaking, low blood presure, weight change, skin reactions, jaundice or blood changes, loss of sexual function may occur.
Caution: in nursing mothers or in patients suffering from heart disease, thyroid disease, epilepsy, diabetes, adrenal tumour, urinary retention, glaucoma, some other psychiatric conditions. Your doctor may advise regular blood tests.
Not to be used for: children, pregnant women, or for patients suffering from heart attacks, liver disease, heart block, heart rhythm disturbances, other heart disorders.
Caution needed with: alcohol, sedatives, ANTICHOLINERGICS, ADRENALINE,

MAOIS, BARBITURATES, other antidepressants, blood-pressure lowering drugs, CIMETIDINE, oestrogens, some local anaesthetics, CARBAMAZEPINE, PHENYTOIN.
Contains: PROTRIPTYLINE hydrochloride.
Other preparations:

Condyline
(Nycomed)

A solution with applicators used to treat warts on the penis and the external female genitalia.

Dose: apply twice a day for 3 days and repeat after 7 days if needed. Maximum treatment period 5 weeks.
Availability: NHS and private prescription.
Side effects: irritation.
Caution:
Not to be used for: children or on open wounds.
Caution needed with:
Contains: PODOPHYLLOTOXIN.
Other preparations: WARTICON, WARTICON-FEM.

conjugated oestrogens *see* Premarin, Prempak-C

Conotrane
(Yamanouchi)

A cream used as an antiseptic for protecting the skin from water, nappy rash, bed sores.

Dose: apply to the affected area several times a day.
Availability: NHS, private prescription, over the counter.
Side effects:
Caution:
Not to be used for:
Caution needed with:
Contains: BENZALKONIUM CHLORIDE, DIMETHICONE.
Other preparations:

Conova 30
(Gold Cross)

A white tablet used as an oestrogen, progestogen contraceptive.

Dose: 1 tablet a day for 21 days starting on day 5 of the period.

Availability: NHS and private prescription.
Side effects: enlarged breasts, bloating and fluid retention, cramps, leg pains, mood change, reduction in sexual desire, headaches, nausea, vaginal erosion, discharge, and bleeding, weight gain, skin changes, rarely thrombosis, raised blood pressure, jaundice.
Caution: in patients suffering from high blood pressure, diabetes, vascular disorders, asthma, depression, kidney disease, multiple sclerosis, womb diseases. Your doctor may advise you not to smoke, to have regular examinations. You should stop treatment at the first sign of serious symptoms such as severe headache or jaundice. Treatment should be stopped before surgery.
Not to be used for: pregnant women, or for patients suffering from sickle-cell anaemia, history of heart disease or thrombosis, liver disorders, some cancers, undiagnosed vaginal bleeding, some ear, skin, and kidney disorders.
Caution needed with: RIFAMPICIN, TETRACYCLINE ANTIBIOTICS, GRISEOFULVIN, BARBITURATES, PHENYTOIN, PRIMIDONE, CARBAMAZEPINE, ETHOSUXIMIDE, CHLORAL HYDRATE.
Contains: ETHINYLOESTRADIOL, ETHYNODIOL DIACETATE.
Other preparations:

Contraflam *see* mefenamic acid capsules
(Berk)

Convulex
(Pharmacia)

A soft, coated capsule supplied at strengths of 150 mg, 300 mg, 500 mg, and used as an anticonvulsant to treat epilepsy.

Dose: 15 mg per kilogram bodyweight a day in divided doses at first, increasing by 5-10 mg/kg a day until control is achieved.
Availability: NHS, private prescription.
Side effects: liver poisoning, coagulation, stomach upsets, nervous disorder, rarely pancreatitis, hair loss.
Caution: in pregnant women. Liver function and coagulation tests should be carried out before treatment, when dose is increased, and at regular intervals.
Not to be used for: patients suffering from liver disorder.
Caution needed with: BARBITURATES, other anticonvulsants, antidepressants, tranquillizers, alcohol, ANTICOAGULANTS.
Contains: VALPROIC ACID.
Other preparations:

---

copper acetate *see* **Cuplex**

Coracten *see* **nifedipine modified release capsules**
(Evans)

Cordarone X *see* **amiodarone tablets**
(Sanofi Winthrop)

Cordilox *see* **verapamil tablets**
(Baker Norton)

Corgard
(Sanofi Winthrop)

A pale-blue tablet supplied at strengths of 40 mg, 80 mg and used as a ß-BLOCKER to treat heart rhythm disturbances, angina, high blood pressure, additional treatment in thyroid disease, migraine.

Dose: 40 mg a day at first increasing to 160 mg a day as required in heart rhythm treatment or 240 mg a day for angina. High blood pressure 80 mg a day at first, then 80-240 mg a day. Thyroid disease 80-160 mg once a day. Migraine 40 mg once a day at first, increasing to 80-160 mg a day as needed.
Availability: NHS and private prescription.
Side effects: cold hands and feet, sleep disturbances, slow heart rate, tiredness, wheezing, heart failure, stomach upset, dry eyes, rash.
Caution: in pregnant women, nursing mothers, and in patients suffering from diabetes, kidney or liver disorders, asthma. May need to be withdrawn before surgery. Withdraw gradually. Your doctor may advise additional treatment with DIURETICS or DIGOXIN.
Not to be used for: children or for patients suffering from heart block or failure.
Caution needed with: VERAPAMIL, CLONIDINE withdrawal, some anti-arrhythmic drugs and anaesthetics, RESERPINE, some blood-pressure lowering drugs, ERGOTAMINE, antidiabetics, CIMETIDINE, sedatives, SYMPATHOMIMETICS, INDOMETHACIN.
Contains: NADOLOL.
Other preparations:

Corgaretic 40
(Sanofi Winthrop)

A white, mottled, scored tablet used as a ß-BLOCKER/thiazide DIURETIC combination drug to treat high blood pressure.

Dose: 1-2 tablets a day.
Availability: NHS and private prescription.
Side effects: cold hands and feet, sleep disturbances, slow heart rate, tiredness, wheezing, heart failure, stomach upset, low blood potassium, rash, sensitivity to light, blood changes, gout, dry eyes.
Caution: in pregnant women or nursing mothers, or patients suffering from asthma, gout, diabetes, kidney or liver disorders. May need to be withdrawn before surgery. Withdraw gradually. Your doctor may advise additional treatment with DIGOXIN or DIURETICS.
Not to be used for: children or for patients suffering from heart block or failure, severe kidney failure, or liver disease.
Caution needed with: VERAPAMIL, CLONIDINE withdrawal, some anti-arrhythmic drugs and anaesthetics, RESERPINE, antidiabetics, CIMETIDINE, sedatives, SYMPATHOMIMETICS, INDOMETHACIN, LITHIUM, DIGOXIN, some blood-pressure lowering drugs, ERGOTAMINE, other diuretics.
Contains: NADOLOL, BENDROFLUAZIDE.
Other preparations: Corgaretic 80.

Corlan
(Evans)

A pellet supplied at a strength of 2.5 mg and used as a STEROID to treat mouth ulcers.

Dose: 1 pellet allowed to dissolve in the mouth touching the ulcer 4 times a day.
Availability: NHS, private prescription, over the counter.
Side effects:
Caution: in pregnant women.
Not to be used for: patients suffering from untreated mouth infections.
Caution needed with:
Contains: HYDROCORTISONE.
Other preparations:

Coro-Nitro
(Boehringer Mannheim)

An pump spray used as a NITRATE for the treatment and prevention of angina.

Dose: 1-2 sprays on to or under the tongue before exertion or when an attack begins to a maximum of 3 doses per attack.
Availability: NHS, private prescription, over the counter.

Side effects: headache, flushes, dizziness.
Caution: do not inhale spray.
Not to be used for: children.
Caution needed with:
Contains: GLYCERYL TRINITRATE.
Other preparations: DEPONIT, GLYCERYL TRINITRATE TABLETS, GLYTRIN, NITROCONTIN, NITRO-DUR, NITROLINGUAL, PERCUTOL, SUSCARD BUCCAL, SUSTAC, TRANSIDERM-NITRO.

Corsodyl
(SmithKline Beecham)

A solution used as an antibacterial treatment for gingivitis, mouth ulcers, thrush, and for mouth hygiene.

Dose: rinse with 10 ml for 1 minute twice a day.
Availability: NHS, private prescription, over the counter.
Side effects: local irritation, stained tongue or teeth, may affect taste.
Caution:
Not to be used for:
Caution needed with:
Contains: CHLORHEXIDINE gluconate.
Other preparations: Corsodyl Gel, Corsodyl Spray.

---

corticosteroid *see* steroid

---

cortisone *see* Cortisyl

Cortisyl
(Hoechst Roussel)

A white tablet supplied at strength of 25 mg and used as a STEROID to treat Addison's disease, and as replacement therapy after removal of the adrenal glands.

Dose: usually 12.5-37.5 mg a day, up to a maximum of 300 mg a day.
Availability: NHS and private prescription.
Side effects: high blood pressure, fluid retention, potassium loss, muscle weakness, weight gain, high blood sugar levels, thinning of bones, mood changes, stomach ulcer.
Caution: in pregnant women, in patients who have had recent bowel surgery, or who are suffering from inflamed veins, psychiatric disorders, virus infections, some cancers, some kidney diseases, thinning of the

bones, ulcers, tuberculosis, other infections, high blood pressure, glaucoma, epilepsy, diabetes, underactive thyroid, liver disease, stress. Withdraw gradually.
Not to be used for: children.
Caution needed with: PHENYTOIN, PHENOBARBITONE, EPHEDRINE, RIFAMPICIN, DIURETICS, ANTICHOLINESTERASES, DIGOXIN, antidiabetic drugs, ANTICOAGULANTS, NON-STEROIDAL ANTI-INFLAMMATORY DRUGS.
Contains: CORTISONE acetate.
Other preparations:

Corwin
(Stuart)

A yellow tablet supplied at a strength of 200 mg and used as a heart muscle stimulant to treat heart failure.

Dose: 1 tablet once or twice a day.
Availability: NHS and private prescription.
Side effects: stomach upset, headache, dizziness, muscle cramp, palpitations, rash.
Caution: in patients suffering from some lung and kidney disease, heart muscle and valve disease, or deterioration of the heart failure (withdraw).
Not to be used for: children, pregnant women, nursing mothers, or patients suffering from sudden heart failure, rapid heart rate, low blood pressure, fluid retention, breathlessness or tiredness without activity.
Caution needed with:
Contains: XAMOTEROL fumarate.
Other preparations:

Cosalgesic *see* co-proxamol tablets
(Cox)

Cosuric *see* allopurinol tablets
(DDSA)

Coversyl
(Servier)

A white tablet supplied at strengths of 2 mg, 4 mg and used as an ACE INHIBITOR to treat high blood pressure, or as an additional treatment for congestive heart failure.

Dose: initially 2 mg a day, increasing to 4-8 mg a day; elderly 2 mg a day.

Availability: NHS and private prescription.
Side effects: rash, itching, flushing, severe allergy, swelling, low blood pressure, alteration of taste, nausea, stomach pain, tiredness, feeling of being unwell, headache, mild cough, blood changes, protein in the urine.
Caution: in patients suffering from kidney disease, or undergoing surgery, dialysis, or anaesthesia.
Not to be used for: children, pregnant women, or nursing mothers.
Caution needed with: other blood-pressure lowering drugs, potassium supplements, some DIURETICS, LITHIUM, antidepressants.
Contains: PERINDOPRIL tertbutylamine.
Other preparations:

Cozaar
(MSD)

A white, film-coated tablet supplied at a strength of 50 mg and used as a blood-pressure lowering drug to treat raised blood pressure.

Dose: 1 tablet once a day, up to a maximum of 2 tablets once a day if needed; elderly ½-2 tablets once a day.
Availability: NHS, private prescription.
Side effects: dizziness, low blood pressure on standing; rarely rash.
Caution: in patients suffering from liver damage, kidney disorders, low blood volume. Blood potassium levels should be checked regularly in the elderly and in patients with kidney damage.
Not to be used for: children, pregnant women, nursing mothers.
Caution needed with: some DIURETICS.
Contains: LOSARTAN POTASSIUM.
Other preparations: Cozaar Half-Strength.

Cremalgin
(Rhône-Poulenc Rorer)

A balm used as an ANALGESIC rub to treat rheumatism, fibrositis, lumbago, sciatica.

Dose: massage into the affected area 2-3 times a day.
Availability: NHS, private prescription, over the counter.
Side effects: may be irritant.
Caution:
Not to be used for: areas near the eyes, or on broken or inflamed skin, or on membranes (such as the mouth).
Caution needed with:
Contains: METHYL NICOTINATE, GLYCOL SALICYLATE, CAPSICUM OLEORESIN.
Other preparations:

Creon
(Solvay Healthcare)

A brown/yellow capsule used to supply pancreatic enzymes in the treatment of pancreatic exocrine insufficiency.

Dose: 1-2 capsules with meals at first, then usually 5-15 capsules a day according to response.
Availability: NHS, private prescription, over the counter.
Side effects: perianal irritation, stomach block (when the drug should be withdrawn).
Caution:
Not to be used for:
Caution needed with:
Contains: PANCREATIN.
Other preparations: Creon Sachets, Creon 25000. NUTRIZYM GR, PANCREASE, PANCREX V.

Cromogen *see* sodium cromoglycate inhaler
(Baker-Norton)

---

crotamiton *see* Eurax, Eurax-Hydrocortisone

---

crystal violet paint BP 1980

A purple solution used as a disinfectant to treat burns, boils, ulcers, and some skin infections, where the skin is not broken.

Dose: use undiluted as directed.
Availability: NHS, private prescription, over the counter.
Side effects:
Caution: stains skin and clothing.
Not to be used for: application to mucous membranes or broken skin.
Caution needed with:
Contains: crystal violet (GENTIAN VIOLET).
Other preparations:

Cuplex
(Smith and Nephew Healthcare)

A gel used as a skin softener to treat warts, corns, and calluses.

Dose: at night apply 1-2 drops of gel to the wart after soaking in water and

C

drying, remove the film in the morning and repeat the process, rubbing the area with a pumice stone between treatments.

Availability: NHS, private prescription, over the counter.

Side effects:

Caution: do not apply to healthy skin; keep away from the eyes.

Not to be used for: warts on the anal or genital areas, or on the face.

Caution needed with:

Contains: SALICYLIC ACID, LACTIC ACID, COPPER ACETATE.

Other preparations: DUOFILM, SALACTOL, SALATAC.

Cusilyn *see* sodium cromoglycate eye drops
(Cusi)

Cutivate
(Glaxo)

A cream used as a strong STEROID to treat eczema and dermatitis.

Dose: apply sparingly to the affected area once a day.

Availability: NHS, private prescription.

Side effects: thinning, spotting, and streaking of the skin, suppression of the adrenal glands, flushing, hair growth.

Caution: in infants, especially if wearing nappies or plastic pants. Do not use on children or on the face for more than 5 days. If used for psoriasis, regular checks are needed. Withdraw slowly after prolonged use.

Not to be used for: prolonged used in pregnant women, for long-term prevention, or for patients suffering from acne, scabies, leg ulcers, skin disorders around the mouth, or infected skin conditions.

Caution needed with:

Contains: FLUTICASONE PROPIONATE.

Other preparations: Cutivate ointment (used twice a day).

CX Powder
(Bio-Medical)

A powder used as a disinfectant to clean and disinfect the skin and prevent infection.

Dose: apply to the affected area 3 times a day.

Availability: NHS, private prescription, over the counter.

Side effects:

Caution:

Not to be used for:

Caution needed with:

Contains: CHLORHEXIDINE acetate.
Other preparations:

---

cyanocobalamin *see* Cytamen, vitamin B₁₂

---

cyclizine *see* Diconal, Migril, Valoid

Cyclo-Progynova 1 mg
(Schering Healthcare)

A beige tablet and a brown tablet used as an oestrogen and progestogen treatment for senile vaginitis, post-menopausal osteoporosis, menopausal symptoms.

Dose: 1 beige tablet a day for 11 days then 1 brown tablet a day for 10 days followed by 7 days without tablets. Begin on the fifth day of the period if present.
Availability: NHS and private prescription.
Side effects: enlarged breasts, fluid retention, nausea, vaginal bleeding, weight gain, headache, dizziness. Rarely jaundice, raised blood pressure, thrombosis.
Caution: in patients suffering from high blood pressure, diabetes, epilepsy, womb diseases, gall bladder disorder, migraine, multiple sclerosis, PORPHYRIA, liver disorders, some ear disorders, or a history or increased risk of breast disorders (including cancer) and thrombosis. Your doctor may advise you to have regular examinations.
Not to be used for: children, pregnant women, nursing mothers, or for patients suffering from thombosis, severe liver, kidney, or heart disorders, some cancers, undiagnosed vaginal bleeding, endometriosis.
Caution needed with: ACE INHIBITORS, ANTICOAGULANTS, BARBITURATES, ß-BLOCKERS, CARBAMAZEPINE, PHENYTOIN, RIFAMPICIN.
Contains: OESTRADIOL valerate; OESTRADIOL valerate and LEVONORGESTREL.
Other preparations: Cyclo-Progynova 2 mg, NUVELLE.

Cyclodox *see* doxycycline capsules
(Berk)

Cyclogest
(Hoechst Roussel)

A suppository supplied at strengths of 200 mg, 400 mg and used as a progesterone treatment for premenstrual syndrome, puerperal depression.

Dose: 200-400 mg 1-2 times a day in the rectum or the vagina from the twelfth or fourteenth day of the cycle until the period begins.
Availability: NHS and private prescription.
Side effects: altered menstrual pattern, soreness, diarrhoea, wind.
Caution: in patients suffering from liver disease. Avoid contact with barrier contraceptives.
Not to be used for: children or for patients suffering from abnormal vaginal bleeding or a history of blood clotting disorders.
Caution needed with:
Contains: PROGESTERONE.
Other preparations:

Cyclomin *see* minocycline tablets
(Berk)

---

cyclopenthiazide *see* Navidrex, Navispare, Trasidrex

---

cyclopentolate hydrochloride *see* Cyclopentolate Minims, Mydrilate

---

Cyclopentolate Minims
(Chauvin)

Drops used as an ANTICHOLINERGIC agent in ophthalmic procedures to dilate the pupil and paralyse the eye muscle.

Dose: 1 or more drops into the eye as needed.
Availability: NHS and private prescription.
Side effects:
Caution:
Not to be used for: newborn infants, or for patients suffering from narrow-angle glaucoma.
Caution needed with:
Contains: CYCLOPENTOLATE HYDROCHLORIDE.
Other preparations: MYDRILATE.

---

cycloserine capsules

A red/grey capsule supplied at a strength of 250 mg and used with other drugs to treat tuberculosis when other treatments have failed.

Dose: adults, 1 capsule every 12 hours for 2 weeks, increasing if necessary to a maximum of 2 capsules every 12 hours; children, 10 mg per kilogram of bodyweight per day at first.
Availability: NHS and private prescription.
Side effects: headache, vertigo, drowsiness, dizziness, hands shaking, convulsions, mental disorder, rash, anaemia, liver changes.
Caution: in pregnant women and nursing mothers, and in patients who develop rash or symptoms noted above. Your doctor may advise regular blood, liver, and kidney function tests.
Not to be used for: alcoholics, or for patients suffering from severe kidney failure, epilepsy, depression or other mental disorders, PORPHYRIA.
Caution needed with: ISONIAZID, PHENYTOIN.
Contains: CYCLOSERINE.
Other preparations:

---

cyclosporin *see* Sandimmun

Cyklokapron
(Pharmacia)

A white, oblong, scored tablet supplied at a strength of 500 mg and used as a blood-clotting agent to treat heavy periods and other heavy bleeding states.

Dose: 2-3 tablets 3-4 times a day for 3-4 days for a maximum of 3 cycles, or as advised by doctor.
Availability: NHS and private prescription.
Side effects: stomach upset, disturbances in colour vision (stop taking the drug if this occurs).
Caution: in patients with kidney disease, or blood in the urine. Your doctor may advise some patients to have regular eye tests.
Not to be used for: patients with a history of blood clotting disorders.
Caution needed with:
Contains: TRANEXAMIC ACID.
Other preparations: Cyklokapron Injection, Cyklokapron Syrup.

Cymevene
(Roche)

A green capsule used as an antiviral treatment to treat retinitis.

Dose: adults 12 capsules a day in divided doses with food; children as advised by the physician.
Availability: NHS, private prescription.

Side effects: blood changes, stomach upset, loss of appetite, rash, headache, itching, fever, abnormal liver function tests.
Caution: in patients suffering from kidney damage. Your doctor will advise regular blood tests.
Not to be used for: pregnant women or nursing mothers. Sexually active patients must take adequate contraceptive precautions.
Caution needed with: drugs that suppress blood cell production, ZIDOVUDINE, DIDANOSINE, imipenem.
Contains: GANCICLOVIR.
Other preparations:

---

cyproheptadine hydrochloride *see* Periactin

---

cyproterone acetate *see* Androcur, Dianette

Cystrin
(Pharmacia)

A white tablet supplied at strengths of 3 mg, 5 mg and used as an antispasmodic and ANTICHOLINERGIC treatment for incontinence, urgency or frequency of urination, or night-time incontinence in children.

Dose: adults, 5 mg 2-3 times a day, to a maximum of 20 mg a day; elderly 3 mg twice a day at first; children over 5 years, 3 mg twice a day, increasing to 5 mg 2-3 times a day if needed.
Availability: NHS and private prescription.
Side effects: anticholinergic effects, flushing of the face.
Caution: in pregnant women, and in patients suffering from liver or kidney disease, heart disorders, overactive thyroid, enlarged prostate, hiatus hernia or existing disturbance of normal bodily functions.
Not to be used for: children under 5 years, nursing mothers, or for patients suffering from blockage in the bowel or bladder, severe ulcerative colitis, other intestinal disorders, MYASTHENIA GRAVIS, or glaucoma.
Caution needed with: sedatives, AMANTADINE, LEVODOPA, DIGOXIN, TRICYCLIC ANTIDEPRESSANTS, other anticholinergics, HALOPERIDOL, BENPERIDOL, DROPERIDOL.
Contains: OXYBUTYNIN hydrochloride.
Other preparations: DITROPAN.

Cytacon
(Goldshield Healthcare)

A white tablet supplied at a strength of 50 micrograms as a source of VITAMIN B_{12} to treat undernourishment, vitamin deficiencies, some types of anaemia, vitamin B$_{12}$ deficiency after stomach surgery.

Dose: adults1-3 tablets a day up to a maximum of six tablets a day for pernicious anaemia; children use liquid.
Availability: NHS (only when prescribed as a generic), private prescription, over the counter.
Side effects: rarely allergy.
Caution:
Not to be used for:
Caution needed with: PARA-AMINOSALICYLIC ACID, METHYLDOPA, COLCHICINE, CHOLESTYRAMINE, NEOMYCIN, some antidiabetic drugs, POTASSIUM CHLORIDE, CIMETIDINE.
Contains: VITAMIN B$_{12}$ (also known as CYANOCOBALAMIN).
Other preparations: Cytacon Liquid (not available on NHS), CYTAMEN injection.

Cytamen
(Evans)

An injection supplied at a strength of 1000 micrograms per 1 ml ampoule and used as a source of vitamin B$_{12}$ to treat megaloblastic and other anaemias.

Dose: 250-1000 mcg on alternate days for 1-2 weeks, then 250 mcg a week until blood count is normal; maintenance, 1000 mcg a month.
Availability: NHS (when prescribed as a generic), private prescription.
Side effects: rarely allergy.
Caution:
Not to be used for:
Caution needed with: CHLORAMPHENICOL, the contraceptive pill.
Contains: VITAMIN B$_{12}$ (CYANOCOBALAMIN).
Other preparations: CYTACON (tablet and liquid preparations).

Cytotec
(Searle)

A white, hexagonal tablet supplied at a strength of 200 micrograms and used as a PROSTAGLANDIN for the prevention and treatment of ulcers caused by NON-STEROIDAL ANTI-INFLAMMATORY DRUGS.

Dose: 4 tablets a day with meals and at bedtime for 4-8 weeks; prevention 1 tablet 2-4 times a day when using non-steroidal anti-inflammatory drugs.
Availability: NHS and private prescription.
Side effects: diarrhoea, abdominal pain, stomach upset, menstrual disturbance, vaginal bleeding, rash, dizziness.

Caution: in patients suffering from circulatory disorders of the brain, heart, or peripheral vessels. Women of child-bearing age must use contraception.
Not to be used for: nursing mothers, pregnant women, or those planning a pregnancy.
Caution needed with:
Contains: MISOPROSTOL.
Other preparations:

---

d-alpha-tocopheryl acetate *see* **Vita-E, vitamin E**

Daktacort
(Janssen-Cilag)

A cream used as a STEROID, antifungal, and antibacterial treatment for skin infections where there is also inflammation.

Dose: apply to the affected area 2-3 times a day.
Availability: NHS and private prescription.
Side effects: fluid retention, suppression of adrenal glands, thinning, streaking, or spotting of the skin may occur.
Caution: use for short periods of time only, especially in pregnant women or on the face.
Not to be used for: patients suffering from acne or any other skin infections caused by tuberculosis, ringworm, viruses, or fungi, leg ulcers, scabies, or continuously especially in pregnant women.
Caution needed with:
Contains: MICONAZOLE nitrate, HYDROCORTISONE.
Other preparations: Daktacort Ointment.

Daktarin Cream
(Janssen-Cilag)

A cream used as an antifungal treatment for infections of the skin and nails.

Dose: apply 1-2 times a day until 10 days after the wounds have healed. Nails, apply sparingly once a day and cover.
Availability: NHS, private prescription, over the counter.
Side effects:
Caution:
Not to be used for:
Caution needed with:
Contains: MICONAZOLE nitrate.

Other preparations: Daktarin Twin Pack, Daktarin Spray Powder, Daktarin Powder.

Daktarin Oral Gel
(Janssen-Cilag)

A gel used as an antifungal treatment for fungal infections of the mouth and pharynx.

Dose: adults hold 5-10 ml of gel in the mouth 4 times a day; children under 2 years use 2.5 ml gel twice a day, 2-6 years 5 ml gel twice a day, over 6 years 5 ml gel 4 times a day.
Availability: NHS, private prescription, over the counter.
Side effects: mild stomach upset.
Caution:
Not to be used for:
Caution needed with: WARFARIN.
Contains: MICONAZOLE.
Other preparations: DUMICOAT.

Dalacin C
(Upjohn)

A lavender capsule or a maroon/lavender capsule according to strengths of 75 mg, 150 mg and used as an antibiotic treatment for serious infections.

Dose: adults150-450 mg every 6 hours; children under 12 years use Dalacin C Paediatric.
Availability: NHS and private prescription.
Side effects: stomach disturbances including colitis, jaundice, blood disorders.
Caution: in patients suffering from kidney or liver disease. The treatment should be stopped if diarrhoea and colitis develop.
Not to be used for: patients suffering from sensitivity to LINCOMYCIN.
Caution needed with: some drugs used during anaesthesia.
Contains: CLINDAMYCIN hydrochloride.
Other preparations: Dalacin C Paediatric Liquid, Dalacin C Phosphate injection.

Dalacin Cream
(Upjohn)

A cream supplied with applicators and used as an antibiotic to treat

D

bacterial infections of the vagina.

Dose: 1 applicatorful inserted into the vagina at night for 7 days.
Availability: NHS, private prescription.
Side effects: stomach upset, vaginal irritation, diarrhoea or colitis
(discontinue treatment at once).
Caution: patients should be advised that barrier contraceptives may be
less effective.
Not to be used for: children or for patients allergic to lincomycin.
Caution needed with: barrier contraceptives (*see* above).
Contains: CLINDAMYCIN phosphate.
Other preparations: DALACIN-C (capsule treatment for general infection),
DALACIN-T (skin solution to treat acne).

D

Dalacin T
(Upjohn)

A solution used as an antibiotic treatment for acne.

Dose: apply to the affected area twice a day for up to 12 weeks.
Availability: NHS and private prescription.
Side effects: dry skin, inflammation, inflammation of the follicles, possible
diarrhoea or colitis (discontinue immediately).
Caution: keep out of the eyes, mouth, and nose.
Not to be used for: patients sensitive to LINCOMYCIN.
Caution needed with: skin-softening agents.
Contains: CLINDAMYCIN phosphate.
Other preparations: Dalacin T Lotion.

Dalivit
(Eastern)

Drops used as a multivitamin preparation to prevent vitamin deficiency.

Dose: 0-1 year 7 drops a day, over 1 year 14 drops a day.
Availability: NHS, private prescription, over the counter.
Side effects:
Caution:
Not to be used for: pregnant women.
Caution needed with: LEVODOPA.
Contains: VITAMINS A, B_1, B_2, B_3, B_6, C, D.
Other preparations: ABIDEC.

Dalmane
(Roche)

A grey/yellow capsule or a black/grey capsule according to strengths of 15 mg, 30 mg and used as a sleeping capsule for the short-term treatment of severe sleeplessness.

Dose: elderly 15 mg before going to bed; adults 15-30 mg before going to bed.
Availability: private prescription only.
Side effects: light headedness, drowsiness, lack of co-ordination, confusion, vertigo, stomach upset, low blood pressure, rash, changes in vision and sexual function, retention of urine. Rarely blood disorders, jaundice. Risk of addiction.
Caution: in the elderly, nursing mothers, pregnant women, and in patients suffering from lung, kidney, or liver disorders. Avoid long-term use. Withdraw gradually.
Not to be used for: children or for patients suffering from lung disease or some obsessional and psychotic disorders.
Caution needed with: alcohol, other tranquillizers, anticonvulsants.
Contains: FLURAZEPAM.
Other preparations:

---

danazol *see* danazol capsules, Danol

---

danazol capsules

A capsule supplied at strengths of 100 mg, 200 mg and used as a hormone inhibitor to treat endometriosis (a womb and menstrual disorder), heavy periods, non-malignant breast disorders.

Dose: 200-800 mg a day in divided doses according to condition.
Availability: NHS and private prescription.
Side effects: nausea, dizziness, rash, backache, flushing, muscle spasm, reduction in size of breasts, weight gain, male hormone effects, fluid retention, hair loss, headache, emotional disturbance, blood changes, visual disturbances, jaundice.
Caution: in the elderly and in patients suffering from heart, liver, or kidney disorder, epilepsy, migraine, diabetes, a tendency to gain weight, high blood pressure or other circulatory disorders.
Not to be used for: children, pregnant women, nursing mothers, or for patients suffering from PORPHYRIA, severe kidney, liver, or heart disease, blocked blood vessels, some tumours, undiagnosed vaginal bleeding.
Caution needed with: contraceptive pill, ANTICOAGULANTS, CARBAMAZEPINE, antidiabetics, blood-pressure lowering drugs, CYCLOSPORIN, STEROIDS.

Contains: DANAZOL.
Other preparations: DANOL.

Daneral SA
(Hoechst Roussel)

An orange, long-acting tablet supplied at a strength of 75 mg and used as an ANTIHISTAMINE treatment for allergies.

Dose: 1-2 tablets at night.
Availability: NHS, private prescription, over the counter.
Side effects: drowsiness, reduced reactions.
Caution: in nursing mothers.
Not to be used for: children.
Caution needed with: sedatives, MAOIS, alcohol.
Contains: PHENIRAMINE maleate.
Other preparations:

Danol *see* danazol capsules
(Sanofi Winthrop)

danthron *see* Codalax, co-danthramer capsules and suspension, co-danthrusate capsules, Normax

Dantrium
(Procter & Gamble)

An orange/light brown capsule supplied at strengths of 25 mg, 100 mg and used as a muscle relaxant to treat chronic or severe spasticity.

Dose: 25 mg a day at first increasing as needed to a maximum of 100 mg 4 times a day.
Availability: NHS and private prescription.
Side effects: weakness, tiredness, drowsiness, diarrhoea.
Caution: in pregnant women and in patients suffering from lung or heart disease. Your doctor may advise that your liver should be checked before and 6 weeks after treatment.
Not to be used for: children or for patients suffering from liver disease or where spasticity is useful for movement.
Caution needed with: alcohol, sedatives.
Contains: DANTROLENE SODIUM.
Other preparations:

dantrolene sodium *see* **Dantrium**

Daonil *see* **glibenclamide tablets**
(Hoechst Roussel)

---

dapsone *see* **dapsone tablets, Maloprim**

---

dapsone tablets

A tablet supplied at strengths of 50 mg, 100 mg and used as an anti-leprotic treatment for leprosy.

Dose: 1-2 mg per kg body weight a day.
Availability: NHS and private prescription.
Side effects: liver disease, nausea, headache, dizziness, rapid heart rate, sleeplessness, rash, blood changes.
Caution: in pregnant women and in patients suffering from heart or lung disease, anaemia, glucose 6PD deficiency (an inherited disorder). This treatment should only be given under specialist advice.
Not to be used for: patients suffering from PORPHYRIA.
Caution needed with: RIFAMPICIN, PROBENECID.
Contains: DAPSONE.
Other preparations:

Daranide
(M.S.D.)

A yellow, scored tablet supplied at a strength of 50 mg used as a fluid balance medication in additonal treatment for glaucoma.

Dose: 2-4 tablets at first then 2 tablets every 12 hours, reducing to ½-1 tablet 1-3 times a day.
Availability: NHS and private prescription.
Side effects: stomach upset, loss of weight, constipation, frequent need to urinate, headache, itch, lassitude, prickly sensation, blood changes.
Caution: in pregnant women, the elderly. Potassium supplements may be needed.
Not to be used for: children or for patients suffering from liver or kidney disease, adrenocortical weakness, low sodium or potassium levels, high blood chloride levels, severe blockage of the lungs.
Caution needed with: STEROIDS, DIGOXIN, antidiabetic drugs, ANTICOAGULANTS, local anaesthetics, anticonvulsants, TRIMETHOPRIM, ASPIRIN, METHOTREXATE.

Contains: DICHLORPHENAMIDE.
Other preparations:

Daraprim
(Wellcome)

A white, scored tablet supplied at a strength of 25 mg and used as an antimalarial drug for the prevention of malaria for residents in malarial areas.

Dose: adults and children over 10 years 1 tablet a week; children 5-10 years half adult dose. Continue for 4 weeks after leaving area.
Availability: NHS, private prescription, over the counter.
Side effects: rash, anaemia.
Caution: in pregnant women, nursing mothers, and in patients suffering from liver or kidney disease.
Not to be used for: children under 5 years. Travellers use alternative measures.
Caution needed with: CO-TRIMOXAZOLE, LORAZEPAM.
Contains: PYRIMETHAMINE.
Other preparations: FANSIDAR, MALOPRIM.

DDAVP
(Ferring)

A white scored tablet supplied at strengths of 0.1 mg, 0.2 mg, and used as a hormone to treat diabetes insipidus (a fluid balance disorder), excessive thirst and urination after surgical removal of the pituitary gland, bedwetting.

Dose: diabetes insipidus, 0.1 mg 3 times a day at first, then 0.1-0.2 mg 3 times a day; excessive thirst and urination after surgery, as required; bedwetting, patients 5-65 years 0.2 mg at bedtime at first, increasing if needed to o.4 mg.
Availability: NHS and private prescription.
Side effects: headache, stomach pain, nausea.
Caution: pregnant women and in patients suffering from kidney disorder, circulatory disease, cystic fibrosis.
Not to be used for: patients suffering from weak heart, high blood pressure
Caution needed with: INDOMETHACIN, CHLORPROMAZINE, CARBAMAZEPINE, TRICYCLIC ANTIDEPRESSANTS.
Contains: DESMOPRESSIN.
Other preparations: DDAVP Nasal Solution.

De-Nol
(Yamanouchi)

A white liquid used as a cell-surface protector to treat gastric and duodenal ulcer.

Dose: adults 10 ml diluted with 15 ml water twice a day 30 minutes before meals, for 28-56 days.
Availability: NHS, private prescription, over the counter.
Side effects: black colour to tongue and stools.
Caution:
Not to be used for: children or for patients suffering from kidney failure.
Caution needed with:
Contains: TRI-POTASSIUM DIC!TRATO BISMUTHATE.
Other preparations: DE-NOLTAB.

De-Noltab *see* De-Nol
(Yamanouchi)

Debrisan
(Pharmacia)

A powder used as an absorbant to treat weeping wounds including ulcers.

Dose: wash the wound with a saline solution and, without drying first, coat with 3 mm of powder, and cover with a perforated plastic sheet; repeat before the sheet is saturated.
Availability: NHS, private prescription, over the counter.
Side effects:
Caution:
Not to be used for:
Caution needed with:
Contains: DEXTRANOMER.
Other preparations: Debrisan Paste, Debrisan Pads.

---

debrisoquine sulphate *see* Declinax

Decadron *see* dexamethasone tablets
(M.S.D.)

Declinax
(Roche)

A white, scored tablet supplied at a strength of 10 mg, and used as an ANTIHYPERTENSIVE drug to treat high blood pressure.

Dose: 10-20 mg once or twice a day at first, increasing to 120 mg a day if needed.
Availability: NHS and private prescription.
Side effects: low blood pressure when standing up, general feeling of being unwell, headache, failure of ejaculation.
Caution: in patients suffering from kidney disease.
Not to be used for: children or for patients suffering from PHAEOCHROMOCYTOMA (a disease of the adrenal glands) or recent heart attack.
Caution needed with: TRICYCLIC ANTIDEPRESSANTS, SYMPATHOMIMETICS.
Contains: DEBRISOQUINE SULPHATE.
Other preparations:

Decortisyl *see* prednisone tablets
(Hoechst Roussel)

Delfen
(Janssen-Cilag)

A spermicidal foam supplied in an aerosol with applicator and used with barrier methods as a means of contraception.

Dose: 1 applicatorful of foam inserted into the vagina before intercourse.
Availability: NHS, private prescription, over the counter.
Side effects: possibly sensitivity.
Caution:
Not to be used for: children.
Caution needed with:
Contains: NONOXYNOL-9.
Other preparations:

Deltacortril *see* prednisolone tablets
(Pfizer)

Deltastab *see* prednisolone tablets
(Knoll)

D

Delvas *see* **co-amilozide tablets**
(Berk)

---

demeclocycline *see* **Ledermycin**

Demix *see* **doxycycline capsules**
(Ashbourne)

Dentomycin
(Lederle)

A gel used as an antibacterial to treat moderate to severe gum inflammation.

Dose: fill the pocket between the gum and tooth with gel, and repeat 2-3 times at 14-day intervals. Treatment not to be repeated within 6 months
Availability: NHS and private prescription.
Side effects: irritation.
Caution: in pregnant women, nursing mothers, and in patients with severe liver or kidney disorders. Avoid cleaning teeth, eating, drinking, or rinsing mouth for 2 hours after treatment.
Not to be used for: patients with complete kidney failure.
Caution needed with: ANTICOAGULANTS.
Contains: MINOCYCLINE hydrochloride.
Other preparations:

Depixol
(Lundbeck)

A yellow tablet supplied at a strength of 3 mg and used as a sedative to treat schizophrenia and other mental disorders, especially withdrawal or apathy.

Dose: usually 1-3 tablets a day, up to a maximum of 6 tablets a day.
Availability: NHS and private prescription.
Side effects: muscle spasms, restlessness, hands shaking, dry mouth, blocked nose, constipation, blurred vision, urine retention, palpitations, low blood pressure, weight gain, changes in sexual function, low body temperature, breast swelling, menstrual changes, jaundice, blood and skin changes, drowsiness, tiredness, rarely fits.
Caution: in the elderly, and in patients suffering from kidney, liver, heart, or lung disease, Parkinson's disease, or anyone who is intolerant of those drugs taken by mouth.

Not to be used for: children, pregnant women, nursing mothers, or for very excitable or overactive patients.
Caution needed with: alcohol, sedatives, tranquillizers, pain killers, blood-pressure lowering drugs, antidepressants, anticonvulsants, antidiabetic drugs, LEVODOPA.
Contains: FLUPENTHIXOL dihydrochloride.
Other preparations: Depixol Injection, Depixol-Conc, FLUANXOL.

Depo-Medrone
(Upjohn)

An injection supplied at a strength of 40 mg/ml, and used as a CORTICOSTEROID to treat seasonal allergic rhinitis, asthma, rheumatoid arthritis, osteoarthritis, collagen diseases, and some skin disorders.

D

Dose: as advised by the physician.
Availability: NHS, private prescription.
Side effects: raised blood sugars, osteoporosis, depression, stomach ulcer, weight gain, flushing, hair growth, raised blood pressure, mental disturbances.
Caution: in pregnant women and in patients suffering from stress, underactive thyroid, cirrhosis of the liver, diabetes, epilepsy, glaucoma, raised blood pressure, chickenpox, tuberculosis, stomach ulcer, osteoporosis, kidney disorders, measle-like illnesses, mental disorders, thrombophlebitis, or who have undergone recent stomach surgery. Patients exposed to chicken pox should seek medical advice immediately.
Not to be used for: intravenous injection or where there is infection near the proposed injection site.
Caution needed with: PHENYTOIN, PHENOBARBITONE, EPHEDRINE, RIFAMPICIN, DIURETICS, ANTICHOLINESTERASES, some antidiabetic drugs, ANTICOAGULANTS taken by mouth, NON-STEROIDAL ANTI-INFLAMMATORY DRUGS, DIGOXIN.
Contains: METHYLPREDNISOLONE acetate.
Other preparations: Depo-Medrone with Lidocaine (including anaesthetic for pain relief).

Depo-Provera
(Upjohn)

An injection supplied at a strength of 150 mg/ml and used to provide contraception after family planning advice.

Dose: 1 injection during the first 5 days of the cycle, then repeat at 12-weekly intervals. Immediately after childbirth, 1 injection within the first 5 days if not breastfeeding, or after 6 weeks if breastfeeding.
Availability: NHS, private prescription.

Side effects: temporary infertility after ceasing treatment, changes in the period for the first 2 or 3 cycles, headache, stomach pain, dizziness, weakness, weight gain, fluid retention.
Caution: in patients suffering from undiagnosed vaginal bleeding, diabetes, severe depression.
Not to be used for: children, pregnant women, or for patients suffering from some cancers.
Caution needed with:
Contains: MEDROXYPROGESTERONE acetate.
Other preparations:

Deponit
(Schwarz)

Self-adhesive patches supplied in strengths of 5 mg, 10 mg and used as a NITRATE preparation for the prevention of angina.

Dose: apply a 5 mg patch at first increasing to 10 mg if required with each subsequent patch applied to a different part of the skin.
Availability: NHS, private prescription, over the counter.
Side effects: headache, rash, dizziness.
Caution: reduce use of this treatment by replacing with oral nitrates.
Not to be used for: children.
Caution needed with:
Contains: GLYCERYL TRINITRATE.
Other preparations: CORO-NITRATE, GLYCERYL TRINITRATE TABLETS, GLYTRIN, MINITRAN, NITROCONTIN, NITRO-DUR, NITROLINGUAL, PERCUTOL, SUSCARD BUCCAL, SUSTAC, TRANSIDERM NITRO.

Derbac-C Shampoo
(Seton Healthcare)

A shampoo used as a pediculicide to treat head lice.

Dose: use as a shampoo, applying twice and then leaving the second treatment for 5 minutes before rinsing, combing, and then drying. Repeat twice at 3-day intervals.
Availability: NHS, private prescription.
Side effects:
Caution: keep out of the eyes.
Not to be used for: infants under 6 months.
Caution needed with:
Contains: CARBARYL.
Other preparations: Derbac-C Liquid. CARYLDERM, CLINICIDE, SULEO-C.

Derbac-M
(Seton Healthcare)

A liquid used as a pediculicide and scabicide to treat scabies, lice of the head and pubic areas.

Dose: apply liberally and then shampoo after 12 hours for lice, 24 hours for scabies.
Availability: NHS, private prescription, over the counter.
Side effects:
Caution: keep out of the eyes.
Not to be used for: infants under 6 months.
Caution needed with:
Contains: MALATHION.
Other preparations: PRIODERM, SULEO-M.

D

Dermalex
(Sanofi Winthrop)

A lotion used as an antiseptic emollient to prevent and treat rashes (including incontinence rash) and to prevent bedsores.

Dose: apply sparingly every 4-6 hours.
Availability: NHS, private prescription, over the counter.
Side effects:
Caution:
Not to be used for: children under 2 years, pregnant women, nursing mothers, or on broken skin or mucous membranes.
Caution needed with:
Contains: SQUALENE, HEXACHLOROPHANE, ALLANTOIN.
Other preparations:

Dermamist
(Yamanouchi)

A spray used as an emollient to treat eczema, scaly skin conditions, and itching.

Dose: after bathing spray on to clean dry skin.
Availability: NHS, private prescription, over the counter.
Side effects:
Caution:
Not to be used for: the face or on broken skin.
Caution needed with:
Contains: WHITE SOFT PARAFFIN, LIQUID PARAFFIN, COCONUT OIL.

Other preparations:

Dermovate
(Glaxo)

A cream used as a STEROID treatment for psoriasis, eczema, other skin disorders where there is inflammation

Dose: apply a small quantity to the affected area once or twice a day for up to 4 weeks.
Availability: NHS and private prescription.
Side effects: fluid retention, suppression of adrenal glands, thinning of the skin may occur.
Caution: adults check after 4 weeks; children check after 5 days; use for short periods of time only.
Not to be used for: patients suffering from acne or any other skin infections caused by tuberculosis, ringworm, viruses, or fungi, leg ulcers, scabies, or continuously especially in pregnant women.
Caution needed with:
Contains: CLOBETASOL PROPIONATE.
Other preparations: Dermovate Ointment, Dermovate Scalp Application, Dermovate-NN (for infected conditions).

Deseril
(Sandoz)

A white tablet supplied at a strength of 1 mg and used as an anti-spasmodic treatment for diarrhoea associated with carcinoid disease, migraine, severe headache.

Dose: for diarrhoea 12-20 tablets a day in divided doses. For migraine 1-2 tablets 2-3 times a day with food.
Availability: NHS and private prescription.
Side effects: nausea and other stomach disturbances, drowsiness, dizziness, lassitude, fluid retention, arterial spasm, retroperitonital, membrane thickening (discontinue treatment), leg cramps, weight gain, rash, hair loss, disturbance of nervous system.
Caution: in patients suffering from or with a history of stomach ulcer.
Not to be used for: children, pregnant women, nursing mothers, or patients suffering from severe high blood pressure, collagen disorders, heart or blood vessel disease, liver or kidney disease, weight loss, sepsis, lung disease, cellulitis.
Caution needed with: medicines affecting blood vessels, alcohol, sedatives, ERGOTAMINE.
Contains: METHYSERGIDE.

Other preparations:

---

desipramine *see* **Pertofran**

---

desmopressin *see* **DDAVP, Desmospray, Desmotabs**

Desmospray
(Ferring)

A nasal spray used as a hormone treatment for cranial diabetes insipidus (a fluid-balance disorder), bedwetting, testing kidney function.

Dose: adults diabetes insipidus 1-2 sprays into the nose once or twice a day, kidney testing 2 sprays into each nostril, children diabetes insipidus as adult; kidney testing 1-15 years 1 spray into each nostril, adults 2 sprays in each nostril. Adults and children over 5 years primary bed wetting 1-2 sprays into each nostril before going to bed, for up to 3 months.
Availability: NHS and private prescription.
Side effects: headache, stomach pain, nausea.
Caution: in pregnant women and in patients suffering from kidney disease, multiple sclerosis, cardiovascular disease. Patients should not drink excessively after dose taken for testing or bedwetting.
Not to be used for: children under 5 years (bedwetting).
Caution needed with: CARBAMAZEPINE, TRICYCLIC ANTIDEPRESSANTS, INDOMETHACIN, CHLORPROMAZINE.
Contains: DESMOPRESSIN.
Other preparations:

Desmotabs
(Ferring)

A white scored tablet supplied at a strength of 0.2 mg and used as a hormone supplement to treat bedwetting.

Dose: patients aged 5-65 years, 1 tablet before going to bed at first, increasing only if necessary to 2 tablets. Reduce fluid intake before bedtime, and reassess after 3 months of treatment.
Availability: NHS, private prescription.
Side effects: headache, nausea, stomach ache.
Caution: in pregnant women and in patients suffering from cystic fibrosis, heart or circulatory disease, kidney damage. Treatment should not start on patients suffering from abnormal thirst or alcohol abuse until these

conditions have ceased.
Not to be used for: patients suffering from weak heart, raised blood pressure.
Caution needed with: TRICYCLIC ANTIDEPRESSANTS, CHLORPROMAZINE, INDOMETHACIN, CARBAMAZEPINE.
Contains: DESMOPRESSIN acetate.
Other preparations:

---

desogestrel *see* **Marvelon, Mercilon**

---

desoxymethasone *see* **Stiedex**

Destolit
(Marion Merrell Dow)

A white, scored tablet supplied at a strength of 150 mg and used as a bile acid to dissolve gallstones.

Dose: 3-4 tablets a day in divided doses after meals with 1 dose always after the evening meal. Continue for 3-4 months after stones dissolve.
Availability: NHS and private prescription.
Side effects: diarrhoea.
Caution:
Not to be used for: children, for women who are not taking contraceptive precautions, or for patients with a non-functioning gall bladder, active stomach ulcers, liver disorder, or certain diseases of the intestine.
Caution needed with: the contraceptive pill, oestrogens, treatments to reduce cholesterol levels.
Contains: URSODEOXYCHOLIC ACID.
Other preparations: URSOFALK.

Deteclo
(Lederle)

A blue, film-coated tablet used as a TETRACYCLINE ANTIBIOTIC, to treat infections of the ear, nose, throat, chest, digestive tract, and soft tissues.

Dose: 1 tablet every 12 hours.
Availability: NHS and private prescription.
Side effects: stomach upset, allergy, additional infections, raised pressure in the brain.
Caution: in the elderly, and in patients suffering from liver disorders.
Not to be used for: children, pregnant women, nursing mothers, or for

patients suffering from LUPUS or kidney disorder.
Caution needed with: milk, ANTACIDS, the contraceptive pill, PENICILLIN and similar antibiotics, ANTICOAGULANTS.
Contains: CHLORTETRACYCLINE hydrochloride, TETRACYCLINE hydrochloride, DEMECLOCYCLINE hydrochloride.
Other preparations:

Dexa-Rhinaspray
(Boehringer Ingelheim)

An aerosol used as a STEROID, antibiotic, and SYMPATHOMIMETIC treatment for allergic rhinitis.

Dose: adults 1 spray into each nostril no more than 6 times a day; children 5-12 years 1 spray into each nostril no more than twice a day.
Availability: NHS and private prescription.
Side effects: itching nose.
Caution: do not use for extended periods.
Not to be used for: children under 5 years.
Caution needed with:
Contains: TRAMAZOLINE hydrochloride, DEXAMETHASONE-21 ISONICOTINATE, NEOMYCIN sulphate.
Other preparations:

---

dexamethasone see Decadron, dexamethasone tablets, Dexa-Rhinaspray, Maxidex, Maxitrol, Otomize, Sofradex, Sofradex Ointment

---

dexamethasone tablets

A tablet supplied at a strength of 0.5 mg and used as a STEROID treatment for rheumatic or inflammatory conditions, shock, allergy.

Dose: as prescribed by your doctor.
Availability: NHS and private prescription.
Side effects: high blood sugar, thin bones, mood changes, ulcers.
Caution: in pregnant women, in patients who have had recent bowel surgery, or who are suffering from inflamed veins, psychiatric disorders, virus infections, some cancers, some kidney diseases, thinning of the bones, stomach ulcers, tuberculosis, other infections, high blood pressure, glaucoma, epilepsy, diabetes, underactive thyroid, liver disease, stress. Withdraw gradually. Avoid contact with chickenpox during treatment and for 3 months afterwards.
Not to be used for:

Caution needed with: PHENYTOIN, PHENOBARBITONE, EPHEDRINE, RIFAMPICIN, DIURETICS, ANTICHOLINESTERASES, DIGOXIN, antidiabetic agents, ANTICOAGULANTS taken by mouth, NON-STEROIDAL ANTI-INFLAMMATORY DRUGS, ASPIRIN, anticonvulsants.
Contains: DEXAMETHASONE.
Other preparations: DECADRON.

---

dexamphetamine *see* Dexedrine

Dexedrine
(Evans)

A white, scored tablet supplied at a strength of 5 mg and used as a SYMPATHOMIMETIC to stimulate the central nervous system.

Dose: adults 1 tablet twice a day at first increasing every 7 days by 2 tablets a day to a maximum of 12 tablets a day; elderly 1 tablet a day at first increasing every 7 days by 1 tablet a day; children 3-5 years ½ tablet a day at first increasing every 7 days by ½ tablet a day, 6-12 years 1-2 tablets a day at first increasing every 7 days by 1 tablet a day to a maximum of 4 tablets a day.
Availability: controlled drug; NHS and private prescription.
Side effects: sleeplessness, restlessness, slowing of growth, mood changes, dry mouth, loss of appetite, stomach upset, sweating, rapid heart rate, raised blood pressure, addiction.
Caution: in pregnant women.
Not to be used for: infants under 3 years, for patients with a history of drug abuse, or for patients suffering from high blood pressure, heart or circulatory disorders, overactive thyroid gland, hyperexcitability, glaucoma.
Caution needed with: MAOIS, GUANETHIDINE.
Contains: DEXAMPHETAMINE sulphate.
Other preparations:

---

dexfenfluramine *see* Adifax

---

dextran *see* Tears Naturale

---

dextranomer *see* Debrisan

---

dextromoramide tartrate *see* Palfium

---

dextropropoxyphene *see* **co-proxamol tablets, Cosalgesic, Doloxene, Doloxene Co.**

Dextrostix
(Bayer Diagnostics)

A plastic reagent strip used, either visually or – more accurately – in conjunction with a meter, to detect blood glucose levels. Blood-glucose monitoring enables individual patients suffering from diabetes accurately to control blood glucose and manage their condition.

DF 118 *see* **dihydrocodeine tablets**

DHC Continus *see* **dihydrocodeine tablets**
(Napp)

---

di-isobutylphenoxy-polyethoxyethanol *see* **Ortho-Gynol**

Diabetamide *see* **glibenclamide tablets**
(Ashbourne)

Diabinese *see* **chlorpropamide tablets**
(Pfizer)

Diabur Test 5000
(Boehringer Mannheim Diagnostics)

A plastic reagent strip used for the detection of glucose in the urine. This gives an approximate estimate of blood glucose levels which may be adequate for the management of Type II diabetes.

Dialar *see* **diazepam tablets**
(Lagap)

Diamicron
(Servier)

A white, scored tablet supplied at a strength of 80 mg and used as an antidiabetic treatment for diabetes.

Dose: ½-1 tablet a day increasing if needed to a maximum of 4 a day in 2 divided doses.
Availability: NHS and private prescription.
Side effects: allergy, including skin rash.
Caution: in the elderly and in patients suffering from kidney failure.
Not to be used for: children, pregnant women, nursing mothers, during surgery, or for patients suffering from juvenile diabetes, severe liver or kidney disorders, stress, hormone disorders, infections.
Caution needed with: ß-BLOCKERS, MAOIS, STEROIDS, DIURETICS, alcohol, ANTICOAGULANTS, lipid-lowering agents, ASPIRIN, some antibiotics (RIFAMPICIN, sulphonamides, CHLORAMPHENICOL), GLUCAGON, cyclophosphamide, the contraceptive pill.
Contains: GLICLAZIDE.
Other preparations:

---

diamorphine hydrochloride *see* diamorphine tablets

---

diamorphine tablets

A tablet supplied at a strength of 10 mg and used as an opiate ANALGESIC to relieve moderate to severe pain, and acute swelling of the lungs.

Dose: as prescribed by your doctor.
Availability: controlled drug, NHS and private prescription.
Side effects: nausea, vomiting, constipation, drowsiness, breathing difficulties, low blood pressure – especially on standing, depression, difficulty in urinating, dry mouth, sweating, headache, itch, flushing, vertigo, shaking, heart rhythm disturbance, severe coldness, mental changes.
Caution: children, the elderly, pregnant women, nursing mothers, and in patients suffering from low blood pressure, underactive thyroid, asthma, breathing difficulties, liver and kidney failure.
Not to be used for: children under 1 year, or for patients with head injury.
Caution needed with: alcohol, sedatives, ANTICOAGULANTS, MAOIS, SILEGILINE, CIMETIDINE.
Contains: DIAMORPHINE HYDROCHLORIDE.
Other preparations: diamorphine injection, linctus.

Diamox *see* acetazolamide tablets
(Storz)

Dianette
(Schering Healthcare)

A beige tablet used as an anti-androgen and oestrogen to treat severe acne in women, hairiness.

Dose: 1 tablet a day for 21 days beginning on day 1 of the cycle, then 7 days without tablets.
Availability: NHS and private prescription.
Side effects: enlarged breasts, bloating and fluid retention, cramps, leg pains, mood change, reduction in sexual desire, headaches, nausea, vaginal erosion, discharge, and bleeding, weight gain, skin changes. The tablet also functions as an oral contraceptive.
Caution: in patients suffering from high blood pressure, diabetes, vascular disorders, asthma, depression, kidney disease, multiple sclerosis, womb diseases. Your doctor may advise you not to smoke, to have regular examinations. You should stop treatment at the first sign of serious symptoms such as severe headache or jaundice. Treatment should be stopped before surgery.
Not to be used for: children, males, pregnant women, or for patients suffering from sickle-cell anaemia, history of heart disease or thrombosis, liver disorders, some cancers, undiagnosed vaginal bleeding, some ear, skin, and kidney disorders.
Caution needed with: RIFAMPICIN, TETRACYCLINE ANTIBIOTICS, GRISEOFULVIN, BARBITURATES, PHENYTOIN, PRIMIDONE, CARBAMAZEPINE, ETHOSUXIMIDE, CHLORAL HYDRATE.
Contains: CYPROTERONE ACETATE, ETHINYLOESTRODIOL.
Other preparations:

Diarrest
(Galen)

A liquid supplied in 200 ml bottles and used as an opiate, anti-spasmodic, and electrolyte to treat diarrhoea.

Dose: adults 20 ml 4 times a day with water; children 4-5 years 5 ml 4 times a day; children 6-9 years 10 ml 4 times a day; children 10-13 years 15 ml 4 times a day.
Availability: NHS and private prescription.
Side effects: sedation.
Caution: in patients suffering from thyroid disease, heart failure, kidney or liver disease, glaucoma, ulcerative colitis.
Not to be used for: children under 4 years, or for patients suffering from pseudomembranous colitis (a bowel disorder), diverticular disease.
Caution needed with: MAOIS.
Contains: CODEINE PHOSPHATE, DICYCLOMINE hydrochloride, POTASSIUM

CHLORIDE, SODIUM CHLORIDE, SODIUM CITRATE.
Other preparations:

Diastix
(Bayer Diagnostics)

A plastic reagent strip used for the detection of glucose in the urine. This gives an approximate estimate of blood glucose levels which may be adequate for the management of Type II diabetes.

diazepam *see* diazepam tablets, Diazepam Rectubes, Rimapam, Stesolid, Tensium, Valclair, Valium

diazepam tablets

A tablet supplied at strengths of 2 mg, 5 mg, 10 mg and used as a tranquillizer to treat anxiety.

Dose: elderly 7.5-15 mg a day; adults 15-30 mg a day; children 1-5 mg a day.
Availability: NHS and private prescription.
Side effects: drowsiness, confusion, unsteadiness, low blood pressure, rash, changes in vision, changes in sexual function, retention of urine, occasionally headache, vertigo, stomach upset, blood changes, jaundice. Risk of addiction increases with dose and length of treatment. May impair judgement.
Caution: in the elderly, pregnant women, nursing mothers, and in patients suffering from lung disorders, muscle weakness, kidney or liver disorders, or a history of drug or alcohol abuse. Avoid long-term use and withdraw gradually.
Not to be used for: children, or for patients suffering from acute lung diseases, some chronic lung diseases, some obsessional and psychotic diseases.
Caution needed with: alcohol, sedatives, other tranquillizers, anticonvulsants, RIFAMPICIN, ISONIAZID, CIMETIDINE.
Contains: DIAZEPAM.
Other preparations: diazepam suppositories. DIALAR syrup, RIMAPAM, TENSIUM, VALIUM (all available on NHS only if prescribed as generics). STESOLID.

Diazepam Rectubes *see* Stesolid
(CP Pharmaceuticals)

diazoxide *see* **Eudemine**

Dibenyline
(Forley)

A red/white capsule supplied at a strength of 10 mg and used as an anti-ADRENALINE drug to treat high blood pressure associated with PHAEOCHROMOCYTOMA (a disease of the adrenal glands).

Dose: adults 1 capsule a day at first increasing by 1 capsule a day as necessary; children 1-2 mg per kg bodyweight per day in divided doses.
Availability: NHS and private prescription.
Side effects: low blood pressure when standing, dizziness, rapid heart rate, failure of ejaculation, vision changes.
Caution: in the elderly, and in patients suffering from congestive heart failure, cardiovascular or kidney disease.
Not to be used for: patients suffering strokes or heart attacks.
Caution needed with:
Contains: PHENOXYBENZAMINE.
Other preparations:

---

dichlorphenamide *see* **Daranide**

---

diclofenac *see* **Arthrotec, diclofenac tablets, Dicloflex, Diclomax, Diclozip, Flamrase, Isclofen, Motifene, Rhumalgan, Valenac, Volraman, Voltarol**

---

diclofenac tablets

A tablet, coated to protect the stomach, supplied at strengths of 25 mg, 50 mg and used as a NON-STEROIDAL ANTI-INFLAMMATORY DRUG to treat bone or muscular problems, rheumatoid arthritis, osteoarthritis, ankylosing spondylitis, acute gout, chronic juvenile arthritis. (Slow-releasing forms at higher strengths are also available.)

Dose: adults 75-150 mg a day in 2-3 divided doses; children 1-3 mg per kg body weight a day in divided doses.
Availability: NHS and private prescription.
Side effects: stomach pain, nausea, diarrhoea, dizziness, vertigo, hearing disturbance, headache, rash, fluid retention, rarely blood changes, stomach ulcer, abnormal liver or kidney function.
Caution: in pregnant women, nursing mothers, the elderly, or patients suffering from kidney, liver, or heart weakness, blood abnormalities,

PORPHYRIA, history of gastro-intestinal disorders. Your doctor may advise regular check-ups.
Not to be used for: patients suffering from asthma, stomach ulcer, or allergy to ASPIRIN/non-steroidal anti-inflammatory drugs, rectal inflammation.
Caution needed with: SALICYLATES, METHOTREXATE, LITHIUM, DIGOXIN, DIURETICS, CYCLOSPORIN, blood-pressure lowering drugs, other non-steroidal anti-inflammatory drugs, some antibiotics, some antidiabetics, ß-BLOCKERS, STEROIDS, ANTACIDS.
Contains: DICLOFENAC sodium.
Other preparations: diclofenac retard. DICLOFLEX, DICLOMAX, DICLOZIP, FLAMRASE, ISCLOFEN, MOTIFENE, RHUMALGAN, VALENAC, VOLRAMAN, VOLTAROL. (Many available as long-acting preparations, and some as suppositories.)

Dicloflex *see* diclofenac tablets
(Pharmacia)

Dicloflex Retard *see* diclofenac tablets
(Pharmacia)

Diclomax Retard *see* diclofenac tablets
(Parke-Davis Medical)

Diclomax SR *see* diclofenac tablets
(Parke Davis Research)

Diclozip *see* diclofenac tablets
(Ashbourne)

Diconal
(Wellcome)

A pink, scored tablet used as an opiate and anti-emetic to control pain.

Dose: 1 tablet at first and then as advised by physician.
Availability: controlled drug; NHS and private prescription.
Side effects: tolerance, dependence, drowsiness, dry mouth, blurred vision.
Caution: in pregnant women and in patients suffering from liver or kidney disease.

Not to be used for: children or for patients suffering from respiratory depression or blocked airways.
Caution needed with: MAOIS, alcohol, sedatives.
Contains: DIPIPANONE hydrochloride, CYCLIZINE hydrochloride.
Other preparations:

---

dicyclomine *see* **Diarrest, Kolanticon, Merbentyl**

Dicynene
(Delandale)

D

An oval, white tablet supplied at a strength of 500 mg and used as a blood-clotting agent to treat heavy periods.

Dose: 1 tablet 4 times a day until bleeding stops.
Availability: NHS and private prescription.
Side effects: headache, rash, nausea.
Caution:
Not to be used for: children.
Caution needed with:
Contains: ETHAMSYLATE.
Other preparations: Dicynene Injection.

---

didanosine *see* **Videx**

Didronel
(Procter & Gamble)

A white, rectangular tablet supplied at a strength of 200 mg and used as a calcium-lowering agent to treat Paget's disease.

Dose: Paget's disease 5 mg per kg body weight a day as 1 dose 2 hours before and after food for up to 6 months.
Availability: NHS and private prescription.
Side effects: nausea, diarrhoea.
Caution: in pregnant women, nursing mothers, and in patients suffering from enterocolitis, moderate kidney disease. Kidney function should be checked regularly, and calcium and VITAMIN D levels should be maintained.
Not to be used for: children or for patients suffering from severe kidney disease.
Caution needed with:
Contains: ETIDRONATE DISODIUM.

Other preparations: DIDRONEL PMO – contains calcium supplement and used to treat osteoporosis.

Didronel PMO *see* **Didronel**
(Procter & Gamble)

---

dienoestrol *see* **Ortho-Dienoestrol**

---

diethylamine salicylate *see* **Algesal**

Difflam
(3M Healthcare)

A cream used as an NON-STEROIDAL ANTI-INFLAMMATORY and ANALGESIC rub to relieve muscular and skeletal pain.

Dose: massage gently into the affected area 3-6 times a day.
Availability: NHS, private prescription, over the counter.
Side effects: may be irritant.
Caution:
Not to be used for: areas near the eyes or on broken or inflamed skin, or on membranes (such as the mouth).
Caution needed with:
Contains: BENZYDAMINE hydrochloride.
Other preparations:

Difflam Oral Rinse
(3M Healthcare)

A solution used as an ANALGESIC and NON-STEROIDAL ANTI-INFLAMMATORY treatment for painful inflammations of the throat and mouth.

Dose: rinse or gargle with 15 ml every 90 minutes-3 hours.
Availability: NHS, private prescription, over the counter.
Side effects: numb mouth.
Caution:
Not to be used for: children.
Caution needed with:
Contains: BENZYDAMINE hydrochloride.
Other preparations: Difflam Spray (suitable for children).

Diflucan
(Pfizer)

A blue/white, blue, or purple-white capsule according to strengths of 50 mg, 150 mg, 200 mg and used as an antifungal treatment for vaginal or oral thrush, and general fungal infections.

Dose: adults 150 mg as a single dose for vaginal thrush; 50-100 mg a day for oral thrush; up to 400 mg a day for general infections. Children use suspension.
Availability: NHS and private prescription.
Side effects: stomach upset.
Caution: in patients suffering from kidney disease where more than a single dose is prescribed.
Not to be used for: pregnant women, or nursing mothers.
Caution needed with: ANTICOAGULANTS, antidiabetics taken by mouth, THEOPHYLLINE, CYCLOSPORIN, PHENYTOIN, RIFAMPICIN.
Contains: FLUCONAZOLE.
Other preparations: Diflucan Oral Suspension. Diflucan One (available over the counter only to treat vaginal thrush).

---

diflucortolone valerate *see* Nerisone

---

diflunisal *see* Dolobid

Diftavax
(Pasteur Merieux MSD)

A vaccination used to provide active immunization against diphtheria and tetanus in adults and children over 10 years of age.

Dose: 3 injections of 0.5 ml at at least 4-week intervals, then booster after 10 years.
Availability: NHS, private prescription.
Side effects: local reactions, fever, headache, acute allergic reactions including shock, general feeling of being unwell.
Caution: in pregnant women, nursing mothers, and in adults who have previously been vaccinated against diphtheria and tetanus. Adults needing diphtheria immunization should receive low-dose vaccine.
Not to be used for: children under 10 years, patients who have been immunized in the previous month with either diphtheria or tetanus toxoid, or who are suffering from acute infections.
Caution needed with:

D

Contains: diphtheria and tetanus toxoids.
Other preparations: adsorbed diphtheria and tetanus vaccine.

---

digitoxin tablets

Tablets supplied at a strength of 100 micrograms and used as a heart muscle stimulant similar to DIGOXIN treatment, especially for heart failure, abnormal rhythms.

Dose: adults 1-2 tablets a day.
Availability: NHS and private prescription.
Side effects: loss of appetite, nausea, vomiting, diarrhoea, stomach pain, disturbance of vision, headache, tiredness, confusion, delirium, hallucinations, heart disturbances.
Caution: in the elderly, and in patients suffering from underactive thyroid, kidney damage, or recent heart attack.
Not to be used for: patients suffering from some types of heart disorder.
Caution needed with: NON-STEROIDAL ANTI-INFLAMMATORY DRUGS, RIFAMPICIN, BARBITURATES, ß-BLOCKERS, DIURETICS, AMINOGLUTETHIMIDE, SUCRALFATE, other drugs affecting heart rhythm, blood pressure or angina, anticonvulsants, some antifungals, ACE INHIBITORS, AMPHOTERACIN, STEROIDS.
Contains: digitoxin.
Other preparations:

---

digoxin *see* digoxin tablets, Lanoxin

---

digoxin tablets

A tablet supplied at strengths of 62.5 micrograms, 125 micrograms, and 250 micrograms used as a heart muscle stimulant for heart failure and heart rhythm disturbances.

Dose: adults maintenance 62.5 mcg-0.5 mg a day; elderly 125 mcg a day; children as advised by the physician.
Availability: NHS and private prescription.
Side effects: stomach upset, headache, tiredness, drowsiness, confusion, visual changes, and heart rhythm changes, loss of appetite, hallucinations.
Caution: the elderly and in patients suffering from potassium deficiency, kidney and thyroid disorders, recent heart attack.
Not to be used for: patients suffering from some types of heart disorder.
Caution needed with: calcium supplements, some DIURETICS, QUININE, LITHIUM, ACE INHIBITORS, MEFLOQUINE, ß-BLOCKERS, some antibiotics, some antifungals, some antimalarials, other heart muscle stimulants, other drugs affecting heart rhythm, blood pressure, or angina, NON-STEROIDAL ANTI-

INFLAMMATORY DRUGS, STEROIDS.
Contains: DIGOXIN.
Other preparations: Lanoxin (also available as a paediatric solution).

---

dihydrocodeine *see* co-dydramol, DF 118, DHC Continus, dihydrocodeine tablets, Galake, Remedeine

---

dihydrocodeine tablets

A white tablet supplied at a strength of 30 mg and used as an opiate to control pain; for cough use elixir.

Dose: adults1 tablet every 4-6 hours after meals; children 4-12 years 0.5-1 mg per kg body weight every 4-6 hours.
Availability: NHS and private prescription.
Side effects: constipation, nausea, headache, vertigo, vomiting, dizziness, difficulty passing urine, dry mouth, sweating, flushing, altered heart rate, low blood pressure on standing, low body temperature, mood changes, itching, rash, addiction, vision disturbances.
Caution: in pregnant women, nursing mothers, the elderly, and in patients suffering from liver or kidney disease, underactive thyroid gland, low blood pressure, asthma, breathing disorder.
Not to be used for: children under 4 years, or for patients suffering from head injury or raised brain pressure.
Caution needed with: alcohol, sedatives, MAOIS, SILEGILINE.
Contains: DIHYDROCODEINE tartrate.
Other preparations: DF118 FORTE TABLETS (not available on the NHS), DHC CONTINUS (a long-acting preparation for adults only).

---

dihydrotachysterol *see* AT 10

---

diltiazem *see* Adizem, Angiozem, Angitil, Britiazim, Calcicard CR, diltiazem tablets, Dilzem, Slozem, Tildiem

---

diltiazem tablets/diltiazem long-acting tablets

A tablet supplied at a strength of 60 mg and used as a calcium antagonist to treat and prevent angina and high blood pressure. (Long-acting tablets and capsules available in strengths of 90 mg, 120 mg, 180 mg, 240 mg, 300 mg.)

Dose: initially 180 mg a day (in three divided doses), increasing to a maximum of 360-480 mg a day. (Doses may be given as a single daily dose or two divided doses for long-acting preparations.) Lower doses may be given to elderly patients.

Availability: NHS and private prescription.

Side effects: nausea, headache, rash, slow heart rate, swollen ankles, heart conduction block, tiredness, low blood pressure, flushes, liver disorder, depression.

Caution: in patients with heart disease, kidney disorders, liver disease.

Not to be used for: children, pregnant women, nursing mothers, or for patients suffering from slow heart rate or heart block.

Caution needed with: ß-BLOCKERS, DIGOXIN, blood-pressure lowering drugs, AMIODARONE, CARBAMAZEPINE, CYCLOSPORIN, RIFAMPICIN, THEOPHYLLINE, CIMETIDINE, LITHIUM, TRICYCLIC ANTIDEPRESSANTS, PHENYTOIN, PHENOBARBITONE, MEFLOQUINE, MIDAZOLAM.

Contains: DILTIAZEM hydrochloride.

Other preparations: ADIZEM, ANGIOZEM, BRITIAZEM, TILDIEM. (Long-acting preparations: ADIZEM SR, ADIZEM XL, Angitil SR, DILZEM, SLOZEM, TILDIEM LA — some available in capsule form.)

Dilzem SR *see* **diltiazem long-acting tablets**
(Elan Pharma)

Dilzem XL *see* **diltiazem long-acting tablets**
(Elan Pharma)

---

dimenhydrenate *see* **Dramamine**

---

dimethicone *see* **Altacite Plus, Asilone, Cobadex, Conotrane, Diovol, Kolanticon, Sprilon, Timodine**

---

dimethyl sulphoxide *see* **Herpid, Virudox**

Dimetriose
(Hoechst Roussel)

A white capsule used to treat endometriosis (a womb and menstrual disorder).

Dose: 1 capsule twice a week, on days 1 and 4 of cycle, then on the same 2 days each week for the rest of the treatment.

Availability: NHS and private prescription.

Side effects: vaginal bleeding (spotting), acne, weight gain, stomach upset, cramp, depression, voice changes, hair growth.
Caution: in patients suffering from diabetes or high blood lipids. Ensure effective contraception (barrier methods must be used).
Not to be used for: children, pregnant women, nursing mothers, or for patients with heart, kidney, or liver disorder, blood vessel disease, or disturbance of metabolism.
Caution needed with: anticonvulsants, the contraceptive pill, RIFAMPICIN.
Contains: GESTRINONE.
Other preparations:

Dimotane Expectorant
(Whitehall)

A liquid used as an ANTIHISTAMINE, expectorant, and SYMPATHOMIMETIC treatment for cough.

Dose: adults 5-10 ml 3 times a day; children 2-6 years 2.5 ml 3 times a day, 6-12 years 5 ml 3 times a day.
Availability: private prescription and over the counter.
Side effects: anxiety, hands shaking, rapid or abnormal heart rate, dry mouth, brain stimulation, drowsiness.
Caution: in patients suffering from diabetes.
Not to be used for: children under 2 years, or for patients suffering from cardiovascular problems, overactive thyroid gland.
Caution needed with: MAOIS, TRICYCLIC ANTIDEPRESSANTS, sedatives, alcohol, ANTICHOLINERGICS.
Contains: BROMPHENIRAMINE maleate, GUAIPHENESIN, PSEUDOEPHEDRINE hydrochloride.
Other preparations: Dimotane Co, Dimotane Co Paediatric.

Dimotane Plus
(Wyeth)

A liquid used as an ANTIHISTAMINE and SYMPATHOMIMETIC treatment for allergic rhinitis.

Dose: adults 10 ml 3 times a day; children 6-12 years 5 ml 3 times a day (children 2-6 years use paediatric elixir).
Availability: NHS, private prescription, over the counter.
Side effects: drowsiness, reduced reactions, rarely stimulant effects (usually in children).
Caution: in pregnant women and in patients suffering from bronchial asthma, diabetes.
Not to be used for: patients suffering from glaucoma, comatose states,

brain damage, epilepsy, retention of urine, cardiovascular problems, overactive thyroid, high blood pressure.
Caution needed with: sedatives, MAOIS, TRICYCLIC ANTIDEPRESSANTS, ANTICHOLINERGICS, alcohol, NON-STEROIDAL ANTI-INFLAMMATORY DRUGS, DIGOXIN.
Contains: BROMPHENIRAMINE maleate, PSEUDOEPHEDRINE hydrochloride.
Other preparations: Dimotane Plus Paediatric, Dimotane LA, Dimotane Tablets, Dimotane Elixir. (DIMOTANE EXPECTORANT, Dimotane Co, and Dimotane Co Paediatric also available over the counter but not on the NHS.)

Dimotapp LA
(Whitehall)

A brown tablet used as an ANTIHISTAMINE and SYMPATHOMIMETIC treatment for catarrh, allergic rhinitis, sinusitis.

Dose: adults 1 tablet night and morning; children use elixir.
Availability: private prescription and over the counter.
Side effects: drowsiness, reduced reactions, rarely stimulant effects, heart rhythm disturbance, dry mouth.
Caution: in nursing mothers and in patients suffering from bronchial asthma, diabetes, overactive thyroid, high blood pressure, heart disease, raised pressure in the eyes, enlarged prostate.
Not to be used for: children (use elixir).
Caution needed with: sedatives, MAOIS, other sympathomimetics, TRICYCLIC ANTIDEPRESSANTS, ANTICHOLINERGICS, alcohol, FURAZOLIDONE, drugs to reduce the appetite.
Contains: BROMPHENIRAMINE maleate, PHENYLEPHRINE hydrochloride, PHENYLPROPANOLAMINE hydrochloride.
Other preparations: Dimotapp Elixir, Dimotapp Elixir Paediatric.

Dindevan
(Goldshield Healthcare)

A white or a green, scored tablet according to strengths of 10 mg, 25 mg, 50 mg and used as an ANTICOAGULANT to prevent blood from clotting.

Dose: 200 mg a day at first, 100 mg the following day, then 50-150 mg a day.
Availability: NHS and private prescription.
Side effects: rash, fever, blood changes, diarrhoea, hepatitis, kidney damage, discoloration of urine.
Caution: in elderly and very ill patients, and for patients suffering from high blood pressure, weight changes, kidney disease, vitamin K deficiency.

Not to be used for: children, within 24 hours of surgery or labour, for pregnant women, nursing mothers, and for patients suffering from severe liver or kidney disease or bleeding conditions.
Caution needed with: NON-STEROIDAL ANTI-INFLAMMATORY DRUGS, antidiabetics, QUINIDINE, some antibiotics, PHENFORMIN, CIMETIDINE, drugs affecting the liver chemistry, STEROIDS.
Contains: PHENINDIONE.
Other preparations:

Diocaps *see* loperamide capsules
(Berk)

Dioctyl
(Schwartz)

A yellow/white capsule supplied at a strength of 100 mg and used as a faecal softener to treat constipation.

Dose: adults up to 500 mg a day in divided doses; children over 2 years 12.5-25 mg 3 times a day; 6 months-2 years 12.5 mg 3 times a day using syrup.
Availability: NHS, private prescription, over the counter.
Side effects:
Caution:
Not to be used for:
Caution needed with:
Contains: DOCUSATE sodium.
Other preparations: Dioctyl Paediatric Solution, Dioctyl Adult Solution.

Dioderm *see* hydrocortisone cream
(Dermal)

Dioralyte
(Rhône-Poulenc Rorer)

Plain, citrus-, or blackcurrant-flavoured powder supplied as sachets and used as a fluid and electrolyte replacement to treat acute watery diarrhoea including gastroenteritis.

Dose: 1-2 sachets in 200-400 ml water after each occasion of diarrhoea; infants substitute equivalent volume of reconstituted powder to feeds; children 1 sachet after each occasion of diarrhoea.
Availability: NHS, private prescription, and over the counter.

Side effects:
Caution:
Not to be used for:
Caution needed with:
Contains: SODIUM CHLORIDE, POTASSIUM CHLORIDE, SODIUM ACID CITRATE, GLUCOSE.
Other preparations: Dioralyte Effervescent Tablets, ELECTROLADE; GLUCO-
LYTE; REHIDRAT (formulas may vary slightly between brands).

Diovol
(Pharmax)

A white, mint-flavoured suspension used as an ANTACID and anti-wind
preparation to treat ulcers, hiatus hernias, wind, and acidity.

Dose: adults 5-10 ml 3 times a day, or as needed.
Availability: NHS, private prescription, over the counter.
Side effects: occasionally constipation.
Caution:
Not to be used for: children.
Caution needed with: tablets coated to protect the stomach, some
antibiotics, iron.
Contains: ALUMINIUM HYDROXIDE, MAGNESIUM HYDROXIDE, DIMETHICONE.
Other preparations:

Dipentum
(Pharmacia)

A caramel-coloured capsule supplied at a strength of 250 mg used as a
salicylate to treat ulcerative colitis.

Dose: 4-12 capsules a day with food.
Availability: NHS and private prescription.
Side effects: stomach upset, rash, headache, joint pains, blood changes.
Caution: you should report any unexplained bleeding, bruising, or illness
to your physician.
Not to be used for: children, pregnant women, or for patients suffering
from ASPIRIN allergy or kidney disease.
Caution needed with:
Contains: OLSALAZINE SODIUM.
Other preparations:

---

diphenhydramine hydrochloride *see* **Caladryl, Nytol**

---

diphenoxylate *see* **Lomotil, Lotharin, Tropergen**

---

diphtheria vaccine

Diphtheria vaccine provides active immunization against the disease by stimulating the body's production of an antitoxin. (Used only after contact with the disease.)

Dose: initial vaccination for children over 2 months by three injections at 4-week intervals, if no previous vaccination given. (For previously vaccinated children, one single booster dose is given.)
Side effects: local reactions, headache, fever, generalized feeling of illness.
Not to be used for: adults or children over 10 years, or for treating acute diphtheria infections.
Other preparations: diphtheria vaccine for adults and adolescents.

---

diphtheria and tetanus vaccine

Diphtheria and tetanus vaccine provides active immunization against the diseases by stimulating the body's production of an antitoxin.

Dose: initial vaccination for children over 2 months by three injections at 4-week intervals, followed by a booster at 4-5 years (at least 3 years after initial course).
Side effects: local reactions, headache, fever, generalized feeling of illness.
Not to be used for: adults or children over 10 years, or for children with acute infections.
Other preparations: diphtheria and tetanus vaccine for adults and adolescents. Diftavax.

---

diphtheria, tetanus, and pertussis (DTP) vaccine

Diphtheria, tetanus, and pertussis (DTP) vaccine provides active immunization against diptheria, tetanus, and pertussis (whooping cough) by stimulating the body's production of an antitoxin.

Dose: initial vaccination for children over 2 months by three injections at 4-week intervals, followed by a diphtheria and tetanus booster at 4-5 years (at least 3 years after initial course).
Side effects: poor appetite, mood changes, crying, fever.
Caution: in patients with a history of allergy, convulsions, or who have brain damage, disease, or injury, or whose close relatives have epilepsy.
Not to be used for: adults or children over 10 years, or for children with

acute feverish infections, or who have suffered from a severe reaction to the vaccination.

---

dipipanone *see* **Diconal**

---

dipivefrin *see* **Propine**

---

dipotassium hydrogen phosphate *see* **Glandosane**

---

dipotassium phosphate *see* **Salivace**

Diprobase
(Schering-Plough)

A cream used as an emollient to soften skin.

Dose: apply sparingly when required.
Availability: NHS, private prescription, over the counter.
Side effects:
Caution:
Not to be used for:
Caution needed with:
Contains: LIQUID PARAFFIN, WHITE SOFT PARAFFIN, CETOMACROGOL, CETOSTEARYL ALCOHOL.
Other preparations: Diprobase Ointment, LIPOBASE, ULTRABASE.

Diprobath
(Schering-Plough)

A bath emulsion used to treat dry or thickening skin conditions.

Dose: adults, 2½ capsful added to the bath, and soak for 20 minutes; children, 1 capful per bath.
Availability: NHS, private prescription, over the counter.
Side effects:
Caution:
Not to be used for:
Caution needed with:
Contains: light LIQUID PARAFFIN, ISOPROPYL MYRISTATE.
Other preparations: HYDROMOL (bath additive and emollient cream).

Diprosalic
(Schering-Plough)

An ointment used as a strong STEROID and skin softener to treat hard skin and dry skin disorders.

Dose: apply lightly to the affected area 1-2 times a day.
Availability: NHS and private prescription.
Side effects: fluid retention, suppression of adrenal glands, thinning, streaking, or spotting of the skin may occur.
Caution: use for short periods of time only, especially in children or on the face.
Not to be used for: patients suffering from acne or any other skin infections caused by tuberculosis, ringworm, viruses, or fungi, leg ulcers, scabies, or continuously especially in pregnant women.
Caution needed with:
Contains: BETAMETHASONE dipropionate, SALICYLIC ACID.
Other preparations: Diprosalic Scalp Application.

Diprosone *see* Betnovate
(Schering-Plough)

dipyridamole *see* dipyridamole tablets, Persantin

dipyridamole tablets

A coated tablet supplied at strengths of 25 mg, 100 mg and used as an anti-platelet drug in addition to oral ANTICOAGULANTS or ASPIRIN to prevent thrombosis.

Dose: adults 300-600 mg a day in 3-4 doses before meals; children 5 mg per kg body weight a day in divided doses.
Availability: NHS and private prescription.
Side effects: headache, dizziness, stomach upset, rash, low blood pressure.
Caution: care in patients suffering from rapidly worsening angina, some other heart conditions, low blood pressure, migraine.
Not to be used for:
Caution needed with: ANTACIDS, ANTICOAGULANTS.
Contains: DIPYRAMIDOLE.
Other preparations: CEREBROVASE, MODAPLATE, PERSANTIN.

Dirythmin SA *see* **disopyramide capsules**
(Astra)

Disipal
(Yamanouchi)

A yellow tablet supplied at a strength of 50 mg and used as an
ANTICHOLINERGIC drug to treat Parkinson's disease.

Dose: 1 tablet 3 times a day at first increasing by 1 tablet a day every 2-3
days usually to 2-6 tablets a day and a maximum of 8 tablets a day.
Availability: NHS and private prescription.
Side effects: euphoria, anticholinergic effects, and confusion, agitation,
and rash at high dose.
Caution: in patients suffering from heart problems or stomach obstruction.
Reduce dose slowly.
Not to be used for: children, or for patients suffering from glaucoma,
enlarged prostate, some movement disorders.
Caution needed with: some sedative drugs, ANTIHISTAMINES,
antidepressants.
Contains: ORPHENADRINE hydrochloride.
Other preparations: Disipal Injection, BIORPHEN (liquid).

---

disopyramide *see* **Dirythmin, disopyramide capsules,
Rythmodan**

---

disopyramide capsules

A capsule supplied at strengths of 100 mg, 150 mg and used as an anti-
arrhythmic drug to treat abnormal heart rhythm.

Dose: 300-800 mg a day in divided doses.
Availability: NHS and private prescription.
Side effects: stomach upset, low blood pressure, dry mouth, blurred
vision, constipation, palpitations, heart block, mental disorders, heart
muscle depression, retention of urine, low blood sugar.
Caution: in the elderly, pregnant women, and nursing mothers and in
patients suffering from mild heart block, enlarged prostate, glaucoma,
retention of urine, low potassium levels, heart failure, kidney or liver failure.
Not to be used for: children or for patients suffering from some types of
heart block, heart muscle disease or shock.
Caution needed with: other similar drugs, some antibiotics,
PHENOBARBITONE, PHENYTOIN, PRIMIDONE, ASTEMIZOLE, TERFENADINE, VERAPAMIL,
some DIURETICS, ß-BLOCKERS, potassium-lowering drugs, some drugs used

for mental disorders and sickness, GLYCERYL TRINITRATE and other NITRATES.
Contains: DISOPYRAMIDE phosphate.
Other preparations: DIRYTHMIN, RYTHMODAN (both available as long-acting preparations).

Disprin CV
(Reckitt & Colman)

A white capsule-shaped, sustained-release, scored tablet supplied at strengths of 100 mg, 300 mg and used as an anti-platelet drug to reduce risk of heart attack in patients suffering from angina or who have had previous heart attack; to reduce the risk of stroke in patients with a history of attacks; to prevent the closure of grafts following heart bypass surgery.

Dose: 100-300 mg once a day.
Availability: NHS, private prescription, over the counter.
Side effects: stomach upset, asthma, or other allergic reactions.
Caution: in pregnant women and in patients with a history of bronchial spasm or allergy to ASPIRIN or anti-inflammatory drugs.
Not to be used for: patients suffering from asthma, haemophilia, or stomach ulcer.
Caution needed with: some ANTICOAGULANTS, some anti-inflammatory drugs, METHOTREXATE, SPIRONOLACTONE, CORTICOSTEROIDS, drugs that increase the amount of uric acid in the urine, some antidiabetic drugs.
Contains: ASPIRIN.
Other preparations: ASPIRIN TABLETS, CAPRIN, NU-SEALS ASPIRIN, POSTMI.

Disprol Paediatric *see* Calpol Paediatric
(Reckitt & Colman)

Distaclor *see* cefaclor capsules
(Eli Lilly)

Distalgesic *see* co-proxamol tablets
(Eli Lilly)

Distamine
(Eli Lilly)

A white tablet or a white, scored tablet according to strengths of 125 mg, 250 mg and used as an anti-arthritic drug and binding agent to treat severe active rheumatoid arthritis, cystinuria, Wilson's disease (inherited disorders), heavy metal poisoning, liver disease.

Dose: for arthritis, adults 125-250 mg a day for 4 weeks increasing by
same amount at 4-12 week intervals, usually to 500-750 mg a day or a
maximum of 1.5 g a day; elderly 50-125 mg a day at first increasing to a
maximum of 1 g a day; children 50 mg a day for 4 weeks, increasing every
4 weeks to a usual dose of 15-20 mg per kg body weight a day. Or as
advised.
Availability: NHS and private prescription.
Side effects: nausea, loss of appetite, fever, rash, loss of taste, blood
changes, blood or protein in the urine, kidney changes, muscle disease,
LUPUS, MYASTHENIA GRAVIS.
Caution: in patients suffering from kidney disease, allergy to penicillin.
Your doctor may advise that your blood and urine should be checked
regularly.
Not to be used for: pregnant women, nursing mothers, or for patients
suffering from LUPUS erythematosus, agranulocytosis, thrombocytopenia
(rare blood and multi-system disorders).
Caution needed with: gold salts, anti-malaria or cytotoxic drugs, ANTACIDS,
zinc salts, iron salts.
Contains: PENICILLAMINE.
Other preparations: PENDRAMINE.

---

distigmine *see* **Ubretid**

---

disulfiram *see* **Antabuse**

---

dithranol *see* **Dithrocream, Dithrolan, Psoradrate, Psorin**

Dithrocream
(Dermal)

A cream, available in 5 strengths, and used as an antipsoriatic treatment
for psoriasis.

Dose: apply to the affected area once a day and wash off after ½-1 hour
or apply at night and wash off in the morning. Start with weakest strength
and increase if necessary.
Availability: NHS, private prescription. (Weaker strengths also available
over the counter.)
Side effects: irritation, allergy.
Caution: stains skin and clothing.
Not to be used for: patients suffering from acute psoriasis.

Caution needed with:
Contains: DITHRANOL.
Other preparations: Dithrocream Forte, Dithrocream HP, Dithrocream 2%. PSORADRATE.

Dithrolan
(Dermal)

An ointment used as an antipsoriatic and skin softener to treat psoriasis.

Dose: before going to bed, bath and then apply the ointment to the affected area. Use once or twice a week.
Availability: NHS, private prescription, over the counter.
Side effects: irritation, allergy.
Caution: stains skin and clothing.
Not to be used for: patients suffering from acute psoriasis.
Caution needed with:
Contains: DITHRANOL, SALICYLIC ACID.
Other preparations: PSORIN.

Ditropan *see* Cystrin
(Lorex Synthélabo)

Diumide-K Continus
(ASTA Medica)

A white/orange tablet used as a DIURETIC/potassium supplement combination to treat fluid retention including that associated with congestive heart failure, kidney and liver disease where a potassium supplement is needed.

Dose: 1 tablet a day in the morning.
Availability: NHS and private prescription.
Side effects: gout, bowel disturbances.
Caution: in pregnant women, nursing mothers, and in patients suffering from kidney or liver disease, diabetes, enlarged prostate, impaired urination, gout.
Not to be used for: children or for patients suffering from liver cirrhosis, raised potassium levels, Addison's disease.
Caution needed with: some diuretics, LITHIUM, DIGOXIN, some antibiotics, NON-STEROIDAL ANTI-INFLAMMATORY DRUGS, blood-pressure lowering drugs.
Contains: FRUSEMIDE, POTASSIUM CHLORIDE.
Other preparations: LASIKAL, LASIX + K.

D

diuretic

A drug which removes salt and water from the body, thus treating fluid retention. Example FRUSEMIDE *see* frusemide tablets.

Diurexan
(ASTA Medica)

A white, scored tablet supplied at a strength of 20 mg and used as a DIURETIC to treat high blood pressure, congestive heart failure, fluid retention.

Dose: high blood pressure 1 tablet a day in the morning; fluid retention 2 tablets a day in the morning and then 1-4 tablets a day as needed.
Availability: NHS and private prescription.
Side effects: electrolyte disturbances, dizziness, stomach upset, pancreatitis.
Caution: potassium supplements may be needed; care in pregnant women, the elderly, and in patients suffering from gout, kidney or liver disease, diabetes, enlarged prostate, some circulatory disorders.
Not to be used for: children, nursing mothers, or for patients suffering from severe kidney failure or cirrhosis of the liver, Addison's disease.
Caution needed with: DIGOXIN, LITHIUM, STEROIDS, AMPHOTERACIN, laxatives, antidiabetics.
Contains: XIPAMIDE.
Other preparations:

Dixarit
(Boehringer Ingelheim)

A blue tablet supplied at a strength of 25 micrograms and used as a blood vessel antispasmodic drug to treat migraine, headache, menopausal flushing.

Dose: 2-3 tablets morning and evening.
Availability: NHS and private prescription.
Side effects: sedation, dry mouth, dizziness, sleeplessness.
Caution: in nursing mothers or in patients suffering from depression.
Not to be used for: children.
Caution needed with: blood-pressure lowering drugs, alcohol, sedatives.
Contains: CLONIDINE hydrochloride.
Other preparations:

---

dl-methionine *see* Lipotriad

---

dl-threonine *see* **Cicatrin**

---

docosahexaenoic acid *see* **Maxepa**

---

docusate *see* **Capsuvac, co-danthrusate capsules, Dioctyl, Fletchers' Enemette, Norgalax, Normax, Waxsol**

Dolmatil
(Delandale)

D

A white, scored tablet supplied at a strength of 200 mg and used as a sedative to treat schizophrenia.

Dose: over 14 years 2-4 tablets a day at first in 2 divided doses, then 1-6 tablets twice a day as needed.
Availability: NHS and private prescription.
Side effects: muscle spasms, restlessness, hands shaking, dry mouth, urine retention, palpitations, low blood pressure, weight gain, changes in sexual function, low body temperature, breast swelling, menstrual changes, jaundice, blood and skin changes, drowsiness, rarely fits.
Caution: in pregnant women or for patients suffering from hypomania, kidney disease, or epilepsy.
Not to be used for: for children under 14 years or for patients suffering from PHAEOCHROMOCYTOMA (a disease of the adrenal glands), severe liver, kidney, or blood diseases.
Caution needed with: alcohol, sedatives, tranquillizers, pain killers, blood-pressure lowering drugs, antidepressants, ANTICOAGULANTS, antidiabetic drugs, LEVODOPA, ANTACIDS, anticonvulsants, drugs that affect heart rhythm, ASTEMIZOLE, TERFENADINE, ß-BLOCKERS, LITHIUM, METOCLOPRAMIDE.
Contains: SULPIRIDE.
Other preparations: SULPITIL.

Dolobid
(Morson)

A peach tablet or an orange tablet according to strengths of 250 mg, 500 mg and used as an ANALGESIC to treat pain, rheumatoid arthritis, osteoarthritis.

Dose: usually 500-1000 mg a day; maximum 1500 mg a day.
Availability: NHS and private prescription.
Side effects: stomach pain, nausea, vomiting, indigestion, diarrhoea, rash, headache, dizziness, tinnitus, drowsiness, sleeplessness.

Caution: in the elderly and in patients suffering from kidney, heart, or liver disease or with a history of stomach bleeding or ulcers.
Not to be used for: children, pregnant women, nursing mothers or for patients suffering from anti-inflammatory-induced allergy, asthma, or stomach ulcer.
Caution needed with: alcohol, ASPIRIN, CODEINE, METHOTREXATE, CYCLOSPORIN, INDOMETHACIN, ANTICOAGULANTS, ANTACIDS.
Contains: DIFLUNISAL.
Other preparations:

Doloxene
(Eli Lilly)

An orange capsule supplied at a strength of 60 mg and used as an opiate to control pain.

Dose: 1 capsule 3-4 times a day.
Availability: NHS (when prescribed as a generic), private prescription.
Side effects: tolerance, dependence, drowsiness, constipation, rash, dizziness, nausea.
Caution: in pregnant women, the elderly, and in patients suffering from liver or kidney disease.
Not to be used for: children
Caution needed with: alcohol, sedatives, anticonvulsants, ANTICOAGULANTS.
Contains: DEXTROPROPOXYPHENE.
Other preparations:

Doloxene Co.
(Eli Lilly)

A red/grey capsule used as an opiate to control pain.

Dose: 1 capsule 3-4 times a day.
Availability: private prescription only.
Side effects: tolerance, dependence, drowsiness, constipation, dizziness, nausea, rash.
Caution: in pregnant women, nursing mothers, the elderly, and in patients suffering from kidney, heart, or liver disease, anti-inflammatory induced allergy, or a history of bronchospasm.
Not to be used for: children or for patients suffering from stomach ulcer, haemophilia, and blood clotting disorders.
Caution needed with: alcohol, sedatives, ANTICOAGULANTS, antidiabetics, uric acid-lowering drugs, anticonvulsants.
Contains: DEXTROPROPOXYPHENE napsylate, ASPIRIN, CAFFEINE.
Other preparations: DOLOXENE (containing only DEXTROPROPOXYPHENE,

available on NHS only if prescribed as a generic).

Domical *see* **amitriptyline tablets**
(Berk)

---

domperidone *see* **Motilium**

Dopamet *see* **methyldopa tablets**
(Berk)

Doralese
(Bencard)

A yellow, triangular tablet supplied at a strength of 20 mg and used as an alpha-blocker to treat urine obstruction due to prostate disease.

Dose: 1 tablet twice a day (low dose in the elderly).
Availability: NHS and private prescription.
Side effects: dry mouth, nose blockage, weight gain, drowsiness, ejaculation failure.
Caution: in patients suffering from poor heart function, kidney or liver disease, Parkinson's disease, epilepsy, depression.
Not to be used for: children, or for patients suffering from heart failure.
Caution needed with: MAOIS, blood-pressure lowering drugs, alcohol, sedatives.
Contains: INDORAMIN.
Other preparations: BARATOL.

---

dornase alfa *see* **Pulmozyme**

---

dorzolamide *see* **Trusopt**

Dostinex
(Pharmacia)

A white, capsule-shaped, scored tablet supplied at a strength of 0.5 mg and used as a hormone blocker to suppress breast milk production in women, and as a treatment for some types of infertility.

Dose: to suppress milk 2 tablets on the first day after childbirth, ½ tablet every 12 hours for 2 days if milk already produced; to treat infertility 1 tablet a week in 1-2 doses increasing if necessary by 1 tablet a week at monthly intervals to a maximum of 9 tablets a week – usual maintenance 2 tablets a week.

Availability: NHS, private prescription.

Side effects: dizziness, vertigo, headache, tiredness, breast pain, stomach upset, hot flushes, depression, weakness, pins and needles; rarely palpitations, nosebleed, vision disturbances.

Caution: in patients suffering from kidney, liver, or heart disease, Raynaud's syndrome, stomach ulcer or bleeding, raised blood pressure, mental disorders. Before treatment pituitary function should be tested. Your doctor will advise regular blood tests. Stop treatment at least a month before trying to conceive. Use only non-hormonal methods of contraception.

Not to be used for: children under 16 years, pregnant women, or for patients suffering from weak liver function, toxaemia of pregnancy, raised blood pressure during pregnancy, some mental disorders.

Caution needed with: tranquillizers, blood-pressure lowering drugs, ERGOTAMINE, some antibiotics, METOCLOPRAMIDE, DOMPERIDONE, PROCHLORPERAZINE.

Contains: CABERGOLINE.

Other preparations:

Dothapax *see* **dothiepin capsules**
(Ashbourne)

---

dothiepin *see* **Dothapax, dothiepin capsules, Prepadine, Prothiaden**

---

dothiepin capsules

A capsule supplied at a strength of 25 mg and used as a TRICYCLIC ANTIDEPRESSANT to treat depression.

Dose: 3-6 capsules a day (elderly 2-3 capsules a day).

Availability: NHS and private prescription.

Side effects: dry mouth, constipation, urine retention, blurred vision, palpitations, drowsiness, sleeplessness, dizziness, hands shaking, low blood presure, weight change, skin reactions, jaundice or blood changes, interference with sexual function, weakness, lack of co-ordination, convulsions, stomach upset, heart irregularities.

Caution: in the elderly, pregnant women, nursing mothers or in patients suffering from heart disease, thyroid disease, epilepsy, diabetes, retention of urine, liver disorder, adrenal tumour, PORPHYRIA, some other psychiatric

conditions. Your doctor may advise regular blood tests.
Not to be used for: children, or for patients suffering from recent heart attacks, heart rhythm disturbance, liver disease, heart block, mania.
Caution needed with: alcohol, sedatives, ANTICHOLINERGICS, ADRENALINE, ASTEMIZOLE, TERFENADINE, MAOIS, BARBITURATES, other antidepressants, anticonvulsants, CIMETIDINE, other drugs affecting heart rhythm.
Contains: DOTHIEPIN hydrochloride.
Other preparations: dothiepin tablets (higher strength). DOTHAPAX, PROTHIADEN, PREPADINE.

Dovonex
(Leo)

An ointment used to treat mild to moderate psoriasis.

Dose: apply twice a day, not more than 100 g per week.
Availability: NHS and private prescription.
Side effects: irritation, dermatitis, sensitivity to light, worsening of psoriasis.
Caution: in pregnant women and nursing mothers. Avoid the face.
Not to be used for: children, or for patients suffering from disorders of calcium metabolism.
Caution needed with:
Contains: CALCIPOTRIOL.
Other preparations: Dovonex Cream, Dovonex Scalp Solution.

---

doxazosin *see* Cardura

---

doxepin *see* Sinequan

---

doxycycline capsules

A capsule supplied at strengths of 50 mg, 100 mg, and used as a TETRACYCLINE ANTIBIOTIC to treat acne, respiratory, and other infections.

Dose: adults 200 mg on the first day, then 100-200 mg a day. (Dose for acne 50 mg a day.) The capsules should be swallowed whole with food or drink while sitting or standing.
Availability: NHS and private prescription.
Side effects: stomach disturbances, reddening of the skin, additional infections, oesophagitis, allergy, sensitivity to light, raised blood pressure in the brain.
Caution: in patients suffering from liver disease. Swallow the capsules

with plenty of fluid while standing or sitting.

Not to be used for: children, pregnant women, and nursing mothers or for patients suffering from PORPHYRIA or LUPUS.

Caution needed with: ANTACIDS, BARBITURATES, ANTICOAGULANTS, CYCLOSPORIN, iron supplements, the contraceptive pill, zinc supplements.

Contains: DOXYCYCLINE hydrochloride.

Other preparations: CYCLODOX, DEMIX, DOXYLAR, NORDOX, RAMYSIS, VIBRAMYCIN (also available as dispersible tablets).

---

doxycycline hydrochloride *see* Cyclodox, Demix, doxycycline capsules, Doxylar, Nordox, Ramysis, Vibramycin

---

Doxylar *see* doxycycline capsules
(Lagap)

Dozic *see* haloperidol tablets
(Rosemont)

Dramamine
(Searle)

A white, scored tablet supplied at a strength of 50 mg and used as an ANTIHISTAMINE treatment for vertigo, nausea, vomiting, travel sickness.

Dose: adults 1-2 tablets 2-3 times a day; children 1-6 years ¼-½ tablet, 7-12 years ½-1 tablet 2-3 times a day.

Availability: NHS, over the counter, private prescription.

Side effects: drowsiness, reduced reactions, dry mouth, blurred vision, allergy, blood changes, rarely skin eruptions.

Caution: in pregnant women, nursing mothers, and in patients suffering from liver or kidney disease, glaucoma, enlarged prostate, epilepsy. If you become drowsy, do not drive or operate machinery.

Not to be used for: infants under 1 year.

Caution needed with: alcohol, sedatives, some antidepressants (MAOIS), ANTICHOLINERGICS.

Contains: DIMENHYDRENATE.

Other preparations:

Drapolene
(Warner Wellcome Consumer)

A cream used as an antiseptic to treat nappy rash.

Dose: apply twice a day or each time the nappy is changed.
Availability: NHS, private prescription, over the counter.
Side effects:
Caution:
Not to be used for:
Caution needed with:
Contains: BENZALKONIUM CHLORIDE, CETRIMIDE.
Other preparations:

Driclor
(Stiefel)

A solution in a roll-on bottle used as an antiperspirant to treat excessive
sweating from the hands, feet, and armpits.

Dose: dry the affected areas and apply solution; wash off in the morning.
Reduce the treatment as the sweating decreases.
Availability: NHS, private prescription, over the counter.
Side effects: skin irritation.
Caution: make sure that the area to be treated is dry and has not been
shaved either 24 hours before or after treatment. Use only on the feet in
children. Avoid contact with clothes or jewellery.
Not to be used for: inflamed or broken skin.
Caution needed with:
Contains: ALUMINIUM CHLORIDE hexahydrate.
Other preparations:

Droleptan
(Janssen-Cilag)

A yellow, scored tablet supplied at a strength of 10 mg and used as a
sedative to treat manic agitation.

Dose: adults 5-20 mg every 4-8 hours; children 0.5-1 mg a day.
Availability: NHS and private prescription.
Side effects: muscle spasms, restlessness, hands shaking, dry mouth,
urine retention, palpitations, low blood pressure, weight gain, changes in
sexual function, low body temperature, breast swelling, menstrual
changes, jaundice, blood and skin changes, drowsiness, rarely fits.
Caution: in pregnant women, nursing mothers and in patients suffering
from severe liver disease, shaking and stiffness, Parkinson's disease,
epilepsy.
Not to be used for: unconscious patients or patients suffering from
severe clinical depression.
Caution needed with: alcohol, sedatives, tranquillizers, pain killers,

blood-pressure lowering drugs, antidepressants, anticonvulsants, antidiabetic drugs, LEVODOPA.
Contains: DROPERIDOL.
Other preparations: Droleptan Liquid, Droleptan Injection.

droperidol *see* Droleptan

Dryptal *see* frusemide tablets
(Berk)

Dubam
(Norma)

An aerosol used as a topical ANALGESIC to relieve muscular pain.

Dose: spray on to the affected area for 2 seconds up to 4 times a day.
Availability: private prescription, over the counter.
Side effects: may be irritant.
Caution:
Not to be used for: areas near the eyes, or on broken or inflamed skin, or on mucous membranes (such as the mouth).
Caution needed with:
Contains: GLYCOL SALICYLATE, METHYL SALICYLATE, ETHYL SALICYLATE, METHYL NICOTINATE.
Other preparations: Dubam Cream.

Dulco-Lax *see* bisacodyl tablets
(Boehringer Ingelheim)

Dumicoat
(Dumex)

An antifungal denture lacquer used to treat fungal dental infections.

Dose: clean, disinfect, and dry the upper denture, then apply the contents of 1 bottle to upper surface and allow to dry. Repeat once a week.
Availability: NHS and private prescription.
Side effects:
Caution:
Not to be used for: children.
Caution needed with:
Contains: MICONAZOLE.

Other preparations: DAKTARIN ORAL GEL.

___

Duofilm
(Stiefel)

A liquid used as a skin softener to treat warts.

Dose: apply the liquid to the wart once a day, allow to dry, and cover, rubbing down between applications.
Availability: NHS, private prescription, over the counter.
Side effects:
Caution: do not apply to healthy skin.
Not to be used for: warts on the face or anal and genital areas.
Caution needed with:
Contains: SALICYLIC ACID, LACTIC ACID.
Other preparations: CUPLEX, SALACTOL, SALATAC.

___

Duovent
(Boehringer Ingelheim)

An aerosol used as a BRONCHODILATOR to treat blocked airways.

Dose: adults 1-2 sprays 3-4 times a day; children over 6 years 1 spray 3 times a day.
Availability: NHS and private prescription.
Side effects: headache, dry mouth, dilation of the blood vessels.
Caution: in patients suffering from glaucoma, enlarged prostate, high blood pressure,overactive thyroid gland, heart muscle disease, angina, abnormal heart rhythms.
Not to be used for: children under 6 years.
Caution needed with: SYMPATHOMIMETICS.
Contains: FENOTEROL hydrobromide, IPRATROPIUM bromide.
Other preparations: Duovent Autohaler (breath-actuated device), Duovent UDVs (solution for nebulization).

___

Duphalac *see* lactulose solution
(Solvay Healthcare)

___

Duphaston
(Solvay Healthcare)

A white, scored tablet supplied at a strength of 10 mg and used as a progestogen to treat period pain, habitual and threatened abortion, endometriosis (a womb disorder), infertility, premenstrual syndrome, and as an additional treatment to oestrogen in hormone replacement.

Dose: period pain 1 tablet twice a day from the fifth to the twenty-fifth day of the cycle; endometriosis 1 tablet 2-3 times a day from the fifth to the twenty-fifth day or continuously; premenstrual syndrome 1 tablet twice a day from the twelfth to the twenty-sixth day; hormone replacement 1-2 tablets a day for the last 14 days of the cycle.
Availability: NHS and private prescription.
Side effects: irregular bleeding, breast discomfort, acne, headache, bloating, dizziness, skin disorder.
Caution: in patients suffering from high blood pressure or tendency to thrombosis, migraine, liver abnormalities, ovarian cysts.
Not to be used for: children, pregnant women, women having suffered a previous ectopic pregnancy, or for patients suffering from severe heart or kidney disease, benign liver tumours, undiagnosed vaginal bleeding.
Caution needed with: BARBITURATES, PHENYTOIN, PRIMIDONE, CARBAMAZEPINE, CHLORAL HYDRATE, ETHOSUXIMIDE, RIFAMPICIN, MEPROBAMATE, GRISEOFULVIN.
Contains: DYDROGESTERONE.
Other preparations: DUPHASTON-HRT (packed specifically for hormone replacement treatment).

Duphaston-HRT *see* Duphaston
(Solvay Healthcare)

Duragel
(LRC)

A spermicidal gel (applicator available) used with barrier methods as a means of contraception.

Dose: apply to the barrier device before intercourse.
Availability: NHS, private prescription, over the counter.
Side effects: possibly allergy.
Caution:
Not to be used for: children.
Caution needed with:
Contains: NONOXYNOL-9.
Other preparations: GYNOL-II.

Durogesic
(Janssen-Cilag)

A skin patch supplied at strengths of 25, 50, 75, 100 micrograms and used as an opiate ANALGESIC to control severe chronic pain.

Dose: as advised by physician; apply to non-hairy areas of chest or upper arm, and replace the patch every 72 hours.
Availability: controlled drug; NHS, private prescription.
Side effects: breathing difficulties, constipation, low blood pressure, sleepiness, hallucinations, nausea, excitement, itch, retention of urine, tolerance, dependence.
Caution: in the elderly or debilitated, and in patients suffering from breathing difficulty, chronic lung disease, raised brain pressure, brain tumour, slow and irregular heartbeat, kidney or liver damage, fever, or patients exposed to direct heat. Used patches should be disposed of carefully.
Not to be used for: children, pregnant women, nursing mothers, or to control acute pain.
Caution needed with: sedatives.
Contains: FENTANYL.
Other preparations:

Duromine
(3M Health Care)

A grey/green capsule or a grey/maroon capsule according to strengths of 15 mg, 30 mg and used as an appetite suppressant to treat obesity.

Dose: 15-30 mg once a day at breakfast.
Availability: controlled drug; NHS and private prescription.
Side effects: tolerance, addictions, mental disturbances, restlessness, nervousness, agitation, dry mouth, heart palpitations, raised blood pressure, fluid retention, hallucinations.
Caution: do not use for prolonged treatments. Care in patients suffering from high blood pressure, angina, abnormal heart rhythm.
Not to be used for: children, pregnant women, nursing mothers, or for patients suffering from hardening of the arteries, overactive thyroid gland, severe high blood pressure, or with a history of mental illness, alcoholism or drug addiction.
Caution needed with: MAOIS, SYMPATHOMIMETICS, METHYLDOPA, GUANETHIDINE, other appetite suppressants, antidepressants, tranquillizers.
Contains: PHENTERMINE.
Other preparations: IONAMIN.

Dutonin
(Bristol-Meyers Squibb)

A white, hexagonal, scored tablet or a yellow, hexagonal, scored tablet according to strengths of 100 mg and 200 mg, and used as an antidepressant to treat depression with anxiety or disturbed sleep.

Dose: 100 mg twice a day at first increasing to 200 mg twice a day after 5-7 days, up to a maximum of 300 mg twice a day; elderly maximum 100-200 mg twice a day.
Availability: NHS, private prescription.
Side effects: weakness, dry mouth, sleepiness, nausea, dizziness, chills, fever, low blood pressure on standing, constipation, confusion, shaking and unsteadiness, impaired eyesight, pins and needles.
Caution: in pregnant women, nursing mothers, and in patients suffering from mania, hypomania, epilepsy, liver or kidney failure, or who are undergoing electric shock treatment.
Not to be used for: persons under 18.
Caution needed with: other antidepressants, BENZODIAZEPINES, LITHIUM, HALOPERIDOL, MAOIS, blood-pressure lowering drugs, general anaesthetics, alcohol, SUMATRIPTAN.
Contains: NEFAZODONE hydrochloride.
Other preparations:

Dyazide see co-triamterzide tablets
(SmithKline Beecham)

---

dydrogesterone *see* **Duphaston, Duphaston-HRT, Femoston**

Dynamin *see* **isosorbide mononitrate tablets**
(Berk)

Dysman *see* **mefenamic acid capsules**
(Ashbourne)

Dyspamet *see* **cimetidine tablets**
(SmithKline Beecham)

Dytac
(Pharmark)

A maroon capsule supplied at a strength of 50 mg and used as a potassium-sparing DIURETIC to treat fluid retention especially when associated with congestive heart failure, liver or kidney disease.

Dose: 3-5 capsules a day in divided doses for 7 days, and then usually every other day.
Availability: NHS and private prescription.
Side effects: nausea, diarrhoea, cramps, weakness, headache, dry mouth, rash, blood changes, reversible kidney failure.
Caution: in pregnant women, nursing mothers, and in patients suffering from kidney or liver disease, gout, electrolyte changes, diabetes.
Not to be used for: children or for patients suffering from raised potassium levels, or progressive kidney or liver failure, Addison's disease (a disease of the adrenal glands).
Caution needed with: potassium supplements, some diuretics, blood-pressure lowering drugs, INDOMETHACIN, ACE INHIBITORS.
Contains: TRIAMTERENE.
Other preparations:

Dytide
(Pharmark)

E

A clear/maroon capsule used as a potassium-sparing DIURETIC to treat fluid retention.

Dose: 2 capsules after breakfast and 1 capsule after lunch at first, then 1 or 2 capsules every other day.
Availability: NHS and private prescription.
Side effects: nausea, diarrhoea, cramps, weakness, headache, dry mouth, rash, blood changes, reversible kidney failure.
Caution: in pregnant women, nursing mothers, and in patients suffering from liver or kidney disease, diabetes, or gout.
Not to be used for: children, or for patients suffering from raised potassium levels, or progressive or severe kidney failure, progressive liver failure, raised calcium levels, Addison's disease (a disease of the adrenal glands), ketoacidosis in diabetes.
Caution needed with: potassium supplements, some diuretics, LITHIUM, DIGOXIN, blood-pressure lowering drugs, INDOMETHACIN, ACE INHIBITORS.
Contains: TRIAMTERENE, BENZTHIAZIDE.
Other preparations:

Ebufac *see* ibuprofen tablets
(DDSA)

Econacort
(Squibb)

A cream used as a STEROID, antifungal, and antibacterial treatment for skin infections where there is also inflammation.

Dose: massage into the affected area night and morning.
Availability: NHS and private prescription.
Side effects: fluid retention, suppression of adrenal glands, thinning, spotting, or streaking of the skin may occur.
Caution: use for short periods of time only, especially on the face or in children.
Not to be used for: patients suffering from acne or any other skin infections caused by tuberculosis, ringworm, viruses, or fungi, leg ulcers, scabies, or continuously especially in pregnant women.
Caution needed with:
Contains: ECONAZOLE nitrate, HYDROCORTISONE.
Other preparations:

---

econazole *see* Econacort, Ecostatin, Ecostatin-1, Gyno-Pevaryl 1, Pevaryl

---

Economycin *see* tetracycline tablets
(DDSA)

Ecostatin
(Squibb)

A cream used as an antifungal, antibacterial treatment for fungal infections of the skin, and some bacterial infections.

Dose: apply to the affected area night and morning.
Availability: NHS, private prescription, over the counter.
Side effects:
Caution: avoid the eyes.
Not to be used for:
Caution needed with:
Contains: ECONAZOLE nitrate.
Other preparations: PEVARYL.

Ecostatin-1
(Squibb)

A pessary plus applicator supplied at a strength of 150 mg and used as an antifungal and antibacterial treatment for thrush of the vulva or vagina. (This product may be purchased without prescription only for the treatment of vaginal thrush.)

Dose: 1 pessary inserted into the vagina at bed time.
Availability: NHS, private prescription, over the counter (*see* above).
Side effects: mild burning or irritation.
Caution: when using applicator in pregnancy.
Not to be used for: children.
Caution needed with:
Contains: ECONAZOLE nitrate.
Other preparations: Ecostatin Pessaries, Ecostatin Cream, Ecostatin Twinpack. GYNO-PEVARYL.

Edecrin
(M.S.D.)

A white, scored tablet supplied at a strength of 50 mg and used as a DIURETIC to treat fluid retention including that associated with congestive heart failure, or kidney or liver disease.

Dose: adults 1 tablet a day after breakfast at first, increasing by ½-1 tablet a day until the minimum effective dose usually of 1-3 tablets a day is found to a maximum of 8 in 2 divided doses; children 2-12 years ½ tablet a day after breakfast, then increasing by ½ tablet a day to the minimum effective dose.
Availability: NHS and private prescription.
Side effects: stomach upset, gout, jaundice, blood changes.
Caution: in pregnant women, and in patients suffering from liver disease, diabetes, enlarged prostate, impaired urination, or gout.
Not to be used for: infants, nursing mothers, or for patients suffering from cirrhosis of the liver, or severe kidney failure, failure of urination.
Caution needed with: LITHIUM, WARFARIN, DIGOXIN, blood-pressure lowering drugs, some antibiotics, CORTICOSTEROIDS, ACETAZOLAMIDE, DICHLORPHENAMIDE.
Contains: ETHACRYNIC ACID.
Other preparations: Edecrin Injection.

Efalith
(Scotia)

An anti-inflammatory ointment used to treat seborrhoeic dermatitis.

Dose: apply thinly and evenly twice a day. Rub in gently.
Availability: NHS and private prescription.
Side effects: irritation.
Caution: in patients suffering from psoriasis. Avoid eyes and mucous membranes.
Not to be used for: children.
Caution needed with:

Contains: LITHIUM SUCCINATE, ZINC SULPHATE.
Other preparations:

Efamast
(Searle)

An oblong, soft capsule supplied at a strength of 40 mg and used to treat breast pain.

Dose: 3-4 capsules twice a day.
Availability: NHS and private prescription.
Side effects: nausea, diarrhoea, headache.
Caution: in patients suffering from epilepsy. Your doctor may suggest detailed breast examination before starting treatment.
Not to be used for: children.
Caution needed with:
Contains: GAMOLENIC ACID.
Other preparations: EPOGAM (used for eczema). Low-strength food supplements containing gamolenic acid are available over the counter (e.g. evening primrose oil, starflower oil).

Efcortelan *see* hydrocortisone cream
(Glaxo)

Efexor
(Wyeth)

A peach-coloured, shield-shaped tablet supplied at strengths of 37.5 mg, 50 mg, 75 mg, and used as an antidepressant to treat depression.

Dose: 37.5 mg twice a day with food increasing if necessary after several weeks to 150 mg a day; severe depression 75 mg twice a day at first increasing to 375 mg a day; reduce according to response.
Availability: NHS, private prescription.
Side effects: nausea, headache, dizziness, constipation, sleeplessness or drowsiness, sweating, low blood pressure on standing, constipation, shaking and unsteadiness, nervousness, impotence, liver changes.
Caution: in patients suffering from liver or kidney damage, or with a history of epilepsy, heart attack, or heart disease, drug abuse. Your doctor will advise regular blood pressure checks and re-evaluation of therapy. Withdraw gradually.
Not to be used for: children, pregnant women, nursing mothers.
Caution needed with: sedatives, MAOIS.
Contains: VENLAFAXINE.

Other preparations:

Effercitrate
(Typharm)

A white, effervescent tablet used as an alkalizing agent to treat cystitis.

Dose: adults and children over 6 years 2 tablets dissolved in water up to 3 times a day with meals; children 1-6 years half adult dose.
Availability: NHS, private prescription, over the counter.
Side effects: raised potassium levels, stomach irritation, mild increase in fluid output.
Caution: in patients suffering from kidney disease.
Not to be used for: infants under 1 year or for patients suffering from ulcerated or blocked small bowel.
Caution needed with: some DIURETICS.
Contains: CITRIC ACID, POTASSIUM CITRATE.
Other preparations: Potassium Citrate Mixture.

---

eicosapentaenoic acid *see* Maxepa

Elantan *see* isosorbide mononitrate tablets
(Schwarz)

Elavil *see* amitriptyline tablets
(DDSA)

Eldepryl *see* selegiline tablets
(Orion Pharma)

Electrolade *see* Dioralyte
(Eastern)

Elocon
(Schering Plough)

An ointment, lotion, or cream used as a strong STEROID treatment for psoriasis and dermatitis.

Dose: apply sparingly to the affected area once a day. Treatment for

children should not last longer than 5 days.
Availability: NHS, private prescription.
Side effects: thinning, spotting, and streaking of the skin, suppression of the adrenal glands, flushing, hair growth.
Caution: in infants, especially if wearing nappies or plastic pants. Do not use on children or on the face for more than 5 days. If used for psoriasis, regular checks are needed. Withdraw slowly after prolonged use.
Not to be used for: prolonged use in pregnant women, for long-term prevention, or for patients suffering from chicken pox, shingles, tuberculosis, syphilis, acne, scabies, leg ulcers, skin disorders around the mouth, or for infected skin conditions.
Caution needed with:
Contains: MOMETASONE FUROATE.
Other preparations:

Eltroxin *see* thyroxine tablets
(Goldshield Healthcare)

Eludril
(Chefaro)

A solution used as an antibacterial treatment for throat and mouth infections, gingivitis, ulcers.

Dose: dilute 10-15 ml with a-third of a glass of warm water and gargle or rinse the mouth 2-3 times a day.
Availability: NHS, private prescription, over the counter.
Side effects:
Caution:
Not to be used for: children under 6 years.
Caution needed with:
Contains: CHLORHEXIDINE digluconate, CHLORBUTOL.
Other preparations: Eludril Spray (not suitable for children).

Elyzol
(Dumex)

A gel in a disposable applicator used as an antibacterial preparation in addition to other treatments for gum disease.

Dose: fill pocket around tooth with gel and repeat treatment after 1 week. Do not repeat treatment for at least 6 months.
Availability: NHS, private prescription.
Side effects: headache, irritation.

Caution: in pregnant women.
Not to be used for: children.
Caution needed with: ANTICOAGULANTS taken by mouth, alcohol, DISULFIRAM.
Contains: METRONIDAZOLE.
Other preparations: METRONIDAZOLE TABLETS.

Emblon *see* tamoxifen tablets
(Berk)

Emcor
(Merck)

An orange, heart-shaped tablet supplied at a strength of 10 mg and used as a ß-BLOCKER to treat angina, high blood pressure.

Dose: 10 mg once a day to a maximum of 20 mg a day.
Availability: NHS and private prescription.
Side effects: cold hands and feet, sleep disturbance, slow heart rate, tiredness, wheezing, heart failure, low blood pressure, stomach upset, dry eyes, rash.
Caution: in pregnant women, nursing mothers, and in patients suffering from diabetes, kidney or liver disorders, asthma. May need to be withdrawn before surgery. Withdraw gradually. Your doctor may advise additional treatment with DIURETICS or DIGOXIN.
Not to be used for: children, or for patients suffering from heart block or failure, low blood pressure, untreated PHAEOCHROMOCYTOMA.
Caution needed with: VERAPAMIL, CLONIDINE withdrawal, some anti-arrhythmic drugs and anaesthetics, some blood-pressure lowering drugs, ERGOTAMINE, CIMETIDINE, sedatives, SYMPATHOMIMETICS, INDOMETHACIN, antidiabetics, RESERPINE.
Contains: BISOPROLOL FUMARATE.
Other preparations: Emcor LS, MONOCOR.

Emeside
(L.A.B.)

An orange capsule supplied at a strength of 250 mg and used as an anticonvulsant to treat epilepsy.

Dose: adults 2 capsules a day at first, increasing by 1 capsule a day every 5-7 days to a maximum of 8 capsules a day; children under 6 years 1 capsule a day at first increasing gradually to a maximum of 4 capsules a day, 6-12 years as adult dose.
Availability: NHS and private prescription.

E

Side effects: stomach and brain disturbances, rash, blood changes,
LUPUS.
Caution: in pregnant women, nursing mothers, and in patients suffering
from kidney or liver disease. Dose should be reduced gradually.
Not to be used for:
Caution needed with:
Contains: ETHOSUXIMIDE.
Other preparations: Emeside Syrup. ZARONTIN.

Emflex
(Merck)

A yellow/orange capsule supplied at a strength of 60 mg and used to treat
rheumatoid arthritis, osteoarthritis, low back pain, pain and inflammation
after operation.

Dose: 2-3 capsules a day in divided doses, with food, milk, or ANTACID.
Availability: NHS and private prescription.
Side effects: stomach upset, headache, dizziness, fluid retention, chest
pain, itching, blood changes, noises in the ears, blurred vision.
Caution: in patients suffering from psychiatric disorder, epilepsy,
Parkinson's disease, liver or kidney disorder, congestive heart failure,
some infections, body fluid imbalance, and in elderly patients. Your doctor
may advise regular examinations.
Not to be used for: children, pregnant women, nursing mothers, or for
patients suffering from stomach ulcer, allergy to ASPIRIN or anti-
inflammatory drugs, severe allergy, or with a history of a stomach/intestinal
disorder.
Caution needed with: ANTICOAGULANTS, some painkillers, PROBENECID,
LITHIUM, TRIAMTERENE, ACE INHIBITORS, HALOPERIDOL, METHOTREXATE, ß-BLOCKERS,
some DIURETICS, some antibiotics.
Contains: ACEMETACIN.
Other preparations:

EMLA
(Astra)

A cream used as a topical anaesthetic for skin and genital areas before
surgical procedures.

Dose: small areas, apply 2 g for 1-5 hours under a dressing; large areas,
apply 1.5-3 g/10 sq. cm for 2-5 hours under a dressing; for genital warts
apply 10 g for 5-10 minutes before surgery.
Availability: NHS, private prescription.
Side effects: temporary skin reactions.

Caution:
Not to be used for: infants, or on wounds, mucous membranes, or for patients suffering from allergic skin disorders.
Caution needed with:
Contains: LIGNOCAINE, PRILOCAINE.
Other preparations:

Emulsiderm *see* Diprobath
(Dermal)

---

emulsifying ointment BP

An ointment used as an emollient to treat dry skin conditions.

Dose: apply as required, or use in place of soap.
Availability: NHS, private prescription, over the counter.
Side effects:
Caution:
Not to be used for:
Caution needed with:
Contains: emulsifying ointment BP.
Other preparations:

En-De-Kay Daily fluoride mouth rinse
(Stafford-Miller)

A blue-coloured mouth rinse used as a fluoride supplement to strengthen tooth enamel to resist decay.

Dose: rinse with 10 ml of rinse for 1 minute each day and then spit out.
Availability: NHS, private prescription, over the counter. (Not available from dentists on NHS.)
Side effects: occasional white flecks on teeth.
Caution: do not swallow; avoid eating, drinking, or rinsing mouth for 15 minutes afterwards. Do not exceed recommended dose.
Not to be used for: children under 6 years, or in areas where drinking water is fluoridated.
Caution needed with:
Contains: SODIUM FLUORIDE.
Other preparations: EN-DE-KAY FLUORINSE. FLUORIGARD DENTAL RINSE.

En-De-Kay Fluorinse
(Stafford-Miller)

A red-coloured mouth rinse used as a fluoride supplement to strengthen tooth enamel to resist decay.

Dose: for daily use dilute 5 drops in 10 ml water, rinse mouth with solution and spit out; for weekly use dilute 20 drops in 10 ml water, rinse, and spit out.
Availability: NHS, private prescription. (Not available from dentists on NHS.)
Side effects: occasional white flecks on teeth.
Caution: do not swallow; avoid eating, drinking, or rinsing mouth for 15 minutes afterwards. Do not exceed recommended dose.
Not to be used for: children under 8 years, or in areas where drinking water is fluoridated.
Caution needed with:
Contains: SODIUM FLUORIDE.
Other preparations: EN-DE-KAY DAILY FLUORIDE MOUTHRINSE. FLUORIGARD DENTAL RINSE.

En-De-Kay Fluodrops
(Stafford-Miller)

Sugar-free drops used as a fluoride supplement for children to strengthen tooth enamel to resist decay.

Dose: children under 2 years 0-7 drops, 2-4 years 7-14 drops, over 4 years 14-28 drops once a day (depending on fluoride content of drinking water).
Availability: NHS, private prescription, over the counter.
Side effects: occasional white flecks on teeth.
Caution: do not exceed recommended dose.
Not to be used for: children in areas where drinking water is fluoridated above 0.7 ppm.
Caution needed with:
Contains: SODIUM FLUORIDE.
Other preparations: EN-DE-KAY FLUOTABS, FLUOR-A-DAY TABLETS, FLUORIGARD DROPS.

En-De-Kay Fluotabs
(Stafford-Miller)

An orange-flavoured tablet available in 2 strengths for ages 2-4 years and over 4 years, and used as a fluoride supplement to strengthen tooth enamel to resist decay.

Dose: ½-1 tablet sucked or dissolved in the mouth, preferably in the evening. (Dose depends on age and water fluoride content.)
Availability: NHS, private prescription, over the counter.
Side effects: occasional white flecks on teeth.
Caution: do not exceed recommended dose.
Not to be used for: patients in areas where drinking water is fluoridated above 0.7 ppm.
Contains: SODIUM FLUORIDE.
Other preparations: EN-DE-KAY FLUODROPS, FLUOR-A-DAY TABLETS, FLUORIGARD DROPS.

---

enalapril maleate *see* Innovace, Innozide

Engerix B
(Smith, Kline & French)

An injection supplied in prefilled vials or syringes and used as a vaccine to provide active immunization against hepatitis B.

Dose: adults 1 ml (children 0.5 ml) by injection repeated 1 month and 6 months later.
Availability: NHS, private prescription.
Side effects: temporary local soreness, mild fever, nausea, dizziness, general feeling of being unwell, reddening or hardening of the skin at the injection site.
Caution: in pregnant women and in patients with reduced immunity or who undergo dialysis.
Not to be used for: patients suffering from severe feverish illness.
Caution needed with:
Contains: HEPATITIS B antigen.
Other preparations: H-B-VAX.

Epanutin *see* phenytoin tablets
(Parke-Davis)

---

ephedrine *see* CAM, ephedrine nasal drops BP, Franol, Haymine

---

ephedrine nasal drops BP

Drops, available in 2 strengths, and used to treat congestion in the nose.

Dose: 1-2 drops in each nostril 3-4 times a day when required.
Availability: NHS, private prescription, over the counter.
Side effects: irritation, congestion, and less effect after excessive use.
Caution: in infants under 3 months. Avoid excessive use.
Not to be used for:
Caution needed with:
Contains: EPHEDRINE hydrochloride.
Other preparations:

Epifoam
(Stafford-Miller)

A foam supplied in an aerosol and used as a STEROID, local anaesthetic treatment for damage to the external genital area.

Dose: apply foam 3-4 times a day with a sterile, non-absorbent pad for up to 7 days.
Availability: NHS and private prescription.
Side effects: fluid retention, suppression of adrenal glands, thinning of skin may occur.
Caution: use for short periods of time only.
Not to be used for: patients suffering from infected wounds, or continuously especially in pregnant women.
Caution needed with:
Contains: HYDROCORTISONE acetate, PRAMOXINE hydrochloride.
Other preparations:

Epilim *see* sodium valproate tablets
(Sanofi Winthrop)

Epipen *see* Min-i-jet adrenaline
(Allerayde)

epoetin alfa *see* Eprex

epoetin beta *see* Recormon

Epogam
(Searle)

An oil-filled capsule supplied at a strength of 40 mg and used to relieve the symptoms of eczema.

Dose: adults 4-6 capsules twice a day; children over 1 year, 2-4 capsules twice a day.
Availability: NHS and private prescription.
Side effects: nausea, headache.
Caution: in patients suffering from epilepsy.
Not to be used for: children under 1 year.
Caution needed with:
Contains: GAMOLENIC ACID.
Other preparations: Epogam Paediatric (higher-strength product designed to be emptied on to food), EFAMAST (used for breast disorders). Low-strength food supplements containing gamolenic acid are available over the counter – e.g. evening primrose oil, starflower oil.

Eppy
(Chauvin)

Drops used as a SYMPATHOMIMETIC to treat glaucoma.

Dose: 1 drop into the eye 1-2 times a day.
Availability: NHS, private prescription.
Side effects: pain in the eye, headache, skin reactions, red eye, rarely SYMPATHOMIMETIC effects.
Caution:
Not to be used for: children, or for patients suffering from absence of the lens, narrow-angle glaucoma.
Caution needed with: MAOIs, TRICYCLIC ANTIDEPRESSANTS
Contains: ADRENALINE.
Other preparations: SIMPLENE.

Eprex
(Janssen-Cilag)

An injection supplied in prefilled syringes and used as a hormone treatment for anaemia associated with chronic kidney failure.

Dose: as advised by your physician.
Availability: NHS, private prescription.
Side effects: raised blood pressure, headache, blood clots, fits, skin reactions, flu-like symptoms.
Caution: in pregnant women and in patients suffering from raised blood pressure, reduced blood flow, or with a history of epilepsy or liver failure. Other forms of anaemia should be corrected, and diet or any dialysis may need correcting. Blood pressure should be monitored throughout

treatment.
Not to be used for: patients suffering from uncontrolled raised blood
pressure.
Caution needed with: CYCLOSPORIN.
Contains: EPOETIN ALFA.
Other preparations:

Equagesic
(Wyeth)

A pink/white/yellow tablet used as an opiate, ANALGESIC, and muscle
relaxant to control pain in muscles or bones.

Dose: 2 tablets 3-4 times a day.
Availability: controlled drug; private prescription only.
Side effects: drowsiness, dizziness, nausea, unsteadiness, rash, blood
changes, low blood pressure, excitement, allergy, stomach bleeding, pins
and needles.
Caution: in the elderly and in patients with a history of epilepsy, or
suffering from depression, suicidal behaviour, or liver or kidney disease,
heart failure.
Not to be used for: children, pregnant women, nursing mothers, or for
patients suffering from PORPHYRIA, alcoholism, stomach ulcer, haemophilia,
kidney failure, allergy to anti-inflammatory drugs or ASPIRIN.
Caution needed with: alcohol, sedatives, ANTICOAGULANTS, antidiabetics,
uric acid-lowering agents, PHENYTOIN, GRISEOFULVIN, RIFAMPICIN, STEROIDS, the
contraceptive pill, TRICYCLIC ANTIDEPRESSANTS, tranquillizers.
Contains: ETHOHEPTAZINE, MEPROBAMATE, ASPIRIN.
Other preparations:

Equanil
(Wyeth)

A white tablet or a white, scored tablet according to strengths of 200 mg,
400 mg and used as a tranquillizer for short-term treatment of anxiety,
muscular tension.

Dose: elderly 200 mg 3 times a day; adults 400 mg 3 times a day and
before going to bed.
Availability: controlled drug; NHS and private prescription.
Side effects: brain and stomach disturbances, low blood pressure, pins
and needles, allergy, excitement, blood disorders.
Caution: in patients with a history of epilepsy or depression, or patients
suffering from liver or kidney disease, weak muscles. Patients should be
warned that the drug is addictive and that it will interfere with judgement

and manual ability.
Not to be used for: children, pregnant women, nursing mothers, alcoholics or for patients suffering from acute intermittent PORPHYRIA.
Caution needed with: alcohol, sedatives, ANTICOAGULANTS, PHENYTOIN, GRISEOFULVIN, RIFAMPICIN, STEROIDS taken by mouth, the contraceptive pill, TRICYCLIC ANTIDEPRESSANTS, tranquillizers.
Contains: MEPROBAMATE.
Other preparations: MEPRATE.

Eradacin
(Sanofi Winthrop)

A red/yellow capsule supplied at a strength of 150 mg and used as an antibiotic to treat acute gonorrhoea.

Dose: 2 capsules as a single dose.
Availability: NHS and private prescription.
Side effects: stomach upset, headache, dizziness, drowsiness.
Caution: in pregnant women and in patients suffering from liver or kidney disease.
Not to be used for: children.
Caution needed with: alcohol, sedatives.
Contains: ACROSOXACIN.
Other preparations:

---

ergocalciferol *see* calcium and ergocalciferol tablets, vitamin D

---

ergotamine tartrate *see* Cafergot, Lingraine, Medihaler-Ergotamine, Migril

---

Ervevax *see* rubella vaccine
(Smith Kline & French)

Erycen *see* erythromycin tablets
(Berk)

Erymax *see* erythromycin tablets
(Elan)

Erythrocin *see* **erythromycin tablets**
(Abbott)

---

erythromycin *see* **Benzamycin, Erycen, Erymax, Erythrocin, erythromycin tablets, Erythroped, Retcin, Rommix, Stiemycin, Tiloryth, Zineryt**

---

erythromycin tablets

A tablet supplied at strengths of 250 mg, 500 mg and used as an antibiotic, especially where there is sensitivity to penicillin, to treat infections such as legionnaire's disease, infections of the respiratory and urinary tract, and acne.

Dose: adults and childen over 8 years 1-2 g a day. Dose may be double in severe infections. (Children under 8 years use reduced dose in the form of mixture.)
Availability: NHS and private prescription.
Side effects: stomach disturbances, allergies. Large doses may cause reversible loss of hearing. Prolonged use may rarely cause jaundice.
Caution: in nursing mothers, and in patients suffering from liver or kidney disease, PORPHYRIA, or some heart rhythm disturbances.
Not to be used for:
Caution needed with: THEOPHYLLINE, DISOPYRAMIDE, ANTICOAGULANTS taken by mouth, CARBAMAZEPINE, DIGOXIN, TERFENADINE, ASTEMIZOLE, CIMETIDINE, CYCLOSPORIN, ERGOTAMINE.
Contains: ERYTHROMYCIN.
Other preparations: erythromycin mixture. ARPIMYCIN, ERYCEN, ERYMAX, ERYTHROPED, ERYTHROPED A, ERYTHROCIN, ILOSONE, RETCIN, ROMMIX, TILORYTH. (Some available in capsule form.)

Erythroped *see* **erythromycin tablets**
(Abbott)

Eskamel
(Goldshield Healthcare)

A cream used as a skin softener to treat acne.

Dose: apply a little to the affected area once a day.
Availability: NHS, private prescription, over the counter.
Side effects: irritation.
Caution: keep out of the eyes, nose, and mouth.

Not to be used for: patients suffering from acute infection in the skin.
Caution needed with:
Contains: RESORCINOL, SULPHUR.
Other preparations:

Eskazole
(SmithKline Beecham)

An orange, rounded, oblong, scored tablet supplied at a strength of 400 mg and used to treat hydatid cysts (an infection from contaminated food).

Dose: adults over 60 kg bodyweight 2 tablets a day in divided doses for 28 days, followed by 14 days without treatment. Maximum of 3 cycles of treatment.
Availability: NHS and private prescription.
Side effects: stomach upset, headache, dizziness, hair loss, rash, fever, blood and liver changes.
Caution: women of child-bearing age must use non-hormonal contraceptive measures during treatment and for 1 month afterwards. Your doctor may advise regular liver and blood tests.
Not to be used for: children, adults under 60 kg, pregnant women, women who may become pregnant.
Caution needed with:
Contains: ALBENDAZOLE
Other preparations:

E

Estracombi
(Ciba)

Circular and goggle-shaped patches used as an oestrogen/progestogen hormone-replacement therapy to treat symptoms of menopause and to prevent osteoporosis after menopause.

Dose: apply circular patch twice a week for 2 weeks, followed by goggle-shaped patch twice a week for 2 weeks. Patches should be applied to clean, non-hairy areas of skin below the waste; each patch to be replaced every 3-4 days and the new patch applied to a different area.
Availability: NHS, private prescription.
Side effects: enlarged breasts, fluid retention, nausea, vaginal bleeding, weight gain, headache, dizziness. Rarely jaundice, raised blood pressure, thrombosis.
Caution: in patients suffering from high blood pressure, diabetes, epilepsy, womb diseases, gall bladder disorder, migraine, multiple sclerosis, PORPHYRIA, liver disorders, some ear disorders, or a history or increased risk of breast disorders (including cancer) and thrombosis. Your

doctor may advise you to have regular examinations.
Not to be used for: children, pregnant women, nursing mothers, or for patients suffering from thombosis, severe liver, kidney, or heart disorders, some cancers, undiagnosed vaginal bleeding, endometriosis.
Caution needed with: ACE INHIBITORS, ANTICOAGULANTS, BARBITURATES, ß-BLOCKERS, CARBAMAZEPINE, PHENYTOIN, RIFAMPICIN.
Contains: OESTRADIOL, NORETHISTERONE.
Other preparations: EVOREL-PAK, TRISEQUENS.

Estraderm
(Ciba)

A patch supplied at strengths of 25 micrograms, 50 micrograms, 100 micrograms and used as an oestrogen in oestrogen replacement therapy during the menopause. (Estraderm 50 used to prevent osteoporosis.)

Dose: apply a 50 microgram patch at first to a clean, hairless area of skin below the waist and replace with a new patch every 3-4 days on a different place. (For menopausal symptoms, adjust the dose as needed after 1 month to a maximum of 100 micrograms a day.)
Availability: NHS and private prescription.
Side effects: enlarged breasts, fluid retention, nausea, vaginal bleeding, weight gain, headache, dizziness. Rarely jaundice, raised blood pressure, thrombosis.
Caution: in patients suffering from high blood pressure, diabetes, epilepsy, womb diseases, gall bladder disorder, migraine, multiple sclerosis, PORPHYRIA, liver disorders, some ear disorders, or a history or increased risk of breast disorders (including cancer) and thrombosis. Your doctor may advise you to have regular examinations.
Not to be used for: children, pregnant women, nursing mothers, or for patients suffering from thombosis, severe liver, kidney, or heart disorders, some cancers, undiagnosed vaginal bleeding, endometriosis.
Caution needed with: ACE INHIBITORS, ANTICOAGULANTS, BARBITURATES, ß-BLOCKERS, CARBAMAZEPINE, PHENYTOIN, RIFAMPICIN.
Contains: OESTRADIOL.
Other preparations: CLIMAVAL, EVOREL, FEMATRIX, MENOREST, OESTROGEL, PROGYNOVA, ZUMENON.

Estrapak
(Ciba)

A patch plus a red tablet supplied at strengths of 50 microgram and 1 mg respectively and used as oestrogen and progestogen in hormone replacement.

Dose: place patch on a clean, hairless are of skin below the waist and replace with a new patch every 3-4 days on a different area. 1 tablet a day from the fifteenth to the twenty-sixth days of each 28 days of oestrogen replacement. Start the treatment on the fifth day of the period if present.
Availability: NHS and private prescription.
Side effects: enlarged breasts, fluid retention, nausea, vaginal bleeding, weight gain, headache, dizziness. Rarely jaundice, raised blood pressure, thrombosis.
Caution: in patients suffering from high blood pressure, diabetes, epilepsy, womb diseases, gall bladder disorder, migraine, multiple sclerosis, PORPHYRIA, liver disorders, some ear disorders, or a history or increased risk of breast disorders (including cancer) and thrombosis. Your doctor may advise you to have regular examinations.
Not to be used for: children, pregnant women, nursing mothers, or for patients suffering from thombosis, severe liver, kidney, or heart disorders, some cancers, undiagnosed vaginal bleeding, endometriosis.
Caution needed with: ACE INHIBITORS, ANTICOAGULANTS, BARBITURATES, ß-BLOCKERS, CARBAMAZEPINE, PHENYTOIN, RIFAMPICIN.
Contains: OESTRADIOL, NORETHISTERONE.
Other preparations: ESTRACOMBI, EVOREL-PAK, TRISEQUENS.

E

Estring
(Pharmacia-Leiras)

A vaginal ring used as an oestrogen hormone replacement therapy to treat post-menopausal vaginitis.

Dose: insert 1 ring high into the vagina and wear continuously for 3 months, then replace with new ring. Maximum continuous treatment period 2 years.
Availability: NHS, private prescription.
Side effects: itch, irritation or ulceration of the vagina, infection of the urogenital tract, stomach discomfort.
Caution: in patients suffering from some womb disorders, blood clots, liver disease, PORPHYRIA, Cushing's disease. Your doctor will advise regular check-ups.
Not to be used for: children, or patients suffering from severely inflamed or ulcerated vagina, undiagnosed vaginal bleeding, some cancers.
Caution needed with: STEROIDS, other preparations inserted into the vagina.
Contains: OESTRADIOL.
Other preparations:

---

ethacrynic acid *see* **Edecrin**

---

ethambutol *see* **Myambutol**

---

ethamsylate *see* **Dicynene**

---

ethinyloestradiol *see* **BiNovum, Brevinor, Cilest, Conova 30, Dianette, ethinyloestradiol tablets, Eugynon 30, Femodene, Femodene ED, Loestrin, Logynon, Logynon ED, Marvelon, Mercilon, Microgynon 30, Minulet, Neocon 1/35, Norimin, Ovran, Ovranette, Ovysmen, PC4, Synphase, Tri-Minulet, Trinordiol, Trinovum, Trinovum-ED**

---

ethinyloestradiol tablets

White, round tablets supplied at strengths of 10 micrograms, 50 micrograms, and 1 mg, and used as an oestrogen treatment for menopausal symptoms, and some blood vessel disorders.

Dose: for menopausal symptoms, 10-20 micrograms a day continuously or for 21 days, repeated after 7 days. Additional progestogen treatment may be necessary. For other conditions, as advised by doctor.
Availability: NHS and private prescription.
Side effects: enlarged breasts, fluid retention, nausea, vaginal bleeding, weight gain, skin changes, liver disorders, jaundice, rashes, vomiting, headaches.
Caution: in patients suffering from high blood pressure, diabetes, heart disease, vascular disorders, asthma, kidney disease, epilepsy, womb diseases, thyroid disorder. Your doctor may advise you to have regular examinations.
Not to be used for: pregnant women, nursing mothers, or for patients suffering from sickle-cell anaemia, thrombosis, liver disorders, some cancers, undiagnosed vaginal bleeding, some ear, skin, and kidney disorders, jaundice, PORPHYRIA, brain blood vessel disease.
Caution needed with: DIURETICS, drugs that induce liver enzymes (eg BARBITURATES, CARBAMAZEPINE, PHENYTOIN, RIFAMPICIN), ACE INHIBITORS, ANTICOAGULANTS, ß-BLOCKERS.
Contains: ETHINYLOESTRADIOL.
Other preparations:

Ethmozine
(Monmouth)

A white, film-coated, oval or capsule-shaped tablet supplied at strengths of 200 mg, 250 mg, and 300 mg, and used to treat heart rhythm disturbance.

Dose: usually 200-300 mg every 8 hours, but adjusting as needed to a maximum of 900 mg a day.
Availability: NHS and private prescription.
Side effects: dizziness, nervousness, pins and needles, dry mouth, sleep or vision disturbances, stomach upset, and chest, muscle, or bone pain, breathing disorder.
Caution: in pregnant women, and in patients suffering from liver or kidney disorder, certain heart disorders or heart failure. Treatment should be started in hospital.
Not to be used for: nursing mothers, or for patients with heart block or shock.
Caution needed with: DIGOXIN, CIMETIDINE, THEOPHYLLINE.
Contains: MORACIZINE hydrochloride.
Other preparations:

---

ethoheptazine *see* **Equagesic**

---

ethosuximide *see* **Emeside, Zarontin**

---

ethyl nicotinate *see* **Transvasin**

---

ethyl salicylate *see* **Dubam**

---

ethynodiol diacetate *see* **Conova 30, Femulen**

---

etidronate disodium *see* **Didronel**

---

etodolac *see* **Lodine**

Eucardic
(Boehringer-Mannheim Pharmaceuticals)

A peach-coloured scored tablet or a white scored tablet according to strengths of 12.5 mg and 25 mg, and used as an alpha/BETA-BLOCKER to treat raised blood pressure.

Dose: 1 weaker strength tablet once a day for the first 2 days, then 2 weaker tablets or 1 stronger tablet a day, up to 50 mg a day if required.
Availability: NHS, private prescription.

Side effects: low blood pressure on standing, slow heart rate, dizziness, tiredness, headache, stomach upset, reduced circulation in the hands and feet, dry eyes, chest pain, skin reactions, intermittent limping.
Caution: in patients with weak hearts or who are suffering from overactive thyroid, diabetes. Patients with some forms of heart disease should have treatment withdrawn gradually.
Not to be used for: children, pregnant women, nursing mothers, or for patients suffering from heart block, very slow heart rate, uncontrolled heart failure, asthma, liver damage, blocked airways.
Caution needed with: general anaesthetics, some anti-arrhythmic drugs, VERAPAMIL, DIGOXIN, RIFAMPICIN.
Contains: CARVEDILOL.
Other preparations:

E

Eudemine
(Farillon)

A white, sugar-coated tablet used as a blood sugar-elevating drug to treat low blood glucose levels.

Dose: initially 5 mg per kilogram body weight daily in divided doses.
Availability: NHS and private prescription.
Side effects: loss of appetite, stomach upset, fluid and electrolyte disorder, heart rhythm disturbance, shaking.
Caution: in pregnant women, children, and in patients with severe kidney failure.
Not to be used for:
Caution needed with: DIURETICS, ANTICOAGULANTS, drugs that lower blood pressure.
Contains: DIAZOXIDE.
Other preparations:

Euglucon *see* glibenclamide tablets
(Hoechst Roussel)

Eugynon 30
(Schering Healthcare)

A white tablet used as an oestrogen, progestogen contraceptive.

Dose: 1 tablet a day for 21 days starting on day 5 of the period.
Availability: NHS and private prescription.
Side effects: enlarged breasts, bloating and fluid retention, cramps, leg pains, mood change, reduction in sexual desire, headaches, nausea,

vaginal erosion, discharge, and bleeding, weight gain, skin changes, rarely thrombosis, raised blood pressure, jaundice.

Caution: in patients suffering from high blood pressure, diabetes, vascular disorders, asthma, depression, kidney disease, multiple sclerosis, womb diseases. Your doctor may advise you not to smoke, to have regular examinations. You should stop treatment at the first sign of serious symptoms such as severe headache or jaundice. Treatment should be stopped before surgery.

Not to be used for: pregnant women, or for patients suffering from sickle-cell anaemia, history of heart disease or thrombosis, liver disorders, some cancers, undiagnosed vaginal bleeding, some ear, skin, and kidney disorders.

Caution needed with: RIFAMPICIN, TETRACYCLINE ANTIBIOTICS, GRISEOFULVIN, BARBITURATES, PHENYTOIN, PRIMIDONE, CARBAMAZEPINE, ETHOSUXIMIDE, CHLORAL HYDRATE.

Contains: ETHINYLOESTRADIOL, LEVONORGESTEROL.

Other preparations: OVRAN 30.

E

Eumovate Cream
(Glaxo)

A cream used as a STEROID treatment for skin disorders that respond to steroids.

Dose: apply to the affected area 1-4 times a day.
Availability: NHS and private prescription.
Side effects: fluid retention, suppression of adrenal glands, thinning, spotting, or streaking of the skin may occur.
Caution: use for short periods of time only, especially on the face or in children.
Not to be used for: patients suffering from acne or any other skin infections caused by tuberculosis, ringworm, viruses, or fungi, leg ulcers, scabies, or continuously especially in pregnant women.
Caution needed with:
Contains: CLOBETASONE BUTYRATE.
Other preparations: Eumovate Ointment.

Eurax
(Zyma Healthcare)

A lotion used as a scabicide to treat scabies and itchy skin conditions.

Dose: scabies: apply to the body apart from the head and face after a hot bath; repeat after 24 hours and wash off the next day. Itching; apply when required.

Availability: NHS, private prescription, over the counter.
Side effects:
Caution: keep out of the eyes, and avoid areas of broken skin.
Not to be used for: patients suffering from acute weeping skin conditions.
Caution needed with:
Contains: CROTAMITON.
Other preparations: Eurax Cream.

Eurax-Hydrocortisone
(Zyma)

A cream used as a STEROID and anti-itch treatment for itching skin disorders.

Dose: apply to the affected area 2-3 times a day for 10-14 days (7 days if on face).
Availability: NHS and private prescription.
Side effects: fluid retention, suppression of adrenal glands, thinning, spotting, or streaking of the skin may occur.
Caution: use for short periods of time only, especially on the face and in children.
Not to be used for: patients suffering from acne or any other skin infections caused by tuberculosis, ringworm, viruses, ulcerated or weeping skin conditions, fungi, leg ulcers, scabies, or continuously especially in pregnant women.
Caution needed with:
Contains: CROTAMITON, HYDROCORTISONE.
Other preparations: Eurax HC (available without prescription only for treating irritant and allergic contact dermatitis, mild to moderate eczema, and reactions to insect bites).

Evorel *see* Estradem
(Janssen-Cilag)

EvorelPak *see* Estrapak
(Janssen-Cilag)

ExacTech
(MediSense Britain)

A reagent strip used in conjunction with an ExacTech meter to detect blood glucose levels. Blood-glucose monitoring enables individual patients

THE CEDAR PRACTICE

John Scott Health Centre

Green Lanes London N4 2NU

Tel: 020 7690 1155 (Appointments Only)

General Enquiries & Out of Hours Emergencies

Tel: 020 7690 1151

Reception open Mon- Fri from:

8.30am-12.30pm&2.30pm-6.30pm

(closed Wednesday afternoon)

Dr Richard Carver   Dr Deborah Shier

Dr Paula Stanley   Dr Asim Rashid

YOUR NEXT APPOINTMENT IS:

Dr. *Baumgarter* Date. 1 6 / 6 / 05 Time. 3 2 0 pm

Dr........................Date.............................Time......................

Dr........................ Date........................Time......................

Dr........................Date.............................Time......................

Dr........................Date.............................Time......................

Please let us know in good time if you are unable to
keep an appointment.   Thank you.

suffering from diabetes accurately to control blood glucose and manage their condition.

Exelderm
(Zeneca)

A cream used as an antifungal treatment for fungal infections of the skin.

Dose: rub into the affected area twice a day and continue for 2-3 weeks after the wounds have healed.
Availability: NHS and private prescription.
Side effects: irritation
Caution: keep out of the eyes; if the area becomes irritated, the treatment should be stopped.
Not to be used for:
Caution needed with:
Contains: SULCONAZOLE nitrate.
Other preparations:

Exirel
(3M Health Care)

A beige/turquoise-blue capsule supplied at a strength of 15 mg, and used as a BRONCHODILATOR to treat bronchial spasm brought on by bronchial asthma, bronchitis, emphysema.

Dose: 15 mg 3-4 times a day up to a maximum of 60 mg a day.
Availability: NHS and private prescription.
Side effects: shaking of the hands, nervous tension, headache, dilation of the blood vessels.
Caution: in pregnant women and in patients suffering from high blood pressure, abnormal heart rhythms, angina, heart muscle disease, overactive thyroid.
Not to be used for: children.
Caution needed with: SYMPATHOMIMETICS.
Contains: PIRBUTEROL hydrochloride.
Other preparations: Exirel Inhaler.

Exocin
(Allergan)

Drops used as an antibiotic to treat bacterial infections of the eye.

Dose: 1-2 drops into the eye every 2-4 hours for the first 2 days, then 1-2

drops 4 times a day for a maximum of 10 days.
Availability: NHS, private prescription.
Side effects: temporary stinging, occasionally headache, nausea, numbness, dizziness.
Caution: in pregnant women and nursing mothers.
Not to be used for: patients who wear soft contact lenses.
Caution needed with:
Contains: OFLOXACIN.
Other preparations:

Exterol
(Dermal)

Drops used as a wax softener to remove ear wax.

Dose: hold 5-10 drops in the ear 1-2 times a day for 3-4 days.
Availability: NHS, private prescription, over the counter.
Side effects: slight fizzing.
Caution: stop the treatment if it causes irritation.
Not to be used for: patients suffering from perforated ear drum.
Caution needed with:
Contains: UREA HYDROGEN PEROXIDE, GLYCERINE.
Other preparations:

---

famciclovir *see* **Famvir**

---

famotidine *see* **Pepcid**

Famvir
(SmithKline Beecham)

A white, film-coated tablet supplied at strengths of 125 mg, 250 mg, and used as an antiviral treatment for shingles and herpes infections of the genital tract.

Dose: shingles, 250 mg 3 times a day (or 750 mg once a day) for 7 days; herpes infection of the genital tract, 250 mg 3 times a day for 5 days for the first outbreak, in recurrence 125 mg twice a day for 5 days.
Availability: NHS, private prescription.
Side effects: headache, nausea.
Caution: in patients suffering from kidney failure.
Not to be used for: children, pregnant women, nursing mothers.
Caution needed with:

Contains: FAMCICLOVIR.
Other preparations:

Fansidar
(Roche)

A white, quarter-scored tablet used to prevent and treat malaria.

Dose: prevention adults and children over 14 years 1 tablet a week, treatment 2-3 tablets as one dose or as advised by the physician; children under 14 years reduced doses.
Availability: NHS and private prescription.
Side effects: rash, inflammation of the pharynx, itch, stomach upset, rare skin and blood changes.
Caution: patients should keep out of the sun. Your doctor may advise regular blood tests if the treatment is prolonged.
Not to be used for: new-born infants, pregnant women, nursing mothers or for patients suffering from severe kidney or liver disease, blood disorders, or allergy to similar drugs.
Caution needed with: TRIMETHOPRIM.
Contains: SULFADOXINE, PYRIMETHAMINE.
Other preparations:

F

Fasigyn
(Pfizer)

A white tablet supplied at a strength of 500 mg and used as an antibiotic for the treament and prevention of infection.

Dose: prevention 4 tablets as a single dose, treatment 4 tablets at first then 2 tablets a day for a maximum of 5-6 days.
Availability: NHS and private prescription.
Side effects: stomach upset, furred tongue, unpleasant taste, swelling and brain disturbances, dark-coloured urine, rash; blood changes, weakness, and numbness on long-term therapy.
Caution: in pregnant women and nursing mothers.
Not to be used for: children or for patients suffering from nervous disorders, blood disorders. Your doctor may advise regular blood tests
Caution needed with: alcohol.
Contains: TINIDAZOLE.
Other preparations:

Faverin
(Solvay Healthcare)

A white, scored tablet or a white, oval, scored tablet according to strengths of 50 mg, 100 mg, and used as an antidepressant to treat depression.

Dose: 100 mg in the evening at first then usually 100-200 mg a day in divided doses, up to a maximum of 300 mg a day if needed.
Availability: NHS and private prescription.
Side effects: nausea, vomiting, dry mouth, stomach pain, indigestion, sleepiness, sleeplessness, diarrhoea, constipation, headache, dizziness, agitation, anorexia, sweating, weakness, general feeling of being unwell, tremor, convulsions
Caution: in pregnant women, nursing mothers, and in patients suffering from liver or kidney disease, or with a history of epilepsy.
Not to be used for: children.
Caution needed with: PROPRANOLOL, THEOPHYLLINE, PHENYTOIN, AMINOPHYLLINE, CARBAMAZEPINE, some tranquillizers, TRICYCLIC ANTIDEPRESSANTS, WARFARIN, MAOIS, alcohol, LITHIUM, TRYPTOPHAN.
Contains: FLUVOXAMINE maleate.
Other preparations:

Fectrim *see* co-trimoxazole tablets
(DDSA)

Feldene *see* piroxicam capsules
(Pfizer)

---

felodipine *see* Plendil

Femapak *see* Fematrix

Fematrix
(Solvay)

A patch supplied at strengths of 40 mg, 80 mg, and used as an oestrogen replacement therapy during the menopause.

Dose: apply a new patch every 3-4 days. (Women with an intact uterus also require progestogen supplements – use Femapak – *see* below.)
Availability: NHS, private prescription.
Side effects: enlarged breasts, fluid retention, nausea, vaginal bleeding,

weight gain, headache, dizziness. Rarely jaundice, raised blood pressure, thrombosis.

Caution: in patients suffering from high blood pressure, diabetes, epilepsy, womb diseases, gall bladder disorder, migraine, multiple sclerosis, PORPHYRIA, liver disorders, some ear disorders, or a history or increased risk of breast disorders (including cancer) and thrombosis. Your doctor may advise you to have regular examinations.

Not to be used for: children, pregnant women, nursing mothers, or for patients suffering from thombosis, severe liver, kidney, or heart disorders, some cancers, undiagnosed vaginal bleeding, endometriosis.

Caution needed with: ACE INHIBITORS, ANTICOAGULANTS, BARBITURATES, ß-BLOCKERS, CARBAMAZEPINE, PHENYTOIN, RIFAMPICIN.

Contains: OESTRADIOL.

Other preparations: ESTRADERM, EVOREL. FEMOSTON and FEMAPAK also includes dydrogesterone tablets, for use in women with an intact uterus.

Femodene
(Schering Healthcare)

A white tablet used as an oestrogen, progestogen contraceptive.

Dose: 1 tablet a day for 21 days starting on day 1 of the period.
Availability: NHS and private prescription.
Side effects: enlarged breasts, bloating and fluid retention, cramps, leg pains, mood change, reduction in sexual desire, headaches, nausea, vaginal erosion, discharge, and bleeding, weight gain, skin changes, rarely thrombosis, raised blood pressure, jaundice.
Caution: in patients suffering from high blood pressure, diabetes, vascular disorders, asthma, depression, kidney disease, multiple sclerosis, womb diseases. Your doctor may advise you not to smoke, to have regular examinations. You should stop treatment at the first sign of serious symptoms such as severe headache or jaundice. Treatment should be stopped before surgery.
Not to be used for: pregnant women, or for patients suffering from sickle-cell anaemia, history of heart disease or thrombosis, liver disorders, some cancers, undiagnosed vaginal bleeding, some ear, skin, and kidney disorders.
Caution needed with: RIFAMPICIN, TETRACYCLINE ANTIBIOTICS, GRISEOFULVIN, BARBITURATES, PHENYTOIN, PRIMIDONE, CARBAMAZEPINE, ETHOSUXIMIDE, CHLORAL HYDRATE.
Contains: ETHINYLOESTRADIOL, GESTODENE.
Other preparations: MINULET.

Femodene ED
(Schering Healthcare)

White tablets use as an oestrogen, progestogen contraceptive.

Dose: 1 tablet a day, starting on day 1 of period.
Availability: NHS and private prescription.
Side effects: enlarged breasts, bloating and fluid retention, cramps, leg pains, mood change, reduction in sexual desire, headaches, nausea, vaginal erosion, discharge and bleeding, weight gain, skin changes, rarely thrombosis, raised blood pressure, jaundice.
Caution: in patients suffering from high blood pressure, diabetes, vascular disorders, asthma, depression, kidney disease, multiple sclerosis, womb diseases. Your doctor may advise you not to smoke, and to have regular examinations. You should stop treatment at the first sign of serious symptoms such as severe headache or jaundice. Treatment should be stopped before surgery.
Not to be used for: pregnant women, or for patients suffering from sickle-cell anaemia, history of heart disease, or thombosis, liver disorders, some cancers, undiagnosed vaginal bleeding, some ear, skin, and kidney disorders.
Caution needed with: RIFAMPICIN, TETRACYCLINE ANTIBIOTICS, GRISEOFULVIN, BARBITURATES, PHENYTOIN, PRIMIDONE, CARBAMAZEPINE, ETHOSUXIMIDE, CHLORAL HYDRATE.
Contains: ETHINYLOESTRADIOL, GESTODENE, LACTOSE.
Other preparations:

Femoston 2/10
(Solvay)

Orange tablets and yellow tablets used as hormone replacement therapy for treating the symptoms of menopause and for the prevention of osteoporosis.

Dose: 1 tablet a day continuously starting with the orange tablets, beginning by the fifth day of menstruation if present or at any time if not. Change to Femoston 2/20 if breakthrough bleeding or inadequate response occurs.
Availability: NHS, private prescription.
Side effects: enlarged breasts, fluid retention, nausea, vaginal bleeding, weight gain, headaches, dizziness. Rarely jaundice, raised blood pressure, thrombosis.
Caution: in patients suffering from high blood pressure, diabetes, epilepsy, womb diseases, gall bladder disorder, migraine, multiple sclerosis, PORPHYRIA, liver disorders, some ear disorders, or a history or increased risk of breast disorders (including cancer) and thrombosis. Your

doctor may advise you to have regular examinations.
Not to be used for: children, pregnant women, nursing mothers, or for patients suffering from thombosis, severe liver, kidney, or heart disorders, some cancers, undiagnosed vaginal bleeding, endometriosis.
Caution needed with: ACE INHIBITORS, ANTICOAGULANTS, BARBITURATES, ß-BLOCKERS, CARBAMAZEPINE, PHENYTOIN, RIFAMPICIN.
Contains: OESTRADIOL, DYDROGESTERONE.
Other preparations: Femoston 2/20, Femosten 1/10 (used only to treat menopause symptoms). FEMAPAK.

Femulen
(Gold Cross)

A white tablet used as a progesterone contraceptive.

Dose: 1 tablet at the same time every day starting on day 1 of the period.
Availability: NHS and private prescription.
Side effects: irregular bleeding, breast discomfort, acne, headache, ovarian cyst, rarely thrombosis, raised blood pressure, jaundice.
Caution: in patients suffering from high blood pressure, tendency to thrombosis, migraine, liver abnormalities, ovarian cysts, some cancers. Your doctor may advise regular check-ups.
Not to be used for: pregnant women, or for patients suffering from severe heart or artery disease, benign liver tumours, vaginal bleeding, previous ectopic pregnancy.
Caution needed with: BARBITURATES, PHENYTOIN, PRIMIDONE, CARBAMAZEPINE, CHLORAL HYDRATE, ETHOSUXIMIDE, RIFAMPICIN, CHLORPROMAZINE, MEPROBAMATE, GRISEOFULVIN.
Contains: ETHYNODIOL DIACETATE.
Other preparations:

Fenbid Spansule *see* ibuprofen tablets
(Goldshield Healthcare)

---

fenbufen *see* fenbufen tablets, Fenbuzip, Lederfen

---

fenbufen tablets

A tablet used as a NON-STEROIDAL ANTI-INFLAMMATORY DRUG to treat rheumatic disorders and other muscle or bone problems.

Dose: either 300 mg in the morning and 600 mg at night or 450 mg twice a day.

Availability: NHS and private prescription.
Side effects: rash and other skin disorders, fluid retention, blood disorders, stomach upset, rarely lung disorders, headaches, dizziness, vertigo, hearing disturbance, LUPUS.
Caution: in the elderly, pregnant women, nursing mothers, and in patients suffering from heart failure, LUPUS, asthma, kidney or liver disorders, or with a history of stomach disorders.
Not to be used for: children or for patients suffering from anti-inflammatory drug/ASPIRIN allergy, stomach ulcer, or history of gastro-intestinal disease.
Caution needed with: other non-steroidal anti-inflammatory drugs, ANTICOAGULANTS, some antibiotics, METHOTREXATE, some antidiabetic drugs, drugs that lower blood pressure, CYCLOSPORIN, LITHIUM, DIGOXIN.
Contains: FENBUFEN.
Other preparations: fenbufen capsules. FENBUZIP, LEDERFEN.

Fenbuzip *see* **fenbufen capsules/tablets**
(Ashbourne)

---

fenchone *see* **Rowatinex**

---

fenfluramine *see* **Ponderax**

---

fenofibrate *see* **Lipantil**

Fenoket *see* **ketoprofen capsules**
(Opus)

---

fenoprofen *see* **Fenopron**

Fenopron
(Dista)

An orange, oval tablet or orange, oblong, scored tablet according to strengths of 300 mg, 600 mg and used as a NON-STEROIDAL ANTI-INFLAMMATORY DRUG to treat pain, rheumatoid arthritis, osteoarthritis, ankylosing spondylitis.

Dose: 300-600 mg 3-4 times a day to a maximum of 3 g a day.
Availability: NHS and private prescription.

Side effects: stomach intolerance, allergy, kidney and liver disorders, blood changes.
Caution: in the elderly, pregnant women, nursing mothers, and in patients with a history of stomach ulcer or stomach bleeding, or suffering from asthma, kidney or liver disease, or heart failure.
Not to be used for: children or for patients suffering from stomach ulcer, severe kidney disease, or allergy to ASPIRIN or anti-inflammatory drugs.
Caution needed with: ANTICOAGULANTS, ASPIRIN, some anticonvulsants, antidiabetics, some antibiotics, some DIURETICS, PHENOBARBITONE.
Contains: FENOPROFEN.
Other preparations: PROGESIC.

---

fenoterol *see* **Berotec, Duovent**

Fentamox *see* **tamoxifen tablets**
(Opus)

---

fentanyl *see* **Durogesic**

Fentazin
(Forley)

A white tablet supplied at strengths of 2 mg, 4 mg and used as a sedative to treat anxiety, tension, chronic mental disorders, schizophrenia, vomiting, nausea, and other psychiatric problems.

Dose: usually 12 mg day in divided doses to a maximum of 24 mg day (lower doses in the elderly).
Availability: NHS and private prescription.
Side effects: muscle spasms, restlessness, hands shaking, blurred vision, dry mouth, blocked nose, constipation, urine retention, palpitations, low blood pressure, weight gain, changes in sexual function, low body temperature, breast swelling, menstrual changes, jaundice, blood and skin changes, drowsiness, tiredness, rarely fits.
Caution: in pregnant women, nursing mothers, and in patients suffering from Parkinson's disease, liver disease, cardiovascular disease, kidney failure, epilepsy, glaucoma, heart or circulation disorder, MYASTHENIA GRAVIS, PHAEOCHROMOCYTOMA, adrenal tumour, enlarged prostate, underactive thyroid.
Not to be used for: children, unconscious patients, or those suffering from bone marrow depression.
Caution needed with: alcohol, sedatives, tranquillizers, pain killers, blood-pressure lowering drugs, antidepressants, anticonvulsants,

antidiabetic drugs, LEVODOPA.
Contains: PERPHENAZINE.
Other preparations: Fentazin Injection.

---

fenticonazole *see* **Lomexin**

Ferfolic SV
(Sinclair)

A pink tablet used as a supplement to treat iron and FOLIC ACID deficiencies, and to prevent deformities in the foetus in pregnant women.

Dose: for iron deficiency, 1 tablet 3 times a day; for prevention of birth defects, 1 tablet a day (continued until the twelfth week of pregnancy).
Availability: NHS and private prescription.
Side effects: nausea, constipation
Caution:
Not to be used for: children, or for patients suffering from megaloblastic anaemia.
Caution needed with: PHENYTOIN, some antibiotics, ANTACIDS, LEVODOPA.
Contains: FOLIC ACID, FERROUS GLUCONATE, VITAMIN C.
Other preparations:

Ferrocontin Continus
(ASTA Medica)

A red tablet supplied at a strength of 100 mg and used as an iron supplement to treat iron deficiency, anaemia.

Dose: 1 tablet a day.
Availability: NHS, private prescription, over the counter.
Side effects:
Caution:
Not to be used for: children under 10 years.
Caution needed with: PENICILLAMINE, zinc, some antibiotics, ANTACIDS, LEVODOPA.
Contains: FERROUS GLYCINE SULPHATE.
Other preparations: PLESMET.

Ferrocontin Folic Continus
(ASTA Medica)

A pale-orange tablet used as an iron supplement to prevent iron and FOLIC

ACID deficiencies in pregnancy.

Dose: 1 tablet a day.
Availability: NHS, private prescription, over the counter.
Side effects:
Caution:
Not to be used for: children.
Caution needed with: PENICILLAMINE, PHENYTOIN, zinc, some antibiotics, ANTACIDS, LEVODOPA.
Contains: FERROUS GLYCINE SULPHATE, FOLIC ACID.
Other preparations:

Ferrograd
(Abbott)

A red tablet supplied at a strength of 325 mg and used as an iron supplement to treat iron deficiency anaemia.

Dose: 1 tablet a day before food.
Availability: NHS, private prescription, and over the counter.
Side effects:
Caution: in patients suffering from slow bowel actions.
Not to be used for: children or for patients suffering from diverticular disease, blocked intestine.
Caution needed with: some antibiotics, ANTACIDS, LEVODOPA.
Contains: FERROUS SULPHATE.
Other preparations: SLOW FE.

Ferrograd Folic
(Abbott)

A yellow/red tablet used as an iron supplement to treat anaemia in pregnancy.

Dose: 1 tablet a day before food.
Availability: NHS, private prescription, over the counter.
Side effects:
Caution: in patients suffering from slow bowel movements.
Not to be used for: children or for patients suffering from diverticular disease, intestinal blockage, VITAMIN B_{12} deficiency.
Caution needed with: PHENYTOIN, some antibiotics, ANTACIDS, LEVODOPA.
Contains: FERROUS SULPHATE, FOLIC ACID.
Other preparations:

F

ferrous fumarate *see* **Fersaday, Fersamal, Folex-350, Galfer, Meterfolic, Pregaday**

---

ferrous gluconate *see* **Ferfolic SV, ferrous gluconate tablets**

---

ferrous gluconate tablets

A red, coated tablet used as an iron supplement to treat and prevent iron deficiency anaemia.

Dose: adults 4-6 tablets a day in divided doses before meals to treat anaemia (2 tablets a day to prevent anaemia); children 6-12 years half adult dose.
Availability: NHS, private prescription, over the counter.
Side effects: nausea, altered bowel habit, discoloration of faeces.
Caution: in the elderly, pregnant women, and in patients suffering from inflammatory bowel disease, or intestinal blockage, diverticulosis, or slow bowel movement.
Not to be used for: children under 6 years.
Caution needed with: some antibiotics, ANTACIDS, LEVODOPA.
Contains: FERROUS GLUCONATE.
Other preparations: Fergon (not available on NHS prescription).

---

ferrous glycine sulphate *see* **Ferrocontin Continus, Ferrocontin Continus Folic, Plesmet**

---

ferrous sulphate *see* **Ferrograd, Ferrograd Folic, ferrous sulphate tablets, Slow-Fe, Slow-Fe Folic**

---

ferrous sulphate tablets

A coated tablet used as an iron supplement to treat and prevent iron deficiency anaemia.

Dose: adults 2-3 tablets a day before meals to treat anaemia (1 tablet a day to prevent anaemia); children use paediatric mixture.
Availability: NHS, private prescription, over the counter.
Side effects: nausea, altered bowel habit, discoloration of faeces.
Caution: in the elderly, pregnant women, and patients suffering from slow bowel movement, inflammatory bowel disease, intestinal blockage, diverticulosis.
Not to be used for:

Caution needed with: some antibiotics, ANTACIDS, LEVODOPA.
Contains: ferrous sulphate.
Other preparations: ferrous sulphate oral solution, paediatric BP.
FERROGRAD, FEOSPAN SPANSULE, SLOW-FE (all available as slow-release forms).
Feospan (not available on NHS prescription).

Fersaday
(Goldshield Healthcare)

A brown tablet supplied at a strength of 100 mg and used as an iron supplement to treat iron deficiency.

Dose: 1 tablet 1-2 times a day.
Availability: NHS, private prescription, over the counter.
Side effects: stomach upset.
Caution: in patients with a history of stomach ulcer.
Not to be used for: children.
Caution needed with: ANTACIDS, some antibiotics, LEVODOPA.
Contains: FERROUS FUMARATE.
Other preparations: FERSAMAL, GALFER.

Fersamal
(Forley)

A brown tablet supplied at a strength of 65 mg and used as an iron supplement to treat iron deficiency.

Dose: adults 1 tablet 3 times a day; children use Fersamal Syrup.
Availability: NHS, private prescription, over the counter.
Side effects: stomach upset.
Caution: in patients with a history of stomach ulcer.
Not to be used for:
Caution needed with: ANTACIDS, some antibiotics, ANTACIDS, LEVODOPA.
Contains: FERROUS FUMARATE.
Other preparations: Fersamal Syrup. FERSADAY, GALFER.

Fertiral
(Hoechst)

An injection supplied at a strength of 500 micrograms per ml, and used as a hormone treatment for the absence of periods and infertility.

Dose: as advised by your physician.
Availability: NHS, private prescription.

Side effects: stomach pain, nausea, headache, vaginal bleeding.
Caution: discontinue treatment after conception or after 6 months.
Not to be used for: children, or for patients suffering from untreated weight-related absent periods, cysts in the womb or ovary.
Caution needed with:
Contains: GONADORELIN.
Other preparations:

Filair *see* **beclomethasone inhaler**
(3M Health Care)

---

finasteride *see* **Proscar**

Flagyl *see* **metronidazole tablets**
(Rhône-Poulenc Rorer)

Flamatrol *see* **piroxicam capsules**
(Berk)

Flamazine
(Smith & Nephew Healthcare)

A cream used as an antibacterial treatment for wounds, burns, infected ulcers of the leg, bed sores, and where skin has been removed for grafting.

Dose: apply a layer up to 0.5 cm thick to the affected area; change dressing 3 times a week (or every day for burns).
Availability: NHS and private prescription.
Side effects:
Caution: in patients suffering from kidney or liver disease.
Not to be used for: infants under 3 months or for pregnant women.
Caution needed with: PHENYTOIN, some antibiotics, antidiabetics, enzyme wound treatments.
Contains: SILVER SULPHADIAZINE.
Other preparations:

Flamrase *see* **diclofenac tablets**
(Berk)

264

flavoxate hydrochloride *see* **Urispas**

---

flecainide *see* **Tambocor**

Fletchers' Arachis Oil
(Pharmax)

A 130 ml, single-dose enema used as a faecal softener to treat faecal impaction.

Dose: 1 enema as required; children in proportion according to age and body weight.
Availability: NHS, private prescription, over the counter.
Side effects:
Caution: warm before use.
Not to be used for:
Caution needed with:
Contains: ARACHIS OIL.
Other preparations:

Fletchers' Enemette
(Pharmax)

A 5 ml, single-dose micro-enema supplied at a strength of 90 mg and used as a faecal softener to treat constipation, and for evacuation of bowels before surgery etc.

Dose: adults and children over 3 years 1 as required.
Availability: NHS, private prescription, over the counter.
Side effects:
Caution:
Not to be used for: children under 3 years.
Caution needed with:
Contains: DOCUSATE sodium.
Other preparations:

Fletchers' Phosphate
(Pharmax)

A 128 ml, single-dose enema used as a bowel evacuator to treat constipation, and for evacuation of the bowels before surgery, examinations, etc.

Dose: adults 1 enema as required; children over 3 years in proportion to age and body weight.
Availability: NHS, private prescription, over the counter.
Side effects:
Caution: in patients with restricted sodium intake.
Not to be used for: children under 3 years, or for patients where the absorptive capacity of the colon is increased.
Caution needed with:
Contains: SODIUM ACID PHOSPHATE, SODIUM PHOSPHATE.
Other preparations:

Flexin Continus *see* **indomethacin capsules**
(Napp)

Flixonase
(A & H)

A nasal spray used as a STEROID to prevent and treat rhinitis, hay fever.

Dose: adults, 2 sprays in each nostril once a day in the morning, to a maximum of 4 sprays in each nostril a day; children over 4 years, 1-2 sprays in each nostril a day.
Availability: NHS and private prescription.
Side effects: irritation of the nose, nose bleed, taste and smell disturbances.
Caution: in pregnant women, nursing mothers, and in patients being transferred from steroids taken orally.
Not to be used for: children under 4 years.
Caution needed with:
Contains: FLUTICASONE PROPIONATE.
Other preparations:

Flixotide
(A&H)

An inhaler, supplied at strengths of 25 micrograms, 50 mcg, 125 mcg, 250 mcg, and used as a CORTICOSTEROID for the prevention of bronchial asthma.

Dose: adults, 100-1000 mcg twice a day; children over 4 years, 50-100 mcg twice a day.
Availability: NHS, private prescription.
Side effects: fungal infections of mouth and throat, hoarseness, bronchial spasm.
Caution: in pregnant women, and in patients suffering from tuberculosis of

the lungs or who are transferring from STEROID tablets/injections.
Not to be used for: children under 4 years.
Caution needed with:
Contains: FLUTICASONE PROPIONATE.
Other preparations: Flixotide Accuhaler, Flixotide Diskhaler.

Florinef
(Squibb)

A pink, scored tablet supplied at a strength of 0.1 mg and used as a
STEROID replacement treatment in Addison's disease, salt-losing
adrenogenital syndrome (adrenal disorders).

Dose: adults ½-3 tablets a day; children in proportion to adult dose
according to age, body weight, and severity of illness.
Availability: NHS and private prescription.
Side effects: high blood pressure, fluid retention, potassium loss, muscle
weakness, weight gain.
Caution: in pregnant women, in patients who have had recent bowel
surgery, or who are suffering from inflamed veins, psychiatric disorders,
virus infections, some cancers, some kidney diseases, thinning of the
bones, ulcers, tuberculosis, other infections, high blood pressure,
glaucoma, epilepsy, diabetes, underactive thyroid, liver disease, stress.
Avoid contact with chickenpox or shingles. Withdraw gradually.
Not to be used for:
Caution needed with: PHENYTOIN, PHENOBARBITONE, EPHEDRINE, RIFAMPICIN,
DIURETICS, ANTICHOLINESTERASES, DIGOXIN, antidiabetic agents, ANTICOAGULANTS,
NON-STEROIDAL ANTI-INFLAMMATORY DRUGS.
Contains: FLUDROCORTISONE acetate.
Other preparations:

Floxapen *see* flucloxacillin capsules
(Beecham Research)

Fluanxol
(Lundbeck)

A red tablet supplied at strengths of 0.5 mg, 1 mg and used as a sedative
for the short-term treatment of depression and anxiety.

Dose: adults 1-2 mg in the morning to a maximum of 3 mg a day in
divided doses; elderly 0.5 mg in the morning to a maximum of 2 mg a day
in divided doses.
Availability: NHS and private prescription.

F

Side effects: muscle spasms, restlessness, hands shaking, blurred vision, dry mouth, urine retention, palpitations, low blood pressure, weight gain, changes in sexual function, low body temperature, breast swelling, menstrual changes, jaundice, blood and skin changes, drowsiness, rarely fits.

Caution: in patients suffering from Parkinson's disease, severe hardening of the arteries, confusion in the elderly, severe kidney, liver, or heart disease.

Not to be used for: children or for excitable, overactive, or severely clinically depressed patients.

Caution needed with: alcohol, sedatives, tranquillizers, pain killers, blood-pressure lowering drugs, antidepressants, anticonvulsants, antidiabetic drugs, LEVODOPA.

Contains: FLUPENTHIXOL dihydrochloride.

Other preparations: DEPIXOL.

Fluarix *see* influenza vaccine
(SmithKline Beecham)

Fluclomix *see* flucloxacillin capsules
(Ashbourne)

---

flucloxacillin *see* Floxapen, Fluclomix, flucloxacillin capsules, Galfloxen, Ladropen, Magnapen, Stafoxil

---

flucloxacillin capsules

A capsule supplied at strengths of 250 mg, 500 mg and used as a penicillin treatment for skin, soft tissue, respiratory, and throat, and other infections.

Dose: adults and children over 10 years 250-500 mg 4 times a day half an hour before food; children 2-10 years half adult dose, under 2 years quarter adult dose.

Availability: NHS and private prescription.

Side effects: allergy which may be severe in very sensitive patients, stomach disturbances, rarely jaundice, blood changes.

Caution: in patients with kidney failure, PORPHYRIA, or with a history of allergy to penicillin.

Not to be used for: patients suffering from penicillin allergy.

Caution needed with: ANTICOAGULANTS, METHOTREXATE, the contraceptive pill.

Contains: FLUCLOXACILLIN sodium.

Other preparations: flucloxacillin oral solution and suspension, injection.

fluconazole *see* **Diflucan**

fludrocortisone *see* **Florinef**

flumethasone *see* **Locorten-Vioform**

flunisolide *see* **Syntaris**

flunitrazepam *see* **Rohypnol**

fluocinolone *see* **Synalar**

fluocinonide *see* **Metosyn**

fluocortolone *see* **Ultralanum Plain Cream, Ultraproct**

Fluor-a-day
(Dental Health)

An chewable tablet available in 2 strengths for ages up to 4 years and over 4 years, and used as a fluoride supplement to prevent dental decay.

Dose: ½-1 tablet a day, preferably in the evening. (Dose depends on age and water fluoride content.)
Availability: NHS, private prescription, over the counter.
Side effects: occasional white flecks on teeth.
Caution: use only if fluoride content of drinking water is less than 0.7 ppm. Do not exceed recommended dose.
Not to be used for:
Contains: SODIUM FLUORIDE.
Other preparations: EN-DE-KAY FLUOTABS.

Fluorescein Minims
(Chauvin)

Drops used as a dye for staining purposes to enable abrasions or foreign bodies in the eye to be found.

Dose: 1 or more drops into the eye as needed.
Availability: NHS, private prescription, over the counter.
Side effects:
Caution:
Not to be used for: patients wearing soft contact lenses.
Caution needed with: soft contact lenses.
Contains: SODIUM FLUORESCEIN.
Other preparations: Fluorescein and Lignocaine Minims.

---

fluorescein *see* **Fluorescein Minims**

FluoriGard Drops
(Colgate-Palmolive)

Sugar-free drops used as a fluoride supplement to prevent dental decay.

Dose: 2-8 drops a day according to age and water fluoride content.
Availability: NHS, private prescription, over the counter.
Side effects: occasional white flecks on teeth.
Caution: use only if fluoride content of drinking water is less than 0.7 ppm.
Do not exceed recommended dose.
Not to be used for:
Caution needed with:
Contains: SODIUM FLUORIDE.
Other preparations: EN-DE-KAY FLUODROPS.

FluoriGard Gelkam
(Colgate-Palmolive)

A gel used as a toothpaste to prevent dental caries and early dental decay.

Dose: use to brush teeth (after normal brushing) at night.
Availability: NHS (not available on NHS from dentists), private prescription, over the counter.
Side effects:
Caution: do not swallow excess gel.
Not to be used for: children under 6 years.

Caution needed with:
Contains: STANNOUS FLUORIDE.
Other preparations:

FluoriGard dental rinse
(Stafford-Miller)

A blue-coloured mouth rinse, available in two strengths (for daily or weekly use), and used as a fluoride supplement to treat early decay and prevent cavities.

Dose: rinse with 10 ml of rinse for 1 minute and then spit out.
Availability: NHS (not available on NHS from dentists), private prescription, over the counter.
Side effects: occasional white flecks on teeth.
Caution: do not swallow; avoid eating drinking, or rinsing mouth for 15 minutes afterwards. Do not exceed recommended dose. Use only if fluoride content of drinking water is less than 0.7 ppm.
Not to be used for: children under 6 years.
Caution needed with:
Contains: SODIUM FLUORIDE.
Other preparations: EN-DE-KAY DAILY FLUORIDE MOUTH RINSE.

F

FluoriGard Tablets
(Colgate-Palmolive)

An purple grape-flavoured tablet or orange, orange-flavoured tablet according to strength, and used as a fluoride supplement to prevent dental decay.

Dose: ½-2 tablets of 0.5 mg strength or ½-1 tablet of 1 mg strength sucked or dissolved in the mouth every day, preferably in the evening. (Dose depends on age and water fluoride content.)
Availability: NHS, private prescription, over the counter.
Side effects: occasional white flecks on teeth.
Caution: use only if fluoride content of water is less than 0.7 ppm. Do not exceed recommended dose.
Not to be used for:
Contains: SODIUM FLUORIDE.
Other preparations: EN-DE-KAY FLUOTABS, FLUOR-A-DAY TABLETS.

---

fluorometholone *see* **FML**

---

fluoxetine *see* **Prozac**

---

flupenthixol *see* **Depixol, Fluanxol**

---

fluphenazine *see* **Moditen, Motipress, Motival**

---

flurandrenolone *see* **Haelan**

---

flurazepam *see* **Dalmane**

---

flurbiprofen *see* **flurbiprofen tablets, Froben, Ocufen**

---

flurbiprofen tablets

A tablet supplied at strengths of 50 mg, 100 mg and used as a NON-STEROIDAL ANTI-INFLAMMATORY DRUG and analgesic to treat mild to moderate pain, period pain, post-operative pain, rheumatoid disease, and other muscle and bone problems.

Dose: 150-200 mg a day in divided doses to a maximum of 300 mg a day.
Availability: NHS and private prescription.
Side effects: stomach upset, rash, blood changes, fluid retention; rarely liver or kidney disorders, headache, tinnitus, vertigo.
Caution: in the elderly, pregnant women, nursing mothers, and in patients suffering from asthma, LUPUS, kidney, liver, or heart disease, or with a history of stomach ulcers.
Not to be used for: children or for patients suffering from stomach ulcer or bleeding, allergy to ASPIRIN or anti-inflammatory drugs.
Caution needed with: some DIURETICS, METHOTREXATE, ANTICOAGULANTS, LITHIUM, drugs used to lower blood pressure, other non-steroidal anti-inflammatory drugs, some antibiotics, some antidiabetics, DIGOXIN, CYCLOSPORIN.
Contains: FLURIBIPROFEN.
Other preparations: flurbiprofen suppositories. FROBEN, FROBEN SR (a long-acting preparation).

---

fluticasone propionate *see* **Cutivate, Flixonase, Flixotide**

---

fluvastatin *see* **Lescol**

Fluvirin *see* **influenza vaccine**
(Evans)

---

fluvoxamine *see* **Faverin**

Fluzone *see* **influenza vaccine**
(Servier)

FML
(Allergan)

Drops used as a STEROID treatment for inflammation of the eye where no infection is present.

Dose: 1-2 drops into the eye 2-4 times a day.
Availability: NHS and private prescription.
Side effects: rise in eye pressure, thinning cornea, fungal infection, cataract.
Caution: in pregnant women and infants – do not use for extended periods – or for patients suffering from glaucoma.
Not to be used for: infants under 2 years, or for patients suffering from viral, fungal, tubercular, or weeping infections, or who wear soft contact lenses.
Caution needed with:
Contains: FLUOROMETHOLONE.
Other preparations: FML-Neo (with NEOMYCIN for infected conditions).

Folex-350
(Shire)

A pink tablet used as an iron supplement for the prevention of iron and FOLIC ACID deficiency in pregnancy.

Dose: 1 tablet a day.
Availability: private prescription, over the counter.
Side effects: nausea, constipation, diarrhoea.
Caution:
Not to be used for: children or for patients suffering from megaloblastic anaemia.

F

Caution needed with: PHENYTOIN, some antibiotics, ANTACIDS, LEVODOPA.
Contains: FERROUS FUMARATE, FOLIC ACID.
Other preparations: GALFER FA, METERFOLIC, PREGADAY.

---

folic acid *see* Ferfolic SV, Ferrocontin Continus Folic, Ferrograd Folic, Folex-350, folic acid tablets, Ketovite, Lexpec, Meterfolic, Preconceive, Pregaday, Slow-Fe Folic

---

folic acid tablets

A tablet supplied at strengths of 400 mcg and 5 mg and used as a FOLIC ACID supplement to treat megaloblastic anaemia (anaemia with large red blood cells), and to treat or prevent other folate deficiencies. In pregnancy it is used to prevent neural tube defects in the foetus.

Dose: adults usually 5 mg a day (rarely up to 15 mg a day); children up to 1 year use syrup, children over 1 year adult dose. To prevent neural tube defects in pregnancy, 400 mcg a day for the first 12 weeks.
Availability: NHS, private prescription, and over the counter provided daily dose does not exceed 500 mcg.
Side effects: nausea, constipation.
Caution:
Not to be used for: megaloblastic anaemia caused by VITAMIN B$_{12}$ deficiency.
Caution needed with: PHENYTOIN.
Contains: FOLIC ACID.
Other preparations: folic acid syrup. LEXPEC.

---

folinic acid *see* Refolinon

Fomac *see* mebeverine tablets

Foradil
(Ciba)

A white powder in a clear capsule, supplied at a strength of 12 micrograms, and used by inhalation as a BRONCHODILATOR for the long-term treatment of asthma and other bronchial obstruction disorders.

Dose: 1-2 capsules inhaled (using the device supplied) twice a day.
Availability: NHS, private prescription.
Side effects: shaking hands, palpitations, headaches; rarely muscle

cramp or pain, heart rhythm disturbance, mouth and throat irritation, low blood potassium levels, breathing difficulty, itching, eye disorders, taste disturbance, stomach upset, anxiety, sleeplessness.
Caution: in patients suffering from severe asthma, overactive thyroid, severe heart or circulation problems, diabetes.
Not to be used for: pregnant women, nursing mothers.
Caution needed with: ß-BLOCKERS, SYMPATHOMIMETICS, drugs affecting heart rhythm, MAOIS, TRICYCLIC ANTIDEPRESSANTS.
Contains: EFORMOTEROL fumarate.
Other preparations:

---

formaldehyde *see* **Veracur**

Fortagesic
(Sanofi Winthrop)

A white tablet used as an opiate ANALGESIC to relieve pain in the bones and muscles.

Dose: children 7-12 years 1 tablet up to 4 times a day; adults 2 tablets up to 4 times a day.
Availability: controlled drug; private prescription only.
Side effects: sedation, dizziness, nausea, psychological effects.
Caution: in pregnant women and in patients suffering from kidney, liver, or respiratory disease, or some blood disorders, PORPHYRIA.
Not to be used for: children under 7 years, or for patients with respiratory difficulty, raised brain pressure, head injuries, or certain brain conditions, or for patients who are addicted to similar drugs.
Caution needed with: MAOIS, some other analgesics, alcohol, other drugs containing PARACETAMOL.
Contains: PENTAZOCINE hydrochloride, PARACETAMOL.
Other preparations:

Fortral *see* **pentazocine tablets/capsules**
(Sanofi Winthrop)

Fosamax
(MSD)

A white tablet supplied at a strength of 10 mg, and used as a treatment for osteoporosis in women after the menopause.

Dose: 1 tablet a day with a full glass of water first thing in the morning, 30

minutes before food or other medicines.
Availability: NHS, private prescription.
Side effects: rash, abdominal pain.
Caution: in patients suffering from upper gastro-intestinal disorders or
calcium/VITAMIN D deficiency.
Not to be used for: children, pregnant women, nursing mothers, or for
patients with kidney impairment.
Caution needed with: calcium, ANTACIDS, NON-STEROIDAL ANTI-INFLAMMATORY
DRUGS.
Contains: ALENDRONATE sodium.
Other preparations:

---

fosfomycin *see* **Monuril**

---

fosinopril *see* **Staril**

---

framycetin *see* **Sofradex Drops, Sofradex Ointment,
Soframycin Drops, Sofratulle**

---

frangula *see* **Normacol Plus**

Franol
(Sanofi Winthrop)

A white tablet used as a BRONCHODILATOR to treat blocked airway brought on
by chronic bronchitis or bronchial asthma.

Dose: 1 tablets 3 times a day and 1 tablet before going to bed if needed.
Availability: NHS, private prescription, over the counter.
Side effects: nausea, stomach upset, headache, sleeplessness, rapid or
abnormal heart rate, flushing, anxiety, tremor.
Caution: in the elderly, nursing mothers, and in patients suffering from
kidney, heart or liver disease, stomach ulcer, agitation, overactive thyroid,
glaucoma, enlarged prostate, fits, PHAEOCHROMOCYTOMA.
Not to be used for: children, pregnant women, or for patients suffering
from some types of angina, PORPHYRIA, coronary heart disease, high blood
pressure.
Caution needed with: CIMETIDINE, ERYTHROMYCIN, CIPROFLOXACIN, MAOIS,
TRICYCLIC ANTIDEPRESSANTS, SYMPATHOMIMETICS, the contraceptive pill.
Contains: EPHEDRINE hydrochloride, THEOPHYLLINE.
Other preparations: Franol Plus.

Frisium
(Hoechst-Roussel)

A blue capsule supplied at a strength of 10 mg and used as a sedative to treat anxiety, tension, agitation, and as an additional treatment for epilepsy.

Dose: elderly 1 tablet twice a day or 2 tablets at night; adults 1 tablet 2-3 times a day or 2-3 tablets at night. Maximum dose 6 tablets a day. Children over 3 years half adult dose.
Availability: NHS (for epilepsy when prescribed as a generic) and private prescription.
Side effects: drowsiness, confusion, unsteadiness, low blood pressure, rash, changes in vision, changes in sexual function, retention of urine, rarely blood changes, jaundice. Risk of addiction increases with dose and length of treatment. May impair judgement.
Caution: in the elderly, pregnant women, nursing mothers, in women during labour, and in patients suffering from lung disorders, kidney or liver disorders. Avoid long-term use and withdraw gradually.
Not to be used for: for patients suffering from acute lung disorders, some chronic lung disorders, some obsessional and psychotic diseases.
Caution needed with: alcohol, other tranquillizers, anticonvulsants, sedatives.
Contains: CLOBAZAM.
Other preparations:

Froben *see* flurbiprofen tablets
(Knoll)

Froop 40 *see* frusemide tablets

Fru-Co *see* co-amilofruse tablets
(Baker Norton)

Frumil *see* co-amilofruse tablets
(Rhône-Poulenc Rorer)

---

frusemide *see* Aridil, Diumide-K Continus, Dryptal, Froop 40, Fru-Co, Frumil, frusemide tablets, Frusene, Frusid, Lasikal, Lasilactone, Lasix, Lasix + K, Lasoride, Rusyde

---

frusemide tablets

A tablet supplied at strengths of 20 mg, 40 mg and used as a DIURETIC to treat fluid retention, reduction in urination caused by kidney failure.

Dose: fluid retention adults 20-80 mg a day or every other day as one dose; children 1-3 mg per kg bodyweight per day; reduction in urination, adults 250 mg a day at first increasing if required.
Availability: NHS and private prescription.
Side effects: reduced blood sodium, potassium, or magnesium levels, low blood pressure, stomach upset, gout, raised blood sugars; rarely rash, sensitivity to light, hearing disturbance.
Caution: in pregnant women, nursing mothers, and in patients suffering from liver or kidney disease, gout, diabetes, enlarged prostate, PORPHYRIA.
Not to be used for: patients suffering from liver cirrhosis, kidney failure with failed urination.
Caution needed with: DIGOXIN, LITHIUM, ASTEMIZOLE, TERFENADINE, STEROIDS, some antibiotics, blood-pressure lowering drugs, NON-STEROIDAL ANTI-INFLAMMATORY DRUGS, drugs affecting heart rhythm, some antidiabetics, CARBAMAZEPINE.
Contains: FRUSEMIDE.
Other preparations: frusemide oral solution, injection. DRYPTAL, FROOP, FRUSID, LASIX, RUSYDE.

Frusene
(Fisons)

A yellow, scored tablet used as a potassium-sparing DIURETIC to treat fluid retention caused by heart or liver problems, and congestive heart failure.

Dose: ½-2 tablets a day (occasionally up to 6 tablets a day).
Availability: NHS and private prescription.
Side effects: stomach upset, feeling of being unwell, rash, gout, blood changes.
Caution: in pregnant women, nursing mothers, and in patients suffering from kidney or liver disease, diabetes, electrolyte disorder, enlarged prostate, impaired urination, gout.
Not to be used for: children or for patients suffering from cirrhosis of the liver, progressive kidney failure, or raised potassium levels.
Caution needed with: potassium supplements, some diuretics, LITHIUM, DIGOXIN, blood-pressure lowering drugs, some antibiotics, some muscle relaxants, THEOPHYLLINE, NON-STEROIDAL ANTI-INFLAMMATORY DRUGS, ACE INHIBITORS.
Contains: FRUSEMIDE, TRIAMTERENE.
Other preparations:

Frusid see frusemide tablets
(DDSA)

Fucibet
(Leo)

A cream used as an antibacterial and strong STEROID treatment for eczema where there is also infection.

Dose: apply to the affected area 2-3 times a day at first and then reduce if possible.
Availability: NHS and private prescription.
Side effects: fluid retention, suppression of the adrenal glands, thinning, spotting, and streaking of the skin may occur.
Caution: use for short periods of time only, especially in children and on the face.
Not to be used for: patients suffering from acne or any other skin infections caused by tuberculosis, ringworm, viruses, or fungi, leg ulcers scabies, or continuously especially in pregnant women.
Caution needed with:
Contains: BETAMETHASONE valerate, FUSIDIC ACID.
Other preparations:

Fucidin Tablets
(Leo)

A white, oval tablet supplied at a strength of 250 mg and used as an antibiotic to treat infections.

Dose: 2 tablets 3 times a day; children use Fucidin Suspension.
Availability: NHS and private prescription.
Side effects: jaundice, stomach disturbances.
Caution: the liver should be checked regularly.
Not to be used for:
Caution needed with:
Contains: SODIUM FUSIDATE.
Other preparations: Fucidin Suspension.

Fucidin Cream
(Leo)

A cream used as an antibacterial treatment for skin infections.

Dose: apply to the affected area 3-4 times a day (or less if dressings used).

Availability: NHS and private prescription.
Side effects:
Caution:
Not to be used for:
Caution needed with:
Contains: FUSIDIC ACID.
Other preparations: Fucidin Gel, Fucidin Ointment.

Fucidin H
(Leo)

An ointment used as a STEROID and antibacterial treatment for eczema and dermatitis where there is inflammation and infection.

Dose: apply to the affected area 3-4 times a day.
Availability: NHS and private prescription.
Side effects: fluid retention, suppression of the adrenal glands, thinning, spotting, or streaking of the skin may occur.
Caution: use for short periods of time only, especially in children or on the face.
Not to be used for: patients suffering from acne or any other skin infections caused by tuberculosis, ringworm, viruses, or fungi, leg ulcers, scabies, or continuously especially in pregnant women.
Caution needed with:
Contains: SODIUM FUSIDATE, HYDROCORTISONE acetate.
Other preparations: Fucidin H Cream, Fucidin H Gel.

Fucidin Intertulle
(Leo)

A sterile, impregnated gauze dressing, supplied at a size of 10 cm square, and used as a dressing for ulcers, wounds, burns, and grafts where there is infection.

Availability: NHS, private prescription.
Contains: SODIUM FUSIDATE.

Fucithalmic
(Leo)

Drops used as an antibacterial treatment for conjunctivitis.

Dose: 1 drop into the eye twice a day.
Availability: NHS and private prescription.

Side effects: temporary irritation, allergy.
Caution:
Not to be used for:
Caution needed with:
Contains: FUSIDIC ACID.
Other preparations:

Fulcin
(Zeneca)

A white, scored tablet or a white tablet according to strengths of 125 mg, 500 mg and used as an anti-fungal treatment for scalp, skin, and nail infections.

Dose: adults 125 mg 4 times a day or 500 mg once a day; children 10 mg per kg body weight in one or divided doses.
Availability: NHS and private prescription.
Side effects: stomach upset, headache, allergy, sensitivity to light, rarely LUPUS, rash, blood changes.
Caution:
Not to be used for: pregnant women or for patients suffering from PORPHYRIA, severe liver disease.
Caution needed with: some ANTICOAGULANTS, BARBITURATES, the contraceptive pill, alcohol.
Contains: GRISEOFULVIN.
Other preparations: Fulcin Suspension. GRISOVIN.

Full Marks
(Seton Healthcare)

An alcohol-based lotion used to treat head and pubic lice.

Dose: rub into hair and leave to dry naturally. Shampoo after 2 hours and comb hair while still wet.
Availability: NHS, private prescription, over the counter.
Side effects:
Caution: in children under 6 months, and in patients suffering from asthma, eczema. Avoid the eyes.
Not to be used for:
Caution needed with:
Contains: PHENOTHRIN.
Other preparations:

F

Fungilin
(Squibb)

A light-brown, scored tablet supplied at a strength of 100 mg and used as an antibiotic to treat intestinal thrush, and for the prevention of vaginal or skin thrush.

Dose: adults 1-2 tablets 4 times a day; children use Suspension.
Availability: NHS and private prescription.
Side effects: stomach upset at high doses.
Caution:
Not to be used for:
Caution needed with:
Contains: AMPHOTERICIN.
Other preparations: FUNGILIN LOZENGES, Fungilin Suspension.

Fungilin Lozenges
(Squibb)

A yellow lozenge supplied at a strength of 10 mg and used as an antifungal treatment for thrush.

Dose: 1 lozenge allowed to dissolve slowly in the mouth 4-8 times a day.
Availability: NHS and private prescription.
Side effects: stomach upset at high doses.
Caution:
Not to be used for:
Caution needed with:
Contains: AMPHOTERICIN.
Other preparations: FUNGILIN, Fungilin Suspension.

Furadantin *see* nitrofurantoin tablets
(Procter & Gamble)

---

fusafungine *see* Locabiotal

---

fusidic acid *see* Fucibet, Fucidin Cream, Fucidin Tablets, Fucithalmic

---

Fybogel
(Reckitt & Colman)

Plain, orange-, or lemon-flavoured, effervescent granules supplied in sachets of 3.5 g and used as a bulking agent in the treatment of diverticular disease, spastic and irritable colon, constipation.

Dose: adults 1 sachet in water evening and morning; children 2.5-5 ml in water evening and morning.
Availability: NHS, private prescription, over the counter.
Side effects:
Caution:
Not to be used for: patients suffering from intestinal obstruction.
Caution needed with:
Contains: ISPAGHULA husk.
Other preparations: Fybogel Orange. ISOGEL, REGULAN.

Fybogel Mebeverine
(Reckitt & Colman)

Effervescent granules in sachets used as an antispasm treatment and bulking agent for irritable bowel syndrome.

Dose: 1 sachet of granules in water morning and evening ½-hour before meals. If necessary an additional sachet may be taken 30 minutes before the midday meal.
Availability: NHS, private prescription.
Side effects:
Caution:
Not to be used for: children, or for patients suffering from severe kidney, heart, or circulation disorders, blocked intestines, or inelastic colon.
Caution needed with:
Contains: MEBEVERINE HYDROCHLORIDE, ISPAGHULA husk.
Other preparations:

---

gabapentin *see* Neurontin

Galake *see* co-dydramol tablets
(Galen)

Galcodine *see* codeine linctus
(Galen)

Galenamet *see* **cimetidine tablets**
(Galen)

Galenamox *see* **amoxycillin capsules**
(Galen)

Galenphol *see* **pholcodine linctus**
(Galen)

Galfer
(Galen)

A green/red capsule supplied at a strength of 305 mg and used as an iron supplement to treat iron-deficiency anaemia.

Dose: adults 1 capsule 1-2 times a day before food; children use syrup.
Availability: NHS, private prescription, over the counter.
Side effects: nausea, constipation.
Caution:
Not to be used for:
Caution needed with: some antibiotics, ANTACIDS, LEVODOPA.
Contains: FERROUS FUMARATE.
Other preparations: Galfer Syrup. FERSADAY, FERSAMAL.

Galfer FA *see* **Folex 350**
(Galen)

Galfloxin *see* **flucloxacillin capsules**
(Galen)

Galpseud
(Galen)

A white tablet supplied at a strength of 60 mg and used as a SYMPATHOMIMETIC to treat congestion of the nose, sinuses, and upper respiratory tract.

Dose: adults 1 tablet 3 times a day; children use linctus.
Availability: NHS, private prescription, over the counter.
Side effects: anxiety, hands shaking, irregular or rapid heart rate, dry mouth, excitement.

G

Caution: in patients suffering from diabetes, overactive thyroid, high blood pressure, enlarged prostate, raised eye pressure, heart disease.
Not to be used for: children under 2 years.
Caution needed with: MAOIS, TRICYCLIC ANTIDEPRESSANTS other SYMPATHOMIMETICS, appetite suppressants, FURAZOLIDONE.
Contains: PSEUDOEPHEDRINE hydrochloride.
Other preparations: Galpseud Linctus. SUDAFED.

Galpseud Plus
(Galen)

A linctus used as a SYMPATHOMIMETIC and ANTIHISTAMINE to treat allergic rhinitis.

Dose: adults, 10 ml 3 times a day; children 2-6 years 2.5 ml 3 times a day, children 6-12 years 5 ml 3 times a day.
Availability: NHS, private prescription, over the counter.
Side effects: drowsiness, reduced reactions.
Caution: in patients suffering from enlarged prostate, bladder disorder, severe kidney or liver disease.
Not to be used for: children under 2 years, or for patients suffering from epilepsy or high blood pressure.
Caution needed with: MAOIS, blood-pressure lowering drugs, other sympathomimetics, alcohol, sedatives.
Contains: PSEUDOEPHEDRINE hydrochloride, CHLORPHENIRAMINE MALEATE.
Other preparations:

G

Gamanil *see* lofepramine tablets
(Merck)

Gammabulin *see* human normal immunoglobulin injection
(Immuno)

---

gamolenic acid *see* Epogam, Efamast

---

ganciclovir *see* Cymevene

Ganda
(Chauvin)

Drops used as a fluid channel drug to treat glaucoma.

Dose: 1 drop into the eye 1-2 times a day.
Availability: NHS and private prescription.
Side effects: pain in the eye, headache, redness, skin reactions, melanosis, increase in eye pressure, drooping of the upper eyelid, inflammation of the cornea.
Caution: your doctor may advise that the conjunctiva and cornea should be checked every 6 months if you are undergoing prolonged treatment.
Not to be used for: patients suffering from narrow-angle glaucoma, absence of the lens.
Caution needed with: MAOIS.
Contains: GUANETHIDINE monosulphate, ADRENALINE.
Other preparations:

Garamycin *see* Cidomycin Drops
(Schering-Plough)

Gastrobid Continus *see* metoclopramide tablets
(Napp)

Gastrocote
(Seton Healthcare)

A white tablet used as an ANTACID and reflux suppressant to treat heartburn, hiatus hernia, oesophagitis

Dose: adults 1-2 tablets chewed 4 times a day and at bedtime, children over 6 years as adult.
Availability: NHS, private prescription, over the counter.
Side effects: occasionally constipation.
Caution:
Not to be used for: children under 6 years.
Caution needed with: tablets coated to protect the stomach, some antibiotics, iron.
Contains: ALGINIC ACID, ALUMINIUM HYDROXIDE, MAGNESIUM TRISILICATE, SODIUM BICARBONATE.
Other preparations: Gastrocote Liquid.

Gastroflux *see* metoclopramide tablets
(Ashbourne)

Gastromax *see* **metoclopramide tablets**
(Pharmacia)

Gastron
(Sanofi Winthrop)

A white tablet used as an ANTACID and reflux suppressant to treat reflux symptoms.

Dose: adults 1-2 tablets chewed 3 times a day after meals and 2 at bedtime.
Availability: NHS, private prescription, over the counter.
Side effects: occasionally constipation.
Caution: in pregnant women, and in patients suffering from high blood pressure, heart or kidney failure.
Not to be used for: children.
Caution needed with: tablets coated to protect the stomach, some antibiotics, iron.
Contains: ALGINIC ACID, ALUMINIUM HYDROXIDE, SODIUM BICARBONATE, MAGNESIUM TRISILICATE.
Other preparations:

G

Gastrozepin
(Knoll)

A white tablet used as an antispasm, ANTICHOLINERGIC treatment for gastric and duodenal ulcers.

Dose: adults 1 tablet twice a day before meals for 4-6 weeks.
Availability: NHS and private prescription.
Side effects: blurred vision, confusion, dry mouth.
Caution:
Not to be used for: children, or for patients with glaucoma, inflammatory bowel disease, intestinal obstruction, or enlarged prostate.
Caution needed with:
Contains: PIRENZEPINE.
Other preparations:

Gaviscon
(Reckitt & Colman)

A tablet used as an ANTACID and reflux suppressant to treat reflux symptoms including indigestion, hiatus hernia, heartburn, oesophagitis.

Dose: adults 1-2 tablets after meals and at night; children half adult dose.

Availability: NHS, private prescription, over the counter.
Side effects:
Caution:
Not to be used for:
Caution needed with: tablets coated to protect the stomach, some antibiotics, iron.
Contains: ALGINIC ACID, ALUMINIUM HYDROXIDE GEL, MAGNESIUM TRISILICATE, SODIUM BICARBONATE.
Other preparations: Gaviscon Liquid, Gaviscon Infant Sachets (to treat reflux and regurgitation in children), Gaviscon-250 tablets (half strength – not available on NHS).

---

gelatin *see* **Orabase**

Gelcosal
(Quinoderm)

A gel used as an antipsoriatic and skin softener to treat psoriasis, dermatitis, when the condition is scaling.

Dose: massage into the affected area twice a day.
Availability: NHS, private prescription, over the counter.
Side effects:
Caution:
Not to be used for:
Caution needed with:
Contains: strong COAL TAR solution, TAR, SALICYLIC ACID.
Other preparations: CAPASAL, IONIL-T.

Gelcotar
(Quinoderm)

A gel used as an antipsoriatic treatment for psoriasis, dermatitis.

Dose: massage into the affected area twice a day.
Availability: NHS, private prescription, over the counter.
Side effects: irritation, sensitivity to light.
Caution:
Not to be used for: patients suffering from acute psoriasis.
Caution needed with:
Contains: strong COAL TAR solution, TAR.
Other preparations: Gelcotar Liquid. CARBO-DOME, CLINITAR, PSORIDERM, PSORIGEL.

Gelkam *see* **Fluorigard Gelkam**

---

gemfibrozil *see* **Lopid**

Genisol
(Roche Consumer Health)

A liquid used as an antipsoriatic and antidandruff treatment for psoriasis or scaly inflammation of the scalp.

Dose: shampoo once a week or as needed.
Availability: NHS, private prescription, over the counter.
Side effects:
Caution: avoid eyes.
Not to be used for:
Caution needed with:
Contains: COAL TAR, SODIUM SULPHOSUCCINATED UNDECYLENIC MONOALKYOLAMIDE.
Other preparations:

---

gentamicin *see* **Cidomycin Cream, Cidomycin Drops, Genticin Drops, Gentamicin Minims, Gentisone HC Drops**

Gentamicin Minims
(Chauvin)

Drops used as an aminoglycoside antibiotic to treat bacterial infections of the eye.

Dose: 1 drop into the eye as needed.
Availability: NHS and private prescription.
Side effects:
Caution:
Not to be used for:
Caution needed with:
Contains: GENTAMICIN sulphate.
Other preparations: CIDOMYCIN DROPS, GARAMYCIN, GENTICIN.

---

gentian mixture

A tonic used to improve appetite.

Dose: 10 ml 3 times a day before meals.

Availability: NHS, private prescription, over the counter.
Side effects:
Caution:
Not to be used for: children.
Caution needed with:
Contains: gentian infusion, hydrochloric acid (in gentian mixture acid), sodium bicarbonate (in gentian mixture alkaline).
Other preparations: gentian mixture, alkaline.

---

gentian violet *see* crystal violet paint

Genticin Drops *see* Cidomycin Drops
(Nicholas)

Gentisone HC Drops
(Roche)

Drops used as an antibiotic, STEROID treatment for inflammation of the outer ear, chronic weeping inflammation of the middle ear.

Dose: 2-4 drops into the ear 3-4 times a day and at night.
Availability: NHS and private prescription.
Side effects: additional infection.
Caution: in pregnant women, infants, and in patients suffering from perforated ear drum. Use for short periods of time only.
Not to be used for:
Caution needed with:
Contains: GENTAMICIN sulphate, HYDROCORTISONE acetate.
Other preparations:

---

gestodene *see* Femodene, Femodene ED, Minulet, Tri-Minulet, Triadene

---

Gestone
(Paines & Byrne)

An injection supplied at strengths 25 mg, 50 mg, 100 mg, and used as a progesterone treatment for abnormal vaginal bleeding and to maintain pregnancy.

Dose: for bleeding, 5-10 mg by injection for 5-10 days until 2 days before menstruation; in pregnancy, 25-100 mg twice a week from day 15 to week

8-16 of pregnancy.
Availability: NHS and private prescription.
Side effects: disturbance of normal menstrual bleeding, breast discomfort, acne, ovarian cyst, headache, stomach upset, fluid retention, rash, depression, tiredness, sleeplessness, rarely jaundice.
Caution: in nursing mothers and in patients suffering from diabetes, epilepsy, migraine, high blood pressure, ovarian cysts, and some cancers, heart or kidney disorders.
Not to be used for: children, or for patients suffering from liver disorder, undiagnosed vaginal bleeding, breast cancer, PORPHYRIA, or with a history of blood clots.
Caution needed with: BARBITURATES, PHENYTOIN, PRIMIDONE, CARBAMAZEPINE, CHLORAL HYDRATE, ETHOSUXIMIDE, RIFAMPICIN, GLUTHETHIMIDE, CHLORPROMAZINE, MEPROBAMATE, GRISEOFULVIN, CYCLOSPORIN.
Contains: progesterone.
Other preparations:

---

gestrinone *see* Dimetriose

Glandosane
(Fresenius)

An aerosol used to provide artificial saliva for dry mouth and throat.

Dose: spray into the mouth and throat for 1-2 seconds as needed.
Availability: NHS, private prescription, over the counter.
Side effects:
Caution:
Not to be used for:
Caution needed with:
Contains: CARBOXYMETHYLCELLULOSE sodium, SORBITOL, POTASSIUM CHLORIDE, SODIUM CHLORIDE, MAGNESIUM CHLORIDE, CALCIUM CHLORIDE, DIPOTASSIUM HYDROGEN PHOSPHATE.
Other preparations:

Glaucol *see* Timoptol Eye Drops
(Baker Norton)

---

glibenclamide *see* Calabren, Daonil, Diabetamide, Euglucon, glibenclamide tablets, Libanil, Malix, Semi-Daonil

---

G

glibenclamide tablets

A tablet supplied at strengths of 2.5 mg, 5 mg and used as an antidiabetic drug to treat diabetes.

Dose: 5 mg (elderly 2.5 mg) a day at breakfast at first increasing if needed to a maximum of 15 mg a day.
Availability: NHS and private prescription.
Side effects: allergy including skin rash, stomach upset, headache; rarely blood disorders.
Caution: in the elderly and in patients suffering from kidney or liver disorders.
Not to be used for: children, pregnant women, nursing mothers, during surgery, or for patients suffering from juvenile diabetes, hormone disorders, stress, infections, PORPHYRIA, severe illness.
Caution needed with: MAOIS, STEROIDS, DIURETICS, alcohol, the contraceptive pill, ASPIRIN, some antibiotics, some antifungals, GLUCAGON, drugs used to lower blood pressure, NON-STEROIDAL ANTI-INFLAMMATORY DRUGS, KETOTIFEN, CIMETIDINE, LITHIUM, ß-BLOCKERS.
Contains: GLIBENCLAMIDE.
Other preparations: CALABREN, DAONIL, DIABETAMIDE, EUGLUCON, LIBANIL, MALIX, SEMI-DAONIL.

G Glibenese
(Pfizer)

A white, oblong, scored tablet supplied at a strength of 5 mg and used as a sulphonylurea to treat diabetes.

Dose: ½-1 tablet a day before breakfast or lunch at first increasing if needed by ½-1 tablet a day every 3-5 days to a maximum of 8 tablets a day in divided doses.
Availability: NHS and private prescription.
Side effects: allergy including skin rash.
Caution: in the elderly and in patients suffering from kidney failure.
Not to be used for: children, pregnant women, nursing mothers, during surgery, or for patients suffering from juvenile diabetes, liver or kidney impairment, hormone disorders, stress, infections.
Caution needed with: ß-BLOCKERS, MAOIS, STEROIDS, DIURETICS, alcohol, ANTICOAGULANTS, lipid-lowering agents, ASPIRIN, some antibiotics (RIFAMPICIN, sulphonamides, CHLORAMPHENICOL), GLUCAGON, cyclophosphamide, the contraceptive pill.
Contains: GLIPIZIDE.
Other preparations: MINODIAB.

---

gliclazide *see* **Diamicron**

---

glipizide *see* **Glibenese, Minodiab**

---

gliquidone *see* **Glurenorm**

Glucagen *see* **Glucagon**
(Novo)

Glucagon
(Lilly)

An injection administered by the subcutaneous, intramuscular, or intravenous route to treat severe low blood glucose levels (eg in diabetics when too much insulin has been used). A similar effect can be achieved by giving the patient sugar by mouth, if conscious.

Dose: adults and children 0.5-1 mg immediately.
Availability: NHS and private prescription.
Side effects: nausea, vomiting, diarrhoea, low blood potassium levels, allergy.
Caution: in pregnant women and nursing mothers. If a suitable response is not seen within 20 minutes of the dose, further treatment is needed urgently.
Not to be used for: patients suffering from adrenal tumour, pancreatic tumour.
Caution needed with: WARFARIN.
Contains: glucagon hydrochloride.
Other preparations: GLUCAGEN.

Glucamet *see* **metformin tablets**
(Opus)

Gluco-lyte *see* **Dioralyte**
(Seton Healthcare)

Glucobay
(Bayer)

An off-white tablet supplied at strengths of 50 mg, 100 mg used to treat diabetes.

Dose: 50 mg chewed with the first mouthful of food or swallowed whole with liquid 3 times a day at first, increasing to 100 mg 3 times a day if needed after 6-8 weeks, up to a maximum of 200 mg 3 times a day.
Availability: NHS, private prescription.
Side effects: wind, bloating, stomach pain, diarrhoea, feeling over-full after eating.
Caution: your doctor may advise regular blood tests.
Not to be used for: children, pregnant women, nursing mothers, or for patients suffering from liver or severe kidney disorder, inflammatory bowel disorders, ulcers of the colon, blocked intestines, digestive disorders, any disorders made worse by wind.
Caution needed with: pancreatic enzymes, NEOMYCIN, CHOLESTYRAMINE, other antidiabetic drugs, KAOLIN, CHARCOAL.
Contains: ACARBOSE.
Other preparations:

Glucophage *see* metformin tablets
(Lipha)

---

glucose *see* Dioralyte, Electrolade, Gluco-lyte, Rehidrat

Glucostix
(Bayer Diagnostics)

A plastic reagent strip used in conjunction with a Glucometer GX meter to detect blood glucose levels. Blood-glucose monitoring enables individual patients suffering from diabetes accurately to control blood glucose and manage their condition.

Glucotide
(Bayer Diagnostics)

A plastic reagent strip used in conjunction with a Glucometer 4 meter to detect blood glucose levels. Blood-glucose monitoring enables individual patients suffering from diabetes accurately to control blood glucose and manage their condition.

Glurenorm
(Sanofi Winthrop)

A white, scored tablet supplied at a strength of 30 mg and used as an antidiabetic to treat diabetes.

Dose: 1½-2 tablets a day in divided doses before food to a maximum of 6 tablets a day.
Availability: NHS and private prescription.
Side effects: allergy including skin rash.
Caution: in the elderly and in patients suffering from kidney failure.
Not to be used for: children, pregnant women, nursing mothers, during surgery, or for patients suffering from juvenile diabetes, liver or kidney impairment, hormone disorders, stress, infections.
Caution needed with: ß-BLOCKERS, MAOIS, STEROIDS, DIURETICS, alcohol, ANTICOAGULANTS, lipid-lowering agents, ASPIRIN, some antibiotics (RIFAMPICIN, sulphonamides, CHLORAMPHENICOL), GLUCAGON, cyclophosphamide, the contraceptive pill.
Contains: GLIQUIDONE.
Other preparations:

---

glutaraldehyde *see* Glutarol, Verucasep

Glutarol
(Dermal)

A solution used as a virucidal, skin-drying agent to treat warts.

Dose: apply the solution to the wart twice a day and rub down hard skin.
Availability: NHS, private prescription, over the counter.
Side effects: staining of the skin.
Caution: do not apply to healthy skin.
Not to be used for: warts on the face or anal and genital areas.
Caution needed with:
Contains: GLUTARALDEHYDE.
Other preparations: VERUCASEP.

G

---

glycerin/glycerol *see* Audax, Exterol, glycerol suppositories, magnesium sulphate paste, Micolette, Relaxit, sodium bicarbonate ear drops, Unguentum Merck

---

glycerol suppositories

Suppositories supplied at strengths of 1 g, 2 g, 4 g and used as a stimulant laxative to treat constipation.

Dose: adults 4 g suppository as necessary; children 2 g suppository, infants 1 g suppository.
Availability: NHS, private prescription, over the counter.

Side effects:
Caution: moisten suppository with water before use.
Not to be used for:
Caution needed with:
Contains: GLYCEROL (GLYCERINE)
Other preparations:

---

glyceryl trinitrate *see* **Coro-Nitro, Deponit, glyceryl trinitrate tablets, Glytrin, GTN, Minitran, Nitrocontin Continus, Nitrodur, Nitrolingual, Percutol, Suscard Buccal, Sustac, Transiderm-Nitro**

---

glyceryl trinitrate tablets

A tablet supplied at strengths of 300 mcg, 500 mcg and used as a NITRATE to treat and prevent angina by dissolving the tablet under the tongue. (Long-acting brands can be swallowed in the usual way.)

Dose: under the tongue 0.3-1 mg as needed; as swallowed doses 2.6-6.4 mg 2-3 times a day; or up to 10 mg 3 times a day for severe angina (as long-acting product).
Availability: NHS, private prescription, over the counter.
Side effects: headache, flushing, dizziness, low blood pressure on standing, rapid pulse.
Caution: in patients suffering from severe liver or kidney damage, underactive thyroid gland, history of heart attack, malnutrition, low body temperature.
Not to be used for: children; or for patients suffering from allergy to nitrates, low blood pressure, some heart conditions, severe anaemia, head injury or brain haemorrhage, closed-angle glaucoma.
Caution needed with: DISOPYRAMIDE, ANTICOAGULANTS, TRICYCLIC ANTIDEPRESSANTS, ANTICHOLINERGICS.
Contains: GLYCERYL TRINITRATE.
Other preparations: preparations for use under the tongue: GTN, CORO-NITRO SPRAY, GLYTRIN SPRAY, NITROLINGUAL SPRAY. Preparations to be swallowed: NITROCONTIN, SUCARD, SUSTAC (all long-acting preparations). Patch products available: DEPONIT, MINITRAN, NITRO-DUR, TRANSIDERM-NITRO. Ointment product: PERCUTOL.

---

glycine *see* **Cicatrin, Titralac**

---

glycol salicylate *see* **Cremalgin, Dubam, Salonair**

Glyconon *see* **tolbutamide tablets**
(DDSA)

Glymese *see* **chlorpropamide tablets**
(DDSA)

Glytrin *see* **Coro-nitro**
(Sterwin Medicines)

---

gonadorelin *see* **Fertiral**

---

gonadotrophin *see* **Gonadotrophon LH, Pregnyl, Profasi**

Gonadotrophon LH
(Ferring)

A powder and solvent supplied in separate vials and used as a hormone treatment for infertility in women and failure of the testicles to descend or reduced sperm production in males.

Dose: as advised by the physician.
Side effects: fluid retention, headache, tiredness, mood changes, allergy, increased sexuality.
Caution: in patients suffering from asthma, epilepsy, migraine, heart or kidney disorders.
Not to be used for: male children under 7 years, female children.
Caution needed with:
Contains: GONADOTROPHIN.
Other preparations: PREGNYL, PROFASI.

Gopten
(Knoll)

A red/yellow capsule, red/orange capsule, or red/red capsule according to strengths of 0.5 mg, 1 mg, 2 mg, and used as an ACE INHIBITOR to treat raised blood pressure.

Dose: 0.5 mg once a day at first, increasing to 1-2 mg once a day for maintenance, but up to a maximum of 4 mg a day.
Availability: NHS, private prescription.
Side effects: cough, headache, weakness, dizziness, rash, low blood

pressure, palpitations, rarely blood changes, severe allergy with swelling. *Caution:* in patients undergoing dialysis, surgery, or general anaesthetics, or who are suffering with liver or kidney failure, congestive heart failure, salt or volume depletion. Your doctor may advise regular kidney tests. Stop using any DIURETICS 2-3 days before starting treatment.

Not to be used for: children, pregnant women, nursing mothers, or for patients suffering from swelling of the blood vessels associated with previous ACE inhibitor treatment, major blood vessel obstruction.

Caution needed with: some diuretics, NON-STEROIDAL ANTI-INFLAMMATORY DRUGS.

Contains: TRANDOLAPRIL.

Other preparations:

---

goserelin *see* **Zoladex**

---

gramicidin *see* **Adcortyl with Graneodin, Graneodin, Neosporin, Sofradex Drops, Sofradex Eye Ointment, Tri-Adcortyl, Tri-Adcortyl Otic**

Graneodin
(Squibb)

An ointment used as an antibiotic to treat skin infections such as impetigo and beard infections, and for the prevention of infections during minor surgery.

Dose: apply 2-4 times a day.
Availability: NHS and private prescription.
Side effects: hearing damage, allergy, kidney damage.
Caution: in patients with large areas of affected skin; do not use with dressings or to the ear canal if the eardrum is perforated.
Not to be used for: fungal, viral, or deep infections.
Caution needed with:
Contains: NEOMYCIN sulphate, GRAMICIDIN.
Other preparations:

Gregoderm
(Unigreg)

An ointment used as a STEROID, antibacterial treatment for psoriasis, itch of the anal and genital area, and other skin disorders where there is also inflammation and infection.

Dose: apply to the affected area 2-3 times a day.
Availability: NHS and private prescription.
Side effects: fluid retention, suppression of the adrenal glands, thinning, spotting, or streaking of the skin may occur.
Caution: use for short periods of time only, especially in children or on the face.
Not to be used for: continuously especially for pregnant women, or for patients suffering from acne or any other tubercular, fungal, viral, or ringworm infections, scabies, or leg ulcers.
Caution needed with:
Contains: NEOMYCIN sulphate, NYSTATIN, POLYMYXIN B SULPHATE, HYDROCORTISONE.
Other preparations:

---

griseofulvin *see* Fulcin, Grisovin

Grisovin
(Glaxo)

A white tablet supplied at strengths of 125 mg, 500 mg and used as an antifungal treatment for infections of the nails, skin, and scalp.

Dose: adults 500 mg-1 g a day in divided doses after meals; children 10 mg per kg body weight a day in divided doses.
Availability: NHS and private prescription.
Side effects: drowsiness, gastric upset, headache, allergies, sensitivity to light, rarely precipitation of LUPUS.
Caution: in pregnant women and in patients on prolonged treatment.
Not to be used for: patients suffering from PORPHYRIA, liver disease, lupus.
Caution needed with: BARBITURATES, some ANTICOAGULANTS, alcohol, sedatives, the contraceptive pill.
Contains: GRISEOFULVIN.
Other preparations: FULCIN.

GTN *see* glyceryl trinitrate tablets
(Martindale)

---

guaiphenesin *see* Dimotane Expectorant

---

guanethidine *see* Ganda, Ismelin Tablets

---

guar gum *see* **Guarem**

Guarem
(Shire)

Dispersible granules in a 5 g sachet used as a bulking agent to treat diabetes and dumping syndrome (abnormal reactions after eating).

Dose: 1 sachet dispersed in 200 ml of liquid immediately before each meal or stirred into food and eaten with 200 ml liquid.
Availability: NHS, private prescription, over the counter.
Side effects: wind, swollen abdomen.
Caution: glucose levels should be checked in diabetics.
Not to be used for: children or for patients suffering from a blocked intestine or oesophageal disease.
Caution needed with: other antidiabetic treatments.
Contains: GUAR GUM.
Other preparations:

Gyno-Daktarin 1
(Janssen-Cilag)

A white vaginal capsule supplied at a strength of 1200 mg and used as an antifungal treatment for thrush of the vulva or vagina.

Dose: 1 capsule inserted high into the vagina as a single dose.
Availability: NHS, private prescription, over the counter.
Side effects: mild burning or irritation.
Caution:
Not to be used for: children.
Caution needed with:
Contains: MICONAZOLE nitrate.
Other preparations: Gyno-Daktarin Pessaries, Gyno-Daktarin CombiPack, Gyno-Daktarin Cream. (All available over the counter to treat vaginal thrush.)

Gyno-Pevaryl 1
(Janssen-Cilag)

A pessary supplied at a strength of 150 mg and used as an antifungal treatment for vaginal thrush.

Dose: 1 pessary inserted into the vagina at night as a single dose.
Availability: NHS, private prescription, over the counter.

Side effects: mild burning or irritation.
Caution:
Not to be used for: children.
Caution needed with:
Contains: ECONAZOLE nitrate.
Other preparations: Gyno-Pevaryl 1CP, Gyno-Pevaryl Cream, Gyno-Pevaryl Pessaries, Gyno-Pevaryl Combipack. (All available over the counter to treat vaginal thrush.)

Gynol II
(Janssen-Cilag)

A non-perfumed, water-based jelly, used with a diaphragm as a spermicidal contraceptive.

Dose: apply to the inner surface and the rim of the diaphragm before intercourse.
Availability: NHS, private prescription, over the counter.
Side effects:
Caution:
Not to be used for: children.
Caution needed with:
Contains: NONOXYNOL-9.
Other preparations: DURAGEL.

Haelan
(Dista)

H

A cream used as a STEROID treatment for skin disorders.

Dose: apply 2-3 times a day.
Availability: NHS and private prescription.
Side effects: fluid retention, suppression of the adrenal glands, thinning, spotting, or streaking of the skin may occur.
Caution: use for short periods of time only, especially on the face or in children.
Not to be used for: continuously especially for pregnant women, or for patients suffering from acne, or any other tubercular, viral, fungal, or ringworm skin infections, leg ulcers, scabies.
Caution needed with:
Contains: FLURANDRENOLONE.
Other preparations: Haelan Ointment, Haelan Tape (not available on NHS), Haelan-C (with CLIOQUINOL for infected conditions).

Halciderm
(Squibb)

A cream used as a STEROID treatment for acute skin disorders, such as eczema, psoriasis.

Dose: apply to the affected area 2-3 times a day.
Availability: NHS and private prescription.
Side effects: fluid retention, suppression of the adrenal glands, thinning, spotting, or streaking of the skin may occur.
Caution: do not dilute the cream. Use for short periods of time only.
Not to be used for: continuously especially for pregnant women, or for patients suffering from other tubercular, fungal, viral, or ringworm infections, scabies, leg ulcers.
Caution needed with:
Contains: HALCINONIDE.
Other preparations:

---

halcinonide *see* **Halciderm**

Haldol *see* **haloperidol tablets**
(Janssen-Cilag)

Half-Beta-Prograne *see* **propanolol tablets**
(Tillomed Laboratories)

Half-Inderal LA *see* **propanolol tablets**
(Zeneca)

Half-Securon SR *see* **verapamil tablets**
(Knoll)

Half Sinemet CR *see* **Sinemet**
(Du Pont)

Halfan
(Smith Kline & French)

A white, scored, capsule-shaped tablet supplied at a strength of 250 mg, and used to treat malaria.

Dose: adults and children over 37 kg in weight, 6 tablets taken in 3 divided doses at 6-hourly intervals. Repeat the dose one week later. Do not take with meals
Availability: NHS and private prescription.
Side effects: stomach upset, abdominal pain, blood changes, irregular heart rate.
Caution: in women of child-bearing age, and in patients suffering from complicated malarial conditions, or malaria involving the brain.
Not to be used for: children under 37 kg body weight, pregnant women, nursing mothers, for patients suffering from some heart disorders, or for preventing malaria.
Caution needed with: QUININE, CHLOROQUINE, MEFLOQUINE, TRICYCLIC ANTIDEPRESSANTS, drugs used to treat heart rhythm disturbances, TERFENADINE, ASTEMIZOLE.
Contains: HALOFANTRINE.
Other preparations:

---

halofantrine *see* **Halfan**

---

haloperidol *see* **Dozic, Haldol, haloperidol tablets, Serenace**

---

haloperidol tablets

A tablet supplied at strengths of 1.5 mg, 5 mg, 10 mg, and 20 mg and used as a sedative to treat mental disorders (including schizophrenia, severe anxiety), persistent hiccups and tics.

Dose: for mental disorders, adults usually 3-15 mg a day (elderly patients use half adult dose). Doses may be increased in severe cases. Children require reduced doses. For hiccups, adults 1.5 mg 3 times a day. For tics and movement disorders, adults usually 0.5-1.5 mg 3 times a day.
Availability: NHS and private prescription.
Side effects: muscle spasms, restlessness, hands shaking, dry mouth, urine retention, palpitations, low blood pressure, weight gain, changes in sexual function, low body temperature, breast swelling, menstrual changes, jaundice, blood and skin changes, drowsiness, rarely fits, sensitivity to light.
Caution: in the elderly, pregnant women, nursing mothers or in patients suffering from liver, lung, or kidney disease, epilepsy, severe cardiovascular disease, Parkinson's disease, thyroid disorders, infections, some blood disorders, prostate disease, glaucoma.
Not to be used for: unconscious patients, or for patients with some blood or bone marrow disorders.
Caution needed with: alcohol, sedatives, tranquillizers, pain killers,

H

blood-pressure lowering drugs, antidepressants, some antidiabetic drugs, LEVODOPA, RIFAMPICIN, LITHIUM, ANTACIDS, drugs affecting heart rhythm, CARBAMAZEPINE, ASTEMIZOLE, TERFENADINE, CIMETIDINE.
Contains: HALOPERIDOL.
Other preparations: DOZIC liquid, HALDOL, SERENACE.

Halycitrol
(LAB)

An emulsion used as a multivitamin preparation to treat VITAMIN A and VITAMIN D deficiencies.

Dose: adults and children over 6 months 5 ml a day; infants under 6 months 2.5 ml a day.
Availability: private prescription and over the counter.
Side effects: vitamin poisoning.
Caution: in pregnant women, and in patients suffering from kidney disease, sarcoidosis (a chest disease that affects calcium levels).
Not to be used for:
Caution needed with: some DIURETICS.
Contains: vitamin A, vitamin D.
Other preparations:

Harmogen
(Upjohn)

An orange, oval, scored tablet supplied at a strength of 1.5 mg and used as an oestrogen to treat menopausal oestrogen deficiency.

Dose: 1-2 tablets a day continuously. (Women with an intact uterus may require additional progestogen treatment.)
Availability: NHS and private prescription.
Side effects: enlarged breasts, fluid retention, nausea, vaginal bleeding, weight gain, headache, dizziness. Rarely jaundice, raised blood pressure, thrombosis.
Caution: in patients suffering from high blood pressure, diabetes, epilepsy, womb diseases, gall bladder disorder, migraine, multiple sclerosis, PORPHYRIA, liver disorders, some ear disorders, or a history or increased risk of breast disorders (including cancer) and thrombosis. Your doctor may advise you to have regular examinations.
Not to be used for: children, pregnant women, nursing mothers, or for patients suffering from thombosis, severe liver, kidney, or heart disorders, some cancers, undiagnosed vaginal bleeding, endometriosis.
Caution needed with: ACE INHIBITORS, ANTICOAGULANTS, BARBITURATES, ß-BLOCKERS, CARBAMAZEPINE, PHENYTOIN, RIFAMPICIN.

Contains: PIPERAZINE OESTRONE SULPHATE.
Other preparations:

Havrix Monodose
(SmithKline Beecham)

A vaccination containing the inactivated virus and used to provide active immunization against hepatitis A.

Dose: adults over 16 years, 1 injection of 1 ml, and then a booster dose of 1 ml 6-12 months later; children use Havrix Junior.
Availability: NHS, private prescription.
Side effects: soreness, reddening and hardening of the skin at the injection site, fever, tiredness, nausea, loss of appetite, general feeling of being unwell.
Caution: in pregnant women and nursing mothers, and in patients on dialysis or suffering from infection or changed immunity.
Not to be used for: patients suffering from severe feverish infections.
Caution needed with:
Contains: inactivated HEPATITIS A virus.
Other preparations: Havrix Junior.

Haymine
(Pharmax)

A yellow tablet used as an ANTIHISTAMINE and SYMPATHOMIMETIC treatment for allergies.

Dose: 1 tablet in the morning and 1 tablet at night if needed.
Availability: NHS, private prescription, over the counter.
Side effects: drowsiness, reduced reactions, dizziness.
Caution:
Not to be used for: children or for patients suffering from overactive thyroid gland, high blood pressure, coronary thrombosis.
Caution needed with: sedatives, MAOIS, alcohol.
Contains: CHLORPHENIRAMINE MALEATE, EPHEDRINE hydrochloride.
Other preparations:

H-B-VAX II
(Pasteur Merieux MSD)

A vaccination used to provide active immunization against hepatitis B.

Dose: adults and children over 10 years, 1 injection of 1 ml, and then repeated doses of 1 ml 1 month and 6 months later; children under 10 years, 1 injection of 0.5 ml, and then repeated doses of 0.5 ml 1 month and 6 months later.

Availability: NHS, private prescription.

Side effects: soreness, reddening and hardening of the skin at the injection site, mild fever, rash, nausea, dizziness, general feeling of being unwell.

Caution: in pregnant women, and in patients suffering from heart or breathing disorders. Patients on dialysis or whose immune systems are weakened may need further doses.

Not to be used for: patients suffering from severe feverish infections.

Caution needed with:

Contains: HEPATITIS B antigen.

Other preparations: ENGERIX B.

Heminevrin
(Astra)

A syrup used as a sedative for the short-term treatment of sleeplessness in the elderly, agitated states, tension and anxiety, daytime sedation in senile mental disorder, confusion, alcohol withdrawal symptoms, severe epilepsy.

Dose: 10 ml in water or fruit juice before going to bed. For sedation 5 ml 3 times a day. (Different doses for alcohol withdrawal. Injection used for toxaemia and epilepsy.)

Availability: NHS and private prescription.

Side effects: blocked and irritating nose, irritating eyes, stomach upset, severe allergy, excitement, confusion, drowsiness, headache, rash.

Caution: in pregnant women, nursing mothers, the elderly, patients suffering from long-term lung weakness, kidney or liver disease, or with a history of drug or alcohol abuse. Patients should be warned of impaired ability and not to continue drinking alcohol while on this treatment.

Not to be used for: children, or patients suffering from acute lung weakness.

Caution needed with: alcohol, sedatives, DIAZOXIDE, PROPRANOLOL, CIMETIDINE.

Contains: CHLORMETHIAZOLE EDISYLATE.

Other preparations: Heminevrin Capsules, Heminevrin IV, Heminevrin Solution.

---

heparinoid *see* **Anacal, Hirudoid, Lasonil**

---

hepatitis A vaccine *see* **Havrix**

---

hepatitis B vaccine *see* **Engerix B, H-B-Vax**

Herpid
(Yamanouchi)

A solution used as an anti-viral treatment for shingles and cold sores.

Dose: apply locally 4 times a day for 4 days.
Availability: NHS and private prescription.
Side effects:
Caution:
Not to be used for: children, pregnant women, nursing mothers.
Caution needed with:
Contains: IDOXURIDINE, DIMETHYL SULPHOXIDE.
Other preparations: IDURIDIN (stronger product also available for once-daily application), VIRUDOX.

---

hexachlorophane *see* **Dermalex, Ster-Zac Powder**

---

hexamine hippurate *see* **Hiprex**

---

hexetidine *see* **Oraldene**

Hexopal
(Sanofi Winthrop)

A white, scored tablet supplied at a strength of 500 mg and used as a vasodilator to treat Raynaud's phenomenon (a condition caused by spasm of the blood vessels), intermittent claudication (difficulty walking caused by circulation disorders).

Dose: 2 tablets 3-4 times a day.
Availability: NHS, private prescription, over the counter.
Side effects:
Caution: in pregnant women.
Not to be used for: children.
Caution needed with:
Contains: INOSITOL nicotinate.

H

Other preparations: Hexopal Forte, Hexopal Suspension.

---

hexyl nicotinate *see* **Transvasin**

Hibiscrub
(Zeneca)

A solution used as a disinfectant for cleansing and disinfecting skin and hands.

Dose: use as a liquid soap.
Availability: NHS, private prescription, over the counter.
Side effects:
Caution:
Not to be used for:
Caution needed with:
Contains: CHLORHEXIDINE gluconate.
Other preparations: HIBISOL, HIBITANE, PHISOMED, UNISEPT.

Hibisol
(Zeneca)

A solution used as a disinfectant for cleansing and disinfecting skin and hands.

Dose: rub vigorously on to the skin until dry.
Availability: NHS, private prescription, over the counter.
Side effects:
Caution:
Not to be used for:
Caution needed with:
Contains: CHLORHEXIDINE gluconate, ISOPROPYL ALCOHOL.
Other preparations: HIBISCRUB, HIBITANE, PHISOMED, UNISEPT.

Hioxyl
(Quinoderm)

A cream used as a disinfectant to treat minor wounds, infections, bed sores, leg ulcers.

Dose: apply freely as needed and cover with a dressing.
Availability: NHS, private prescription, over the counter.
Side effects:

Caution:
Not to be used for:
Caution needed with:
Contains: HYDROGEN PEROXIDE.
Other preparations:

Hiprex
(3M Health Care)

A white, oblong, scored tablet supplied at a strength of 1 g and used as an antibacterial treatment for infections of the urinary tract.

Dose: adults 1 g twice a day; children 6-12 years half adult dose.
Availability: NHS, private prescription, over the counter.
Side effects: stomach upset, rash, bladder irritation.
Caution:
Not to be used for: children under 6 years, or for patients suffering from severe dehydration, severe kidney failure, or electrolyte changes.
Caution needed with: some antibiotics, SODIUM BICARBONATE, SODIUM CITRATE, POTASSIUM CITRATE.
Contains: METHENAMINE HIPPURATE (HEXAMINE HIPPURATE).
Other preparations:

Hirudoid
(Panpharma)

A cream used as an anti-inflammatory agent to treat superficial thrombophlebitis, superficial blood clotting, and bruising.

Dose: apply liberally up to 4 times a day.
Availability: NHS, private prescription, over the counter.
Side effects:
Caution:
Not to be used for: children under 5 years, or on open wounds or mucous membranes.
Caution needed with:
Contains: HEPARINOID.
Other preparations: Hirudoid Gel.

Hismanal
(Janssen-Cilag)

A white, scored tablet supplied at a strength of 10 mg and used as an ANTIHISTAMINE treatment for hay fever, allergic rhinitis, skin allergies.

Dose: adults 1 tablet a day 1 hour before food; children 6-12 years half adult dose.
Availability: NHS, private prescription, over the counter.
Side effects: rarely drowsiness or gain in weight, heart rhythm disturbance.
Caution: in patients with some heart rhythm disturbances, liver damage, electrolyte disturbances; women of child-bearing age should take steps to avoid conception during and for some weeks after the treatment.
Not to be used for: children under 6 years, pregnant women, nursing mothers.
Caution needed with: alcohol, sedatives, anti-arrhythmic drugs, TRICYCLIC ANTIDEPRESSANTS, DIURETICS, some tranquillizers, KETOCONAZOLE, ERYTHROMYCIN and similar antibiotics, ITRACONAZOLE, TERFENADINE, SOTALOL.
Contains: ASTEMIZOLE.
Other preparations: Hismanal Suspension (available only on prescription). Pollon-eze.

Histafen *see* terfenadine tablets
(Berk)

---

histamine-H$_2$ antagonist (blocker)
A drug which works on the stomach to reduce acid production by blocking the histamine pathway. Example RANITIDINE *see* Zantac.

Hivid
(Roche)

A beige or grey film-coated tablet according to strengths of 0.375 mg and 0.75 mg and used as an antiviral drug to combat HIV infections where the patient is unable to take ZIDOVUDINE.

Dose: 0.75 mg 3 times a day.
Availability: NHS, private prescription.
Side effects: weakness and numbness in the hands and feet, inflammation of the pancreas, stomach upsets, rash, itching, sweating, rarely lactic acidosis, liver disorders, ulcers of the oesophagus, severe allergic shock.
Caution: in pregnant women, nursing mothers, and in patients suffering from heart failure, liver or kidney damage or with a history of alcohol abuse, or who are at risk of developing weakness or numbness of the hands and feet, or inflamed pancreas. Your doctor will recommend regular blood tests.
Not to be used for: children, or for patients suffering from weakness and numbness of the hands and feet.

Caution needed with: any drugs that may cause weakness and numbness of hands and feet, DIDANOSINE, AMPHOTERICIN, FOSCARNET, some antibiotics.
Contains: ZALCITABINE.
Other preparations:

---

homatropine eye drops

Drops used as an ANTICHOLINERGIC preparation for pupil dilation.

Dose: 1 or more drops into the eye as needed.
Availability: NHS and private prescription.
Side effects: skin problems, closed-angle glaucoma.
Caution: do not drive for 1-2 hours after treatment.
Not to be used for: patients suffering from narrow-angle glaucoma.
Caution needed with: other eye medications.
Contains: HOMATROPINE HYDROBROMIDE.
Other preparations: Minims Homatropine Hydrobromide (packed in single-use containers).

---

homatropine hydrobromide *see* **homatropine eye drops, Homatropine Minims**

Homatropine Minims
(Chauvin)

Drops used as an ANTICHOLINERGIC preparation for pupil dilation.

Dose: 1 or more drops into the eye as needed.
Availability: NHS and private prescription.
Side effects:
Caution:
Not to be used for: patients suffering from narrow-angle glaucoma.
Caution needed with:
Contains: HOMATROPINE HYDROBROMIDE.
Other preparations: Homatropine Eye Drops.

Hormonin
(Shire)

A pink, scored tablet used as an oestrogen treatment for symptoms associated with the menopause, and for prevention of osteoporosis after the menopause.

H

Dose: 1-2 tablets a day; (if uterus still intact, progestogen supplements may also be required).
Availability: NHS and private prescription.
Side effects: enlarged breasts, fluid retention, nausea, vaginal bleeding, weight gain, headache, dizziness. Rarely jaundice, raised blood pressure, thrombosis.
Caution: in patients suffering from high blood pressure, diabetes, epilepsy, womb diseases, gall bladder disorder, migraine, multiple sclerosis, PORPHYRIA, liver disorders, some ear disorders, or a history or increased risk of breast disorders (including cancer) and thrombosis. Your doctor may advise you to have regular examinations.
Not to be used for: children, pregnant women, nursing mothers, or for patients suffering from thombosis, severe liver, kidney, or heart disorders, some cancers, undiagnosed vaginal bleeding, endometriosis.
Caution needed with: ACE INHIBITORS, ANTICOAGULANTS, BARBITURATES, ß-BLOCKERS, CARBAMAZEPINE, PHENYTOIN, RIFAMPICIN.
Contains: OESTRIOL, OESTRONE, OESTRADIOL.
Other preparations:

---

human menopausal gonadotrophin *see* Humegon, Normegon

---

human normal immunoglobulin injection

A vaccination administered by injection prepared from human blood plasma that contains antibodies effective against measles, mumps, chickenpox, hepatitis A, and other viruses.

Dose: prevention of hepatitis A, adult 250 mg, child under 10 years 125 mg (effects last for 2 months; doubling the dose provides up to 5 months' protection); prevention of measles, child under 1 year 250 mg, 1-2 years 500 mg, 3 years and over 750 mg; prevention of rubella in pregnancy 750 mg.
Availability: NHS and private prescription.
Side effects: general feeling of illness, chills, fever, rarely shock and allergy.
Caution:
Not to be use for: patients with known class specific antibody to immunoglobulin.
Caution needed with: live virus vaccines.
Contains: normal immunoglobulin.
Other preparations: GAMMABULIN, KABIGLOBULIN.

Humegon *see* Normegon
(Organon)

Humiderm
(Convatec)

A cream used as an emollient to treat chronic dry skin, thickening of the skin.

Dose: apply to the affected area after bathing.
Availability: NHS, private prescription, over the counter.
Side effects:
Caution:
Not to be used for:
Caution needed with:
Contains: SODIUM PYRROLIDONE CARBOXYLATE.
Other preparations:

Humulin *see* Insulin
(Lilly)

Hydergine
(Sandoz)

A white tablet supplied at strengths of 1.5 mg, 4.5 mg and used as a vasodilator as an additional treatment for elderly patients suffering from dementia.

Dose: 4.5 mg a day.
Availability: NHS and private prescription.
Side effects: stomach upset, flushes, rash, blocked nose, cramps, headache, dizziness, low blood pressure when standing.
Caution: in patients suffering from slow heart rate.
Not to be used for: children
Caution needed with:
Contains: CODERGOCRINE MESYLATE.
Other preparations:

---

hydralazine *see* Apresoline, hydralazine tablets

---

hydralazine tablets

A tablet supplied at strengths of 25 mg, 50 mg and used as a vasodilator for the treatment of moderate to severe high blood pressure.

Dose: 25 mg twice a day at first increasing to 50 mg twice a day if necessary.
Availability: NHS and private prescription.
Side effects: rapid heart rate, fluid retention, headache, flushes, nausea, vomiting, especially if more than 100 mg a day are taken; rarely rashes, fever, liver damage, kidney disorders, changes in blood count, nerve disorders, LUPUS-like disorders.
Caution: in pregnant women, nursing mothers, and in patients suffering from heart or brain circulatory disease, kidney failure.
Not to be used for: children, for patients suffering from certain heart diseases, LUPUS, PORPHYRIA, or during the first half of pregnancy
Caution needed with: antidepressants, MAOIS, blood-pressure lowering drugs, tranquillizers, anaesthetics, DIAZOXIDE, alcohol, NON-STEROIDAL ANTI-INFLAMMATORY DRUGS.
Contains: HYDRALAZINE hydrochloride.
Other preparations: APRESOLINE.

Hydrenox
(Knoll)

A white, scored tablet supplied at a strength of 50 mg and used as a DIURETIC to treat fluid retention, high blood pressure.

Dose: adults fluid retention 1-4 tablets a day as a single dose in the morning, then ½-1 tablet a day every other day, high blood pressure ½-1 tablet a day; children 1 mg per kg bodyweight a day.
Availability: NHS and private prescription.
Side effects: blood changes, stomach upset, rash, sensitivity to light, loss of appetite, impotence, pancreatitis, dizziness.
Caution: in the elderly, in pregnant women, nursing mothers, and in patients suffering from diabetes, liver or kidney disease, gout, SLE; your doctor may advise that a potassium supplement is needed.
Not to be used for: patients suffering from severe kidney or liver failure, Addison's disease, raised calcium levels, allergy to some antibiotics.
Caution needed with: LITHIUM, DIGOXIN, blood-pressure lowering drugs, STEROIDS, CARBENOXOLONE, NON-STEROIDAL ANTI-INFLAMMATORY DRUGS, antidiabetics, BARBITURATES, alcohol, opioid ANALGESICS.
Contains: HYDROFLUMETHIAZIDE.
Other preparations:

Hydrocal *see* **hydrocortisone cream**
(Bioglan)

---

hydrochlorothiazide *see* **Accuretic, Acezide, Amil-Co, Amilmax, Capozide, Carace Plus, Co-Betaloc, Delvas, Dyazide, Hydromet, Hydrosaluric, Kalten, Innozide, Moducren, Moduret 25, Moduretic, Monozide 10, Secadrex, Sotazide, Synuretic, Thyamil, Tolerzide, Triam-Co**

---

hydrocortisone *see* **Actinac, Alphaderm, Alphosyl HC, Anugesic-HC, Anusol HC, Calmurid HC, Canesten-HC, Carbo-Cort, Chloromycetin Hydrocortisone, Cobadex, Colifoam, Corlan, Daktacort, Econacort, Efcortelan, Epifoam, Eurax-Hydrocortisone, Fucidin H, Gentisone HC Drops, Gregoderm, Hydrocal, Hydrocortistab, Hydrocortone, Locoid, Locoid Lipocream, Mildison Lipocream, Neo-Cortef, Nystaform-HC, Otosporin, Perinal, Proctofoam HC, Proctosedyl, Quinocort, Tarcortin, Terra-Cortril, Timodine, Uniroid, Vioform-Hydrocortisone, Xyloproct**

---

hydrocortisone cream

A cream used as a STEROID treatment for eczema, itch, nappy rash, and other skin disorders.

Dose: apply to the affected area 1-4 times a day.
Availability: NHS and private prescription.
Side effects: fluid retention, suppression of adrenal glands, thinning, spotting, or streaking of the skin may occur.
Caution: use for short periods of time only, especially in children or on the face, and in patients suffering from psoriasis.
Not to be used for: continuously especially for pregnant women, or for patients suffering from acne or any other tubercular, viral, fungal, or ringworm skin infections, leg ulcers, scabies.
Caution needed with:
Contains: HYDROCORTISONE.
Other preparations: Hydrocortisone Ointment. DIODERM, EFCORTELAN, HYDROCAL (with added CALAMINE), HYDROCORTISTAB, HYDROCORTISYL, LOCOID (a stronger product), MILDISON LIPOCREAM. (Some other brands available over the counter for the following conditions only: allergic or irritant contact dermatitis, insect bites, mild to moderate eczema. Other restrictions also apply to over-the-counter sales.)

Hydrocortistab Tablets
(Knoll)

A white, scored tablet supplied at a strength of 20 mg and used as a STEROID for replacement treatment in adrenocortical deficiency, acute emergency treatment for severe bronchial asthma, allergy and allergic fluid retention and shock, and severe reaction to the serum used in vaccinations etc.

Dose: replacement therapy, adults 20-30 mg a day; children 10-30 mg a day in divided doses. For other treatments, as advised by the physician.
Availability: NHS and private prescription.
Side effects: high blood sugar, thin bones, mood changes, ulcers, high blood pressure, fluid retention, potassium loss, muscle weakness.
Caution: in pregnant women, in patients who have had recent bowel surgery, or who are suffering from inflamed veins, psychiatric disorders, virus infections, some cancers, some kidney diseases, thinning of the bones, ulcers, tuberculosis, other infections, high blood pressure, glaucoma, epilepsy, diabetes, underactive thyroid, liver disease, stress. Withdraw gradually. Avoid contact with chickenpox or herpes virus.
Not to be used for:
Caution needed with: PHENYTOIN, PHENOBARBITONE, EPHEDRINE, RIFAMPICIN, DIURETICS, ANTICHOLINESTERASES, DIGOXIN, antidiabetic agents, ANTICOAGULANTS, NON-STEROIDAL ANTI-INFLAMMATORY DRUGS.
Contains: HYDROCORTISONE.
Other preparations: Hydrocortistab Injection. HYDROCORTONE.

Hydrocortistab Cream/Ointment *see* hydrocortisone cream
(Knoll)

Hydrocortisyl *see* hydrocortisone cream
(Hoechst Roussel)

Hydrocortone
(M.S.D.)

A white, quarter-scored tablet or a white, scored, oval tablet according to strengths of 10 mg, 20 mg and used as a STEROID replacement treatment in adrenocortical deficiency.

Dose: as advised by the physician.
Availability: NHS and private prescription.
Side effects: high blood sugar, thin bones, mood changes, ulcers, high blood pressure, fluid retention, potassium loss, muscle weakness.

Caution: in pregnant women, in patients who have had recent bowel surgery, or who are suffering from inflamed veins, psychiatric disorders, virus infections, some cancers, some kidney diseases, thinning of the bones, ulcers, tuberculosis, other infections, high blood pressure, glaucoma, epilepsy, diabetes, underactive thyroid, liver disease, stress. Withdraw gradually. Avoid contact with chickenpox or herpes virus.
Not to be used for:
Caution needed with: PHENYTOIN, PHENOBARBITONE, EPHEDRINE, RIFAMPICIN, DIURETICS, ANTICHOLINESTERASES, DIGOXIN, antidiabetic agents, ANTICOAGULANTS, NON-STEROIDAL ANTI-INFLAMMATORY DRUGS.
Contains: HYDROCORTISONE.
Other preparations: HYDROCORTISTAB.

---

hydroflumethiazide *see* **Aldactide, Hydrenox, Spiro-Co 50**

---

hydrogen peroxide *see* **Hioxyl**

Hydromet
(M.S.D.)

A pink tablet used as an DIURETIC treatment for high blood pressure.

Dose: adults 1 tablet twice a day at first increasing at 2-day intervals to a maximum of 12 tablets a day; children as advised by physician.
Availability: NHS and private prescription.
Side effects: sedation, headache, weakness, depression, slow heart rate, low blood pressure, blocked nose, dry mouth, stomach upset, blood changes, kidney disorder, electrolyte and other changes.
Caution: in pregnant women, nursing mothers, patients undergoing anaesthesia, and in patients with a history of liver disease, or in patients suffering from some blood disorders, gout, diabetes, liver or kidney disease. Your doctor may advise that potassium supplements may be needed.
Not to be used for: patients suffering from depression, severe kidney or liver failure, failure to produce urine, raised calcium levels, Addison's disease, PHAEOCHROMOCYTOMA (a disease of the adrenal glands).
Caution needed with: TRICYCLIC ANTIDEPRESSANTS, MAOIS, blood-pressure lowering drugs, STEROIDS, SYMPATHOMIMETICS, NON-STEROIDAL ANTI-INFLAMMATORY DRUGS, LEVODOPA, some tranquillizers, DIGOXIN, LITHIUM.
Contains: METHYLDOPA, HYDROCHLOROTHIAZIDE.
Other preparations:

H

Hydromol *see* **Diprobath**
(Quinoderm)

Hydrosaluric
(M.S.D.)

A white, scored tablet supplied at strengths of 25 mg, 50 mg and used as a DIURETIC to treat fluid retention, high blood pressure.

Dose: adults as a diuretic 25-100 mg once or twice a day, high blood pressure 25-50 mg a day at first, then up to not more than 100 mg a day; infants under 6 months up to 3.5 mg per kg bodyweight a day, 6 months-2 years 12.5-37.5 mg a day, 2-12 years 37.5-100 mg a day all in 2 divided doses.
Availability: NHS and private prescription.
Side effects: low potassium levels, rash, sensitivity to light, blood changes, gout, tiredness.
Caution: in pregnant women and in patients suffering from diabetes, liver or kidney disease, electrolyte imbalance, SLE, or gout. Your doctor may advise that a potassium supplement is needed.
Not to be used for: nursing mothers or for patients suffering from severe kidney or liver failure, raised calcium levels, Addison's disease, failure to produce urine.
Caution needed with: LITHIUM, DIGOXIN, blood-pressure lowering drugs, sedatives, ACE INHIBITORS, STEROIDS, antidiabetics, muscle relaxants, NON-STEROIDAL ANTI-INFLAMMATORY DRUGS.
Contains: HYDROCHLOROTHIAZIDE.
Other preparations:

---

hydrotalcite *see* **Altacite Plus**

---

hydrous ointment BP

A cream used as an emollient to treat dry skin conditions.

Dose: apply as required
Availability: NHS, private prescription, over the counter.
Side effects:
Caution:
Not to be used for:
Caution needed with:
Contains: hydrous ointment BP (oily cream).
Other preparations:

---

hydroxocobalamin *see* **Cobalin-H, Lipoflavonoid, Lipotriad, Neo-Cytamen, vitamin B$_{12}$**

---

hydroxy-progesterone hexanoate *see* **Proluton Depot**

---

hydroxyapatite compound *see* **Ossopan**

---

hydroxychloroquine *see* **Plaquenil**

---

hydroxyethylcellulose *see* **Artificial Tears Minims**

---

hydroxyzine *see* **Atarax**

Hygroton
(Ciba)

A pale-yellow, scored tablet supplied at a strength of 50 mg and used as a DIURETIC to treat high blood pressure, fluid retention.

Dose: adults fluid retention 50 mg a day or 100-200 mg every other day at first, then 50-100 mg 3 times a week as a single dose after breakfast, high blood pressure 25-50 mg a day as a single dose after breakfast; children 2 mg per kg a day maximum.
Availability: NHS and private prescription.
Side effects: abnormal heart rhythm, stomach disturbances, loss of appetite, rash, sensitivity to light, blood changes, gout, tiredness, electrolyte disturbances, visual disturbances, impotence, low blood pressure when standing, dizziness, rarely liver disturbances.
Caution: in the elderly, pregnant women, nursing mothers, and in patients suffering from diabetes, kidney or liver disease, high blood lipids, severe thickening of the arteries, SLE, or gout. Your doctor may advise that a potassium supplement is needed.
Not to be used for: patients suffering from Addison's disease, severe kidney or liver failure, low sodium or potassium levels, high calcium or uric acid levels, sensitivity to some antibiotics.
Caution needed with: LITHIUM, DIGOXIN, blood-pressure lowering drugs, STEROIDS, alcohol, BARBITURATES, CARBENOXOLONE, opiate ANALGESICS, NON-STEROIDAL ANTI-INFLAMMATORY DRUGS, INSULIN, antidiabetics.
Contains: CHLORTHALIDONE.
Other preparations:

H

hyoscine *see* Buscopan, hyoscine eye drops

hyoscine eye drops

Drops usually supplied at a strength of 0.25% and used to dilate the eye pupil.

Dose: as directed by the doctor.
Availability: NHS and private prescription.
Side effects:
Caution: in very young and very old patients.
Not to be used for: patients with some types of glaucoma.
Caution needed with:
Contains: HYOSCINE hydrobromide.
Other preparations:

Hypoguard GA
(Hypoguard)

A plastic reagent strip used, either visually or – more accurately – in conjunction with a Hypocount GA meter, to detect blood glucose levels. Blood-glucose monitoring enables individual patients suffering from diabetes accurately to control blood glucose and manage their condition.

Hypoguard Supreme
(Hypoguard)

A plastic reagent strip used, either visually or – more accurately – in conjunction with a Hypocount Supreme meter, to detect blood glucose levels. Blood-glucose monitoring enables individual patients suffering from diabetes accurately to control blood glucose and manage their condition.

Hypolar Retard *see* nifedipine modified release tablets
(Lagap)

Hypotears
(Ciba Vision Ophthalmics)

Drops used to moisten dry eyes.

Dose: 1-2 drops as needed.
Availability: NHS, private prescription, over the counter.

Side effects:
Caution:
Not to be used for: patients who wear soft contact lenses.
Caution needed with:
Contains: POLYVINYL ALCOHOL.
Other preparations: LIQUIFILM TEARS, SNO TEARS.

Hypovase *see* prazosin tablets
(Invicta)

---

hypromellose *see* hypromellose eye drops, Ilube, Isopto Alkaline, Isopto Atropine, Isopto Carbachol, Isopto Carpine, Isopto Plain, Maxidex, Maxitrol, Tears Naturale

---

hypromellose eye drops

Drops used to treat tear deficiency.

Dose: 1-2 drops 3 times a day or as required.
Availability: NHS, private prescription, over the counter.
Side effects:
Caution:
Not to be used for:
Caution needed with:
Contains: HYPROMELLOSE.
Other preparations: ISOPTO ALKALINE, ISOPTO PLAIN, TEARS NATURALE.

H

Hypurin *see* Insulin
(CP Pharmaceuticals)

Hytrin
(Abbott)

A white, yellow, brown, or blue tablet according to strengths of 1 mg, 2 mg, 5 mg, 10 mg and used as an ANTIHYPERTENSIVE to treat high blood pressure.

Dose: 1 mg at bed time at first, then increase dose at weekly intervals to a usual dose of 2-10 mg once a day.
Availability: NHS and private prescription.
Side effects: fainting with first dose, dizziness, lowered blood pressure on standing, weariness, swelling of the limbs.
Caution: in patients with a history of fainting.

Not to be used for: children.
Caution needed with:
Contains: TERAZOSIN hydrochloride.
Other preparations:

Hytrin BPH
(Abbott)

A white, yellow, brown, or blue tablet according to strengths of 1 mg, 2 mg, 5 mg, 10 mg, used as an alpha-blocker to treat the symptoms of urinary obstruction caused by prostate enlargement.

Dose: 1 mg before going to bed each day at first, increasing at weekly intervals up to 10 mg a day if required.
Availability: NHS, private prescription.
Side effects: first dose may cause fainting; then dizziness, low blood pressure on standing, tiredness, swelling of the hands and feet.
Caution: in patients with a history of fainting.
Not to be used for: children.
Caution needed with: blood-pressure lowering drugs.
Contains: TERAZOSIN hydrochloride.
Other preparations:

Ibufac *see* ibuprofen tablets
(DDSA)

Ibugel *see* Proflex
(Dermal)

Ibuleve *see* Proflex
(Dendron)

---

ibuprofen *see* Apsifen, Arthrofen Brufen, Codafen, Ebufac, Fenbid, Ibufac, Ibugel, Ibuleve, ibuprofen tablets, Ibuspray, Isisfen, Junifen, Lidifen, Motrin, Proflex, Rimafen

---

ibuprofen tablets

A coated tablet supplied at strengths of 200 mg, 400 mg, 600 mg and used as a NON-STEROIDAL ANTI-INFLAMMATORY AND ANALGESIC DRUG to treat pain, fever, period pain, post-surgery pain, rheumatoid arthritis, and other muscle and bone disorders.

Dose: adults 1200-1800 mg a day in 3-4 divided doses, to a maximum of 2400 mg a day; children 20 mg per kilogram of bodyweight a day in divided doses.
Availability: NHS and private prescription (200 and 400 mg tablets may be purchased without a prescription).
Side effects: stomach upset, stomach bleeding, rash, blood changes, fluid retention; rarely liver or kidney disorders, headache, tinnitus, vertigo.
Caution: in pregnant women, nursing mothers, the elderly, and in patients suffering from asthma, LUPUS, liver, kidney, or heart disease, history of stomach ulcers.
Not to be used for: children under 7 kg in weight or for patients suffering from stomach ulcer or bleeding, or with a history of allergy to ASPIRIN or anti-inflammatory drugs.
Caution needed with: ANTICOAGULANTS, other non-steroidal anti-inflammatory drugs, some antibiotics, STEROIDS, LITHIUM, drugs used to lower blood pressure, some antidiabetics, DIGOXIN, CYCLOSPORIN, METHOTREXATE.
Contains: IBUPROFEN.
Other preparations: APSIFEN, ARTHROFEN, BRUFEN, EBUFAC, FENBID, IBUFAC, IBULAR, ISIFEN, LIDIFEN, MOTRIN (additionally available at 800 mg strength), RIMAFEN. (Some brands are long-acting preparations.) JUNIFEN and Brufen available as liquids. Other brands are available without prescription.

Ibuspray *see* Proflex
(Dermal)

Ichthopaste
(Smith & Nephew Healthcare)

A medicated bandage supplied at a size of 7.5 cm x 6 m, and used to treat leg ulcers, varicose eczema, and chronic skin disorders.

Availability: NHS, private prescription, over the counter. (Also available on a trial basis from nurses.)
Contains: ZINC PASTE, ICHTHAMMOL.

Icthaband
(Smith & Nephew Healthcare)

A medicated bandage supplied at a size of 7.5 cm x 6 m, and used, in conjunction with a compression bandage, to treat varicose and gravitational ulcers, and skin disorders where the patient is sensitive to tar.

Availability: NHS, private prescription, over the counter. (Also available on a trial basis from nurses.)
Contains: ZINC PASTE, ICHTHAMMOL.

---

ichthammol *see* **Ichthopaste, Icthaband**

---

idoxuridine *see* **Iduridin, Herpid, Virudox**

Iduridin *see* **Herpid**
(Ferring)

Ikorel
(Rhône-Poulenc Rorer)

A white scored tablet supplied at strengths of 10 mg and 20 mg, and used for the prevention and treatment of angina.

Dose: 5-10 mg twice a day at first, increasing if necessary to a maximum of 30 mg twice a day; usual maintenance 10-20 mg twice a day.
Availability: NHS, private prescription.
Side effects: headache, dilation of the blood vessels, vomiting, dizziness, low blood pressure and/or rapid heart rate at high doses, weakness.
Caution: in patients with a history of headaches.
Not to be used for: children, pregnant women, nursing mothers, or for patients suffering from heart shock or failure, low blood pressure, fluid on the lungs, decrease in blood volume.
Caution needed with: blood-pressure lowering drugs.
Contains: NICORANDIL.
Other preparations:

Ilosone *see* **erythromycin tablets**
(Dista)

Ilube
(Cusi)

Drops used to moisten dry eyes.

Dose: 1-2 drops into the eye 3-4 times a day.
Availability: NHS and private prescription.
Side effects:

Caution:
Not to be used for: patients who wear soft contact lenses.
Caution needed with:
Contains: ACETYLCYSTEINE, HYPROMELLOSE.
Other preparations:

Imbrilon *see* indomethacin capsules
(Berk)

Imdur *see* isosorbide mononitrate tablets
(Astra)

Imigran
(Glaxo)

A pink or white, capsule-shaped tablet according to strengths of 50 mg, 100 mg, and used to treat migraine.

Dose: 50-100 mg soon after onset of attack. If migraine responds but then recurs, repeat the dose, to a maximum of 300 mg in 24 hours. Repeat doses should not be used if migraine did not respond initially.
Availability: NHS and private prescription.
Side effects: tiredness, dizziness, feelings of heaviness and weakness, throat symptoms or chest pain (stop treatment), liver disorder; rarely fits, low blood pressure, slow heart rate, serious circulatory disorders, severe allergy, pain.
Caution: in pregnant women, nursing mothers, and in patients suffering from liver or kidney disorder, heart disease, allergy to some antibiotics, or with a history of epilepsy or mental disorders. Your doctor may warn you not to drive or operate machinery.
Not to be used for: children, or for patients suffering from certain heart disease disorders, or uncontrolled high blood pressure, some circulatory disorders.
Caution needed with: MAOIS, LITHIUM, ERGOTAMINE, some antidepressants.
Contains: SUMATRIPTAN.
Other preparations: Imigran Subject Injection (also used to treat cluster headache).

---

imipramine *see* imipramine tablets, Tofranil

---

imipramine tablets

A coated tablet supplied at strengths of 10 mg, 25 mg and used as a TRICYCLIC ANTIDEPRESSANT to treat depression, night-time bed wetting in children

Dose: adults 75 mg a day at first, increasing to 200 mg if needed (elderly, 10-50 mg a day); children 7 years 25 mg, 8-11 years 25-50 mg, over 11 years 50-75 mg before going to bed, for up to 3 months. (Full examination recommended before further treatment.)
Availability: NHS and private prescription.
Side effects: dry mouth, tinnitus, tiredness, constipation, urine retention, blurred vision, nausea, palpitations, drowsiness, sleeplessness, dizziness, hands shaking, low blood pressure, weight change, sweating, fever, behavioural changes in children, confusion in the elderly, skin reactions, jaundice or blood changes, interference with sexual function.
Caution: in the elderly, pregnant women, nursing mothers, and in patients suffering from heart disease, liver and kidney disorders, thyroid disease, adrenal tumours, epilepsy, diabetes, glaucoma, PORPHYRIA, constipation, some other psychiatric conditions. Your doctor may advise regular blood tests.
Not to be used for: children under 7 years, children under 16 years to treat depression, or for patients suffering from recent heart attacks, heart rhythm disturbance, severe liver disease, heart block, or mania.
Caution needed with: alcohol, sedatives, ANTICHOLINERGICS, ADRENALINE, MAOIS, BARBITURATES, ASTEMIZOLE, TERFENADINE, other antidepressants, CIMETIDINE, drugs affecting heart rhythm, anticonvulsants.
Contains: IMIPRAMINE hydrochloride.
Other preparations: TOFRANIL (liquid form available).

Immunoprin *see* azathioprine tablets
(Ashbourne)

Imodium *see* loperamide capsules
(Centra Healthcare)

Imtack
(Astra)

An aerosol used as a NITRATE to treat and prevent angina.

Dose: 1-3 doses sprayed under the tongue (while holding breath) at start of an attack or before exertion.
Availability: NHS, private prescription, over the counter.

Side effects: flushes, headache, dizziness.
Caution: do not inhale the spray.
Not to be used for: for children.
Caution needed with:
Contains: ISOSORBIDE DINITRATE.
Other preparations: CEDOCARD, ISOKET RETARD, ISORDIL, ISOSORBIDE DINITRATE TABLETS, SONI-SLO, SORBICHEW, SORBID-SA, SORBITRATE.

Imunovir
(Leo)

A white tablet supplied at a strength of 500 mg and used as an anti-viral treatment for genital herpes, warts, and other herpes-type infections.

Dose: herpes 8 tablets a day for 7-14 days; warts 6 tablets a day for 14-28 days.
Availability: NHS and private prescription.
Side effects: increased levels of uric acid.
Caution: in patients suffering from kidney disease, gout, raised uric acid levels.
Not to be used for: children.
Not to be used with:
Contains: INOSINE PRANOBEX.
Other preparations:

Imuran *see* azathioprine tablets
(Wellcome)

Inadine
(Johnson & Johnson Patient Care)

A slow-release, impregnated, non-sticky dressing, supplied at a size of 5 cm square and 9.5 cm square, and used as a dressing for leg ulcers, burns, minor skin injuries.

Availability: NHS, private prescription, over the counter.
Contains: POVIDINE IODINE.

---

indapamide hemihydrate *see* indapamide tablets, Natrilix

---

indapamide tablets

A tablet supplied at a strength of 2.5 mg and used as a DIURETIC to treat high blood pressure.

Dose: 1 tablet a day in the morning.
Availability: NHS and private prescription.
Side effects: low potassium level, nausea, headache, dizziness, tiredness, muscle cramps, diarrhoea, constipation, indigestion, rash, loss of appetite. Rarely low blood pressure on standing, high blood sugar levels, pins and needles, electrolyte changes, sensitivity to light, kidney disorder, visual disturbance.
Caution: in the elderly, pregnant women, nursing mothers, and in patients suffering from severe kidney or liver disease, gout. Rarely, raised blood sugar levels, sensitivity to light, impotence, kidney disorder, blood and vision changes.
Not to be used for: children, or for patients suffering from severe liver failure or who have recently suffered a stroke.
Caution needed with: other diuretics, anti-arrhythmics, DIGOXIN, STEROIDS, laxatives, LITHIUM, NON-STEROIDAL ANTI-INFLAMMATORY DRUGS, some antibiotics, some antidiabetics, CARBAMAZEPINE, TERFENADINE, calcium supplements, VITAMIN D.
Contains: INDAPAMIDE HEMIHYDRATE.
Other preparations: NATRAMID, NATRILIX.

Inderal *see* propranolol tablets
(Zeneca)

Inderal LA *see* propranolol tablets
(Zeneca)

Inderetic
(Zeneca)

A white capsule used as a ß-BLOCKER and DIURETIC to treat high blood pressure.

Dose: 1 capsule twice a day.
Availability: NHS and private prescription.
Side effects: cold hands and feet, sleep disturbance, slow heart rate, tiredness, wheezing, heart failure, stomach upset, low blood potassium, rash, sensitivity to light, blood changes, gout, dry eyes.
Caution: in pregnant women, nursing mothers, and in patients suffering from diabetes, high blood lipids, overactive thyroid, kidney or liver

disorders, asthma, gout. May need to be withdrawn before surgery. Withdraw gradually. Your doctor may advise additional treatment with DIURETICS or DIGOXIN, blood tests.

Not to be used for: children or for patients suffering from heart block or failure, severe kidney failure, low blood pressure, untreated PHAEOCHROMOCYTOMA.

Caution needed with: VERAPAMIL, CLONIDINE withdrawal, some anti-arrhythmic drugs, some blood-pressure lowering drugs, anaesthetics, RESERPINE, CIMETIDINE, sedatives, SYMPATHOMIMETICS, INDOMETHACIN, other diuretics, antidiabetics, ERGOTAMINE, LITHIUM, NON-STEROIDAL ANTI-INFLAMMATORY DRUGS, DIGOXIN, ALLOPURINOL, AMANTADINE.

Contains: PROPANOLOL HYDROCHLORIDE, BENDROFLUAZIDE.

Other preparations: INDEREX (double strength).

Inderex *see* **Inderetic**
(Zeneca)

Indocid *see* **indomethacin capsules**
(Morson)

Indolar SR *see* **indomethacin capsules**
(Lagap)

Indomax *see* **indomethacin capsules**
(Ashbourne)

---

indomethacin *see* **Artracin, Flexin Continus, Imbrilon, Indocid, Indolar, Indomax, indomethacin capsules, Indomod, Indotard, Maximet, Rheumacin, Rimacid**

---

indomethacin capsules

A capsule supplied at strengths of 25 mg, 50 mg and used as a NON-STEROIDAL ANTI-INFLAMMATORY DRUG to treat acute rheumatoid arthritis, other joint and muscle disorders, acute gout, painful periods.

Dose: 50-200 mg a day in divided doses with food. (Up to 75 mg a day used to treat painful periods.)

Availability: NHS and private prescription.

Side effects: stomach upset or bleeding, fluid retention, headache, corneal deposits, disturbances of the retina, dizziness, brain effects; rarely sleeplessness, high blood pressure, fainting, fits, blood changes, kidney disorder, blood in the urine, noises in the ears, rash, inflammation of blood vessels, liver disorder.

Caution: in the elderly, pregnant women, nursing mothers, and in patients suffering from liver or kidney disease, brain disorders, LUPUS, asthma, heart failure, epilepsy, parkinsonism, or a history of stomach ulcers. Your doctor may advise regular eye and blood tests.

Not to be used for: children, or for patients suffering from stomach ulcer or allergy to ASPIRIN or anti-inflammatory drugs.

Caution needed with: ANTICOAGULANTS, LITHIUM, STEROIDS, DIURETICS, DIGOXIN PROBENECID, METHOTREXATE, other NON-STEROIDAL ANTI-INFLAMMATORY DRUGS, drugs that lower the blood pressure, some antibiotics, some antidiabetics, CYCLOSPORIN.

Contains: INDOMETHACIN.

Other preparations: ARTRACIN, FLEXIN, IMBRILON, INDOCID, INDOLAR, INDOMAX, INDOMOD, INDOTARD, MAXIMET, RHEUMACIN, RIMACID (some available as long-acting preparations and liquids).

Indomod *see* indomethacin capsules
(Pharmacia)

---

indoramin *see* Baratol, Doralese

Indotard MR *see* indomethacin capsules
(Bartholomew Rhodes)

Infacol
(Pharmax)

A liquid supplied with a dropper for administration, and used as an anti-wind preparation to treat colic and griping pain in infants.

Dose: 0.5-1 ml before feeds.
Availability: NHS, private prescription, over the counter.
Side effects:
Caution:
Not to be used for:
Caution needed with:
Contains: DIMETHICONE.
Other preparations:

---

influenza vaccine

An inactivated vaccine administered by injection and recommended only for people at high risk, including the elderly, especially those suffering from chronic respiratory disease, chronic heart disease, kidney failure, diabetes, etc.

Dose: 0.5 ml by injection as a single dose if previously vaccinated, otherwise repeated after 4-6 weeks.
Availability: NHS and private prescription.
Side effects: flu-like symptoms, local reaction, headache, fever, tiredness, general feeling of illness.
Caution: in pregnant women.
Not to be used for: patients suffering from feverish illness or with allergy to eggs or chicken.
Caution needed with: WARFARIN, PHENYTOIN, THEOPHYLLINE.
Contains: influenza vaccine.
Other preparations: FLUARIX, FLUVIRON, FLUZONE, INFLUVAC.

Influvac *see* influenza vaccine
(Solvay)

Innovace
(M.S.D.)

A round white tablet, a white scored, or red or peach, triangular tablet according to strengths of 2.5 mg, 5 mg, 10 mg, 20 mg and used as an ACE INHIBITOR to treat congestive heart failure, high blood pressure, and for the prevention of heart attack.

Dose: heart failure adults 2.5 mg at first in hospital, then increase if necessary to a maximum of 40 mg a day. High blood pressure 5 mg a day at first, then increase to a maximum of 40 mg once a day; elderly or patients suffering from kidney disease or being treated with DIURETICS start with 2.5 mg a day.
Availability: NHS and private prescription.
Side effects: low blood pressure, kidney failure, swelling, rash, headache, tiredness, dizziness, stomach upset, and rarely a cough.
Caution: fluid depletion may cause a marked drop in blood pressure. Dose of DIURETIC given may need to be reduced. Care in patients suffering from some kidney diseases, severe heart failure, and in nursing mothers and patients being anaesthetized.
Not to be used for: children, pregnant women, or for patients suffering from some heart defects.
Caution needed with: other blood-pressure lowering drugs, LITHIUM, potassium supplements, some DIURETICS.

Contains: ENALAPRIL MALEATE.
Other preparations:

Innozide
(MSD)

A yellow, scored tablet used as an ACE INHIBITOR and DIURETIC to treat mild to moderate high blood pressure.

Dose: 1-2 tablets once a day.
Availability: NHS and private prescription.
Side effects: dizziness, tiredness, headache, cramp, weakness, low blood pressure, cough, impotence, chest pain, rash, kidney failure, severe allergy, swelling, liver disorder, pancreatitis.
Caution: in nursing mothers, and in patients suffering from body fluid imbalance, blood vessel disease in the heart or brain, diabetes, gout, liver or kidney disease, and during anaesthesia or dialysis.
Not to be used for: children, pregnant women, or for patients suffering from inability to produce urine, or with a history of severe allergy to ACE inhibitors or some antibiotics.
Caution needed with: LITHIUM, NON-STEROIDAL ANTI-INFLAMMATORY DRUGS, some diuretics, potassium supplements, sedatives, antidiabetics, STEROIDS.
Contains: ENALPRIL MALEATE, HYDROCHLOROTHIAZIDE.
Other preparations:

---

inosine pranobex *see* Imunovir

---

inositol *see* Hexopal, Ketovite, Lipoflavonoid, Lipotriad

Insulatard *see* insulin
(Novo Nordisk)

---

insulin

An injectable liquid used to treat diabetes.

Dose: usually by subcutaneous injection (occasionally intramuscular or intravenous, depending on type of insulin), according to patient's requirements.
Availability: NHS, private prescription, over the counter.
Side effects: allergy at injection site, alteration in fat at injection site. Low blood sugar if too much insulin given.

Caution: in patients transferring from other types of insulin, in pregnant women, and in patients suffering from infection, emotional distress, or liver or kidney disease.
Not to be used for:
Caution needed with: ß-BLOCKERS, MAOIS, STEROIDS, DIURETICS, the contraceptive pill, alcohol.
Contains: (*see* table below)
Other preparations: (*see* table below)

Humaject *see* Humulin M, I, S
(Lilly)

Human Actrapid
(Novo Nordisk)

Ingredients: human neutral insulin.
Duration of action: short-acting.

Human Insulatard
(Novo Nordisk)

Ingredients: human isophane insulin.
Duration of action: intermediate-acting.

Human Insulatard ge (formerly known as Human Protaphane)
(Novo Nordisk)

Ingredients: human isophane insulin.
Duration of action: intermediate-acting.

Human Mixtard
(Novo Nordisk)

Ingredients: human neutral insulin, human isophane insulin.
Duration of action: biphasic (mixed effect).

Human Mixtard ge (formerly known as Human Actraphane)
(Novo Nordisk)

Ingredients: human neutral insulin, human isophane insulin.
Duration of action: biphasic (mixed effect).

Human Monotard
(Novo Nordisk)

Ingredients: human insulin zinc suspension (mixed).
Duration of action: intermediate-acting.

I

Human Ultratard
(Novo Nordisk)

Ingredients: human insulin zinc suspension (crystalline).
Duration of action: long-acting.

Human Velosulin
(Novo Nordisk)

Ingredients: human neutral insulin.
Duration of action: short-acting.

Humulin I
(Lilly)

Ingredients: human isophane insulin.
Duration of action: intermediate-acting.

Humulin Lente
(Lilly)

Ingredients: human insulin zinc suspension (mixed).
Duration of action: intermediate-acting.

Humulin M1, M2, M3, M4, M5
(Lilly)

Ingredients: human neutral insulin, human isophane insulin.
Duration of action: biphasic (mixed effect).

Humulin S
(Lilly)

Ingredients: human neutral insulin.
Duration of action: short-acting.

Humulin Zn
(Lilly)

Ingredients: human insulin zinc suspension (crystalline).
Duration of action: intermediate-acting.

Hypurin Isophane
(CP Pharmaceuticals)

Ingredients: beef isophane insulin.
Duration of action: intermediate-acting.

Hypurin Lente
(CP Pharmaceuticals)

Ingredients: beef insulin zinc suspension.
Duration of action: long-acting.

Hypurin Neutral
(CP Pharmaceuticals)

Ingredients: beef neutral insulin.
Duration of action: short-acting.

Hypurin Protamine Zinc
(CP Pharmaceuticals)

Ingredients: beef protamine zinc insulin.
Duration of action: long-acting.

Lentard MC
(Novo Nordisk)

Ingredients: beef and pork insulin zinc suspensions (mixed).
Duration of action: intermediate-acting.

Pork Insulatard (formerly known as Insulatard)
(Novo Nordisk)

Ingredients: pork isophane insulin.
Duration of action: intermediate-acting.

Pork Mixtard 30 (formerly known as Mixtard 30/70)
(Novo Nordisk)

Ingredients: pork neutral insulin, pork isophane insulin.
Duration of action: biphasic (mixed effect).

Pork Velosulin (formerly known as Velosulin)
(Novo Nordisk)

Ingredients: pork neutral insulin.
Duration of action: short-acting.

Rapitard MC
(Novo Nordisk)

Ingredients: pork neutral insulin, beef crystalline insulin.
Duration of action: biphasic (mixed effect).

I

Semitard MC
(Novo Nordisk)

Ingredients: pork insulin zinc suspension (amorphous).
Duration of action: intermediate-acting

Intal *see* sodium cromoglycate inhaler
(Fisons)

Intralgin
(3M Health Care)

A gel used as an ANALGESIC rub to treat muscle strains, sprains.

Dose: massage gently into the affected area as needed.
Availability: NHS, private prescription, and over the counter.
Side effects: may be irritant.
Caution:
Not to be used for: areas near the eyes or on broken or inflamed skin or on mucous membranes (such as the mouth).
Caution needed with:
Contains: SALICYLAMIDE, BENZOCAINE.
Other preparations:

Iodoflex
(Perstorp)

A paste on a removable carrier gauze supplied in 5 g, 10 g, 17 g sachets, and used as an absorbent anti-bacterial treatment for chronic weeping leg ulcers.

Dose: apply up to 50 g of paste and cover with a dressing; change 3 times a week or when paste is saturated. Do not exceed 150 g of paste in any 1 week and do not continue treatment for more than 3 months at a time.
Availability: NHS, private prescription.
Side effects:
Caution: in patients suffering from thyroid disorders.
Not to be used for: children under 2 years, pregnant women, nursing mothers, or in patients suffering from some thyroid disorders.
Caution needed with: LITHIUM, some antidiabetics.
Contains: CADEXOMER IODINE.
Other preparations:

Iodosorb
(Perstorp)

Powder in a sachet used as an absorbant, antibacterial treatment for leg ulcers and moist wounds.

Dose: apply a 3 mm coating and cover with a dressing; repeat the treatment before the dressing is saturated.
Availability: NHS and private prescription.
Side effects:
Caution: in patients suffering from thyroid disorders.
Not to be used for: pregnant women, nursing mothers, or for patients suffering from some thyroid disorders.
Caution needed with: LITHIUM, some antidiabetics.
Contains: CADEXOMER IODINE.
Other preparations: Iodosorb Ointment. IODOFLEX.

Ionamin *see* Duromine
(Torbet)

Ionax
(Novex)

An gel used as an abrasive, antibacterial preparation to clean the skin in the treatment of acne.

Dose: wet the face, then rub in once or twice a day, and rinse.
Availability: NHS, private prescription, over the counter.
Side effects:
Caution:
Not to be used for: children.
Caution needed with:
Contains: POLYETHYLENE GRANULES, BENZALKONIUM CHLORIDE.
Other preparations:

Ionil T
(Novex)

A shampoo used as an antipsoriatic treatment for scaly inflammation of the scalp, psoriasis.

Dose: shampoo once or twice a week.
Availability: NHS, private prescription, over the counter.
Side effects: irritation, sensitivity to light.

Caution:
Not to be used for: patients suffering from acute psoriasis.
Caution needed with:
Contains: SALICYLIC ACID, BENZALKONIUM CHLORIDE, COAL TAR solution.
Other preparations: CAPASAL, GELCOSAL.

Iopidine
(Alcon)

An eye drop (with or without preservative) used to treat glaucoma. (The preservative-free product is used to control eye pressure after laser surgery.)

Dose: 1 drop into the eye three times a day.
Availability: NHS, private prescription.
Side effects: allergic reactions of the eye, dry mouth and disturbances of taste.
Caution: in pregnant women, nursing mothers, and in patients suffering from kidney or liver disorder.
Not to be used for: children, or for patients with a history of heart or circulation disease, or who wear soft contact lenses.
Caution needed with: MAOIS, some SYMPATHOMIMETICS, sedatives, blood-pressure lowering drugs, CLONIDINE, DIGOXIN, TRICYCLIC ANTIDEPRESSANTS.
Contains: APRACLONIDINE hydrochloride.
Other preparations:

Ipral *see* trimethoprim tablets
(Squibb)

ipratropium *see* Atrovent, Combivent, Duovent, Rinatec, Steri-Neb Ipratropium

iron-sorbitol/citric acid complex *see* Jectofer

Isclofen *see* diclofenac tablets
(Isis)

Isib *see* isosorbide mononitrate tablets
(Ashbourne)

Isisfen *see* ibuprofen tablets
(Isis)

Ismelin Tablets
(Ciba)

A white tablet or a pink tablet according to strengths of 10 mg, 25 mg and used as an ANTIHYPERTENSIVE treatment for high blood pressure.

Dose: 10 mg a day at first increasing by 10 mg at a time at weekly intervals if needed. (Usual dose 25-50 mg a day.)
Availability: NHS and private prescription.
Side effects: low blood pressure on standing up, diarrhoea, failure of ejaculation, fluid retention, blood changes, slow heartbeat, stuffy nose.
Caution: in pregnant women and in patients undergoing anaesthesia or suffering from kidney disease, stomach ulcer, asthma, or hardening of the arteries.
Not to be used for: children, or for patients suffering from PHAEOCHROMOCYTOMA (a disease of the adrenal glands), kidney or heart failure.
Caution needed with: TRICYCLIC ANTIDEPRESSANTS, SYMPATHOMIMETICS, MAOIS, DIURETICS, RESERPINE-like drugs, anti-arrhythmics, DIGOXIN, sedatives, blood-pressure lowering drugs, the contraceptive pill, antidiabetics.
Contains: GUANETHIDINE.
Other preparations:

ISMO *see* isosorbide mononitrate tablets
(Boehringer Mannheim)

isocarboxazid tablets

A pink, scored tablet supplied at a strength of 10 mg and used as an MAOI to treat depression.

Dose: adults 3 tablets a day at first, then 1-2 tablets a day; elderly half adult dose.
Availability: NHS and private prescription.
Side effects: severe high blood pressure reactions with certain foods and medicines, sleeplessness, low blood pressure, dizziness, drowsiness, weakness, dry mouth, constipation, stomach upset, blurred vision, urinary difficulties, ankle swelling, rash, jaundice, weight gain, confusion, sexual desire changes.
Caution: in the elderly and in patients suffering from epilepsy.
Not to be used for: children, or for patients suffering from liver disease,

blood disorders, heart disease, PHAEOCHROMOCYTOMA (a disease of the adrenal glands), overactive thyroid, brain artery disease.

Caution needed with: amphetamines or similar SYMPATHOMIMETIC drugs, LEVODOPA, other MAOIS, antidepressants, ANTICHOLINERGICS, drugs used to treat high blood pressure, BUSPIRONE, PETHIDINE and other opiates, some cough mixtures and appetite suppressants containing SYMPATHOMIMETICS. BARBITURATES, sedatives, alcohol, antidiabetics. Cheese, Bovril, Oxo, meat extracts, broad beans, banana, Marmite, yeast extracts, wine, beer, other alcohol, pickled herrings, vegetable proteins. (Up to 14 days after cessation.)

Contains: ISOCARBOXAZID.

Other preparations:

---

isoconazole nitrate *see* Travogyn

Isogel
(Charwell)

Granules used as a bulking agent to treat constipation, diarrhoea, irritable colon, and for colostomy control.

Dose: adults 10 ml in water once or twice a day with meals; children half adult dose.

Availability: NHS, private prescription, over the counter.

Side effects:

Caution:

Not to be used for:

Caution needed with:

Contains: ISPAGHULA husk.

Other preparations: FYBOGEL, REGULAN.

Isoket Retard *see* isosorbide dinitrate tablets
(Schwarz)

---

isometheptene mucate *see* Midrid

---

isoniazid *see* isoniazid tablets, Rifater, Rifinah, Rimactazid

---

isoniazid tablets

Tablets supplied at strengths of 50 mg, 100 mg, and used in combination with other drugs to treat and prevent tuberculosis.

Dose: usually adults, 300 mg a day; children, 10 mg/kg body weight per day.
Availability: NHS and private prescription.
Side effects: nausea, vomiting, allergy including rashes, nerve inflammation, convulsions, mental disturbances, blood changes, liver disorder.
Caution: in nursing mothers, or in patients suffering from kidney or liver damage, alcoholism, PORPHYRIA, epilepsy, or a history of mental disorder.
Not to be used for: patients suffering from drug-induced liver disease.
Caution needed with: ANTACIDS, anti-epileptics, DIAZEPAM, THEOPHYLLINE.
Contains: ISONIAZID.
Other preparations: isoniazid elixir.

---

isoprenaline *see* Medihaler-Iso, Saventrine

---

isopropyl alcohol *see* Hibisol, Manusept

---

isopropyl myristate *see* Diprobath, Emulsiderm, Hydromol

Isopto Alkaline *see* hypromellose eye drops
(Alcon)

Isopto Atropine
(Alcon)

Eye drops used as an ANTICHOLINERGIC and lubricant to treat uveitis (inflammation in the eye) and used to prepare the eye for examination.

Dose: for uveitis, 1 drop 3 times a day. For examination, adults, 1-2 drops 1 hour before examination; children 1 drop twice a day for 1-2 days before examination.
Availability: NHS and private prescription.
Side effects: stinging, dry mouth, blurred vision, intolerance to light, rapid heart rate, headache, mental or behavioural changes.
Caution: in infants.
Not to be used for: patients suffering from some types of glaucoma, or who wear soft contact lenses.

Caution needed with:
Contains: ATROPINE SULPHATE, HYPROMELLOSE.
Other preparations: ATROPINE MINIMS, ATROPINE SULPHATE EYE DROPS.

Isopto Carbachol
(Alcon)

Drops used as a cholinergic and lubricant treatment for glaucoma.

Dose: 2 drops into the eye 3 times a day.
Availability: NHS and private prescription.
Side effects:
Caution:
Not to be used for: children or for patients suffering from damaged cornea, acute iritis, or who wear soft contact lenses.
Caution needed with:
Contains: CARBACHOL, HYPROMELLOSE.
Other preparations:

Isopto Carpine
(Alcon)

Drops used as a cholinergic, lubricant treatment for glaucoma.

Dose: 2 drops into the eye 3 times a day.
Availability: NHS and private prescription.
Side effects:
Caution:
Not to be used for: patients suffering from acute iritis or who wear soft contact lenses.
Caution needed with:
Contains: PILOCARPINE, HYPROMELLOSE.
Other preparations: PILOCARPINE MINIMS, SNO PILO, OCUSERT PILO, PILOCARPINE EYE DROPS.

Isopto Frin
(Alcon)

Drops used as a SYMPATHOMIMETIC and lubricant to relieve redness of the eye caused by minor irritations.

Dose: 1-2 drops into the eye up to 4 times a day.
Availability: NHS, private prescription, over the counter.
Side effects:

Caution: in infants and patients suffering from narrow angle glaucoma.
Not to be used for: patients who wear soft contact lenses.
Caution needed with:
Contains: PHENYLEPHRINE hydrochloride, HYPROMELLOSE.
Other preparations: PHENYLEPHRINE EYE DROPS.

Isopto Plain *see* hypromellose eye drops
(Alcon)

Isordil *see* isosorbide dinitrate tablets
(Monmouth)

isosorbide dinitrate *see* Cedocard, Cedocard Retard, Imtack, Isoket Retard, Isordil, isosorbide dinitrate tablets, Soni-Slo, Sorbichew, Sorbid SA, Sorbitrate

isosorbide dinitrate tablets

A tablet supplied at strengths of 10 mg, 20 mg and used as a NITRATE to prevent and treat angina, and to treat heart failure.

Dose: 30-160 mg a day in divided doses up to a maximum of 240 mg a day if necessary.
Availability: NHS, private prescription, over the counter.
Side effects: headache, flushing, dizziness, low blood pressure on standing, rapid pulse.
Caution: in patients suffering from severe liver or kidney damage, underactive thyroid gland, history of heart attack, malnutrition, low body temperature.
Not to be used for: children, or for patients suffering from allergy to nitrates, low blood pressure, some heart conditions, severe anaemia, head injury or brain haemorrhage, closed-angle glaucoma.
Caution needed with: DISOPYRAMIDE, ANTICOAGULANTS, TRICYCLIC ANTIDEPRESSANTS, ANTICHOLINERGICS.
Contains: ISOSORBIDE DINITRATE.
Other preparations: CEDOCARD, ISOKET, ISORDIL, JERIDIN, SONI-SLO, SORBICHEW, SORBID, SORBITRATE (some available as long-acting preparations). Also IMTACK (a spray for use under the tongue).

I

isosorbide mononitrate *see* **Angeze, Angitate, Dynamin, Elantan, Imdur, Isib, ISMO, isosorbide mononitrate tablets, Isotrate, MCR-50, Monit, Mono-Cedocard, Nitromon**

isosorbide mononitrate tablets

A tablet supplied at strengths of 10 mg, 20 mg, 40 mg and used as a NITRATE treatment for the prevention and treatment of angina, and in addition to other treatments for congestive heart failure.

Dose: 40-80 mg a day at first (20 mg if nitrates not previously used), then up to 120 mg a day if needed.
Availability: NHS, private prescription, and over the counter.
Side effects: headache, flushing, dizziness, low blood pressure on standing, rapid pulse.
Caution: in patients suffering from severe liver or kidney damage, underactive thyroid gland, history of heart attack, malnutrition, low body temperature.
Not to be used for: children; or for patients suffering from allergy to nitrates, low blood pressure, some heart conditions, severe anaemia, head injury or brain haemorrhage, closed-angle glaucoma.
Caution needed with: DISOPYRAMIDE, ANTICOAGULANTS, TRICYCLIC ANTIDEPRESSANTS, ANTICHOLINERGICS.
Contains: ISOSORBIDE MONONITRATE.
Other preparations: ANGEZE, ANGITATE, DYNAMIN, ELANTAN, IMDUR, ISIB, ISMO, ISOTRATE, MCR-50, MONIT, MONO-CEDOCARD, NITROMON (some available as long-acting preparations).

Isotrate *see* **isosorbide mononitrate**
(Bioglan)

isotretinoin *see* **Roaccutane, Isotrex**

Isotrex
(Stiefel)

A gel used to treat acne.

Dose: apply once or twice a day, sparingly, for a minimum of 6-8 weeks. Do not apply to angles of the nose.
Availability: NHS and private prescription.
Side effects: irritation.
Caution: avoid mouth, eyes, mucous membranes, damaged or sunburned

skin. Avoid ultraviolet light.
Not to be used for: pregnant women, nursing mothers, children, or patients with a history of skin cancer.
Caution needed with: skin-softening agents (eg BENZOYL PEROXIDE).
Contains: ISOTRETINOIN.
Other preparations: ROACCUTANE.

---

ispaghula *see* **Fybogel, Fybogel-Mebeverine, Isogel, Konsyl, Regulan**

---

isradipine *see* **Prescal**

Istin
(Pfizer)

White tablets supplied at strengths of 5 mg, 10 mg, and used to treat high blood pressure and poor blood supply to the heart (when associated with angina).

Dose: 5-10 mg once a day.
Availability: NHS and private prescription.
Side effects: headache, fluid retention, tiredness, nausea, flushing, dizziness, palpitations, sleepiness, stomach pain.
Caution: in pregnant women, nursing mothers, and in patients suffering from liver disorder.
Not to be used for: children.
Caution needed with:
Contains: AMLODIPINE besylate.
Other preparations:

---

itraconazole *see* **Sporanox**

J

Jectofer
(Astra)

An injection supplied in a 2 ml ampoule equivalent to a strength of 50 mg/ml, and used as an iron supplement to treat iron-deficiency anaemia.

Dose: 1.5 mg per kilogram bodyweight as a single daily injection up to a maximum of 100 mg per injection. Treatment as advised by your physician.
Availability: NHS, private prescription.

Side effects: irregular heart rate.
Caution:
Not to be used for: children under 3 kg bodyweight, women in early pregnancy, or for patients suffering from severe kidney or liver damage, untreated urinary tract infections. Not effective for some kinds of anaemia or in leukaemia
Caution needed with:
Contains: IRON-SORBITOL/CITRIC ACID complex.
Other preparations:

Jelonet
(Smith & Nephew Healthcare)

A sterile, impregnated gauze dressing, supplied at a size of 10 cm square, and used as a dressing for burns, open wounds, and sensitive areas.

Availability: NHS, private prescription, over the counter. (Also available on a trial basis from nurses.)
Contains: white soft paraffin.

Junifen
(Crookes)

An orange-flavoured, sugar-free suspension used as a NON-STEROIDAL ANTI-INFLAMMATORY DRUG to treat pain and fever in children.

Dose: 1-2 years 2.5 ml, 3-7 years 5 ml, 8-12 years 10 ml, all 3-4 times a day.
Availability: NHS, private prescription, over the counter.
Side effects: stomach upset or bleeding, rash, blood changes.
Caution: in patients suffering from asthma, gastro-intestinal disease, heart failure, liver or kidney disorder.
Not to be used for: children under 1 year, or weighing less than 7 kg, or suffering from stomach ulcer or allergy to ASPIRIN or anti-inflammatory drugs.
Caution needed with: ANTICOAGULANTS, some DIURETICS, some antibiotics.
Contains: IBUPROFEN.
Other preparations: BRUFEN syrup, IBUPROFEN TABLETS.

K-Y
(Johnson and Johnson)

A non-irritating jelly and lubricating pessary used to provide additional vaginal lubrication.

Dose: apply a little jelly to the vagina, or insert a pessary high into the vagina.
Availability: NHS, private prescription, over the counter.
Side effects:
Caution: allow 10 minutes for pessary to melt.
Not to be used for:
Caution needed with:
Contains:
Other preparations:

Kabiglobulin *see* human normal immunoglobulin injection
(Pharmacia)

Kalspare
(Cusi)

An orange, scored tablet used as a DIURETIC combination to treat high blood pressure, fluid retention.

Dose: high blood pressure 1 tablet a day in the morning increasing to 2 tablets if needed, fluid retention 1 tablet a day in the morning increasing to 2 a day after 7 days if the condition fails to respond.
Availability: NHS and private prescription.
Side effects: rash, sensitivity to light, blood changes, gout, cramps.
Caution: in pregnant women, nursing mothers, and in patients suffering from diabetes, electrolyte changes, gout, kidney or liver disease.
Not to be used for: children, and for patients suffering from progressive or severe kidney failure, raised potassium levels, failure to urinate.
Caution needed with: potassium supplements, some diuretics, LITHIUM, DIGOXIN, blood-pressure lowering drugs, ACE INHIBITORS.
Contains: CHLORTHALIDONE, TRIAMTERENE.
Other preparations:

Kalten
(Stuart)

A red and cream capsule used as a ß-BLOCKER and DIURETIC combination to treat high blood pressure.

Dose: 1 capsule a day
Availability: NHS and private prescription.
Side effects: cold hands and feet, sleep disturbance, slow heart rate, tiredness, wheezing, heart failure, low blood pressure, stomach upset, rash, sensitivity to light, blood changes, gout, cramps, dry eyes.

K

Caution: in pregnant women, nursing mothers, and in patients suffering from diabetes, electrolyte changes, gout, kidney or liver disease, asthma, or undergoing general anaesthesia. Withdraw gradually.

Not to be used for: children, or for patients suffering from progressive or severe kidney or liver failure, raised potassium levels, heart block or failure.

Caution needed with: potassium supplements, some diuretics, LITHIUM, DIGOXIN, blood-pressure lowering drugs, ACE INHIBITORS, VERAPAMIL, CLONIDINE withdrawal, some anti-arrhythmic drugs and anaesthetics, RESERPINE, ERGOTAMINE, CIMETIDINE, sedatives, SYMPATHOMIMETICS, INDOMETHACIN.

Contains: ATENOLOL, HYDROCHLOROTHIAZIDE, AMILORIDE hydrochloride

Other preparations:

Kaltogel
(Convatec)

A sterile, alginate dressing used to treat wounds such as leg ulcers and bed sores which are weeping.

Availability: NHS, private prescription, over the counter.
Contains: alginate.
Other preparations: KALTOSTAT, SORBSAN, TEGAGEL.

Kaltostat
(Convatec)

A sterile, alginate dressing, supplied at sizes of 5 cm square and 7.5 cm square, and used as a dressing for leg ulcers, bed sores, bleeding, post-operative, and fungating wounds.

Availability: NHS, private prescription, over the counter. (Also available on a trial basis from nurses.)
Contains: alginate.
Other preparations: KALTOGEL, SORBSAN, TEGAGEL.

Kamillosan
(Norgine)

An ointment used as an emollient to treat chapped skin, sore nipples, nappy rash.

Dose: apply twice a day or after breastfeeding. For nappy rash, apply at each nappy change.
Availability: NHS, private prescription, over the counter.

Side effects:
Caution:
Not to be used for:
Caution needed with:
Contains: CAMOMILE oil, CAMOMILE extract.
Other preparations:

---

kaolin *see* Kaopectate

Kaopectate
(Upjohn)

A suspension used as an adsorbent to treat diarrhoea.

Dose: adults, 10-30 ml every 4 hours; children under 1 year 5 ml, 1-5 years 10 ml, over 5 years as adult, all every 4 hours.
Availability: NHS, private prescription, over the counter.
Side effects: stomach block.
Caution:
Not to be used for: patients with blocked intestines.
Caution needed with:
Contains: KAOLIN.
Other preparations: KAOLIN MIXTURE BP.

Kapake Tablets *see* Tylex Capsules
(Galen)

Kay-Cee-L
(Geistlich)

A syrup used as a potassium supplement to treat potassium deficiency.

Dose: adults, 10-50 ml a day in divided doses after food; children as advised by doctor.
Availability: NHS, private prescription, over the counter.
Side effects:
Caution:
Not to be used for: patients suffering from kidney damage or dehydration.
Caution needed with:
Contains: POTASSIUM CHLORIDE.
Other preparations: SLOW-K.

K

Keflex *see* **cephalexin capsules**
(Eli Lilly)

Kelfizine W
(Pharmacia)

A white tablet supplied at a strength of 2 g and used as a sulphonamide antibiotic to treat bronchitis, urine infections.

Dose: 1 tablet a week.
Availability: NHS and private prescription.
Side effects: anaemia, stomach disturbances, sore tongue, rash, blood changes when used for an extended period of treatment.
Caution: in patients suffering from liver or kidney disease, blood disorders. Your doctor may advise that blood should be checked regularly for patients on extended periods of treatment.
Not to be used for: children, pregnant women, nursing mothers.
Caution needed with: TRIMETHOPRIM, antidiabetics taken by mouth, METHOTREXATE.
Contains: SULFAMETOPYRAZINE.
Other preparations:

Kemadrin *see* **procyclidine tablets**
(Wellcome)

Kenalog
(Squibb)

An injection available in 2 volumes, and used as a STEROID for treating joint pain and swelling due to conditions, such as arthritis, and to treat allergic states, such as hayfever, and other disorders requiring steroid supplement.

Dose: as advised by a doctor.
Availability: NHS and private prescription.
Side effects: high blood sugar, thinning of bones, mood changes, stomach ulcers, high blood pressure, water retention, loss of potassium, weak muscles.
Caution: in pregnant women, and in patients who have had recent bowel surgery, or who suffer from inflamed veins, psychiatric disorders, some cancers, some kidney diseases, thin bones, stomach ulcers, infections, high blood pressure, glaucoma, epilepsy, diabetes, underactive thyroid, liver disease, stress. Withdraw gradually. Avoid contact with chicken pox and shingles during treatments and for 3 months afterwards.

Not to be used for: children under 6 years.
Caution needed with: PHENYTOIN, PHENOBARBITONE, EPHEDRINE, RIFAMPICIN, DIURETICS, ANTICHOLINESTERASES, DIGOXIN, antidiabetics, ANTICOAGULANTS, NON-STEROIDAL ANTI-INFLAMMATORY DRUGS.
Contains: TRIAMCINOLONE acetonide.
Other preparations: ADCORTYL, LEDERCORT (tablet form), LEDERSPAN.

Keri
(Westwood)

A lotion used as an emollient to treat dry, itchy skin conditions.

Dose: massage in to the affected area 3 times a day or as needed.
Availability: NHS, private prescription, over the counter.
Side effects:
Caution:
Not to be used for:
Caution needed with:
Contains: LIQUID PARAFFIN.
Other preparations: ALCODERM.

Kerlone
(Lorex)

A white, scored tablet supplied at a strength of 20 mg and used as a ß-BLOCKER to treat high blood pressure.

Dose: 1 tablet a day; elderly ½ tablet a day at first.
Availability: NHS and private prescription.
Side effects: cold hands and feet, sleep disturbance, slow heart rate, tiredness, wheezing, heart failure, low blood pressure, stomach upset, dry eyes, rash.
Caution: in pregnant women, nursing mothers, and in patients suffering from diabetes, kidney or liver disorders, asthma. May need to be withdrawn before surgery. Withdraw gradually. Your doctor may advise additional treatment with DIURETICS or DIGOXIN.
Not to be used for: children or for patients suffering from heart block or failure, low blood pressure, untreated PHAEOCHROMOCYTOMA.
Caution needed with: VERAPAMIL, CLONIDINE withdrawal, some anti-arrhythmic drugs and anaesthetics, RESERPINE, some blood-pressure lowering drugs, ERGOTAMINE, CIMETIDINE, sedatives, SYMPATHOMIMETICS, INDOMETHACIN, antidiabetics.
Contains: BETAXOLOL hydrochloride.
Other preparations:

K

Ketocid *see* **ketoprofen capsules**
(Trinity)

---

ketoconazole *see* **Nizoral, Nizoral Cream**

Ketonal *see* **ketoprofen capsules**
(Lagap)

---

ketoprofen *see* **Alrheumat, Fenoket, Ketonal, ketoprofen capsules, Ketosaid, Ketovail, Ketozip, Larafen, Orudis, Oruvail, Powergel**

---

ketoprofen capsules

A capsule used as a NON-STEROIDAL ANTI-INFLAMMATORY DRUG to treat mild pain and inflammation in rheumatoid arthritis, other muscle, bone, and joint disorders, after orthopaedic surgery, painful periods, and gout.

Dose: 100-200 mg a day in 2-4 divided doses with food.
Availability: NHS and private prescription.
Side effects: stomach upset, rash, allergic reactions, headache, dizziness, vertigo, hearing disturbance, blood changes, fluid retention, kidney disorder, liver disorder.
Caution: in the elderly, pregnant women, nursing mothers and in patients suffering from asthma, kidney, heart, or liver disease, history of gastro-intestinal disease.
Not to be used for: children or for patients suffering from severe kidney disease, stomach ulcer or a history of recurring ulcer, asthma, allergy to ASPIRIN/non-steroidal anti-inflammatory drugs. (Suppositories not to be used for patients with inflammation of the anus or rectum.
Caution needed with: ANTICOAGULANTS, some antibiotics, DIGOXIN, STEROIDS, METHOTREXATE, drugs which lower blood pressure, other non-steroidal anti-inflammatory drugs, LITHIUM, some antidiabetics, some DIURETICS, PROBENICID.
Contains: KETOPROFEN.
Other preparations: ketoprofen SR. ALRHEUMAT, FENOKET, KETONAL, KETOVAIL, KETOZIP, LARAFEN, ORUDIS, ORUVAIL (some available in slow-release forms or as suppositories). External products: Oruvail gel (available over the counter only to treat pain and swelling in sports injuries, sprains, strains, and rheumatic pain), POWERGEL.

---

ketorolac trometamol *see* **Toradol**

Ketostix
(Bayer Diagnostics)

A plastic reagent strip used to test for the presence of ketones in the urine. Raised ketone levels indicate an imbalance in the metabolism of fat in the body, such as occurs when a patient is suffering from diabetes.

---

ketotifen *see* Zaditen

Ketovail *see* ketoprofen capsules
(A.P.S.)

Ketovite
(Paines & Byrne)

A sugar-free yellow tablet used as a multivitamin supplement in artificial diets.

Dose: 1 tablet 3 times a day plus 5 ml of Ketovite Liquid a day.
Availability: NHS, private prescription.
Side effects:
Caution:
Not to be used for:
Caution needed with: LEVODOPA, PHENYTOIN, some DIURETICS.
Contains: tablet: ACETOMENAPHTHONE, VITAMINS B_1, B_2, B_3, B_5, B_6, C, E, H, INOSITOL, FOLIC ACID; liquid: VITAMINS A, B_{12}, D, CHOLINE.
Other preparations: Ketovite Liquid (available over the counter).

Ketozip *see* ketoprofen capsules
(Ashbourne)

Ketur Test
(Boehringer Mannheim Diagnostics)

A plastic reagent strip used to test for the presence of ketones in the urine. Raised ketone levels indicate an imbalance in the metabolism of fat in the body, such as occurs when a patient is suffering from diabetes.

K

Kinidin Durules
(Astra)

A white tablet supplied at a strength of 250 mg and used as an anti-arrhythmic drug to treat abnormal heart rhythm.

Dose: 1 tablet at first, then 2-5 tablets twice a day.
Availability: NHS and private prescription.
Side effects: allergies, stomach upset, abnormal heart rhythm, low blood pressure, quinine excess.
Caution: in patients with low blood pressure, slow heart rate, low potassium levels, blocked oesophagus.
Not to be used for: children, pregnant women, or for patients suffering from acute infection, MYASTHENIA GRAVIS (a muscle disorder), severe heart disease, DIGOXIN overdose, heart failure, heart block.
Caution needed with: DIGOXIN, DIGITOXIN, ANTICOAGULANTS, blood-pressure lowering drugs, CIMETIDINE, RIFAMPICIN, BARBITURATES, PHENYTOIN, VERAPAMIL, AMIODARONE, NIFEDIPINE, DESIPRAMINE, IMIPRAMINE, METOPROLOL, PROCAINAMIDE.
Contains: QUINIDINE bisulphate
Other preparations:

Klaricid
(Abbott)

A yellow, oval tablet supplied at strengths of 250 mg, 500 mg, and used as an antibiotic to treat infections of the respiratory tract, skin, and soft tissues, acute middle ear inflammation, and as an additional treatment for infection in patients with stomach ulcer.

Dose: 250 mg twice a day for 7 days; severe infections 500 mg twice a day for up to 14 days; stomach infection 500 mg 3 times a day for 14 days with OMEPRAZOLE. Children use paediatric syrup.
Availability: NHS and private prescription.
Side effects: nausea, vomiting, diarrhoea, abdominal pain, headache, rash, some temporary brain effects.
Caution: in pregnant women, nursing mothers, and in patients suffering from kidney or liver damage.
Not to be used for:
Caution needed with: THEOPHYLLINE, ANTICOAGULANTS, DIGOXIN, CARBAMAZEPINE, TERFENADINE.
Contains: CLARITHROMYCIN.
Other preparations: Klaricid Paediatric Syrup.

Kliofem
(Novo Nordisk)

A yellow tablet used as an oestrogen/progestogen hormone-replacement therapy to treat symptoms of menopause and to prevent osteoporosis after menopause.

Dose: for women over 54 years old or 1 year after last period, 1 tablet a day.
Availability: NHS, private prescription.
Side effects: enlarged breasts, fluid retention, nausea, vaginal bleeding, weight gain, headache, dizziness. Rarely jaundice, raised blood pressure, thrombosis.
Caution: in patients suffering from high blood pressure, diabetes, epilepsy, womb diseases, gall bladder disorder, migraine, multiple sclerosis, PORPHYRIA, liver disorders, some ear disorders, or a history or increased risk of breast disorders (including cancer) and thrombosis. Your doctor may advise you to have regular examinations.
Not to be used for: children, pregnant women, nursing mothers, or for patients suffering from thombosis, severe liver, kidney, or heart disorders, some cancers, undiagnosed vaginal bleeding, endometriosis.
Caution needed with: ACE INHIBITORS, ANTICOAGULANTS, BARBITURATES, ß-BLOCKERS, CARBAMAZEPINE, PHENYTOIN, RIFAMPICIN.
Contains: OESTRADIOL, NORETHISTERONE.
Other preparations:

Kloref
(Cox)

A white, effervescent tablet used as a potassium supplement to treat potassium deficiency.

Dose: adults 1-2 tablets in water 3 times a day, increasing if needed; children as advised by the physician.
Availability: NHS, private prescription, and over the counter.
Side effects:
Caution: in patients suffering from kidney disease.
Not to be used for: patients suffering from increased chloride levels or other rare metabolic disorders.
Caution needed with:
Contains: BETAINE HYDROCHLORIDE, POTASSIUM BENZOATE, POTASSIUM BICARBONATE, POTASSIUM CHLORIDE.
Other preparations: Kloref-S (granules).

K

Kolanticon
(Marion Merrell Dow)

A gel used as an ANTACID, antispasm, and ANTICHOLINERGIC treatment for bowel/stomach spasm, acidity, wind, ulcers.

Dose: adults 10-20 ml every 4 hours.
Availability: NHS, over the counter, private prescription.
Side effects: occasionally constipation, blurred vision, confusion, dry mouth.
Caution: in patients suffering from enlarged prostate or glaucoma.
Not to be used for: children or for patients suffering from blocked urinary tract, intestinal obstruction, severe ulcerative colitis, MYASTHENIA GRAVIS.
Caution needed with: tablets coated to protect the stomach, TETRACYCLINE ANTIBIOTICS, iron.
Contains: ALUMINIUM HYDROXIDE, MAGNESIUM OXIDE, DICYCLOMINE hydrochloride, DIMETHICONE.
Other preparations:

Konakion
(Roche)

A white tablet supplied at a strength of 10 mg and used as a VITAMIN K derivative to treat blood disorders which result in bleeding tendency.

Dose: up to 40 mg in 24 hours; children use injectable form.
Availability: NHS, private prescription.
Side effects: flushing, sweating, poor oxygen supply (resulting in bluish colour to skin and mucous membranes).
Caution: in the elderly.
Not to be used for:
Caution needed with:
Contains: vitamin K.
Other preparations: Konakion Injection, Konakion MM.

Konsyl *see* Fybogel
(Eastern)

---

l-cysteine *see* Cicatrin

---

labetolol *see* labetolol tablets, Labrocol, Trandate

---

labetolol tablets

A tablet supplied at strengths of 100 mg, 200 mg, 400 mg and used as a ß-BLOCKER, to treat high blood pressure (including high blood pressure with angina, in pregnancy, and after heart attack).

Dose: 100 mg twice a day with food at first increasing as needed every 14 days to a maximum of 2.4 g a day in 3-4 divided doses; elderly 50 mg twice a day at first.
Availability: NHS and private prescription.
Side effects: cold hands and feet, low blood pressure on standing, sleep disturbance, slow heart rate, tiredness, weakness, headache, wheezing, heart failure, stomach upset, dry eyes, skin rash, tingling scalp, difficulty urinating, liver damage.
Caution: in pregnant women, nursing mothers, and in patients suffering from diabetes, kidney or liver disorders, shock, myasthenia gravis. May need to be withdrawn before surgery. Withdraw gradually. Your doctor may advise additional treatment with DIURETICS or DIGOXIN.
Not to be used for: children or for patients suffering from heart block or failure, asthma, blocked airways disease.
Caution needed with: VERAPAMIL, DILTIAZEM, CLONIDINE, some anti-arrhythmic drugs, some blood-pressure lowering drugs, ERGOTAMINE, CIMETIDINE, sedatives, antidiabetics, SYMPATHOMIMETICS, NON-STEROIDAL ANTI-INFLAMMATORY DRUGS, MEFLOQUINE, STEROIDS.
Contains: LABETOLOL hydrochloride.
Other preparations: TRANDATE, LABROCOL.

Labrocol *see* labetolol tablets
(Lagap)

---

lacidipine *see* Motens

Lacri-Lube
(Allergan)

An ointment used for lubricating the eyes and protecting the cornea.

Dose: apply into the eye as needed.
Availability: NHS, private prescription, over the counter.
Side effects:
Caution:
Not to be used for:
Caution needed with:
Contains: LIQUID PARAFFIN, WOOL FAT, WHITE SOFT PARAFFIN.

L

Other preparations:

---

lactic acid *see* **Calmurid, Calmurid HC, Cuplex, Duofilm, Lacticare, Salactol, Salatac, Tampovagan**

Lacticare
(Stiefel)

A lotion used as an emollient to treat chronic dry skin conditions.

Dose: massage in to the affected area as needed.
Availability: NHS, private prescription, over the counter.
Side effects:
Caution:
Not to be used for:
Caution needed with:
Contains: LACTIC ACID, SODIUM PYRROLIDONE CARBOXYLATE.
Other preparations:

Lactitol
(Zyma)

Powder supplied in 10 g sachets and used as a laxative to treat constipation, brain disease due to liver problems.

Dose: constipation adults, 2 sachets a day initially, then 1 sachet a day; children ¼-2 sachets a day according to age, adjusted according to response. Other conditions 0.5-0.7 g/kg body weight a day in 3 divided doses with meals. Mix powder with food or in a drink.
Availability: NHS and private prescription.
Side effects: stomach discomfort, wind, bloating, itching around the anus.
Caution: in pregnant women, the elderly, or debilitated patients. Adequate fluid intake must be maintained.
Not to be used for: patients suffering from galactosaemia (an inherited disorder), or blocked intestine.
Caution needed with: ANTACIDS, NEOMYCIN.
Contains: LACTITOL.
Other preparations:

L

---

lactose *see* **Logynon ED, Femodene ED, Trinovum ED**

Lactugal *see* lactulose solution
(Galen)

---

lactulose *see* Duphalac, Lactugal, lactulose solution, Laxose

---

lactulose solution

A solution used as a laxative to treat constipation, brain disease due to liver problems.

Dose: children 0-1 year 2.5 ml twice a day; 1-5 years 5 ml twice a day; 5-10 years 10 ml twice a day (children's dose gradually reduced); adults15-50 ml 2-3 times a day, according to response and condition being treated.
Availability: NHS, private prescription, over the counter.
Side effects: wind, stomach cramps and pain.
Caution: in patients sensitive to lactose.
Not to be used for: patients suffering from galactosaemia (an inherited disorder), blocked intestine.
Caution needed with: ANTACIDS, NEOMYCIN.
Contains: LACTULOSE.
Other preparations: DUPHALAC, LACTUGAL, LAXOSE (some available in sachet form), REGULOSE.

Ladropen *see* flucloxacillin capsules
(Berk)

---

laevulose *see* Rehidrat

Lamictal
(Wellcome)

A yellow tablet supplied at strengths of 25 mg, 50 mg, 100 mg, 200 mg, and used as an anticonvulsant to treat epilepsy.

Dose: 25 mg once a day for the first 2 weeks, then 50 mg once a day for the next 2 weeks, increasing usually to 100-200 mg a day, up to 500 mg a day if needed. Dose may need adjustment if other anticonvulsants are also taken. Children over 2 years as advised by a physician.
Availability: NHS and private prescription.
Side effects: rash, severe allergy, double or blurred vision, dizziness, drowsiness, headache, stomach upset, confusion, irritability, aggression, weakness, shaking, sleeplessness.

L

Caution: in pregnant women, nursing mothers, and in patients suffering from rash, fever, influenza, drowsiness, or worsening of symptoms. Must be withdrawn gradually. Your doctor may advise regular check-ups.
Not to be used for: children under 2 years, the elderly, or for patients suffering from liver damage.
Caution needed with: alcohol, sedatives, PHENYTOIN, CARBAMAZEPINE, PHENOBARBITONE, PRIMIDONE, SODIUM VALPROATE.
Contains: LAMOTRIGINE.
Other preparations:

Lamisil
(Sandoz)

A white, scored tablet supplied at a strength of 250 mg and used as an antifungal treatment for fungal infections of skin and nails.

Dose: athlete's foot, 1 tablet a day for 2-6 weeks. Groin infection, 1 tablet a day for 2-4 weeks. Body infection, 1 tablet a day for 4 weeks. Fingernail infection, 1 tablet a day for 6 weeks-3 months. Toenail infection, 1 tablet a day for 3-6 months.
Availability: NHS and private prescription.
Side effects: upset stomach, taste changes, nausea, allergic skin reactions, headache, joint or muscle pains; rarely liver changes.
Caution: in pregnant women, nursing mothers, and in patients suffering from severe liver disorder, kidney damage.
Not to be used for: children.
Caution needed with: drugs affecting liver enzymes (eg BARBITURATES, CARBAMAZEPINE, PHENYTOIN, PRIMIDONE, RIFAMPICIN, ALLOPURINOL, CIMETIDINE, CIPROFLOXACIN, ERYTHROMYCIN).
Contains: TERBINAFINE.
Other preparations: Lamisil Cream.

---

lamotrigine *see* Lamictal

Lamprene
(Ciba)

A brown capsule supplied at a strength of 100 mg and used as an anti-leprotic drug to treat leprosy.

Dose: as advised by the physician.
Availability: NHS and private prescription.
Side effects: skin, hair, faeces and urine discoloration, dry skin, itch, stomach disturbance.

Caution: in pregnant women, nursing mothers, or in patients suffering from stomach pain, diarrhoea, kidney or liver disease.
Not to be used for:
Caution needed with:
Contains: CLOFAZIMINE.
Other preparations:

---

lanolin oil *see* **Alpha Keri**

Lanoxin *see* **digoxin tablets**
(Wellcome)

---

lansoprazole *see* **Zoton**

Larafen *see* **ketoprofen capsules**
(Lagap)

Laraflex *see* **naproxen tablets**
(Lagap)

Laratrim *see* **co-trimoxazole tablets**
(Lagap)

Largactil *see* **chlorpromazine tablets**
(Rhône-Poulenc Rorer)

Lariam
(Roche)

A white, quarter-scored tablet supplied at a strength of 250 mg, and used to treat and prevent malaria.

Dose: for prevention adults, 1 tablet a week; children, up to1 tablet a week according to bodyweight. Start one week before departure and continue for 4 weeks after return. Maximum use 3 months. For treatment, as advised by doctor.
Availability: NHS and private prescription.
Side effects: dizziness, nausea, vomiting, stomach upset, loss of appetite, headache, slow pulse rate, skin changes, psychological changes.

L

Caution: in patients suffering from heart conduction disorders, epilepsy. Women must use reliable contraception during treatment and for 3 months afterwards. Your doctor may advise you not to drive or operate machinery when used for treatment.

Not to be used for: pregnant women, nursing mothers, or for patients suffering from liver or kidney damage, or history of psychiatric disorder or convulsions, or who are allergic to quinine.

Caution needed with: QUININE, SODIUM VALPROATE, TYPHOID vaccination, halofantrine.

Contains: MEFLOQUINE hydrochloride.

Other preparations:

Larodopa
(Cambridge)

A white, quarter-scored tablet supplied at a strength of 500 mg and used as an anti-parkinsonian drug to treat Parkinson's disease.

Dose: ¼ tablet twice a day after meals at first increasing after 7 days to ¼ tablet 4-5 times a day, then increasing every 7 days by ¾ tablet a day to 5-16 tablets a day in 4-5 divided doses.

Availability: NHS and private prescription.

Side effects: nausea, vomiting, loss of appetite, low blood pressure on standing up, involuntary movments, heart and brain disturbances, discoloration of urine.

Caution: in pregnant women and in patients suffering from heart, liver, kidney, lung, or endocrine disease, stomach ulcer, and wide-angle glaucoma. Your doctor may advise that blood and liver, kidney, and cardiovascular systems should be checked regularly.

Not to be used for: children, adults aged under 25, or for patients suffering from severe mental disorder, narrow-angle glaucoma, or a history of malignant melanoma.

Caution needed with: MAOIS, VITAMIN B$_6$, blood-pressure lowering drugs, SYMPATHOMIMETICS, FERROUS SULPHATE, some other similar drugs.

Contains: LEVODOPA.

Other preparations: BROCADOPA.

Lasikal
(Hoechst Roussel)

A white/yellow, double-layered tablet used as a DIURETIC and potassium supplement to treat fluid retention where a potassium supplement is needed.

Dose: 2 tablets a day as a single dose in the morning, then up to 4 tablets

a day in 2 doses if needed, or 1 tablet a day.
Availability: NHS and private prescription.
Side effects: stomach upset, rash, gout.
Caution: in pregnant women, nursing mothers, or in patients suffering from liver or kidney disease, enlarged prostate, diabetes, or impaired urination.
Not to be used for: children, or for patients suffering from cirrhosis of the liver, raised potassium levels, or Addison's disease.
Caution needed with: some diuretics, DIGOXIN, LITHIUM, some antibiotics, NON-STEROIDAL ANTI-INFLAMMATORY DRUGS, blood-pressure lowering drugs.
Contains: FRUSEMIDE, POTASSIUM CHLORIDE.
Other preparations: DIUMIDE-K, LASIX + K.

Lasilactone
(Hoechst Roussel)

A blue/white capsule used as a DIURETIC combination to treat fluid retention, some types of high blood pressure.

Dose: 1-4 capsules a day.
Availability: NHS and private prescription.
Side effects: stomach upset, gout, rash, blood changes, breast swelling.
Caution: in pregnant women, nursing mothers, young patients, or in patients suffering from enlarged prostate, impaired urination, diabetes, kidney or liver disease, gout.
Not to be used for: children, or for patients suffering from severe or progressive kidney failure, liver cirrhosis, raised potassium levels, Addison's disease.
Caution needed with: potassium supplements, some diuretics, blood-pressure lowering drugs, DIGOXIN, LITHIUM, some antibiotics, NON-STEROIDAL ANTI-INFLAMMATORY DRUGS, ACE INHIBITORS.
Contains: FRUSEMIDE, SPIRONOLACTONE.
Other preparations:

Lasix *see* frusemide tablets
(Hoechst Roussel)

Lasix + K
(Hoechst Roussel)

Ten white, scored tablets plus 20 pale-yellow tablets supplied at strengths of 40 mg plus 750 mg and used as a DIURETIC and potassium supplement.

Dose: 1 white tablet a day in the morning and 2 pale-yellow tablets a day

at noon and in the evening.
Availability: NHS and private prescription.
Side effects: stomach upset, rash, gout.
Caution: in pregnant women, nursing mothers, and in patients suffering from liver or kidney disease, enlarged prostate, diabetes, gout, impaired urination.
Not to be used for: patients suffering from liver cirrhosis, raised potassium levels, Addison's disease.
Caution needed with: some diuretics, DIGOXIN, LITHIUM, some antibiotics, NON-STEROIDAL ANTI-INFLAMMATORY DRUGS, blood-pressure lowering drugs.
Contains: FRUSEMIDE plus POTASSIUM CHLORIDE.
Other preparations: DIUMIDE-K, LASIKAL.

Lasma
(Pharmax)

A white, elongated, scored, long-acting tablet supplied at a strength of 300 mg and used as a BRONCHODILATOR to treat brochial spasm brought on by asthma, bronchitis, emphysema.

Dose: 1 tablet every 12 hours increasing by ½ tablet if needed, or 2 tablets a day as a single dose, increasing to 3 tablets after 7 days if needed.
Availability: NHS, private prescription, over the counter.
Side effects: rapid heart rate, nausea, stomach upset, headache, abnormal heart rhythms.
Caution: in pregnant women, nursing mothers, and in patients suffering from heart or liver disease, or stomach ulcer.
Not to be used for: children.
Caution needed with: CIMETIDINE, ERYTHROMYCIN, CIPROFLOXACIN, STEROIDS, DIURETICS, other bronchodilators.
Contains: THEOPHYLLINE.
Other preparations: NUELIN SA, SLO-PHYLLIN, THEO-DUR, UNIPHYLLIN-CONTINUS (some available as capsule forms).

Lasonil
(Bayer)

An ointment used as an anti-inflammatory preparation to treat bruises, sprains, soft tissue injuries.

Dose: apply 2-3 times a day.
Availability: NHS, private prescription, over the counter.
Side effects:
Caution:

Not to be used for: if there are open or infected wounds.
Caution needed with:
Contains: HEPARINOID.
Other preparations:

Lasoride *see* co-amilofruse
(Hoechst Roussel)

---

lauromacrogol *see* Anacal, Balneum Plus

Laxoberal *see* sodium picosulphate elixir
(Windsor Healthcare)

Laxose *see* lactulose solution
(Berk)

Ledercort
(Lederle)

A blue, oblong, scored tablet or a white, oblong, scored tablet according to strengths of 2 mg, 4 mg and used as a STEROID treatment for rheumatoid arthritis, allergies, SLE, Crohn's disease, colitis, asthma.

Dose: as advised by physician.
Availability: NHS and private prescription.
Side effects: raised blood sugar levels, thinning of the bones, mood changes, stomach ulcer.
Caution: in pregnant women, in patients who have had recent bowel surgery or who are suffering from inflamed veins, psychiatric disorders, virus infections, some cancers, some kidney diseases, thinning of the bones, ulcers, tuberculosis, other infections, high blood pressure, glaucoma, epilepsy, diabetes, underactive thyroid, liver disease, stress. Withdraw gradually. Avoid contact with chickenpox or herpes virus.
Not to be used for:
Caution needed with: PHENYTOIN, PHENOBARBITONE, EPHEDRINE, RIFAMPICIN, DIURETICS, ANTICHOLINESTERASES, DIGOXIN, antidiabetics, ANTICOAGULANTS, NON-STEROIDAL ANTI-INFLAMMATORY DRUGS.
Contains: TRIAMCINOLONE.
Other preparations: ADCORTYL, KENALOG, LEDERSPAN (injectable forms)

L

Lederfen *see* **fenbufen tablets**
(Lederle)

Ledermycin
(Lederle)

A dark-red/pale-red capsule supplied at a strength of 150 mg and used as a TETRACYCLINE to treat respiratory and soft tissue infections.

Dose: 2 capsules twice a day or 1 capsule 4 times a day.
Availability: NHS and private prescription.
Side effects: stomach disturbances, sensitivity to light, additional infections, pressure on the brain.
Caution: in patients suffering from liver or kidney disease.
Not to be used for: children, pregnant women, nursing mothers.
Caution needed with: milk, ANTACIDS, mineral supplements, contraceptive pill, penicillins, ANTICOAGULANTS.
Contains: DEMECLOCYCLINE.
Other preparations:

Lederspan 20 mg
(Lederle)

An injection supplied at a strength of 20 mg/ml, and used as a STEROID treatment for arthritis, bursitis, and tendinitis.

Dose: an injection of 2-30 mg according to the severity of the condition and the size of the joint at intervals of not less than 3-4 weeks, or as advised by the physician.
Availability: NHS, private prescription.
Side effects: raised blood sugars, osteoporosis, euphoria, depression, stomach ulcer, weight gain, flushing, hair growth, raised blood pressure, mental disturbances.
Caution: in pregnant women and in patients suffering from stress, underactive thyroid, cirrhosis of the liver, diabetes, epilepsy, glaucoma, raised blood pressure, chickenpox, tuberculosis, stomach ulcer, osteoporosis, kidney disorders, measle-like illnesses, mental disorders, thrombophlebitis, or who have undergone recent stomach surgery.
Not to be used for: intravenous injection or where there is infection near the proposed injection site.
Caution needed with: PHENYTOIN, PHENOBARBITONE, EPHEDRINE, RIFAMPICIN, DIURETICS, ANTICHOLINESTERASES, some antidiabetic drugs, ANTICOAGULANTS taken by mouth, NON-STEROIDAL ANTI-INFLAMMATORY DRUGS, DIGOXIN.
Contains: TRIAMCINOLONE hydrochloride.
Other preparations: ADCORTYL, KENALOG, LEDERCORT (tablet form).

L

lemon bioflavonoid complex *see* **Lipoflavonoid**

Lenium
(Janssen-Cilag)

An anti-dandruff preparation.

Dose: twice a week for the first two weeks, once a week for two further weeks, then once every 3-6 weeks.
Availability: NHS, private prescription, over the counter.
Side effects:
Caution: keep out of the eyes and any areas of broken skin; do not use within 48 hours of waving or colouring substances.
Not to be used for:
Caution needed with:
Contains: SELENIUM SULPHIDE.
Other preparations: SELSUN.

Lentard *see* insulin
(Novo Nordisk)

Lentizol *see* amitriptyline tablets
(Parke-Davis)

Lescol
(Sandoz)

A red-brown/pale yellow capsule or a red-brown/orange-yellow capsule according to strengths of 20 mg, 40 mg, and used as a drug to reduce cholesterol levels in patients with high cholesterol that have not responded to changes in diet.

Dose: 20-40 mg once a day at night.
Availability: NHS, private prescription.
Side effects: stomach upset, sinusitis, weakness, urinary tract infections, sleeplessness, tooth problems; rarely liver disorders, muscle problems.
Caution: in patients with a history of liver disease or alcoholism. Your doctor may advise regular check-ups. You should report any muscle problems to your physician.
Not to be used for: children under 18 years, pregnant women, nursing mothers, or for patients suffering from severe kidney failure, liver disorders, some blood disorders.
Caution needed with: NICOTINIC ACID, ERYTHROMYCIN, RIFAMPICIN, GEMFIBROZIL

L

and related drugs, drugs the suppress the immune system
Contains: FLUVASTATIN.
Other preparations:

---

leuprorelin *see* **Prostap SR**

---

levobunolol *see* **Betagan**

---

levodopa *see* **Brocadopa, Half Sinemet, Larodopa, Madopar, Sinemet**

---

levonorgestrel *see* **Cyclo-Progynova 1mg, Eugynon 30, Logynon, Logynon ED, Microgynon 30, Microval, Mirena, Norgeston, Norplant, Nuvelle, Ovran, Ovranette, PC4, Trinordiol.** *See also* **norgestrel.**

Lexotan
(Roche)

A lilac, hexagonal, scored tablet or a pink, hexagonal, scored tablet according to strengths of 1.5 mg, 3 mg and used for the short-term treatment of anxiety.

Dose: elderly 1.5-9 mg a day in divided doses, adults 3-18 mg a day in divided doses.
Availability: private prescription only.
Side effects: drowsiness, confusion, unsteadiness, weakness, vertigo, stomach upset, low blood pressure, rash, changes in vision, changes in sexual function, retention of urine. Risk of addiction increases with dose and length of treatment. May impair judgement.
Caution: in the elderly, pregnant women, nursing mothers, in women during labour, and in patients suffering from lung disorders, kidney or liver disorders. Avoid long-term use and withdraw gradually.
Not to be used for: children or for patients suffering from acute lung diseases, some chronic lung diseases, some obsessional and psychotic diseases.
Caution needed with: alcohol, sedatives, and other tranquillizers and anticonvulsants.
Contains: BROMAZEPAM.
Other preparations:

Lexpec
(Rosemont)

A syrup used as a FOLIC ACID supplement to treat megaloblastic anaemia (anaemia with large red blood cells).

Dose: adults 20-40 ml a day for 14 days then 5-20 ml a day; children 10-30 ml a day.
Availability: NHS and private prescription.
Side effects: nausea, constipation, mottled teeth.
Caution: mottled teeth can be minimized by drinking syrup through a straw.
Not to be used for: megaloblastic anaemia caused by VITAMIN B_{12} deficiency.
Caution needed with: TETRACYCLINE ANTIBIOTICS, PHENYTOIN.
Contains: FOLIC ACID.
Other preparations: Lexpec with Iron, Lexpec with Iron-M. Folic acid tablets.

Li-liquid *see* Litarex
(Rosemont)

Librium *see* chlordiazepoxide capsules
(Roche)

Lidifen *see* ibuprofen tablets
(Berk)

Lidifen-F *see* ibuprofen tablets
(Berk)

Lignocaine and Fluorescein Minims
(Chauvin)

Drops used as a local anaesthetic and dye for carrying out procedures on the eye.

Dose: 1 or more drops into the eye as needed. Protect eye.
Availability: NHS and private prescription.
Side effects:
Caution:
Not to be used for:

Caution needed with:
Contains: LIGNOCAINE hydrochloride, SODIUM FLUORESCEIN.
Other preparations:

---

lignocaine *see* **Anodesyn, Betnovate Rectal, EMLA, Lignocaine and Fluorescein Minims, Perinal, Xylocaine, Xyloproct**

---

lindane *see* **Quellada**

Lingraine
(Sanofi-Winthrop)

A green tablet supplied at a strength of 2 mg and used as an ergot preparation to treat migraine, headache.

Dose: 1 tablet under the tongue at the beginning of a migraine attack, and repeat if needed ½-1 hour later to a maximum of 3 tablets in 24 hours or 6 tablets in a week.
Availability: NHS and private prescription.
Side effects: nausea, stomach pain, leg cramps.
Caution:
Not to be used for: children, pregnant women, nursing mothers, or for patients suffering from severe high blood pressure, kidney or liver disease, sepsis, overactive thyroid, PORPHYRIA, blood vessel disorders.
Caution needed with: ERYTHROMYCIN, ß-BLOCKERS.
Contains: ERGOTAMINE TARTRATE.
Other preparations: CAFERGOT, MEDIHALER ERGOTAMINE, MIGRIL.

Lioresal *see* **baclofen tablets**
(Ciba)

---

liothyronine *see* **Tertroxin**

Lipantil
(Fournier)

A white capsule supplied at a strength of 100 mg and used as a lipid-lowering agent to lower cholesterol or triglycerides.

Dose: 2-4 capsules a day.

Availability: NHS and private prescription.
Side effects: stomach upset, dizziness, headache, tiredness, rashes.
Rarely altered sexual function and muscle disorder.
Caution: in patients suffering from kidney impairment.
Not to be used for: pregnant women, nursing mothers, or for patients
suffering from severe kidney or liver problems, gall bladder disease.
Caution needed with: ANTICOAGULANTS, antidiabetic drugs taken by mouth.
Contains: FENOFIBRATE.
Other preparations: Lipantil Micro 200 mg.

Lipobase *see* Diprobase
(Yamanouchi)

Lipoflavonoid
(Lewis)

A black/pink capsule used as a multivitamin treatment for VITAMIN B
deficiency.

Dose: 3 capsules 3 times a day for 2-3 months reducing to 2 capsules 3
times a day.
Availability: private prescription and over the counter.
Side effects:
Caution:
Not to be used for: children.
Caution needed with: LEVODOPA.
Contains: CHOLINE BITARTRATE, INOSITOL, METHIONINE, VITAMIN C, LEMON
BIOFLAVONOID COMPLEX, VITAMIN B_1, VITAMIN B_2, VITAMIN B_3, VITAMIN B_6, PANTHENOL,
VITAMIN B_{12}.
Other preparations:

Lipostat
(Squibb)

A pink, oblong tablet supplied at a strength of 10 mg, 20 mg, and used as
a lipid-lowering agent to treat raised cholesterol.

Dose: 10 mg at night initially, increasing to 10-40 mg at night.
Availability: NHS and private prescription.
Side effects: rash, muscle pain, headache, chest pain, nausea, vomiting,
diarrhoea, tiredness.
Caution: in patients with a history of liver disease. Your doctor may advise
regular tests during treatment.
Not to be used for: children under 18 years, pregnant women, nursing

mothers, or for patients suffering from liver disease.
Caution needed with: CHOLESTYRAMINE, COLESTIPOL, VITAMIN B_3, drugs that suppress the immune system, ERYTHROMYCIN, RIFAMPICIN, GEMFIBROZIL.
Contains: PRAVASTATIN.
Other preparations:

Lipotriad
(Lewis)

A clear pink capsule used as a multivitamin treatment for VITAMIN B deficiency.

Dose: 3 capsules 3 times a day for 2-3 months then reducing to 2 capsules 3 times a day.
Availability: private prescription and over the counter.
Side effects:
Caution:
Not to be used for: children.
Caution needed with: LEVODOPA.
Contains: CHOLINE BITARTRATE, INOSITOL, DL-METHIONINE, VITAMIN B_{12}, VITAMIN B_1, VITAMIN B_2, VITAMIN B_3, VITAMIN B_6, PANTHENOL.
Other preparations:

---

liquid paraffin *see* **Alcoderm, Coal tar and salicylic acid ointment, Dermamist, Diprobase, Diprobath, Hydromol, Keri, Lipobase, liquid paraffin and magnesium hydroxide emulsion, Lubrifilm, Oilatum, Oilatum Plus, Polytar Emollient, simple eye ointment, Unguentum Merck**

---

liquid paraffin and magnesium hydroxide emulsion

An emulsion used as a laxative to treat constipation.

Dose: 5-20 ml when required.
Availability: NHS, private prescription, over the counter.
Side effects: colic,
Caution: in the elderly, and in patients who are weak or suffering from kidney or liver damage.
Not to be used for: children, or for sudden, severe symptoms.
Caution needed with:
Contains: LIQUID PARAFFIN, MAGNESIUM HYDROXIDE.
Other preparations:

Liquifilm Tears
(Allergan)

Drops used to lubricate dry eyes.

Dose: 1-2 drops into the eye as needed.
Availability: NHS, private prescription, over the counter.
Side effects:
Caution:
Not to be used for: patients who wear soft contact lenses.
Caution needed with:
Contains: POLYVINYL ALCOHOL.
Other preparations: HYPOTEARS, SNO TEARS.

---

liquorice *see* **Caved-S**

---

lisinopril *see* **Carace, Carace Plus, Zestoretic, Zestril**

Liskonum
(SmithKline Beecham)

A white, scored, oblong tablet supplied at a strength of 450 mg and used as a sedative to treat mania, hypomania, manic depression.

Dose: as judged by blood tests to keep a constant level.
Availability: NHS and private prescription.
Side effects: nausea, diarrhoea, hand tremor, muscular weakness, brain and heart disturbances, weight gain, fluid retention, underactive or over-active thyroid gland, thirst and frequent urination, kidney changes, skin reactions.
Caution: treatment should be started in hospital and a careful check on the functioning of the kidneys and thyroid should be made, as well as ensuring that there is an adequate consumption of salt and fluid. Your doctor may advise blood tests to gauge dose.
Not to be used for: children, for pregnant women, nursing mothers, or for patients suffering from disturbed sodium balance, Addison's disease, kidney or heart disease, or underactive thyroid.
Caution needed with: DIURETICS, NON-STEROIDAL ANTI-INFLAMMATORY DRUGS, CARBAMAZEPINE, PHENYTOIN, HALOPERIDOL, FLUPENTHIXOL, METHYLDOPA, FLUVOXAMINE, FLUOXETINE, METOCLOPRAMIDE.
Contains: LITHIUM carbonate.
Other preparations: CAMCOLIT, LITHONATE, PRIADEL.

L

---

lisuride *see* **Revanil**

Litarex
(Dumex)

A white, oval, scored tablet supplied at a strength of 564 mg and used as a sedative to treat acute mania, and for the prevention of recurring mood changes.

Dose: 1 tablet morning and evening at first and then as advised by the physician.
Availability: NHS and private prescription.
Side effects: nausea, diarrhoea, hand tremor, muscular weakness, brain and heart disturbances, weight gain, fluid retention, underactive or overactive thyroid gland, thirst and frequent urination, skin reactions.
Caution: treatment should be started in hospital, thyroid function should be checked regularly, and there should be an adequate consumption of salt and fluid. Your doctor may advise frequent blood tests to gauge dose.
Not to be used for: children, pregnant women, nursing mothers, the elderly, or for patients suffering from Addison's disease, kidney or cardiovascular disease, underactive thyroid, in cases where there is a disturbed sodium balance.
Caution needed with: DIURETICS, ACE INHIBITORS, ANTACIDS, METRONIDAZOLE, NON-STEROIDAL ANTI-INFLAMMATORY DRUGS, CARBAMAZEPINE, PHENYTOIN, DILTIAZEM, VERAPAMIL, some drugs used to treat MYASTHENIA GRAVIS, DOMPERIDONE, METOCLOPRAMIDE, FLUPENTHIXOL, METHYLDOPA, PHENYTOIN, HALOPERIDOL, antidepressants, antidiabetics, muscle relaxants, SUMATRIPTAN, THEOPHYLLINE.
Contains: LITHIUM CITRATE.
Other preparations: LI-LIQUID.

Lithonate *see* Priadel Tablets
(A.P.S.)

---

lithium *see* Camcolit, Efalith, Li-liquid, Liskonum, Litarex, Priadel

---

Livial
(Organon)

A white tablet supplied at a strength of 2.5 mg, and used to treat symptoms associated with the menopause.

Dose: 1 tablet a day for a minimum of 3 months.

Availability: NHS and private prescription.
Side effects: changes in body weight, dizziness, headache, seborrhoeic dermatitis, vaginal bleeding, stomach upset, liver disorder, hair growth, fluid retention, visual disturbance, skin irritation.
Caution: in patients who have transferred from a similar drug, or who suffer from, or have a history of, kidney disorder, epilepsy, migraine, diabetes, or high cholesterol levels.
Not to be used for: children, pregnant women, nursing mothers, or for patients suffering from some tumours, undiagnosed vaginal bleeding, blood vessel disorder of the brain or heart, severe liver disorders.
Caution needed with: ANTICOAGULANTS, PHENYTOIN, CARBAMAZEPINE, RIFAMPICIN.
Contains: TIBOLONE.
Other preparations:

Locabiotal
(Servier)

An aerosol supplied at a strength of 125 micrograms and used as an anti-inflammatory, antibiotic treatment for infection, inflammation, of the nose, mouth, and throat.

Dose: adults 5 sprays into the mouth or 3 sprays into each nostril 5 times a day; children 3-5 years 2 sprays into the mouth 3 times a day or 1 spray into each nostril 5 times a day, 6-12 years 3 sprays into the mouth 3 times a day or 2 sprays in each nostril 5 times a day, over 12 years 4 sprays into the mouth 3 times a day or 3 sprays in each nostril 5 times a day.
Availability: NHS and private prescription.
Side effects:
Caution:
Not to be used for: children under 3 years.
Caution needed with:
Contains: FUSAFUNGINE.
Other preparations:

Loceryl
(Roche)

A cream used as an antifungal treatment for fungal skin infection.

Dose: apply once a day in the evening, until 3-5 days after apparent cure.
Availability: NHS and private prescription.
Side effects: itching, burning.
Caution: avoid contact with eyes, ears, mucous membranes.
Not to be used for: children, pregnant women, nursing mothers.
Caution needed with:

L

Contains: AMOROLFINE.
Other preparations: Loceryl Lacquer (for nail infections).

Locoid *see* hydrocortisone cream
(Yamanouchi)

Locoid-C
(Yamanouchi)

A cream/ointment used as an antibacterial, antifungal, and strong STEROID to treat eczema, psoriasis, and other skin conditions which are also infected with bacteria or fungi.

Dose: apply 2-4 times a day.
Availability: NHS and private prescription.
Side effects: fluid retention, suppression of adrenal glands, thinning, spotting, or streaking of the skin may occur.
Caution: use for short periods of time only, especially on the face or in children.
Not to be used for: continuous use, especially on pregnant women, or for patients suffering from acne or any other tubercular or viral infection of the skin, scabies, leg ulcers.
Caution needed with:
Contains: HYDROCORTISONE 17-butyrate, CHLORQUINALDOL.
Other preparations:

Locoid Lipocream
(Yamanouchi)

A cream used as a strong STEROID treatment for skin disorders that respond to steroid treatment.

Dose: apply to the affected area 2-3 times a day.
Availability: NHS, private prescription.
Side effects: thinning, spotting, and streaking of the skin, suppression of the adrenal glands, flushing, hair growth.
Caution: in infants, especially if wearing nappies or plastic pants. Do not use on children or on the face for more than 5 days. If used for psoriasis, regular checks are needed. Withdraw slowly after prolonged use.
Not to be used for: prolonged use in pregnant women, for long-term prevention, or for patients suffering from acne, scabies, leg ulcers, skin disorders around the mouth, or for infected conditions.
Caution needed with:
Contains: HYDROCORTISONE 17-BUTYRATE.

Other preparations: LOCOID, Locoid Scalp Lotion, LOCOID-C.

Locorten-Vioform
(Zyma Healthcare)

Drops used as an antibacterial, STEROID treatment for inflammation of the outer ear where secondary infections may be present.

Dose: 2-3 drops into the ear twice a day for 7-10 days.
Availability: NHS and private prescription.
Side effects: irritation, hair discoloration.
Caution: in nursing mothers.
Not to be used for: children under 2 years, or for patients suffering from perforated ear drum or primary infections of the outer ear.
Caution needed with:
Contains: CLIOQUINOL, FLUMETHASONE pivalate.
Other preparations:

Lodine Capsules
(Wyeth)

A dark-grey/light-grey capsule or light grey capsule, marked with 2 red bands supplied at strengths of 200 mg, 300 mg and used as a NON-STEROIDAL ANTI-INFLAMMATORY DRUG to treat rheumatoid arthritis and osteoarthritis.

Dose: 200-300 mg twice a day to a maximum of 600 mg a day.
Availability: NHS and private prescription.
Side effects: nausea, stomach pain, upset, or bleeding, headache, dizziness, tinnitus, rash, swelling, kidney inflammation.
Caution: in the elderly, those on long-term treatment, and in patients suffering from heart, kidney, or liver disease, heart failure.
Not to be used for: children, pregnant women, nursing mothers, or for patients suffering from stomach ulcer, a history of stomach ulcer or gastrointestinal bleeding, allergy to anti-inflammatory drugs/ASPIRIN.
Caution needed with: ANTICOAGULANTS, antidiabetic drugs, some antibiotics.
Contains: ETODOLAC.
Other preparations: Lodine Tablets, Lodine SR.

lodoxamide *see* Alomide

L

Loestrin 20
(Parke-Davis)

A blue tablet used as an oestrogen, progestogen contraceptive.

Dose: 1 tablet a day for 21 days starting on day 5 of the period.
Availability: NHS and private prescription.
Side effects: enlarged breasts, bloating and fluid retention, cramps, leg pains, mood change, reduction in sexual desire, headaches, nausea, vaginal erosion, discharge, and bleeding, weight gain, skin changes, rarely thrombosis, raised blood pressure, jaundice.
Caution: in patients suffering from high blood pressure, diabetes, vascular disorders, asthma, depression, kidney disease, multiple sclerosis, womb diseases. Your doctor may advise you not to smoke, to have regular examinations. You should stop treatment at the first sign of serious symptoms such as severe headache or jaundice. Treatment should be stopped before surgery.
Not to be used for: pregnant women, or for patients suffering from sickle-cell anaemia, history of heart disease or thrombosis, liver disorders, some cancers, undiagnosed vaginal bleeding, some ear, skin, and kidney disorders.
Caution needed with: RIFAMPICIN, TETRACYCLINE ANTIBIOTICS, GRISEOFULVIN, BARBITURATES, PHENYTOIN, PRIMIDONE, CARBAMAZEPINE, ETHOSUXIMIDE, CHLORAL HYDRATE.
Contains: ETHINYLOESTRADIOL, NORETHISTERONE acetate.
Other preparations: Loestrin 30.

Lofensaid *see* diclofenac tablets
(Opus)

lofepramine *see* lofepramine tablets, Gamanil

lofepramine tablets

A tablet supplied at a strength of 70 mg and used as a TRICYCLIC ANTIDEPRESSANT to treat depression.

Dose: 1-3 tablets a day in divided doses.
Availability: NHS and private prescription.
Side effects: dry mouth, tiredness, constipation, urine retention, blurred vision, nausea, palpitations, drowsiness, sleeplessness, dizziness, hands shaking, low blood pressure, weight change, sweating, behavioural changes in children, fits, confusion in the elderly, skin reactions, jaundice or blood changes, interference with sexual function.

Caution: in pregnant women, nursing mothers or in patients suffering from heart disease, thyroid disease, epilepsy, diabetes, glaucoma, adrenal tumour, urinary retention, PORPHYRIA, some other psychiatric conditions. Your doctor may advise regular blood tests.

Not to be used for: children, pregnant women, or for patients suffering from heart attacks, heart block, liver disease, severe kidney disease, heart rhythm disturbance.

Caution needed with: alcohol, sedatives, ANTICHOLINERGICS, ADRENALINE, MAOIS, ASTEMIZOLE, TERFENADINE, other antidepressants, blood-pressure lowering drugs, CIMETIDINE, anaesthetics, drugs affecting heart rhythm, anticonvulsants.

Contains: LOFEPRAMINE hydrochloride.

Other preparations: GAMANIL.

---

lofexidine *see* BritLofex

Logynon
(Schering Healthcare)

A brown tablet, a white tablet, and an ochre tablet used as an oestrogen, progestogen contraceptive.

Dose: 1 tablet a day for 21 days starting on day 1 of the period.

Availability: NHS and private prescription.

Side effects: enlarged breasts, bloating and fluid retention, cramps, leg pains, mood change, reduction in sexual desire, headaches, nausea, vaginal erosion, discharge, and bleeding, weight gain, skin changes, rarely thrombosis, raised blood pressure, jaundice.

Caution: in patients suffering from high blood pressure, diabetes, vascular disorders, asthma, depression, kidney disease, multiple sclerosis, womb diseases. Your doctor may advise you not to smoke, to have regular examinations. You should stop treatment at the first sign of serious symptoms such as severe headache or jaundice. Treatment should be stopped before surgery.

Not to be used for: pregnant women, or for patients suffering from sickle-cell anaemia, history of heart disease or thrombosis, liver disorders, some cancers, undiagnosed vaginal bleeding, some ear, skin, and kidney disorders.

Caution needed with: RIFAMPICIN, TETRACYCLINE ANTIBIOTICS, GRISEOFULVIN, BARBITURATES, PHENYTOIN, PRIMIDONE, CARBAMAZEPINE, ETHOSUXIMIDE, CHLORAL HYDRATE.

Contains: ETHINYLOESTRADIOL, LEVONORGESTREL.

Other preparations: TRINORDIOL.

L

Logynon ED
(Schering Healthcare)

A brown tablet, 2 white tablets, and an ochre tablet used as an oestrogen, progestogen contraceptive.

Dose: 1 tablet a day for 28 days starting on day 1 of the period.
Availability: NHS and private prescription.
Side effects: enlarged breasts, bloating and fluid retention, cramps, leg pains, mood change, reduction in sexual desire, headaches, nausea, vaginal erosion, discharge, and bleeding, weight gain, skin changes, rarely thrombosis, raised blood pressure, jaundice.
Caution: in patients suffering from high blood pressure, diabetes, vascular disorders, asthma, depression, kidney disease, multiple sclerosis, womb diseases. Your doctor may advise you not to smoke, to have regular examinations. You should stop treatment at the first sign of serious symptoms such as severe headache or jaundice. Treatment should be stopped before surgery.
Not to be used for: pregnant women, or for patients suffering from sickle-cell anaemia, history of heart disease or thrombosis, liver disorders, some cancers, undiagnosed vaginal bleeding, some ear, skin, and kidney disorders.
Caution needed with: RIFAMPICIN, TETRACYCLINE ANTIBIOTICS, GRISEOFULVIN, BARBITURATES, PHENYTOIN, PRIMIDONE, CARBAMAZEPINE, ETHOSUXIMIDE, CHLORAL HYDRATE.
Contains: ETHINYLOESTRADIOL, LEVONORGESTREL, LACTOSE.
Other preparations:

Lomexin
(Upjohn)

Soft gelatin pessaries supplied at strengths of 200 mg and 600 mg, and used as an antifungal preparation to treat vaginal thrush.

Dose: 1 600 mg pessary inserted high into the vagina at night, or 1 200 mg pessary inserted on 3 consecutive nights.
Availability: NHS, private prescription.
Side effects: mild irritation.
Caution: in pregnant women and nursing mothers.
Not to be used for: children.
Caution needed with: barrier contraceptives.
Contains: FENTICONAZOLE nitrate.
Other preparations:

Lomotil
(Gold Cross)

A white tablet used to slow down intestinal contents and as an opiate and ANTICHOLINERGIC to treat diarrhoea.

Dose: adults, 4 tablets initially, then 2 every 6 hours; children 4-8 years, 1 tablet 3 times a day, 9-12 years, 1 tablet 4 times a day, 13-16 years, 2 tablets 3 times a day.
Availability: NHS and private prescription.
Side effects: allergy, drowsiness (do not drive or operate machinery if affected), stomach upset, anticholinergic effects, disturbance of brain and spinal cord.
Caution: in pregnant women, nursing mothers, or in patients suffering from liver disorder, dehydration, body fluid imbalance.
Not to be used for: children under 4 years, or for patients suffering from blockage in the intestine, jaundice, colitis.
Caution needed with: MAOIS, sedatives.
Contains: DIPHENOXYLATE hydrochloride, ATROPINE SULPHATE (CO-PHENOTROPE).
Other preparations: Lomotil Liquid. LOTHARIN.

Loniten
(Upjohn)

A white tablet supplied at strengths of 2.5 mg, 5 mg, 10 mg and used as a vasodilator to treat high blood pressure.

Dose: adults 5 mg a day at first increasing at 3-day intervals to up to 10 mg a day and then by 10 mg at a time to a maximum of 50 mg a day; children 0.2 mg per kg of bodyweight a day at first, increasing at 3-day intervals by 0.1-0.2 mg per kg bodyweight to a maximum of 1 mg per kg bodyweight a day.
Availability: NHS and private prescription.
Side effects: hair growth, swelling, rapid heart rate.
Caution: angina or heart attack patients need to be monitored carefully. Other blood-pressure lowering drugs need to be withdrawn (apart from ß-BLOCKERS and DIURETICS). Needs to be given in conjunction with some other antihypertensive drugs.
Not to be used for: patients suffering from PHAEOCHROMOCYTOMA (a disease of the adrenal glands).
Caution needed with:
Contains: MINOXIDIL.
Other preparations: REGAINE – local application for the treatment of baldness (available over the counter).

L

LoperaGen *see* **loperamide capsules**
(Norgine)

---

loperamide *see* Diocaps, LoperaGen, loperamide capsules, Imodium, Norimode

---

loperamide capsules

A capsule supplied at a strength of 2 mg and used to treat acute diarrhoea in adults and children over 4 years (in conjunction with rehydration products) and adults only for chronic diarrhoea.

Dose: acute diarrhoea adults, 2 capsules initially then 1 after each loose bowel motion, to a maximum of 8 capsules a day for up to 5 days; children use liquid forms. Chronic diarrhoea, adults 2-4 capsules a day at first in divided doses, then adjusted according to response.
Availability: NHS, private prescription, over the counter (for adults and children over 12 years) only for the treatments of acute diarrhoea.
Side effects: rash, stomach cramps and bloating, constipation.
Caution: in pregnant women, nursing mothers, and in patients suffering from kidney failure, acute dysentery, blocked intestine.
Not to be used for: children under 4 years, or for patients suffering from swollen abdomen or severe ulcerative colitis.
Caution needed with:
Contains: LOPERAMIDE.
Other preparations: DIOCAPS, IMODIUM, LOPERAGEN. (Liquid forms available for children – only on prescription.)

Lopid
(Parke-Davis)

A white/maroon capsule and white oval tablet supplied at strengths of 300 mg, 600 mg and used as a lipid-lowering agent to treat raised lipid levels in the prevention of coronary heart disease.

Dose: usually 600 mg twice a day to a maximum of 1500 mg a day.
Availability: NHS and private prescription.
Side effects: stomach upset, rashes, impotence, headache, dizziness, painful extremities, muscle aches, blurred vision, jaundice, pancreatitis, fluid retention, abnormal heart rhythm.
Caution: your doctor may advise a lipid check; blood count, and liver function should be checked before treatment; eyes, blood, and serum should be checked regularly.
Not to be used for: pregnant women, nursing mothers, alcoholics, or

patients suffering from gallstones or liver disease.
Caution needed with: ANTICOAGULANTS, COLESTIPOL, other lipid-lowering drugs.
Contains: GEMFIBROZIL.
Other preparations:

Lopranol LA *see* propanolol tablets
(Opus)

---

loprazolam tablets

A tablet supplied at a strength of 1 mg and used as a sleeping tablet for the short-term treatment of sleeplessness or waking at night.

Dose: elderly up to 1 tablet before going to bed; adults 1-2 tablets before going to bed.
Availability: NHS and private prescription.
Side effects: drowsiness, confusion, unsteadiness, low blood pressure, rash, changes in vision, changes in sexual function, retention of urine. Risk of addiction increases with dose and length of treatment. May impair judgement.
Caution: in the elderly, pregnant women, nursing mothers, in women during labour, and in patients suffering from lung disorders, kidney or liver disorders. Avoid long-term use and withdraw gradually.
Not to be used for: children, or for patients suffering from acute lung diseases, some chronic lung diseases, some obsessional and psychotic diseases.
Caution needed with: alcohol, sedatives, other tranquillizers, anticonvulsants.
Contains: loprazolam mesylate.
Other preparations:

Lopresor *see* metoprolol tablets
(Ciba)

---

loratidine *see* Clarityn

---

lorazepam

A tablet supplied at strengths of 1 mg, 2.5 mg and used as a sedative to treat anxiety.

L

Dose: elderly 0.5-2 mg a day in divided doses; adults 1-4 mg a day in divided doses.
Availability: NHS and private prescription.
Side effects: drowsiness, confusion, unsteadiness, low blood pressure, rash, changes in vision, changes in sexual function, retention of urine. Risk of addiction increases with dose and length of treatment. May impair judgement.
Caution: in the elderly, pregnant women, nursing mothers, in women during labour, and in patients suffering from lung disorders, kidney or liver disorders. Avoid long-term use and withdraw gradually.
Not to be used for: children, or for patients suffering from acute lung diseases, some chronic lung diseases, some obsessional and psychotic diseases.
Caution needed with: alcohol, sedatives, other tranquillizers, anticonvulsants.
Contains: lorazepam.
Other preparations: ATIVAN – available on NHS only if prescribed as a generic.

---

lormetazepam

A tablet supplied at strengths of 0.5 mg, 1 mg and used as a sedative to treat sleeplessness.

Dose: elderly 0.5 mg before going to bed; adults 1 mg before going to bed.
Availability: NHS and private prescription.
Side effects: drowsiness, confusion, unsteadiness, low blood pressure, rash, changes in vision, changes in sexual function, retention of urine. Risk of addiction increases with dose and length of treatment. May impair judgement.
Caution: in the elderly, pregnant women, nursing mothers, in women during labour, and in patients suffering from lung disorders, kidney or liver disorders. Avoid long-term use and withdraw gradually.
Not to be used for: children, or for patients suffering from acute lung diseases, some chronic lung diseases, some obsessional and psychotic diseases.
Caution needed with: alcohol, sedatives, other tranquillizers, anticonvulsants.
Contains: lormetazepam.
Other preparations:

L

---

losartan potassium *see* **Cozaar**

Losec
(Astra)

A pink capsule, a pink/brown capsule, or a brown capsule according to strengths of 10 mg, 20 mg, 40 mg, and used as an anti-ulcer drug for ulcers which are difficult to treat, and as a treatment for reflux oesophagitis, acid reflux disease.

Dose: reflux oesophagitis, 20 mg once a day for 4 weeks, then for a further 4-8 weeks if needed; acid reflux disease, 10 mg once a day at first, increasing to 20 mg once a day if needed; ulcer, 20 mg once a day for 4-8 weeks, up to 40 mg a day in severe cases. Up to 120 mg a day may be required for excessive acid production in the stomach.
Availability: NHS and private prescription.
Side effects: constipation, diarrhoea, headache, nausea, rashes.
Caution: your doctor may advise endoscopic checks of the stomach.
Not to be used for: children, pregnant women, nursing mothers.
Caution needed with: DIAZEPAM, PHENYTOIN, WARFARIN, DIGOXIN.
Contains: OMEPRAZOLE.
Other preparations:

Lotharin *see* Lomotil
(Berk)

Lotriderm *see* Betnovate
(Schering-Plough)

Loxapac
(Wyeth)

A yellow/green capsule, light-green/dark-green capsule, or blue/dark-green capsule according to strengths of 10 mg, 25 mg, 50 mg, and used to treat mental disorders.

Dose: 20-50 mg a day in 2 divided doses, increasing to a maximum of 250 mg a day.
Availability: NHS and private prescription.
Side effects: drowsiness, dizziness, faintness, muscle twitching, weakness, confusion, rapid heart beat, low or high blood pressure, changes in heart activity, skin reactions, ANTICHOLINERGIC effects, nausea, vomiting, headache, breathing difficulty, changes in the eye.
Caution: in pregnant women, nursing mothers, and in patients suffering from epilepsy, cardiovascular disease, glaucoma, urine retention. Reduces mental alertness and co-ordination.

L

Not to be used for: children, or for patients in a coma or depressed state because of drugs.
Caution needed with: alcohol, sedatives, ANTICHOLINERGICS.
Contains: LOXAPINE succinate.
Other preparations:

---

loxapine *see* Loxapac

Luborant
(Antigen)

A solution used as an artificial saliva to treat dry mouth.

Dose: 2-3 sprays into the mouth up to 4 times a day.
Availability: NHS, private prescription, over the counter.
Side effects:
Caution:
Not to be used for: children.
Caution needed with:
Contains: CARBOXYMETHYLCELLULOSE.
Other preparations:

Lubrifilm *see* simple eye ointment
(Cusi)

Ludiomil
(Ciba)

A peach tablet, greyish-red tablet, pale-orange tablet, or brownish-orange tablet according to strengths of 10 mg, 25 mg, 50 mg, 75 mg and used as a tetracyclic antidepressant to treat depression.

Dose: adults 25-75 mg a day at first usually at night or in 3 divided doses, then adjusted as needed after 1-2 weeks; elderly 30 mg a day at first at night or in 3 divided doses.
Availability: NHS and private prescription.
Side effects: convulsions, rash, reduced reactions, ANTICHOLINERGIC effects.
Caution: in the elderly, pregnant women, nursing mothers, and in patients suffering from cardiovascular disease, overactive thyroid, schizophrenia.
Not to be used for: children or for patients suffering from mania, severe kidney or liver disease, history of epilepsy, narrow-angle glaucoma, recent heart attack, retention of urine, some heart disorders.
Caution needed with: MAOIS, blood-pressure lowering drugs,

L

SYMPATHOMIMETICS, BARBITURATES, PHENYTOIN, tranquillizers, CIMETIDINE, alcohol, anaesthetics.
Contains: MAPROTILINE hydrochloride.
Other preparations:

lupus

An abbreviated name for various lupus diseases, especially systemic lupus erythematosus (SLE), thought to be an auto-immune reaction causing an allergy-like rash, resulting in thickened areas of skin. Other lupus conditions cause similar skin reactions.

Lurselle
(Marion Merrell Dow)

A white, scored tablet supplied at a strength of 250 mg and used as a lipid-lowering agent to treat elevated lipids.

Dose: 2 tablets twice a day with morning and evening meals.
Availability: NHS and private prescription.
Side effects: diarrhoea, stomach upset, allergy, abnormal heart rhythm.
Caution: in patients suffering from heart disorders. Cease treatment 6 months before a planned pregnancy.
Not to be used for: children, pregnant women, or nursing mothers.
Caution needed with:
Contains: PROBUCOL.
Other preparations:

Lustral
(Invicta)

White, capsule-shaped tablets supplied at strengths of 50 mg, 100 mg, and used to treat the symptoms of depression, and to prevent relapse and further depressive episodes.

Dose: 50 mg once a day after food, increasing if necessary to a maximum of 200 mg a day. Doses of 150 mg or more should be limited to 8 weeks duration
Availability: NHS and private prescription.
Side effects: dry mouth, rash, nausea, diarrhoea, shaking, sweating, stomach discomfort, dizziness, sleeplessness or sleepiness, sexual disturbances, general feeling of being unwell.
Caution: in pregnant women, nursing mothers, patients undergoing electroconvulsive therapy, or suffering from unstable epilepsy or kidney disorder.

L

Not to be used for: children, or for patients suffering from liver disorder.
Caution needed with: MAOIS, LITHIUM, TRYPTOPHAN, SUMATRIPTAN, FENFLURAMINE, DIAZEPAM, TOLBUTAMIDE, CIMETIDINE, WARFARIN.
Contains: SERTRALINE.
Other preparations:

Lyclear Creme Rinse
(Wellcome)

A conditioning lotion applied to the head to treat head lice.

Dose: shampoo hair as usual, rinse and dry with a towel, then apply enough to saturate hair and scalp. Leave for 10 minutes, then rinse and dry.
Availability: NHS, private prescription, over the counter.
Side effects:
Caution: in children under 2 years, pregnant women, and nursing mothers. Avoid eyes.
Not to be used for: infants under 2 months.
Caution needed with:
Contains: PERMETHRIN.
Other preparations: Lyclear Dermal Cream (used to treat scabies).

---

lymecycline *see* Tetralysal

---

lypressin *see* Syntopressin

---

lysuride *see* Revanil

Maalox Plus *see* Asilone
(Rhône-Poulenc Rorer)

Maalox TC Tablets
(Rhône-Poulenc Rorer)

A white tablet used as an ANTACID to treat gastric and duodenal ulcer, gastritis, heartburn, acidity.

Dose: adults 1-3 tablets 4 times a day after meals and at bedtime.
Availability: NHS, private prescription, over the counter.
Side effects: occasionally constipation.

M

Caution:
Not to be used for: children.
Caution needed with: tablets coated to protect the stomach, TETRACYCLINE ANTIBIOTICS, iron.
Contains: ALUMINIUM HYDROXIDE, MAGNESIUM HYDROXIDE.
Other preparations: Maalox, Maalox TC Suspension. MUCOGEL.

Macrobid *see* nitrofurantoin tablets
(Procter & Gamble)

Macrodantin *see* nitrofurantoin tablets
(Procter & Gamble)

Madopar
(Roche)

A blue/grey capsule, blue/pink capsule, or blue/caramel capsule according to strengths of 62.5 mg, 125 mg, 250 mg and used as an anti-parkinsonian combination to treat Parkinson's disease.

Dose: adults over 25 years 1 low-dose capsule 3-4 times a day after meals at first increasing by 2 low-dose capsules a day 1-2 times a week up to 8-16 low-dose capsules (or equivalent) a day in divided doses or as advised by the physician; elderly 1 low-dose capsule once or twice a day at first increasing by 1 low-dose capsule every 3-4 days.
Availability: NHS and private prescription.
Side effects: nausea, vomiting, loss of appetite, low blood pressure on standing, involuntary movements, heart and brain disturbances, discoloration of urine, rarely haemolytic anaemia.
Caution: in patients suffering from cardiovascular, liver, lung, endocrine or kidney disease, stomach ulcer, mental disturbance, wide-angle glaucoma, soft bones. Your doctor may advise that blood, liver, kidney, and cardiovascular systems should be checked regularly.
Not to be used for: children, adults under 25 years, pregnant women, nursing mothers, or for patients suffering from severe mental disorders, narrow-angle glaucoma, history of malignant melanoma.
Caution needed with: MAOIS, blood-pressure lowering drugs, SYMPATHOMIMETICS, FERROUS SULPHATE, other similar drugs.
Contains: LEVODOPA, BENSERAZIDE HYDROCHLORIDE (CO-BENELDOPA).
Other preparations: Madopar Dispersible Tablets, Madopar CR.

M

Magnapen *see* co-fluampicil capsules
(Beecham)

---

magnesium alginate *see* Algicon

---

magnesium carbonate *see* Algicon, Bellocarb, Caved-S, magnesium carbonate aromatic mixture, Topal

---

magnesium carbonate aromatic mixture

A mixture used as an ANTACID to treat indigestion.

Dose: 10 ml 3 times a day in water.
Availability: NHS, private prescription, over the counter.
Side effects: diarrhoea, belching.
Caution: in patients suffering from kidney damage.
Not to be used for: children, or for patients with low phosphate levels in the blood.
Caution needed with: tablets coated to protect the stomach, some antibiotics, iron, ASPIRIN, DIFLUNISAL, QUINIDINE, PHENYTOIN, ITRACONAZOLE, KETOCONAZOLE, FOSINOPRIL, DIPYRIDAMOLE, CHLOROQUINE, HYDROXYCHLOROQUINE, some sedatives, PENICILLAMINE.
Contains: MAGNESIUM CARBONATE, SODIUM BICARBONATE, aromatic cardamom tincture.
Other preparations:

---

magnesium chloride *see* Glandosane

---

magnesium citrate *see* Citramag, Picolax

---

magnesium hydroxide *see* Diovol, liquid paraffin and magnesium hydroxide emulsion, Maalox Plus, magnesium hydroxide mixture, Mucaine

---

magnesium hydroxide mixture

A mixture used as a laxative to treat constipation.

Dose: 25-50 ml when required.
Availability: NHS, private prescription, over the counter.

M

Side effects: colic.
Caution: in the elderly, and in patients who are weak or suffering from kidney or liver damage.
Not to be used for: sudden, severe symptoms.
Caution needed with:
Contains: MAGNESIUM HYDROXIDE.
Other preparations:

---

magnesium oxide *see* Asilone, Kolanticon

---

magnesium sulphate *see* magnesium sulphate (Epsom Salts), magnesium sulphate paste

---

magnesium sulphate (Epsom salts)

An osmotic laxative used to evacuate the bowels quickly.

Dose: adults 5-10 g in water on an empty stomach.
Availability: NHS, private prescription, over the counter.
Side effects:
Caution: in patients suffering from kidney disease.
Not to be used for:
Caution needed with:
Contains: MAGNESIUM SULPHATE.
Other preparations:

---

magnesium sulphate paste

A paste used to treat boils.

Dose: apply under a dressing.
Availability: NHS, private prescription, over the counter.
Side effects:
Caution: stir before use.
Not to be used for:
Caution needed with:
Contains: MAGNESIUM SULPHATE, GLYCEROL, PHENOL.
Other preparations:

---

magnesium trisilicate *see* Bellocarb, Gastrocote, Gastron, Gaviscon, magnesium trisilicate mixture

M

magnesium trisilicate mixture

A white liquid used as an ANTACID to treat acidity, indigestion.

Dose: 10 ml 3 times a day in water.
Availability: NHS, private prescription, over the counter.
Side effects: diarrhoea.
Caution: in patients suffering from kidney impairment.
Not to be used for: children.
Caution needed with: tablets coated to protect the stomach, some antibiotics, iron.
Contains: MAGNESIUM TRISILICATE.
Other preparations: magnesium trisilicate tablets co., magnesium trisilicate powder.

---

malathion *see* **Derbac-M, Prioderm, Suleo-M**

---

malic acid *see* **Aserbine, Salivix**

Maloprim
(Wellcome)

A white, scored tablet used as a sulphone preparation for the prevention of malaria.

Dose: adults and children over 10 years 1 tablet a week; children 5-10 years half adult dose. Continue for 4 weeks after leaving area.
Availability: NHS and private prescription.
Side effects: blood disorders, sensitive skin.
Caution: in pregnant women, nursing mothers, and in patients suffering from liver or kidney disease.
Not to be used for: children under 5 years.
Caution needed with: TRIMETHOPRIM, METHOTREXATE.
Contains: DAPSONE, PYRIMETHAMINE.
Other preparations:

Manerix
(Roche)

A yellow, oblong, film-coated tablet supplied at strengths of 150 mg, 300 mg, and used as an antidepressant to treat serious depression.

Dose: 300 mg a day after meals at first, up to a maximum of 600 mg a day

M

392

in divided doses.
Availability: NHS, private prescription.
Side effects: sleep disturbance, headache, nausea, dizziness, confusion, agitation or excitement.
Caution: in pregnant women, nursing mothers, and in patients suffering from severe liver damage, overactive thyroid, schizophrenia, or where excitement or agitation are main symptoms. Avoid excessive intake of foods such as cheese, meat extract, yeast extract, broad beans, pickled herrings, banana, vegetable proteins.
Not to be used for: children, or for patients suffering from PHAEOCHROMOCYTOMA, acute confusion.
Caution needed with: some other antidepressants, TRAZODONE, some SYMPATHOMIMETICS, CIMETIDINE, PETHIDINE, CODEINE, MORPHINE, FENTANYL, LITHIUM.
Contains: MOCLOBEMIDE.
Other preparations:

Manevac
(Galen)

Granules used as a stimulant and bulking agent to treat constipation.

Dose: adults 5-10 ml at night and before breakfast if needed; children over 5 years 5 ml daily.
Availability: NHS, private prescription, over the counter.
Side effects: wind, distension, diarrhoea.
Caution:
Not to be used for: children under 5 years, or for patients suffering from obstruction of the intestine, coeliac disease.
Caution needed with:
Contains: ISPAGHULA, SENNOSIDES.
Other preparations:

Manusept
(Hough, Hoseason)

A solution used as a disinfectant for cleansing and disinfecting skin and hands before surgery.

Dose: rub into the skin until dry.
Availability: NHS, private prescription, over the counter.
Side effects:
Caution: keep out of the eyes.
Not to be used for:
Caution needed with:
Contains: TRICLOSAN, ISOPROPYL ALCOHOL.

M

Other preparations: AQUASEPT, STER-ZAC BATH CONCENTRATE.

MAOI (mono-amine oxidase inhibitor)
An antidepressant agent which may interact with some foods and other drugs. Example ISOCARBOXAZID *see* ISOCARBOAXAZID TABLETS.

maprotiline *see* Ludiomil

Marevan *see* warfarin tablets
(Goldshield Healthcare)

Marvelon
(Organon)

A white tablet used as an oestrogen, progestogen contraceptive.

Dose: 1 tablet a day for 21 days starting on day 1 or day 5 of the period.
Availability: NHS and private prescription.
Side effects: enlarged breasts, bloating and fluid retention, cramps, leg pains, mood change, reduction in sexual desire, headaches, nausea, vaginal erosion, discharge, and bleeding, weight gain, skin changes, rarely thrombosis, raised blood pressure, jaundice.
Caution: in patients suffering from high blood pressure, diabetes, vascular disorders, asthma, depression, kidney disease, multiple sclerosis, womb diseases. Your doctor may advise you not to smoke, to have regular examinations. You should stop treatment at the first sign of serious symptoms such as severe headache or jaundice. Treatment should be stopped before surgery.
Not to be used for: pregnant women, or for patients suffering from sickle-cell anaemia, history of heart disease or thrombosis, liver disorders, some cancers, undiagnosed vaginal bleeding, some ear, skin, and kidney disorders.
Caution needed with: RIFAMPICIN, TETRACYCLINE ANTIBIOTICS, GRISEOFULVIN, BARBITURATES, PHENYTOIN, PRIMIDONE, CARBAMAZEPINE, ETHOSUXIMIDE, CHLORAL HYDRATE.
Contains: ETHINYLOESTRADIOL, DESOGESTREL.
Other preparations:

Masnoderm *see* clotrimazole cream
(Cusi)

M

Maxepa
(Novex)

A clear, soft capsule used as a lipid-lowering agent to treat elevated lipids.

Dose: 5 capsules twice a day with food.
Availability: NHS, private prescription, over the counter.
Side effects: nausea, belching.
Caution: in patients suffering from bleeding disorders.
Not to be used for: children.
Caution needed with: ANTICOAGULANTS.
Contains: EICOSAPENTAENOIC ACID, DOCOSAHEXAENOIC ACID.
Other preparations: Maxepa Liquid, Maxepa Emulsion.

Maxidex
(Alcon)

Drops used as a STEROID, lubricant treatment for inflammation of the front of the eye.

Dose: 1-2 drops every hour, reducing as inflammation subsides. (Mild disease 4-6 times a day.)
Availability: NHS and private prescription.
Side effects: cataract, thinning cornea, fungal infection, rise in eye pressure.
Caution: in pregnant women and infants – do not use for extended periods.
Not to be used for: patients suffering from viral, fungal, tubercular, or weeping infections, glaucoma, or for patients who wear soft contact lenses.
Caution needed with:
Contains: DEXAMETHASONE, HYPROMELLOSE.
Other preparations:

Maximet *see* indomethacin capsules
(Opus)

Maxitrol
(Alcon)

Drops used as a STEROID, aminoglycoside antibiotic, lubricant, and protein treatment for infected inflammation of the eye.

Dose: 1-2 drops into the eye 4-6 times a day.

M

Availability: NHS and private prescription.
Side effects: rise in eye pressure, fungal infection, thinning cornea, cataract.
Caution: in pregnant women and infants– do not use for extended periods.
Not to be used for: patients suffering from glaucoma, viral, fungal, tubercular, or weeping infections, or for patients who wear soft contact lenses.
Caution needed with:
Contains: DEXAMETHASONE, NEOMYCIN sulphate, HYPROMELLOSE, POLYMYXIN B SULPHATE.
Other preparations: Maxitrol Ointment.

Maxivent *see* salbutamol inhaler
(Ashbourne)

Maxolon *see* metoclopramide tablets
(Monmouth)

Maxtrex
(Pharmacia)

A yellow tablet or a yellow, scored tablet according to strengths of 2.5 mg, 10 mg, and used to treat severe psoriasis.

Dose: as advised by your doctor.
Availability: NHS and private prescription.
Side effects: stomach pain, liver and bone marrow disorder, rash.
Caution: in the elderly and the young, and in patients suffering from blood or gastro-intestinal disorders, mental illness, liver or kidney damage. Your doctor may advise regular tests.
Not to be used for: pregnant women, nursing mothers, or for patients suffering from severe kidney or liver damage, serious blood disorders.
Caution needed with: alcohol, some vaccines, FOLIC ACID, ETRETINATE, anticonvulsants, NON-STEROIDAL ANTI-INFLAMMATORY DRUGS, some other drugs.
Contains: METHOTREXATE.
Other preparations:

MCR-50 *see* isosorbide mononitrate tablets
(Pharmacia)

M

measles vaccine

Measles vaccine has been largely replaced by a combined measles/mumps/rubella vaccine for all children who are eligible. *See* **M-M-R II.**

---

mebendazole *see* Vermox

---

mebeverine *see* Colofac, Fomac, Fybogel-Mebeverine, mebeverine tablets

---

mebeverine tablets

A tablet supplied at a strength of 135 mg and used as an anti-spasm treatment for bowel spasm.

Dose: adults 1 tablet 3 times a day, children over 10 years only adult dose. Take the dose 20 minutes before a meal.
Availability: NHS and private prescription.
Side effects:
Caution: in patients suffering from intestinal block, PORPHYRIA.
Not to be used for: children under 10 years.
Caution needed with:
Contains: MEBEVERINE hydrochloride.
Other preparations: COLOFAC, FOMAC (liquid forms available), FYBOGEL-MEBEVERINE.

Medicoal
(Torbet)

Effervescent granules supplied in sachets, and used as an adsorbent to treat poisoning and overdosing with drugs.

Dose: 1-2 sachets (each suspended in 100 ml water), repeated every 15-20 minutes. Maximum dose 10 sachets.
Availability: NHS, private prescription, over the counter.
Side effects:
Caution:
Not to be used for: poisoning where there is a known antidote or for poisoning by acids, alkalis, iron salts, cyanides, MALATHION, DDT, some antidiabetics.
Caution needed with: drugs taken by mouth, antidotes given by mouth.
Contains: activated CHARCOAL.

M

Other preparations: CARBOMIX.

Medihaler-EPI
(3M Health Care)

An aerosol used as a SYMPATHOMIMETIC additional treatment for sensitivity to drugs or stings due to previous exposure.

Dose: adults at least 20 sprays; children 10-15 sprays.
Availability: NHS and private prescription.
Side effects: nervousness, shaking hands, palpitations, dry mouth, stomach pain.
Caution: in patients suffering from diabetes.
Not to be used for: patients suffering from heart disease, high blood pressure, overactive thyroid, abnormal heart rhythm.
Caution needed with: MAOIS, TRICYCLIC ANTIDEPRESSANTS, other SYMPATHOMIMETICS.
Contains: ADRENALINE acid tartrate.
Other preparations:

Medihaler-Ergotamine
(3M Health Care)

An aerosol used to treat migraine.

Dose: 1 dose repeated if needed after 5 minutes up to a maximum of 6 doses in 24 hours or 15 doses in a week.
Availability: NHS and private prescription.
Side effects: nausea, muscle pain.
Caution:
Not to be used for: children under 10 years, pregnant women, nursing mothers, or for patients suffering from high blood pressure, kidney or liver disease, sepsis, blood vessel disorders.
Caution needed with: ERYTHROMYCIN, ß-BLOCKERS.
Contains: ERGOTAMINE TARTRATE.
Other preparations: CAFERGOT, LINGRAINE, MIGRIL.

Medihaler-Iso
(3M Health Care)

An aerosol used as a BRONCHODILATOR to treat bronchial asthma, chronic bronchitis.

Dose: 1-3 sprays and again after 30 minutes if needed, to a maximum of

M

24 sprays in 24 hours.
Availability: NHS and private prescriptions.
Side effects: rapid or abnormal heart rate, dry mouth, nervousness.
Caution: in pregnant women, and in patients suffering from diabetes, high blood pressure.
Not to be used for: children, or for patients suffering from heart disease, overactive thyroid.
Caution needed with: MAOIS, SYMPATHOMIMETICS, TRICYCLIC ANTIDEPRESSANTS.
Contains: ISOPRENALINE sulphate.
Other preparations: Medihaler Iso Forte. SAVENTRINE.

Medisense G2
(MediSense)

A sensor strip used in conjunction with either a Medisense Companion 2 or a Medisense Pen 2 meter to detect blood glucose levels. Blood-glucose monitoring enables individual patients suffering from diabetes accurately to control blood glucose and manage their condition.

Medomet *see* methyldopa tablets
(DDSA)

Medrone
(Upjohn)

A pink, quarter-scored, oval tablet, a white, quarter-scored, oval tablet, a white, quarter-scored tablet, or a light-blue scored tablet according to strengths of 2 mg, 4 mg, 16 mg, 100 mg and used as a STEROID treatment for inflammatory conditions, such as rheumatoid arthritis, chest complaints, skin disorders.

Dose: as advised by the physician.
Availability: NHS and private prescription.
Side effects: high blood sugar, thin bones, mood changes, ulcers.
Caution: pregnant women, or for patients who have had recent bowel surgery, or who are suffering from inflamed veins, psychiatric disorders, virus infections, some cancers, some kidney diseases, thinning of the bones, ulcers, tuberculosis, other infections, high blood pressure, glaucoma, epilepsy, diabetes, underactive thyroid, liver disease, stress. Withdraw gradually. Avoid contact with chickenpox or herpes virus.
Not to be used for:
Caution needed with: PHENYTOIN, PHENOBARBITONE, EPHEDRINE, RIFAMPICIN, DIURETICS, ANTICHOLINESTERASES, DIGOXIN, antidiabetic agents, ANTICOAGULANTS, NON-STEROIDAL ANTI-INFLAMMATORY DRUGS.
Contains: METHYLPREDNISOLONE.

M

Other preparations:

---

medroxyprogesterone *see* **Depo-Provera, Premique, Provera, Tridestra**

---

mefenamic acid *see* **mefenamic acid capsules, Ponstan Forte**

---

mefenamic acid capsules

A capsule supplied at a strength of 250 mg and used as a NON-STEROIDAL ANTI-INFLAMMATORY DRUG to relieve pain in rheumatoid arthritis, osteoarthritis and related conditions, and to treat period pain.

Dose: adults 2 capsules 3 times a day after food; children over 6 months 25 mg/kg bodyweight in divided doses for a maximum of 7 days except when treating juvenile arthritis.
Availability: NHS and private prescription.
Side effects: diarrhoea, rash, drowsiness, kidney damage, blood changes, liver changes, fluid retention, headache, tinnitus, vertigo, severe allergy.
Caution: in the elderly, in pregnant women, nursing mothers, and in patients suffering from PORPHYRIA, bronchial asthma, allergy, heart failure, or with a history of stomach ulcers, LUPUS, liver or kidney disease.
Not to be used for: infants under 6 months, patients suffering from kidney or liver disease, stomach ulcers, inflammatory bowel disease, allergy to aspirin or non-steroidal anti-inflammatory drugs.
Caution needed with: ANTICOAGULANTS, some antidiabetics, drugs that lower blood pressure, other non-steroidal anti-inflammatory drugs, some antibiotics, DIGOXIN, STEROIDS, CYCLOSPORIN, METHOTREXATE, DIURETICS, LITHIUM.
Contains: MEFENAMIC ACID.
Other preparations: mefenemic acid tablets. CONTRAFLAM, DYSMAN, MEFASAID, MEFLAM, PONSTAN (tablet forms are usually double strength. Some syrup forms available).

Meflam *see* **mefenamic acid capsules**
(Trinity)

---

mefloquine *see* **Lariam**

---

mefruside *see* **Baycaron**

M

Melleril
(Sandoz)

A white tablet supplied at strengths of 10 mg, 25 mg, 50 mg, 100 mg and used as a sedative to treat schizophrenia, manic mental disorders, senile confusion, behavioural disorders, epilepsy in children.

Dose: adults 30-100 mg a day at first increasing to 600 mg a day if needed; children under 5 years 1 mg per kg body weight a day, 5-12 years 75-150 mg a day, to a maximum of 300 mg a day.
Availability: NHS and private prescription.
Side effects: muscle spasms, restlessness, blurred vision, hands shaking, constipation, dry mouth, stuffy nose, urine retention, palpitations, low blood pressure, weight gain, changes in sexual function, low body temperature, breast swelling, menstrual changes, jaundice, blood and skin changes, drowsiness, tiredness, rarely fits.
Caution: in patients suffering from liver disease, kidney disease, cardiovascular disease, epilepsy, glaucoma, MYASTHENIA GRAVIS, enlarged prostate, severe lung disease, parkinsonism, adrenal tumour.
Not to be used for: children under 1 year, pregnant women, nursing mothers, severely depressed or unconscious patients or for patients suffering from blood disorders, severe heart disease.
Caution needed with: alcohol, sedatives, tranquillizers, pain killers, blood-pressure lowering drugs, antidepressants, anticonvulsants, antidiabetic drugs, LEVODOPA.
Contains: THIORIDAZINE hydrochloride.
Other preparations: Melleril Suspension, Melleril Syrup.

Mengivac (A + C)
(Pasteur Merieux MSD)

A vaccination used to provide active immunization against meningitis A and meningitis C.

Dose: adults and children over 18 months old, 1 injection of 0.5 ml.
Availability: NHS, private prescription.
Side effects: mild fever, discomfort at the site of the injection.
Caution: in pregnant women and nursing mothers.
Not to be used for: patients suffering from acute infections or feverish illness.
Caution needed with: drugs that suppress the body's immune system.
Contains: meningococcal polysaccharide vaccine.
Other preparations: AC VAX.

M

Menophase
(Roche)

Five pink tablets, 8 orange tablets, 2 yellow tablets, 3 green tablets, 6 blue tablets, and 4 lavender tablets used as an oestrogen, progestogen treatment for symptoms associated with the menopause, and prevention of thinning of the bones after menopause.

Dose: 1 tablet a day.
Availability: NHS and private prescription.
Side effects: enlarged breasts, fluid retention, nausea, vaginal bleeding, weight gain, headache, dizziness. Rarely jaundice, raised blood pressure, thrombosis.
Caution: in patients suffering from high blood pressure, diabetes, epilepsy, womb diseases, gall bladder disorder, migraine, multiple sclerosis, PORPHYRIA, liver disorders, some ear disorders, or a history or increased risk of breast disorders (including cancer) and thrombosis. Your doctor may advise you to have regular examinations.
Not to be used for: children, pregnant women, nursing mothers, or for patients suffering from thombosis, severe liver, kidney, or heart disorders, some cancers, undiagnosed vaginal bleeding, endometriosis.
Caution needed with: ACE INHIBITORS, ANTICOAGULANTS, BARBITURATES, ß-BLOCKERS, CARBAMAZEPINE, PHENYTOIN, RIFAMPICIN.
Contains: MESTRANOL, NORETHISTERONE,
Other preparations:

Menorest see Estraderm
(Rhône-Poulenc Rorer)

---

menotrophin see Pergonal

---

menthol see Balmosa, Rowachol, Salonair

---

menthone see Rowachol

Menzol see norethisterone tablets
(Schwarz)

---

mepacrine hydrochloride see mepacrine tablets

M

mepacrine tablets

Tablets supplied at a strength of 100 mg and used to treat giardiasis (an intestinal infection).

Dose: adults, 1 tablet every 8 hours; children, 2 mg/kg body weight every 8 hours.
Availability: NHS and private prescription.
Side effects: stomach upset, dizziness, headache, nausea, vomiting, mental disorder, excitation, yellow discoloration of skin and urine, skin disorders, liver disorders, blood changes, changes in vision, discoloured palate and nails.
Caution: in the elderly, and in patients suffering from liver disorder or a history of mental disorder.
Not to be used for: patients suffering from psoriasis.
Caution needed with: primaquin.
Contains: MEPACRINE HYDROCHLORIDE.
Other preparations:

Meprate *see* Equanil
(DDSA)

---

meprobamate *see* Equagesic, Equanil, Meprate

---

meptazinol *see* Meptid

Meptid
(Monmouth)

An orange, oval tablet tablet supplied at a strength of 200 mg and used as an opiate ANALGESIC to relieve pain.

Dose: 1 tablet every 3-6 hours as needed.
Availability: NHS and private prescription.
Side effects: dizziness, nausea.
Caution: in patients with liver or kidney disease or respiratory depression.
Not to be used for: children.
Caution needed with:
Contains: MEPTAZINOL.
Other preparations: Meptid Injection.

M

mepyramine *see* **Anthisan**

---

mequitazine *see* **Primalan**

Merbentyl
(Marion Merrell Dow)

A white tablet supplied at strengths of 10 mg, 20 mg and used as an antispasm, ANTICHOLINERGIC treatment for bowel and stomach spasm.

Dose: children 6 months-2 years 5-10 mg 3-4 times a day before feeds, over 2 years 10 mg 3 times a day, adults 10-20 mg 3 times a day between meals.
Availability: NHS and private prescription.
Side effects: dry mouth, thirst, dizziness, tiredness, drowsiness, blurred vision, headache, nausea, anorexia, rash, constipation, pain and difficulty urinating.
Caution: in patients suffering from glaucoma, enlarged prostate, hiatus hernia with reflux oesophagitis.
Not to be used for: infants under 6 months.
Caution needed with:
Contains: DICYCLOMINE.
Other preparations: Merbentyl syrup.

Mercilon
(Organon)

A white tablet used as an oestrogen, progestogen contraceptive.

Dose: 1 tablet a day for 21 days starting on day 1 or day 5 of the period.
Availability: NHS and private prescription.
Side effects: enlarged breasts, bloating and fluid retention, cramps, leg pains, mood change, reduction in sexual desire, headaches, nausea, vaginal erosion, discharge, and bleeding, weight gain, skin changes, rarely thrombosis, raised blood pressure, jaundice.
Caution: in patients suffering from high blood pressure, diabetes, vascular disorders, asthma, depression, kidney disease, multiple sclerosis, womb diseases. Your doctor may advise you not to smoke, to have regular examinations. You should stop treatment at the first sign of serious symptoms such as severe headache or jaundice. Treatment should be stopped before surgery.
Not to be used for: pregnant women, or for patients suffering from sickle-cell anaemia, history of heart disease or thrombosis, liver disorders, some cancers, undiagnosed vaginal bleeding, some ear, skin, and kidney disorders.

M

Caution needed with: RIFAMPICIN, TETRACYCLINE ANTIBIOTICS, GRISEOFULVIN, BARBITURATES, PHENYTOIN, PRIMIDONE, CARBAMAZEPINE, ETHOSUXIMIDE, CHLORAL HYDRATE.
Contains: ETHINYLOESTRADIOL, DESOGESTREL.
Other preparations:

Merocaine
(Marion Merrell Dow)

A green lozenge used as an antiseptic and local anaesthetic to treat painful infections of the throat and mouth, and as an additional treatment for tonsillitis, pharyngitis, and in dental procedures.

Dose: 1 lozenge allowed to dissolve in the mouth every 2 hours up to a maximum of 8 lozenges in 24 hours.
Availability: NHS, private prescription, over the counter.
Side effects:
Caution:
Not to be used for: children.
Caution needed with:
Contains: CETYLPYRIDINIUM chloride, BENZOCAINE.
Other preparations:

Merocet
(Marion Merrell Dow)

A solution used as an antiseptic to treat infections of the throat and mouth.

Dose: rinse the mouth or gargle with the solution diluted or undiluted every 3 hours or as needed.
Availability: NHS, private prescription, over the counter.
Side effects:
Caution:
Not to be used for: children under 6 years.
Caution needed with:
Contains: CETYLPYRIDINIUM chloride.
Other preparations: Merocets Lozenge

---

mesalazine *see* Asacol, Pentasa, Salofalk

---

mesterolone *see* Pro-Viron

M

Mestinon
(Roche)

A white quarter-scored tablet supplied at a strength of 60 mg and used as a nerve conduction enhancer to treat paralytic ileus, MYASTHENIA GRAVIS (muscular disorders).

Dose: paralytic ileus adults 1-4 tablets as required; children ¼ -1 tablet as required. For myasthenia gravis adults 5-20 tablets a day in divided doses; infants 5-10 mg every 4 hours, under 6 years ½ tablet initially, 6-12 years 1 tablet intitially.
Availability: NHS and private prescription.
Side effects: nausea, salivation, diarrhoea, colic.
Caution: in patients suffering from bronchial asthma, heart disease, low blood pressure, slow heart rate, recent heart attack, epilepsy, Parkinson's disease, kidney disease, stomach ulcer, vagotonia.
Not to be used for: patients with bowel or urinary obstruction.
Caution needed with: some drugs used in anaesthesia.
Contains: PYRIDOSTIGMINE bromide.
Other preparations:

---

mestranol *see* Menophase, Norinyl-1, Ortho-Novin 1/50

Metalpha *see* methyldopa tablets
(Ashbourne)

Meted
(Euroderma)

A liquid used as an antiseptic skin softener to treat psoriasis of the scalp, dandruff, seborrhoeic dermatitis.

Dose: use the liquid as a shampoo at least twice a week.
Availability: NHS, private prescription, over the counter.
Side effects: irritation.
Caution:
Not to be used for:
Caution needed with:
Contains: COLLOIDAL SULPHUR, SALICYLIC ACID.
Other preparations:

M

406

Metenix
(Hoechst Roussel)

A blue tablet supplied at a strength of 5 mg and used as a DIURETIC to treat high blood pressure, fluid retention, swollen abdomen, or toxaemia of pregnancy.

Dose: high blood pressure 5 mg a day at first, then reduce to 5 mg every other day after 3-4 weeks; fluid retention 5-10 mg as a single dose; no more than 80 mg in 24 hours.
Availability: NHS and private prescription.
Side effects: low potassium levels, headache, stomach upset, cramps, rash, sensitivity to light, blood changes, anorexia, dizziness, pancreatitis, changes in sexual function.
Caution: in pregnant women, nursing mothers, the elderly, and in patients suffering from kidney or liver disease, gout, or diabetes, SLE. Potassium supplements may be needed. Your doctor may advise regular blood tests.
Not to be used for: children, or for patients suffering from severe liver or kidney failure, raised calcium levels, Addison's disease, allergy to some antibiotics.
Caution needed with: DIGOXIN, LITHIUM, blood-pressure lowering drugs, STEROIDS, NON-STEROIDAL ANTI-INFLAMMATORY DRUGS, antidiabetics, BARBITURATES, opioid ANALGESICS, alcohol, CARBENOXOLONE.
Contains: METOLAZONE.
Other preparations: XURET.

Meterfolic
(Sinclair)

A grey tablet used as an iron and FOLIC ACID supplement in the prevention of iron and folic acid deficiencies in pregnancy, and to prevent defects in the foetus.

Dose: for deficiency, 1 tablet 1-2 times a day; for prevention of defects, 1 tablet a day, continued until the twelfth week of pregnancy.
Availability: NHS and private prescription.
Side effects: nausea, constipation.
Caution: in patients suffering from haemolytic anaemia, or with a history of stomach ulcer.
Not to be used for: children or for patients suffering from VITAMIN B_{12} deficiency.
Caution needed with: TETRACYCLINE ANTIBIOTICS, PHENYTOIN, some antibiotics, ANTACIDS, LEVODOPA.
Contains: FERROUS FUMARATE, FOLIC ACID.
Other preparations: FOLEX-350, GALFER FA.

M

metformin *see* **Glucamet, Glucophage, metformin tablets, Orabet**

---

metformin tablets

A coated tablet supplied at strengths of 500 mg, 850 mg and used as an antidiabetic to treat diabetes.

Dose: 500 mg every 8 hours or 850 mg twice a day with meals at first increasing gradually if needed to a maximum of 3 g a day.
Availability: NHS and private prescription.
Side effects: allergy including skin rash, loss of appetite, stomach upset, rarely acidosis (a metabolic disorder), decreased vitamin B_{12} absorption.
Caution: in the elderly.
Not to be used for: children, pregnant women, nursing mothers, or for patients suffering from juvenile diabetes, liver or kidney impairment, heart failure, hormone disorders, stress, infections, dehydration, alcoholism.
Caution needed with: ß-BLOCKERS, MAOIS, STEROIDS, DIURETICS, alcohol, CIMETIDINE, lipid-lowering agents, some antibiotics, NON-STEROIDAL ANTI-INFLAMMATORY DRUGS, GLUCAGON, KETOTIFEN, some drugs that lower blood pressure, the contraceptive pill, some antifungals.
Contains: METFORMIN hydrochloride.
Other preparations: GLUCAMET, GLUCOPHAGE, ORABET.

---

methadone *see* **methadone tablets, Physeptone**

---

methadone tablets

A tablet supplied at a strength of 5 mg and used as an opiate to control severe pain.

Dose: 1-2 tablets every 6-8 hours, adjusted according to response.
Availability: controlled drug; NHS and private prescription.
Side effects: dependence, addiction, euphoria, dizziness, sedation, nausea, vomiting, drowsiness, constipation, breathing difficulties, low blood pressure, difficulty passing urine, heart disorders, dry mouth, sweating, flushing, mood changes, itching, rash.
Caution: in the elderly, pregnant women, nursing mothers, and in patients suffering from liver or kidney disease, underactive thyroid, asthma, low blood pressure, or drug dependence.
Not to be used for: children, or for patients with head injury, breathing difficulty, or blocked airways.
Caution needed with: MAOIS, sedatives, alcohol, RIFAMPICIN, SELEGILINE.
Contains: METHADONE hydrochloride.

M

Other preparations: methadone linctus (used to treat severe cough), mixture (used to treat opiate addiction), injection. METHODEX mixture, PHYSEPTONE.

---

methenamine hippurate *see* **Hiprex**

---

methionine *see* **Lipoflavonoid, Lipotriad, Pameton**

---

methocarbamol *see* **Robaxin, Robaxisal Forte**

Methodex Mixture *see* **methadone**
(Link)

---

methotrexate *see* **Maxtrex**

---

methotrimeprazine *see* **Nozinan**

---

methyl nicotinate *see* **Cremalgin, Dubam**

---

methyl salicylate *see* **Balmosa, Dubam, Monphytol, Phytex, Salonair**

---

methyl undecanoate *see* **Monphytol**

---

methylcellulose *see* **Celevac**

---

methylcysteine hydrochloride *see* **Visclair**

---

methyldopa *see* **Aldomet, Hydromet, Medomet, Metalpha, methyldopa tablets**

M

methyldopa tablets

A coated tablet supplied at strengths of 125 mg, 250 mg, and 500 mg, and used in conjunction with a DIURETIC as an ANTIHYPERTENSIVE preparation to treat raised blood pressure.

Dose: 250 mg 2-3 times a day increasing slowly to a maximum of 3 g a day if required; elderly patients 125 mg at first increasing to a maximum of 2 g a day.
Availability: NHS and private prescription.
Side effects: drowsiness, dry mouth, sedation, depression, tiredness, stomach upset, blocked nose, anaemia, parkinsonism, rash, diarrhoea, fluid retention, liver damage, LUPUS, failure to ejaculate.
Caution: in patients suffering from anaemia, kidney disorder, a history of liver disorder, and while using anaesthetics.
Not to be used for: patients suffering from PHAEOCHROMOCYTOMA, liver disease, PORPHYRIA, or with a history of depression.
Caution needed with: alcohol, sedatives, LITHIUM, MAOIS, SYMPATHOMIMETICS anaesthetics, NON-STEROIDAL ANTI-INFLAMMATORY DRUGS, STEROIDS, LEVODOPA, the contraceptive pill, oestrogens, antidepressants.
Contains: METHYLDOPA.
Other preparations: ALDOMET, DOPAMET, HYDROMET, METALPHA, MEDOMET.

---

methylphenidate *see* Ritalin

---

methylphenobarbitone *see* Prominal

---

methylprednisolone *see* Depo-Medrone, Medrone, Neo-Medrone Cream

---

methysergide *see* Deseril

---

metipranolol *see* Metipranolol Minims

Metipranolol Minims
(Chauvin)

Drops used as a ß-BLOCKER to treat high eye pressure, glaucoma in some patients.

Dose: 1 drop into the eye twice a day, or as advised.

M

Availability: NHS and private prescription.
Side effects: slight smarting, temporary headache.
Caution: in pregnant women, and in patients suffering from heart block or slow heart rate.
Not to be used for: patients suffering from heart failure, blocked airways disease, or abnormal heart rhythm.
Caution needed with: VERAPAMIL, other ß-blockers.
Contains: METIPRANOLOL.
Other preparations:

---

metoclopramide *see* **Gastrobid, Gastroflux, Gastromax, Maxolon, metoclopramide tablets, Migravess, Mygdalon, Paramax, Primperan**

---

metoclopramide tablets

A tablet supplied at a strength of 10 mg and used as an anti-sickness, antispasm drug to treat nausea, vomiting, indigestion, and migraine.

Dose: adults over 20 years 10 mg 3 times a day (for migraine, one single dose at onset of symptoms); children and young adults use only for special circumstances such as in sickness caused by cancer treatment (reduced doses).
Availability: NHS and private prescription.
Side effects: occasionally parkinsonian-type symptoms, shaking hands, drowsiness, diarrhoea, restlessness, depression.
Caution: in children, young adults, pregnant women, nursing mothers, and in patients suffering from liver and kidney problems, PHAEOCHROMOCYTOMA, PORPHYRIA.
Not to be used for: where recent gastric or bowel surgery has occurred.
Caution needed with: ANTICHOLINERGICS, some sedatives, ANALGESICS, LEVODOPA, LITHIUM.
Contains: METOCLOPRAMIDE hydrochloride.
Other preparations: metoclopramide oral solution, injection. GASTROBID CONTINUS, GASTROFLUX, GASTROMAX, MAXOLON, MYGDALON, PRIMPERAN.

---

metolazone *see* **Metenix**

Metopirone
(Ciba)

A cream capsule supplied at a strength of 250 mg and used as a hormone blocker to treat Cushing's syndrome, and with glucocorticoids to treat

M

resistant oedema caused by increased aldosterone secretion (adrenal gland disorder).

Dose: adults, Cushing's syndrome 1-24 capsules a day; oedema 12 capsules a day. (Children, reduced doses.)
Availability: NHS and private prescription.
Side effects: nausea, vomiting, low blood pressure, allergies.
Caution: in patients suffering from underactive pituitary gland.
Not to be used for: pregnant women, nursing mothers, or for patients with some hormone deficiencies.
Caution needed with:
Contains: METYRAPONE.
Other preparations:

---

metoprolol *see* Arbralene, Betaloc, Co-Betaloc, Lopresor, metoprolol tablets

---

metoprolol tablets

A tablet supplied at strengths of 50 mg, 100 mg and used as a ß-BLOCKER to treat angina, high blood pressure, and heart rhythm defects. Also used to prevent migraine and as an additional treatment for overactive thyroid

Dose: for angina and heart rhythm defects 50-100 mg 2-3 times a day. High blood pressure 50 mg twice a day at first increasing to 200 mg a day if needed in 1 or 2 doses. Overactive thyroid 50 mg 4 times a day. Migraine 100-200 mg a day.
Availability: NHS and private prescription.
Side effects: cold hands and feet, sleep disturbances, slow heart rate, tiredness, wheezing, heart failure, stomach upset, dry eyes, rash.
Caution: in pregnant women, nursing mothers, and in patients suffering from diabetes, kidney or liver disorders, myasthenia gravis, severe allergic shock. May need to be withdrawn before surgery. Withdraw gradually. Your doctor may advise additional treatment with DIGOXIN and DIURETICS.
Not to be used for: children or for patients suffering from heart block or failure, asthma, blocked airways disease.
Caution needed with: VERAPAMIL, antidiabetics, CLONIDINE, some anti-arrhythmic drugs and anaesthetics, some blood-pressure lowering drugs, ERGOTAMINE, DILTIAZEM, sedatives, SYMPATHOMIMETICS, alcohol, NON-STEROIDAL ANTI-INFLAMMATORY DRUGS, DIGOXIN, STEROIDS.
Contains: METOPROLOL tartrate.
Other preparations: ARBRALENE, BETALOC, LOPRESOR, MEPRANIX.

M

Metosyn
(Stuart)

A cream used as a strong STEROID treatment for allergic and other skin conditions where there is also inflammation.

Dose: massage into the affected area 3-4 times a day at first and then reduce to once or twice a day as soon as possible.
Availability: NHS and private prescription.
Side effects: fluid retention, suppression of adrenal glands, thinning, spotting, or streaking of the skin may occur.
Caution: use for short periods of time only, especially in children or on the face.
Not to be used for: patients suffering from acne or any other skin infections caused by tuberculosis, ringworm, viruses, or fungi, leg ulcers, scabies, or continuously especially in pregnant women.
Caution needed with:
Contains: FLUOCINONIDE.
Other preparations: Metosyn Ointment, Metosyn Scalp Lotion.

Metrodin High Purity
(Serono)

An injection used as an infertility treatment for irregular or absent periods caused by disorder of the hypothalamic pituitary; and to induce ovulation in in-vitro fertilization.

Dose: as advised by the physician.
Availability: NHS, private prescription.
Side effects: overstimulation of the ovaries, multiple pregnancies, allergy.
Caution: hormonal disorders should be treated before therapy.
Not to be used for: children or pregnant women.
Caution needed with:
Contains: UROFOLLITROPHIN.
Other preparations: orgafol.

Metrogel
(Sandoz)

An antibiotic gel used to treat rosacea (a skin disorder of the face).

Dose: apply twice a day for 8-9 weeks.
Availability: NHS and private prescription.
Side effects: irritation.
Caution:

M

Not to be used for: children or for pregnant women
Caution needed with:
Contains: METRONIDAZOLE.
Other preparations:

Metrolyl *see* metronidazole tablets
(Lagap)

---

metronidazole *see* Elyzol, Flagyl, Metrogel, Metrolyl, metronidazole tablets, Rozex, Vaginyl, Zadstat

---

metronidazole tablets

An tablet supplied at strengths of 200 mg, 400 mg and used as an antibiotic treatment for various infections, including some vaginal infections, leg ulcers, ulcerative gingivitis (gum disease), and dental infections.

Dose: adults usually 200-400 mg every 8 hours (some infections require higher doses in short courses); children reduced doses according to age and condition (syrup available).
Availability: NHS and private prescription.
Side effects: stomach upset, furred tongue, unpleasant taste, allergy, rash, swelling, brain disturbances, dark-coloured urine, nerve changes, fits, blood changes, dizziness, drowsiness, headache.
Caution: in patients with brain disorder caused by liver disease. Short-term high-dose treatment should not be used for pregnant women or nursing mothers. Alcohol causes extreme reaction with this preparation, and should not be taken during the treatment or for 48 hours afterwards.
Not to be used for:
Caution needed with: alcohol, PHENOBARBITONE, ANTICOAGULANTS taken by mouth, LITHIUM PHENYTOIN, CIMETIDINE.
Contains: METRONIDAZOLE.
Other preparations: metronidazole suppositories, suspension. FLAGYL, VAGINYL, ZADSTAT. Also ELYZOL (dental product), METROLYL (suppository form).

---

metyrapone *see* Metopirone

---

mexiletine *see* Mexitil

M

Mexitil
(Boehringer Ingelheim)

A red/purple capsule or a red capsule according to strengths of 50 mg, 200 mg and used as an anti-arrhythmic treatment for abnormal heart rhythm.

Dose: 400-600 mg at first, then 2 hours later and thereafter 200-250 mg 3-4 times a day.
Availability: NHS and private prescription.
Side effects: stomach and brain disorders, low blood pressure.
Caution: in patients suffering from nerve conduction defects in the heart, low blood pressure, slow heart rate, heart, liver, or kidney failure, Parkinson's disease.
Not to be used for: children.
Caution needed with:
Contains: MEXILETINE hydrochloride.
Other preparations: Mexitil Perlongets, Mexitil Injection.

MFV-ject *see* influenza vaccine
(Pasteur Merieux MSD)

---

mianserin *see* Bolvidon, mianserin tablets, Norval

---

mianserin tablets

A tablet supplied at a strength of 10 mg, 20 mg, and 30 mg and used as an antidepressant to treat depression.

Dose: adults 30-40 mg a day at first, increasing gradually if needed to 90 mg a day; elderly up to 30 mg a day at first.
Availability: NHS and private prescription.
Side effects: drowsiness, dry mouth, blurred vision, constipation, nausea, difficulty passing urine, heart and circulation disorders, shaking hands, rash, confusion, interference with sexual function, weight change, blood changes, joint disorders, bone marrow depression, jaundice, convulsions, excitement.
Caution: in pregnant women, nursing mothers, the elderly, and in patients suffering from epilepsy, liver disease, heart disease, enlarged prostate, thyroid disease, glaucoma, PORPHYRIA. Your doctor may advise regular blood tests.
Not to be used for: children, or for patients suffering from mania, severe liver disease, heart rhythm disturbance or recent heart attack.
Caution needed with: MAOIS, alcohol, sedatives, ANTICOAGULANTS, other

M

antidepressants, anticonvulsants.
Contains: mianserin hydrochloride.
Other preparations: BOLVIDON, NORVAL.

Micolette
(Cusi)

A micro-enema used as a faecal softener and lubricant to treat constipation, and for the evacuation of bowels before surgery.

Dose: adults and children over 3 years 1-2 enemas.
Availability: NHS, private prescription, over the counter.
Side effects:
Caution:
Not to be used for: children under 3 years or patients suffering from inflammatory or ulcerative bowel disease, or acute stomach conditions.
Caution needed with:
Contains: SODIUM LAURYL SULPHOACETATE, SODIUM CITRATE, GLYCEROL.
Other preparations: RELAXIT.

miconazole *see* Daktacort, Daktarin Cream, Daktarin Oral Gel, Dumicoat, Gyno-Daktarin 1, miconazole cream

miconazole cream

A cream used as an antifungal treatment for fungal infections of the skin and nails.

Dose: apply twice a day until 10 days after the wounds have healed. (For nail infections apply daily under an occlusive dressing.)
Availability: NHS, private prescription, over the counter.
Side effects: occasional irritation, allergy.
Caution:
Not to be used for:
Caution needed with:
Contains: MICONAZOLE nitrate.
Other preparations: DAKTARIN (also available in powder form).

Micralax
(Evans)

A disposable enema used as a faecal softener and lubricant to treat constipation, and for evacuation of bowels

M

Dose: adults and children over 3 years 1 enema.
Availability: NHS, private prescription, over the counter.
Side effects:
Caution:
Not to be used for: children under 3 years, or for patients suffering from inflammatory bowel disease.
Caution needed with:
Contains: SODIUM CITRATE, SODIUM ALKYLSULPHOACETATE, SORBIC ACID.
Other preparations:

Microgynon 30
(Schering Healthcare)

A beige tablet used as an oestrogen, progestogen contraceptive.

Dose: 1 tablet a day for 21 days starting on day 5 of the period.
Availability: NHS and private prescription.
Side effects: enlarged breasts, bloating and fluid retention, cramps, leg pains, mood change, reduction in sexual desire, headaches, nausea, vaginal erosion, discharge, and bleeding, weight gain, skin changes, rarely thrombosis, raised blood pressure, jaundice.
Caution: in patients suffering from high blood pressure, diabetes, vascular disorders, asthma, depression, kidney disease, multiple sclerosis, womb diseases. Your doctor may advise you not to smoke, to have regular examinations. You should stop treatment at the first sign of serious symptoms such as severe headache or jaundice. Treatment should be stopped before surgery.
Not to be used for: pregnant women, or for patients suffering from sickle-cell anaemia, history of heart disease or thrombosis, liver disorders, some cancers, undiagnosed vaginal bleeding, some ear, skin, and kidney disorders.
Caution needed with: RIFAMPICIN, TETRACYCLINE ANTIBIOTICS, GRISEOFULVIN, BARBITURATES, PHENYTOIN, PRIMIDONE, CARBAMAZEPINE, ETHOSUXIMIDE, CHLORAL HYDRATE.
Contains: ETHINYLOESTRADIOL, LEVONORGESTREL.
Other preparations: OVRANETTE.

Micronor
(Janssen-Cilag)

A white tablet used as a progesterone contraceptive.

Dose: 1 tablet at the same time every day starting on day 1 of the period.
Availability: NHS and private prescription.
Side effects: irregular bleeding, breast discomfort, acne, headache, rarely

M

thrombosis, raised blood pressure, jaundice.
Caution: in patients suffering from high blood pressure, tendency to thrombosis, migraine, some cancers, liver abnormalities, ovarian cysts. Your doctor may advise regular check-ups.
Not to be used for: pregnant women, or for patients suffering from severe heart or artery disease, benign liver tumours, vaginal bleeding, previous ectopic pregnancy.
Caution needed with: BARBITURATES, PHENYTOIN, PRIMIDONE, CARBAMAZEPINE, CHLORAL HYDRATE, ETHOSUXIMIDE, RIFAMPICIN, CHLORPROMAZINE, MEPROBAMATE, GRISEOFULVIN.
Contains: NORETHISTERONE.
Other preparations: NORIDAY.

Micronor-HRT
(Janssen-Cilag)

A tablet used as a progestogen for hormone replacement therapy, in addition to an oestrogen.

Dose: 1 tablet a day on days 15-26 of cycle.
Availability: NHS and private prescription.
Side effects: nausea, breast pain, headache.
Caution: in patients suffering from epilepsy, diabetes, high blood pressure, liver disorder, breast disorder, fibroids, gallstones, multiple sclerosis, LUPUS, PORPHYRIA, asthma, some skin cancers.
Not to be used for: children, pregnant women, or for patients suffering from some cancers, liver disease.
Caution needed with: BARBITURATES, CARBAMAZEPINE, MEPROBAMATE, antibiotics, CHARCOAL.
Contains: NORETHISTERONE.
Other preparations:

Microval
(Wyeth)

A white tablet used as a progesterone contraceptive.

Dose: 1 tablet at the same time every day starting on day 1 of the period.
Availability: NHS and private prescription.
Side effects: irregular bleeding, breast discomfort, acne, headache, rarely thrombosis, raised blood pressure, jaundice.
Caution: in patients suffering from high blood pressure, tendency to thrombosis, migraine, some cancers, liver abnormalities, ovarian cysts. Your doctor may advise regular check-ups.
Not to be used for: pregnant women, or for patients suffering from severe

M

heart or artery disease, benign liver tumours, vaginal bleeding, previous
ectopic pregnancy.
Caution needed with: BARBITURATES, PHENYTOIN, PRIMIDONE, CARBAMAZEPINE,
CHLORAL HYDRATE, ETHOSUXIMIDE, RIFAMPICIN, CHLORPROMAZINE, MEPROBAMATE,
GRISEOFULVIN.
Contains: LEVONORGESTREL.
Other preparations: NORGESTON.

Mictral
(Sanofi Winthrop)

Granules in a sachet used as an antiseptic to treat cystitis and some
infections of the urinary tract.

Dose: the contents of 1 sachet dissolved in water 3 times a day for 3 days.
Availability: NHS and private prescription.
Side effects: stomach problems, disturbed vision, brain disturbances,
rash, fits, anaemia, blood changes, sensitivity to light.
Caution: in pregnant women, nursing mothers, and in patients suffering
from liver disease. Keep out of sunlight.
Not to be used for: children or patients suffering from kidney disease,
with a history of convulsions, or PORPHYRIA.
Caution needed with: ANTICOAGULANTS, antibacterials, melphalan,
PROBENECID.
Contains: NALIDIXIC ACID, SODIUM CITRATE, CITRIC ACID, SODIUM BICARBONATE.
Other preparations: NEGRAM, URIBEN.

Midamor *see* amiloride tablets
(Morson)

Midrid
(Shire)

A red capsule used as an ANALGESIC to treat migraine.

Dose: 2 capsules at the beginning of the migraine attack, then 1 capsule
every hour to a maximum of 5 capsules in 12 hours.
Availability: NHS, private prescription, over the counter.
Side effects: dizziness.
Caution: in pregnant women and nursing mothers.
Not to be used for: children, or for patients suffering from severe kidney,
liver, or heart disease, gastritis, severe high blood pressure, or glaucoma.
Caution needed with: MAOIS, other medicines containing PARACETAMOL.
Contains: ISOMETHEPTENE MUCATE, paracetamol.

M

Other preparations:

Migraleve
(Charwell Healthcare)

A pink tablet and a yellow tablet according to strength and contents and used as an ANALGESIC, ANTIHISTAMINE treatment for migraine.

Dose: adults 2 pink tablets at the beginning of the attack, and then 2 yellow tablets every 4 hours if needed to a maximum of 2 pink tablets and 6 yellow tablets in 24 hours; children 10-14 years half adult dose.
Availability: NHS, private prescription, over the counter.
Side effects: drowsiness.
Caution: in patients suffering from kidney or liver disease.
Not to be used for: children under 10 years.
Caution needed with: alcohol, sedatives, other medicines containing PARACETAMOL.
Contains: pink: BUCLIZINE HYDROCHLORIDE, paracetamol, CODEINE PHOSPHATE; yellow: paracetamol, codeine phosphate.
Other preparations:

Migravess
(Bayer)

A white, effervescent tablet used as an anti-emetic and ANALGESIC to treat migraine.

Dose: adults 2 tablets dissolved in water at the beginning of the attack, then up to a maximum of 6 tablets in 24 hours; children 12-15 years half adult dose.
Availability: NHS and private prescription.
Side effects: extrapyramidal reactions (shaking and rigidity), drowsiness, diarrhoea.
Caution: in pregnant women or in patients suffering from kidney or liver disease, asthma.
Not to be used for: children under 12 years or for patients suffering from stomach ulcer, haemophilia or other bleeding disorders, or allergy to ASPIRIN or anti-inflammatory drugs.
Caution needed with: ANTICHOLINERGICS, alcohol, some sedatives, ANTICOAGULANTS, antidiabetics and uric acid-lowering agents, METHOTREXATE, DIURETICS, STEROIDS, NON-STEROIDAL ANTI-INFLAMMATORY DRUGS.
Contains: METOCLOPRAMIDE hydrochloride, ASPIRIN.
Other preparations: Migravess Forte.

Migril
(Wellcome)

A white, scored tablet used as an ergot preparation to treat migraine.

Dose: 1 tablet at the beginning of an attack, then ½-1 tablet every ½ hour if needed to a maximum of 4 tablets for any 1 attack. Do not repeat within 4 days. Maximum of 6 tablets a week.
Availability: NHS and private prescription.
Side effects: rebound headache, poor circulation, abdominal pain, drowsiness, dry mouth.
Caution: in patients suffering from sepsis, anaemia, overactive thyroid.
Not to be used for: children, pregnant women, nursing mothers, or for patients suffering from coronary, peripheral, or occlusive vascular disease, severe high blood pressure, kidney or liver disease.
Caution needed with: ERYTHROMYCIN, ß-BLOCKERS, alcohol, sedatives.
Contains: ERGOTAMINE TARTRATE, CYCLIZINE hydrochloride, CAFFEINE hydrate.
Other preparations: CAFERGOT, LINGRAINE, MEDIHALER ERGOTAMINE.

Mildison Lipocream
(Yamanouchi)

An oily cream used as a STEROID treatment for eczema and other skin disorders.

Dose: apply a small quantity to the affected area 2-3 times a day.
Availability: NHS and private prescription.
Side effects: fluid retention, suppression of adrenal glands, thinning, spotting, or streaking of the skin may occur.
Caution: do not use for children or for facial conditions for longer than 5 days.
Not to be used for: with covering dressings or for patients suffering from bacterial, fungal, or viral infections, leg ulcers, scabies, or for extended treatments in pregnant women.
Caution needed with:
Contains: HYDROCORTISONE.
Other preparations: DIODERM, EFCORTELAN, HYDROCAL, HYDROCORTISONE CREAM, HYDROCORTISTAB, HYDROCORTISYL, LOCOID. Some other brands available over the counter for certain conditions only.

mineral oil *see* Alpha Keri

M

Min-i-jet adrenaline
(IMS)

A ready-to-use injection of a SYMPATHOMIMETIC drug, used for emergency treatment of severe allergy. (Also used by trained medical personnel to treat heart attack.)

Dose: for severe allergy, 0.05 ml-1 ml injected by the intramuscular route (according to age), and repeated if necessary every 10 minutes.
Availability: NHS and private prescription.
Side effects: anxiety, shaking, rapid heart beat, heart beat irregularity, dry mouth, cold hands and feet.
Caution: in the elderly, and in patients suffering from overactive thyroid, diabetes, heart disease, high blood pressure.
Not to be used for:
Caution needed with: anaesthetics, antidepressants, blood-pressure lowering drugs, ß-BLOCKERS, breathing stimulants, other sympathomimetics, MAOIS.
Contains: ADRENALINE.
Other preparations: Adrenaline Injection, EPIPEN, MEDIHALER-EPI.

Minitran *see* Transiderm-Nitro
(3M Health Care)

Minocin *see* minocycline tablets
(Lederle)

Minocin 50 *see* minocycline tablets
(Lederle)

---

minocycline *see* Aknemin, Cyclomin, Dentomycin, Minocin, Minocin 50, minocycline tablets, Minogal

---

minocycline tablets

A tablet supplied at strength of 50 mg, 100 mg, and used as a tetracycline antibiotic treatment for chronic bronchitis and other infections including acne.

Dose: 50-100 mg twice a day, for at least 6 weeks in the case of acne.
Availability: NHS and private prescription.
Side effects: stomach disturbances, allergies, ear disorder, additional

M

infections, dizziness, vertigo, pigmentation, liver disorder, headache, inflamed pancreas, sensitivity to light.

Caution: in patients suffering from liver disease and kidney disorders.

Not to be used for: children, pregnant women, nursing mothers, or for patients suffering from LUPUS.

Caution needed with: ANTACIDS, the contraceptive pill, ANTICOAGULANTS, calcium, zinc, or iron supplements.

Contains: MINOCYCLINE hydrochloride.

Other preparations: minocycline capsules. AKNEMIN, CYCLOMIN, MINOCIN, MINOCIN MR, MINOGAL. (Long-acting preparations available.)

Minodiab
(Pharmacia)

A white tablet supplied at strengths of 2.5 mg, 5 mg and used as an antidiabetic treatment for diabetes.

Dose: 2.5-5 mg a day in divided doses at first increasing by 2.5 or 5 mg a day every 7 days, then usually 2.5-30 mg a day to a maximum of 40 mg a day, taken in divided doses 15-20 minutes before food.

Availability: NHS and private prescription.

Side effects: allergy, including skin rash.

Caution: in the elderly and in patients suffering from kidney failure.

Not to be used for: children, pregnant women, nursing mothers, during surgery, or for patients suffering from juvenile diabetes, liver or kidney disorders, endocrine disorders, stress, infections.

Caution needed with: ß-BLOCKERS, MAOIS, STEROIDS, DIURETICS, ANTICOAGULANTS, lipid-lowering agents, BEZAFIBRATE, CLOFIBRATE, ASPIRIN, some antibiotics (RIFAMPICIN, sulphonamides, CHLORAMPHENICOL), GLUCAGON, cyclophosphamide, the contraceptive pill.

Contains: GLIPIZIDE.

Other preparations: GLIBENESE.

Minogal *see* minocycline tablets
(Galen)

---

minoxidil *see* Loniten, Regaine

Mintec
(Monmouth)

A green/ivory capsule (coated to protect the stomach) used as an anti-spasm treatment for irritable bowel syndrome, spastic colon.

M

Dose: adults 1-2 capsules 3 times a day before meals.
Availability: NHS, over the counter, private prescription.
Side effects:
Caution:
Not to be used for: children.
Caution needed with: ANTACIDS.
Contains: PEPPERMINT OIL.
Other preparations: COLPERMIN.

Mintezol
(M.S.D.)

An orange, scored, chewable tablet supplied at a strength of 500 mg and used to treat worms and other associated conditions and infections.

Dose: under 60 kg body weight 25 mg per kg twice a day with food; over 60 kg body weight 1.5 g twice a day with food.
Availability: NHS and private prescription.
Side effects: reduced alertness, stomach and brain disturbances, allergy, liver damage, changes to sight and hearing, low blood pressure, bed wetting.
Caution: in patients suffering from liver or kidney disease.
Not to be used for: pregnant women, nursing mothers, or for patients suffering from mixed infections with roundworms.
Caution needed with: CHOLINE THEOPHYLLINATE, AMINOPHYLLINE.
Contains: THIABENDAZOLE.
Other preparations:

Minulet
(Wyeth)

A white tablet used as an oestrogen, progestogen contraceptive.

Dose: 1 tablet a day for 21 days starting on day 1 of the period.
Availability: NHS and private prescription.
Side effects: enlarged breasts, bloating and fluid retention, cramps, leg pains, mood change, reduction in sexual desire, headaches, nausea, vaginal erosion, discharge, and bleeding, weight gain, skin changes, rarely thrombosis, raised blood pressure, jaundice.
Caution: in patients suffering from high blood pressure, diabetes, vascular disorders, asthma, depression, kidney disease, multiple sclerosis, womb diseases. Your doctor may advise you not to smoke, to have regular examinations. You should stop treatment at the first sign of serious symptoms such as severe headache or jaundice. Treatment should be stopped before surgery.

M

Not to be used for: pregnant women, or for patients suffering from sickle-cell anaemia, history of heart disease or thrombosis, liver disorders, some cancers, undiagnosed vaginal bleeding, some ear, skin, and kidney disorders.
Caution needed with: RIFAMPICIN, TETRACYCLINE ANTIBIOTICS, GRISEOFULVIN, BARBITURATES, PHENYTOIN, PRIMIDONE, CARBAMAZEPINE, ETHOSUXIMIDE, CHLORAL HYDRATE.
Contains: ETHINYLOESTRADIOL, GESTODENE.
Other preparations: FEMODENE.

Mirena
(Pharmacia-Leiras)

A progestogen form of intra-uterine device, used to provide contraception.

Dose: insertion within 7 days of the onset of menstruation (or 6 weeks after birth of a baby), then left in place for 3 years.
Availability: NHS and private prescription.
Side effects: nausea, breast pain, headache, back pain, abdominal pain, abnormal menstrual bleeding, skin problems, ovarian cysts.
Caution: in nursing mothers and in patients suffering from diabetes, heart valve disorder, or with a history of ovarian cysts, blood clots or ectopic pregnancy.
Not to be used for: children, pregnant women, or for patients suffering from some cancers, blood disorders, undiagnosed vaginal bleeding, inflamed pelvis, abnormal uterus, blood vessel disorders.
Caution needed with: RIFAMPICIN, CIMETIDINE, BARBITURATES, GRISEOFULVIN, anticonvulsants.
Contains: LEVONORGESTREL.
Other preparations:

---

misoprostol *see* Arthrotec, Cytotec, Napratec

Mixtard *see* insulin
(Novo Nordisk)

M-M-R II
(Pasteur Merieux MSD)

A vaccination used to provide active immunization for children, and adults at risk of contracting measles, mumps, or rubella (German measles).

Dose: 1 injection of 0.5 ml.

M

Availability: NHS, private prescription.
Side effects: rash, fever, nausea, local irritation and allergic reactions, temporary joint paint, general feeling of being unwell, swollen glands; very rarely, brain inflammation.
Caution: in patients suffering from acute infections, or who have a history of feverish convulsions, or brain injury. Do not administer within 1 month of other live vaccines, or within 3 months of blood transfusion or immunoglobulin vaccinations. Patients should not become pregnant within 3 months of vaccination.
Not to be used for: pregnant women, or for patients who have impaired immune systems, sensitivity to eggs, kanamycin, or neomycin, or who have a history of severe allergic shock from eggs.
Caution needed with:
Contains: live vaccines of measles, mumps, rubella, NEOMYCIN.
Other preparations: MR vaccine (measles and rubella only).

Mobiflex
(Roche)

A brown, five-sided tablet supplied at a strength of 20 mg and used as a NON-STEROIDAL ANTI-INFLAMMATORY DRUG to treat osteoarthritis, rheumatoid arthritis, soft-tissue injuries.

Dose: 1 tablet a day.
Availability: NHS and private prescription.
Side effects: stomach disturbances, swelling, headache, rash, blood changes, liver changes, disturbances of the eyesight.
Caution: in the elderly or in patients suffering from liver or kidney disease, heart failure.
Not to be used for: children, pregnant women, patients with a history of or suffering from stomach ulcer, gastro-intestinal bleeding, gastritis, allergy to ASPIRIN or anti-inflammatory drugs.
Caution needed with: ANTICOAGULANTS, antidiabetics taken by mouth, other non-steroidal anti-inflammatory drugs, LITHIUM.
Contains: TENOXICAM.
Other preparations: Mobiflex Milk, Mobiflex Effervescent, Mobiflex Injection.

---

moclobemide *see* Manerix

Modalim
(Sanofi Winthrop)

A white, capsule-shaped, scored tablet supplied at a strength of 100 mg and used to treat high blood lipid levels which cannot be controlled by diet alone.

Dose: 1 tablet a day.
Availability: NHS and private prescription.
Side effects: headache, vertigo, rash, stomach upset, muscle pain, impotence, hair loss, dizziness, drowsiness.
Caution: in patients suffering from liver or kidney disease, underactive thyroid. Your doctor may recommend regular liver tests.
Not to be used for: children, pregnant women, nursing mothers, or for patients suffering from severe liver or kidney disease.
Caution needed with: alcohol, sedatives, ANTICOAGULANTS, antidiabetics, the contraceptive pill, some other lipid-lowering drugs.
Contains: CIPROFIBRATE.
Other preparations:

Modaplate *see* **dipyridamole tablets**
(Berk)

Moditen
(Sanofi Winthrop)

A pink tablet, yellow tablet, or white tablet according to strengths of 1 mg, 2.5 mg, 5 mg and used as a sedative to treat schizophrenia, behavioural problems, anxiety, agitation, mania, and other similar disorders.

Dose: adults 2-10 mg a day adjusted if needed (maximum 20 mg a day); senile elderly use lower doses.
Availability: NHS and private prescription.
Side effects: muscle spasms, restlessness, constipation, blurred vision, hands shaking, dry mouth, urine retention, palpitations, low blood pressure, weight gain, changes in sexual function, low body temperature, breast swelling, menstrual changes, jaundice, blood and skin changes, drowsiness, tiredness, stuffy nose, rarely fits, heart disorders.
Caution: in the elderly, pregnant women, nursing mothers, and in patients suffering from tremor or rigidity, liver, lung, or heart disorder, thyroid disorder, epilepsy, glaucoma, MYASTHENIA GRAVIS, or enlarged prostate.
Not to be used for: children or for patients suffering from PHAEOCHROMOCYTOMA (a disease of the adrenal glands), kidney or liver failure, poor brain circulation, severe heart weakness, severe depression or coma, blood disorders.
Caution needed with: alcohol, sedatives, tranquillizers, pain killers, blood-pressure lowering drugs, antidepressants, anticonvulsants, antidiabetic drugs, LEVODOPA.
Contains: FLUPHENAZINE hydrochloride.

M

Other preparations:

Modrasone
(Schering-Plough)

A cream used as a STEROID treatment for skin disorders.

Dose: apply to the affected area 2-3 times a day.
Availability: NHS and private prescription.
Side effects: fluid retention, suppression of adrenal glands, thinning, spotting, or streaking of the skin may occur.
Caution: use for short periods of time only, especially on the face or in children.
Not to be used for: patients suffering from acne or any other skin infections caused by tuberculosis, ringworm, viruses, or fungi, leg ulcers, scabies, or continuously especially in pregnant women.
Caution needed with:
Contains: ALCLOMETASONE DIPROPRIONATE.
Other preparations: Modrasone Ointment.

Modrenal
(Wanskerne)

Capsules supplied at strengths of 60 mg, 120 mg and used as an adrenal inhibitor when the adrenal glands are overactive.

Dose: 60 mg 4 times a day for the first 3 days, then adjust as needed up to a maximum of 960 mg a day.
Availability: NHS and private prescription.
Side effects: flushing, nausea, running nose, diarrhoea.
Caution: in patients suffering from kidney or liver disease, stress. Your doctor may wish to ensure there is no tumour of the adrenal glands.
Not to be used for: children, pregnant women, or for patients suffering from severe kidney or liver disease.
Caution needed with: AMILORIDE, TRIAMTERENE, potassium supplements, SPIRONOLACTONE.
Contains: TRILOSTANE.
Other preparations:

Moducren
(Morson)

A blue, scored, square tablet used as a ß-BLOCKER/DIURETIC/potassium-sparing diuretic combination to treat high blood pressure.

Dose: 1-2 tablets a day.
Availability: NHS and private prescription.
Side effects: cold hands and feet, sleep disturbance, slow heart rate, tiredness, wheezing, heart failure, stomach upset, low blood pressure, rash, sensitivity to light, blood changes, gout, cramps, dry eyes.
Caution: in pregnant women, nursing mothers, and in patients suffering from diabetes, electrolyte changes, gout, kidney or liver disease, high blood lipids.
Not to be used for: children, and for patients suffering from progressive or severe kidney failure, raised potassium levels, low blood pressure, untreated PHAEOCHROMOCYTOMA, failure of the kidneys to produce urine, heart block or failure, asthma.
Caution needed with: potassium supplements, potassium-sparing diuretics, LITHIUM, DIGOXIN, blood-pressure lowering drugs, ACE INHIBITORS, VERAPAMIL, CLONIDINE withdrawal, some anti-arrhythmic drugs and anaesthetics, RESERPINE, ERGOTAMINE, CIMETIDINE, sedatives, SYMPATHOMIMETICS, INDOMETHACIN, antidiabetics, ALLOPURINOL, AMANTADINE.
Contains: HYDROCHLOROTHIAZIDE, AMILORIDE hydrochloride, TIMOLOL maleate.
Other preparations:

Moduret 25 *see* **co-amilozide tablets**
(Du Pont)

Moduretic *see* **co-amilozide tablets**
(Du Pont)

Mogadon *see* **nitrazepam tablets**
(Roche)

Molcer
(Wallace)

Drops as a wax softener to soften ear wax.

Dose: fill ear with the drops and plug with cotton wool on 2 consecutive nights and then clean out.
Availability: NHS, private prescription, over the counter.
Side effects:
Caution:
Not to be used for: patients suffering from perforated ear drum.
Caution needed with:
Contains: sodium DOCUSATE.

M

Other preparations: DIOCTYL EAR DROPS, WAXSOL.

Molipaxin
(Marion Merrell Dow)

A pink, scored tablet supplied at a strength of 150 mg and used as a sedative to treat depression and anxiety.

Dose: 1-4 tablets daily. (Elderly maximum 2 tablets a day.)
Availability: NHS and private prescription.
Side effects: drowsiness, dizziness, headache, nausea, low blood pressure on standing, blood changes, penile erection, liver disorder.
Caution: in patients suffering from epilepsy, severe kidney, liver, or heart disease.
Not to be used for: children.
Caution needed with: anaesthetics, alcohol, sedatives, MAOIS, CLONIDINE, DIGOXIN, PHENYTOIN.
Contains: TRAZODONE hydrochloride.
Other preparations: Molipaxin Capsules, Molipaxin CR, Molipaxin Liquid.

---

mometasone furoate *see* Elocon

Monit *see* isosorbide mononitrate tablets
(Lorex Synthélabo)

---

mono-amine oxidase inhibitor *see* MAOI

Mono-Cedocard *see* isosorbide mononitrate tablets
(Pharmacia)

Monocor
(Lederle)

A pink tablet or a white tablet according to strengths of 5 mg, 10 mg and used as a ß-BLOCKER to treat angina, high blood pressure.

Dose: 10 mg once a day to a maximum of 20 mg a day.
Availability: NHS and private prescription.
Side effects: cold hands and feet, sleep disturbance, slow heart rate, tiredness, wheezing, heart failure, low blood pressure, stomach upset, dry eyes, rash.

M

Caution: in pregnant women, nursing mothers, and in patients suffering from diabetes, kidney or liver disorders, asthma. May need to be withdrawn before surgery. Withdraw gradually. Your doctor may advise additional treatment with DIURETICS or DIGOXIN.
Not to be used for: children or for patients suffering from heart block or failure, low blood pressure, untreated PHAEOCHROMOCYTOMA.
Caution needed with: VERAPAMIL, CLONIDINE withdrawal, some anti-arrhythmic drugs and anaesthetics, RESERPINE, some blood-pressure lowering drugs, ERGOTAMINE, CIMETIDINE, sedatives, antidiabetics, SYMPATHOMIMETICS, INDOMETHACIN.
Contains: BISOPROLOL fumarate.
Other preparations: EMCOR.

Monotard *see* insulin
(Novo Nordisk)

Monotrim *see* trimethoprim tablets
(Solvay Healthcare)

Monovent
(Lagap)

A syrup used as a BRONCHODILATOR to treat bronchial spasm brought on by asthma, bronchitis, or emphysema.

Dose: adults 10-15 ml twice a day or every 8 hours; children reduced doses.
Availability: NHS and private prescription.
Side effects: shaking of the hands, tension, headache, palpitations, low potassium levels, rash, muscle spasm, sleep or behavioural changes in children.
Caution: in pregnant women and in diabetics, or in patients suffering from some heart disorders, overactive thyroid gland.
Not to be used for: children under 2 years
Caution needed with: SYMPATHOMIMETICS, ß-BLOCKERS, drugs that lower potassium levels.
Contains: TERBUTALINE sulphate.
Other preparations: BRICANYL.

Monozide 10
(Lederle)

A white, film-coated tablet used as a ß-BLOCKER and DIURETIC to treat high blood pressure.

M

Dose: 1 tablet a day.
Availability: NHS, private prescription.
Side effects: cold hands and feet, sleep disturbances, slow heart rate, fatigue, bronchial spasm, heart failure, low blood pressure, stomach upsets, dry eyes, rash, gout, sensitivity to light, blood changes.
Caution: in pregnant women, nursing mothers, and in patients suffering from diabetes, raised lipid levels, liver or kidney disorders, raised acidity, gout, history of bronchial spasm. Weak heart should be controlled before treatment.
Not to be used for: children, or for patients suffering from heart block, slow heart rate, some other heart conditions, low blood pressure, untreated PHAEOCHROMOCYTOMA, severe kidney failure, failure of the kidneys to produce urine.
Caution needed with: LITHIUM, DIGOXIN, potassium supplements, some diuretics, VERAPAMIL, SYMPATHOMIMETICS, INDOMETHACIN, sedatives, CIMETIDINE, ERGOTAMINE, other blood-pressure lowering drugs, RESERPINE, some antidiabetic drugs, CLONIDINE withdrawal, some anaesthetics, ALLOPURINOL, AMANTADINE.
Contains: BISOPROLOL FUMARATE, HYDROCHLOROTHIAZIDE.
Other preparations:

Monphytol
(L.A.B.)

A paint used as an anti-fungal treatment for athlete's foot.

Dose: paint on to the affected area twice a day at first then once a week.
Availability: NHS, private prescription, over the counter.
Side effects:
Caution:
Not to be used for: children or pregnant women.
Caution needed with:
Contains: CHLORBUTOL, METHYL UNDECOANATE, SALICYLIC ACID, METHYL SALICYLATE, PROPYL SALICYLATE, PROPYL UNDECOANATE.
Other preparations:

Monuril
(Pharmax)

Granules in a sachet used as an antibacterial preparation to treat urinary tract infections and to prevent such infections during diagnostic and surgical procedures.

Dose: treatment: 1 dose of 3 g at night or 1 hour before or 2 hours after meal; prevention: 3 g 3 hours before procedure and repeat once 24 hours after procedure. Children use paediatric granules

M

Availability: NHS, private prescription.
Side effects: stomach upset, rash.
Caution: in the elderly, pregnant women, nursing mothers, and in patients suffering from kidney disorder.
Not to be used for: children, patients over 75 years, or with severe kidney damage.
Caution needed with: METOCLOPRAMIDE.
Contains: FOSFOMYCIN trometamol.
Other preparations: Monuril Paediatric.

Moracizine *see* Ethmozine

---

morphine *see* morphine suppositories, MST Continus, Oramorph, Sevredol

---

morphine suppositories

A suppository supplied at strengths of 15 mg, 30 mg, and used as an opiate ANALGESIC to control chronic severe pain.

Dose: 15-30 mg every 4 hours.
Availability: controlled drug; NHS and private prescription.
Side effects: nausea, vomiting, constipation, drowsiness, euphoria, mental detachment, breathing difficulties, low blood pressure, difficulty in urinating, sweating, headache, flushing, vertigo, rapid pulse, palpitations, low blood pressure on standing, cold hands and feet, itch, rash, mental disturbances, dry mouth.
Caution: in children, pregnant women, nursing mothers, the elderly and debilitated, and in patients suffering from low blood pressure, underactive thyroid, asthma, liver failure, breathing difficulties, kidney disorders.
Not to be used for: patients suffering from head injury or with raised pressure on the brain.
Caution needed with: alcohol, antidepressants, tranquillizers, sedatives, SELEGILINE, CIMETIDINE.
Contains: MORPHINE hydrochloride or sulphate.
Other preparations

Motens
(Boehringer Ingelheim)

A white film-coated tablet supplied at strengths of 2 mg, 4 mg, used to treat raised blood pressure.

M

Dose: 2 mg once a day at first increasing after 3-4 weeks to 6 mg once a day (elderly to 4 mg once a day after 4 weeks). Usual maintenance dose 4 mg once a day.
Availability: NHS, private prescription.
Side effects: headache, dizziness, flushing, fluid retention, increased frequency of urination, rash, palpitations, chest pain (withdraw immediately), weakness, swollen gums.
Caution: in patients suffering from liver disease, poor heart reserve, some heart conditions.
Not to be used for: children, pregnant women, nursing mothers.
Caution needed with: CIMETIDINE.
Contains: LACIDIPINE.
Other preparations:

Motilium
(Sanofi Winthrop)

A white tablet supplied at a strength of 10 mg and used as an anti-emetic drug to treat acute nausea and vomiting, and indigestion.

Dose: adults 10-20 mg every 4-8 hours (maximum of 3 times a day for indigestion); children use in rare situations in reduced doses.
Availability: NHS and private prescription.
Side effects: blood changes, rash, shaking.
Caution:
Not to be used for: pregnant women.
Caution needed with:
Contains: DOMPERIDONE.
Other preparations: Motilium Suspension, Motilium Suppositories.

Motipress
(Sanofi Winthrop)

A yellow, triangular tablet used as a sedative and TRICYCLIC ANTIDEPRESSANT to treat a mixture of anxiety and depression.

Dose: 1 tablet a day at bedtime for up to 3 months.
Availability: NHS and private prescription.
Side effects: muscle spasms, restlessness, sleeplessness, dizziness, hands shaking, dry mouth, constipation, stuffy nose, blurred vision, urine retention, palpitations, low blood pressure, weight change, changes in sexual function, low body temperature, breast swelling, menstrual changes, jaundice, blood and skin changes, drowsiness, tiredness, rarely fits, heart disorders.
Caution: in patients with a history of epilepsy or brain damage, nursing

M

mothers, and in patients suffering from heart disease, glaucoma, adrenal tumour, urinary retention, thyroid disease, epilepsy, diabetes, some other psychiatric conditions. Your doctor may advise regular blood and liver tests.

Not to be used for: children, pregnant women or for patients suffering from epilepsy or brain damage, liver disease, heart block, kidney disease, weak heart, blood disorders.

Caution needed with: alcohol, sedatives, ANTICHOLINERGICS, ADRENALINE, MAOIS, BARBITURATES, tranquillizers, pain killers, blood-pressure lowering drugs, antidepressants, anticonvulsants, antidiabetic drugs, LEVODOPA, CIMETIDINE, oestrogen, local anaesthetics.

Contains: FLUPHENAZINE hydrochloride, NORTRIPTYLINE

Other preparations: MOTIVAL (a weaker-strength product).

Motival *see* Motipress
(Sanofi Winthrop)

Motrin *see* ibuprofen tablets
(Upjohn)

Movelat
(Panpharma)

A cream and a gel used as an anti-inflammatory rub to relieve pain and inflammation from muscles and joints, such as sprains and strains.

Dose: massage gently into the affected area up to 4 times a day.
Availability: NHS, private prescription, over the counter.
Side effects:
Caution:
Not to be used for: children, women in early or late pregnancy, or for patients suffering from allergy to ASPIRIN, anti-inflammatory preparations, asthma.
Caution needed with:
Contains: SALICYLIC ACID, MUCOPOLYSACCHARIDE POLYSULPHATE.
Other preparations:

MST Continus
(Napp)

A long-acting white tablet, brown tablet, light-green tablet, purple tablet, orange tablet, grey tablet, or green tablet according to strengths of 5 mg, 10 mg, 15 mg, 30 mg, 60 mg, 100 mg, 200 mg and used as an opiate for

M

the prolonged relief of severe pain.

Dose: adults 30 mg every 12 hours at first, then as advised by physician; children 0.2-0.8 mg per kilogram bodyweight every 12 hours at first, then as advised by physician.
Availability: controlled drug; NHS and private prescription.
Side effects: tolerance, addiction, constipation, nausea, vomiting.
Caution: in the elderly and in patients suffering from kidney or liver disease, underactive thyroid, raised pressure on the brain.
Not to be used for: pregnant women, or for patients suffering from breathing disorder or blocked airways, acute liver disease, or 24 hours either side of surgery.
Caution needed with: MAOIS, sedatives, alcohol.
Contains: MORPHINE sulphate.
Other preparations: MST Continus Suspension. ORAMORPH (also available in liquid form), SEVREDOL (not a long-acting formula).

Mucaine
(Wyeth)

A white liquid used as an ANTACID plus local anaesthetic to treat oesophagitis and hiatus hernia.

Dose: adults 5-10 ml 3-4 times a day before meals and at bedtime.
Availability: NHS and private prescription.
Side effects: occasional constipation.
Caution:
Not to be used for: children.
Caution needed with: tablets coated to protect the stomach, some antibiotics, iron.
Contains: OXETHAZAINE, ALUMINIUM HYDROXIDE, MAGNESIUM HYDROXIDE.
Other preparations:

---

mucin *see* **Saliva Orthana**

Mucodyne
(Rhône Poulenc Rorer)

A syrup supplied at a strength of 250 mg/5 ml and used as a mucus softener to clear phlegm, running nose, glue ear in children.

Dose: adults 15 ml 3 times a day reducing to 10 ml; children over 2 years use paediatric syrup.
Availability: NHS (as a generic only if for a child with tracheostomy),

private prescription.
Side effects: stomach disturbance, nausea, rash.
Caution: in pregnant women and in patients with a history of stomach ulcer.
Not to be used for: children under 2 years or for patients suffering from stomach ulcer.
Caution needed with:
Contains: CARBOCISTEINE.
Other preparations: Mucodyne Capsules, Mucodyne Paediatric.

Mucogel *see* Maalox
(Pharmax)

Multiload Cu 250
(Organon)

A copper-bearing coil used as an intra-uterine device to prevent conception.

Dose: as advised. Replace after 3 years.
Availability: NHS, private prescription.
Side effects: pelvic infection, pain, abnormal bleeding, perforation of the uterus. On insertion, persistent low heart rate, asthma attack, epileptic attack.
Caution: in patients suffering from anaemia, heavy periods, diabetes, epilepsy, or who have had inflammatory heart conditions or pelvic inflammatory disease or who are risk from sexually transmitted diseases. Patients should be checked 3 months after insertion and then annually.
Not to be used for: children, pregnant women, or for patients suffering from allergy to copper, abnormal uterus, severe infections, acute pelvic inflammatory disease, endometrial disease, abnormal vaginal bleeding, or some other urinogenital tract disorders, or with a history of ectopic pregnancies.
Caution needed with: ANTICOAGULANTS.
Contains: copper wire.
Other preparations: Multiload Cu 250 Short, Multiload Cu 375. NOVA-T, NOVAGARD, ORTHO-GYNE-T.

Mumpsvax
(Pasteur Merieux MSD)

An injection used to provide active immunization against mumps.

Dose: adults and children over 12 months old, 1 injection.

M

Availability: NHS, private prescription.
Side effects: fever, inflammation of the parotid glands.
Caution: in patients suffering from acute infections.
Not to be used for: pregnant women or within 3 months of pregnancy, or for patients allergic to eggs or penicillin, or with poor immunity.
Caution needed with: other live vaccines, blood transfusions, immunuglobulins.
Contains: mumps virus, NEOMYCIN.
Other preparations: MMR and MR VACCINES (combined vaccines).

---

mupirocin *see* **Bactroban Nasal**

Myambutol
(Lederle)

A yellow tablet or a grey tablet according to strengths of 100 mg, 400 mg and used as an anti-tubercular, additional treatment and preventive drug for tuberculosis.

Dose: adults 15 mg per kg body weight once a day; children treatment 25 mg per kg body weight once a day for 60 days, then 15 mg per kg body weight once a day; prevention 15 mg per kg body weight once a day.
Availability: NHS and private prescription.
Side effects: visual changes, eye inflammation.
Caution: in pregnant women, nursing mothers and in patients suffering from kidney disease. Eyes should be checked regularly.
Not to be used for: patients suffering from inflammation of the optic nerve.
Caution needed with:
Contains: ETHAMBUTOL.
Other preparations:

---

myasthenia gravis
a progressive form of muscle weakness, commonly affecting the muscles used for speaking, eating, and moving the eyes, making these actions difficult.

Mycardol
(Sanofi Winthrop)

A white, scored tablet supplied at a strength of 30 mg and used as a NITRATE in addition to GLYCERYL TRINITRATE in the treatment of angina.

Dose: 2 tablets 3-4 times a day.

M

Availability: NHS, private prescription, over the counter.
Side effects: headache, flushes, dizziness, rapid heart rate, rash,
tiredness, nausea, vomiting.
Caution: in pregnant women and in patients suffering from glaucoma or
who are subject to low blood pressure.
Not to be used for: children or for patients suffering from coronary
thrombosis, bleeding in the brain, head injury, anaemia.
Caution needed with:
Contains: PENTAERYTHRITOL TETRANITRATE.
Other preparations:

Mycifradin
(Upjohn)

A tablet supplied at a strength of 500 mg and used as an aminoglycoside
antibiotic to sterilize the bowel before surgery.

Dose: 2 tablets every 4 hours.
Availability: NHS and private prescription.
Side effects: hearing damage, kidney disorder, intestinal disorder.
Caution: in the young, the elderly, and in patients suffering from kidney or
liver failure. Not for prolonged use.
Not to be used for: pregnant women, or for patients suffering from
MYASTHENIA GRAVIS.
Caution needed with: ANTICOAGULANTS, NEOSTIGMINE, PYRIDOSTIGMINE,
CYCLOSPORIN, some DIURETICS.
Contains: NEOMYCIN sulphate.
Other preparations: NEOMYCIN ELIXIR, NIVEMYCIN.

Mycobutin
(Pharmacia)

A red-brown capsule supplied at a strength of 150 mg and used as anti-
tubercular drug for the prevention and treatment of some mycobacterial
infections and tuberculosis of the lungs.

Dose: 1-4 capsules a day depending on condition.
Availability: NHS, private prescription.
Side effects: stomach upset, anaemia, discoloration of the skin, urine,
and other secretions, blood changes, joint pain.
Caution: in patients suffering from severe liver or kidney disorders. Your
doctor may advise regular blood tests.
Not to be used for: children, pregnant women, and nursing mothers, or
for patients who wear soft contact lenses.
Caution needed with: the contraceptive pill, ANTICOAGULANTS, ANALGESICS,

M

CORTICOSTEROIDS, CYCLOSPORIN, DIGOXIN, DAPSONE, antidiabetics taken by mouth, PHENYTOIN, some antibiotics, some antifungals, ZIDOVUDINE, QUINIDINE.
Contains: RIFABUTIN.
Other preparations:

Mydriacyl
(Alcon)

Drops used as an ANTICHOLINERGIC pupil dilator for eye examinations.

Dose: 1-2 drops into the eye with 1-5 minutes between each drop, then a further drop into the eye after 30 minutes if needed.
Availability: NHS and private prescription.
Side effects: temporary smarting, dry mouth, blurred vision, aversion to light, rapid heart rate, headache, mental and behavioural changes.
Caution: in infants and in patients where the eye pressure is not known.
Not to be used for: patients suffering from narrow-angle glaucoma or who wear soft contact lenses.
Caution needed with:
Contains: TROPICAMIDE.
Other preparations: NODS TROPICAMIDE, TROPICAMIDE MINIMS.

Mydrilate
(Boehringer Ingelheim)

Drops available in 2 strengths, and used as an ANTICHOLINERGIC pupil dilator for eye examinations and to treat eye inflammation.

Dose: adults 1 drop into the eye, repeated 15 minutes later if needed (for uveitis 1 or 2 drops may be used when needed); children reduced dose.
Availability: NHS and private prescription.
Side effects: blurred vision, confusion, dry mouth.
Caution: in patients suffering from inflamed eye.
Not to be used for: patients suffering from glaucoma.
Caution needed with:
Contains: CYCLOPENTOLATE HYDROCHLORIDE.
Other preparations:

Mygdalon *see* metoclopramide tablets
(DDSA)

M

nadolol *see* **Corgard, Corgaretic 40**

nafarelin *see* **Synarel**

naftidrofuryl oxalate *see* **Praxilene, Stimlor**

Nalcrom
(Fisons)

A clear capsule supplied at a strength of 100 mg and used as an anti-allergy drug to treat allergies to foods.

Dose: adults 2 capsules 4 times a day before meals; children over 2 years 1 capsule 4 times a day before meals. Maximum for adults and children 40 mg per kilogram body weight a day.
Availability: NHS and private prescription.
Side effects: rash, pain in the joints, nausea.
Caution:
Not to be used for: infants under 2 years.
Caution needed with:
Contains: SODIUM CROMOGLYCATE.
Other preparations:

nalidixic acid *see* **Mictral, nalidixic acid tablets, Negram, Uriben**

nalidixic acid tablets

A tablet supplied at a strength of 500 mg and used as an antibiotic to treat urinary infections.

Dose: adults acute infections 2 tablets 4 times a day for 7 days, chronic infections 1 tablet 4 times a day; children 3 months-12 years use suspension.
Availability: NHS and private prescription.
Side effects: stomach upset, disturbed vision, rash, blood changes, fits, sensitivity to light, pins and needles, headache, rash, itching, allergy, disturbed sleep, blood and liver changes.
Caution: in pregnant women, nursing mothers and in patients suffering from liver or kidney disease. Keep out of strong sunlight.
Not to be used for: infants under 3 months or for patients suffering from PORPHYRIA, or a history of convulsions.

Caution needed with: ANTICOAGULANTS, PROBENECID, melphalan, NON-STEROIDAL ANTI-INFLAMMATORY DRUGS, some antidiabetics.
Contains: NALIDIXIC ACID.
Other preparations: MICTRAL, NEGRAM, URIBEN (suspension).

Nalorex
(Du Pont)

A mottled, orange, scored tablet supplied at a strength of 50 mg and used as an opiate antagonist as a treatment for patients who have been detoxified from opioid dependency.

Dose: ½ tablet a day at first, then 1 tablet a day for 3 months (treatment should be started in a drug addiction rehabilitation centre).
Availability: NHS and private prescription.
Side effects: vomiting, drowsiness, dizziness, stomach cramps, joint and muscle pain.
Caution: in patients suffering from liver or kidney disease.
Not to be used for: children, or for patients suffering from acute liver disease, liver failure, or current dependence on opiates.
Caution needed with: alcohol, sedatives.
Contains: NALTREXONE HYDROCHLORIDE.
Other preparations:

---

naltrexone hydrochloride *see* Nalorex

Napratec
(Searle)

Yellow, oblong, scored tablets and white, hexagonal scored tablets supplied together in one pack to treat rheumatoid arthritis, osteoarthritis, and ankylosing spondylitis where the stomach also needs protecting against the effects of the medication.

Dose: 1 of each tablet twice a day with food.
Availability: NHS and private prescription.
Side effects: stomach upset, diarrhoea, stomach pain, vaginal bleeding, heavy periods, rash, itching, severe allergy, headache, dizziness, noise in the ears, vertigo, blood changes.
Caution: in the elderly, and in patients suffering from asthma, liver or kidney damage, disorders affecting blood vessels. Women of child-bearing age must use effective contraception.
Not to be used for: children, pregnant women, nursing mothers, or for patients suffering from allergy to ASPIRIN or anti-inflammatory drugs, or stomach ulcer.

Caution needed with: ANTICOAGULANTS, PHENYTOIN, some antidiabetics, sulphonamide antibiotics, DIURETICS, LITHIUM, ß-BLOCKERS, PROBENECID, METHOTREXATE.
Contains: NAPROXEN (yellow tablets), MISOPROSTOL (white tablets).
Other preparations:

Naprosyn *see* naproxen tablets
(Roche)

---

naproxen *see* Arthrosin, Arthroxen, Laraflex, Napratec, Naprosyn, naproxen tablets, Nycopren, Prosaid, Rimoxyn, Synflex, Timpron

---

naproxen tablets

A tablet supplied at strengths of 250 mg, 500 mg and used as a NON-STEROIDAL ANTI-INFLAMMATORY DRUG to treat rheumatoid arthritis, and other muscle, joint, and bone disorders, acute gout.

Dose: adults 500 mg-1 g a day in divided doses; for gout 750 mg at first then 250 mg every 8 hours. Children 5-16 years 10 mg per kg body weight a day in 2 divided doses.
Availability: NHS and private prescription.
Side effects: rash, stomach upset, headache, tinnitus, vertigo, blood changes, severe allergy, fluid retention. Rarely liver or kidney disorders.
Caution: in the elderly, pregnant women, nursing mothers, and in patients suffering from heart, kidney, or liver disease, LUPUS, asthma, a history of stomach ulcers.
Not to be used for: children under 5 years, or for patients suffering from stomach ulcer, or allergy to ASPIRIN or anti-inflammatory drugs.
Caution needed with: ANTICOAGULANTS, some antidiabetics, ß-BLOCKERS, METHOTREXATE, PROBENECID, drugs that lower blood pressure, other non-steroidal anti-inflammatory drugs, some antibiotics, LITHIUM.
Contains: NAPROXEN.
Other preparations: ARTHROSIN, ARTHROXEN, LARAFLEX, NAPROSYN, NYCOPREN, PROSAID, RIMOXYN, SYNFLEX, TIMPRON. (Long-acting preparations, liquids, and suppository forms available. Some brands are coated to protect the stomach – do not take these with ANTACIDS)

Nardil
(Parke-Davis)

An orange tablet supplied at a strength of 15 mg and used as an MAOI to treat depression, phobias.

Dose: 1 tablet 3 times a day at first reducing gradually according to response.

Availability: NHS and private prescription.

Side effects: severe high blood pressure reactions with certain foods and medicines, sleeplessness, low blood pressure, dizziness, drowsiness, weakness, dry mouth, constipation, stomach upset, blurred vision, urinary difficulties, ankle swelling, rash, jaundice, weight gain, confusion, sexual desire changes.

Caution: in the elderly and in patients suffering from epilepsy.

Not to be used for: children, or for patients suffering from liver disease, PORPHYRIA, blood disorders, heart disease, PHAEOCHROMOCYTOMA, overactive thyroid, brain artery disease.

Caution needed with: amphetamines or similar SYMPATHOMIMETIC drugs, some drugs that lower blood pressure, other antidepressants, other MAOIS, GUANETHIDINE, DEXTROMETHORPHAN, opiate ANALGESICS, alcohol, PETHIDINE and other opiate analgesics, some cough/cold remedies and appetite supressants containing sympathomimetics. BARBITURATES, sedatives, alcohol, and antidiabetics may be enhanced. Cheese, Bovril, Oxo, meat extracts, broad beans, banana, Marmite, yeast extracts, wine, beer, other alcohol, pickled herrings, vegetable proteins. (Up to 14 days after cessation.)

Contains: PHENELZINE SULPHATE.

Other preparations:

Narphen
(Napp)

A white, scored tablet supplied at a strength of 5 mg and used as an opiate to control severe, prolonged pain including biliary and pancreatic pain.

Dose: 1 tablet every 4-6 hours either swallowed or under the tongue. No single dose should exceed 4 tablets.

Availability: controlled drug; NHS and private prescription.

Side effects: tolerance, addiction, nausea, dizziness, constipation.

Caution: in the elderly, women in labour, or patients suffering from underactive thyroid, or liver or kidney disease.

Not to be used for: children, pregnant women, or for patients in coma, or suffering from breathing difficulty, blocked airways, acute alcoholism, epilepsy, severe underactive thyroid.

Caution needed with: MAOIS, sedatives, alcohol.

Contains: PHENAZOCINE HYDROBROMIDE.

Other preparations:

Naseptin
(Zeneca)

A cream used as an antibacterial treatment for infections of the nose.

Dose: apply into each nostril 2-4 times a day.
Availability: NHS and private prescription.
Side effects: sensitive skin.
Caution: avoid prolonged use.
Not to be used for:
Caution needed with:
Contains: CHLORHEXIDINE hydrochloride, NEOMYCIN sulphate.
Other preparations:

Natramid *see* indapamide tablets
(Trinity)

Natrilix *see* indapamide tablets
(Servier)

Navidrex
(Ciba)

A white, scored tablet supplied at a strength of 0.5 mg and used as a DIURETIC to treat heart failure, fluid retention, high blood pressure.

Dose: adults ½-2 tablets a day; children as advised by physician.
Availability: NHS and private prescription.
Side effects: rash, sensitivity to light, blood changes, anorexia, impotence, stomach upset, pancreatitis, headache, dizziness, electrolyte and metabolic disturbances.
Caution: the elderly, pregnant women, nursing mothers, and in patients suffering from diabetes, kidney or liver disease, gout, SLE. Potassium supplements may be needed.
Not to be used for: patients suffering from inability to produce urine or severe kidney or liver failure, Addison's disease, high calcium levels, sensitivity to some antibiotics.
Caution needed with: DIGOXIN, LITHIUM, STEROIDS, CARBENOXOLONE, NON-STEROIDAL ANTI-INFLAMMATORY DRUGS, antidiabetics, alcohol, BARBITURATES, opioid ANALGESICS.
Contains: CYCLOPENTHIAZIDE.
Other preparations:

Navispare
(Ciba)

A yellow tablet used as a potassium-sparing DIURETIC to treat high blood pressure.

Dose: 1-2 tablets once a day in the morning.
Availability: NHS and private prescription.
Side effects: rash, sensitivity to light, blood changes, gout, tiredness, stomach upset.
Caution: in pregnant women, nursing mothers, and in patients suffering from diabetes, liver or kidney damage, gout, high acidity in the blood, high blood lipid levels.
Not to be used for: children, or for patients suffering from severe kidney or liver failure, failure of the kidneys to produce urine, high potassium levels, Addison's disease, diabetic kidney disorders, persistent low potassium or sodium levels or high calcium levels.
Caution needed with: DIGOXIN, LITHIUM, some other diuretics, other blood-pressure lowering drugs, ACE-INHIBITORS, potassium supplements.
Contains: CYCLOPENTHIAZIDE, AMILORIDE.
Other preparations:

Nebuhaler
(Astra)

A one-piece 750 ml large volume reservoir chamber device for use as a spacer device with BRICANYL or PULMICORT refill canisters.

---

nedocromil *see* Rapitil

---

nefazodone *see* Dutonin

---

nefopam hydrochloride *see* Acupan

Negram *see* nalidixic acid tablets
(Sanofi Winthrop)

Neo-Bendromax *see* bendrofluazide tablets
(Ashbourne)

Neo-Cortef
(Cusi)

Drops used as an antibiotic, STEROID treatment for inflammation of the outer ear or infected inflammation of the eye.

Dose: 1-2 drops into the eye up to 6 times a day or 2-3 drops into the ear 3-4 times a day.
Availability: NHS and private prescription.
Side effects: additional infection, sensitization, fungal infection, thinning cornea, cataract, rise in eye pressure.
Caution: in pregnant women and infants – avoid using over extended periods.
Not to be used for: patients suffering from perforated ear drum, or viral, tubercular, fungal, or acute weeping infections, glaucoma.
Caution needed with:
Contains: NEOMYCIN sulphate, HYDROCORTISONE acetate.
Other preparations: Neo-Cortef Ointment.

Neo-Cytamen
(Evans)

An injection supplied at a strength of 1000 micrograms per ml, and used as a VITAMIN B$_{12}$ supplement to treat various anaemias, Leber's disease, poor eyesight caused by tobacco.

Dose: as advised by a physician.
Availability: NHS (when prescribed as a generic), private prescription.
Side effects: rarely allergy.
Caution:
Not to be used for:
Caution needed with: CHLORAMPHENICOL, the contraceptive pill.
Contains: hydroxocobalamin.
Other preparations:

Neo-Medrone Cream
(Upjohn)

A cream used as an antibacterial, STEROID treatment for allergic and other skin disorders where there is also inflammation and infection.

Dose: apply to the affected area 1-3 times a day.
Availability: NHS and private prescription.
Side effects: fluid retention, suppression of adrenal glands, thinning, spotting, or streaking of the skin may occur.

Caution: use for short periods of time only, especially in children or on the face.
Not to be used for: patients suffering from acne or any other skin infections caused by tuberculosis, ringworm, viruses, or fungi, leg ulcers, scabies, or continuously especially in pregnant women.
Caution needed with:
Contains: METHYLPREDNISOLONE acetate, NEOMYCIN sulphate.
Other preparations:

Neo-Mercazole
(Roche)

A pink tablet supplied at strengths of 5 mg, 20 mg and used as an antithyroid treatment for overactive thyroid.

Dose: adults 20-60 mg a day at first in 2-3 divided doses, then 5-15 mg a day for 6-18 months, or continue with 20-60 mg a day with THYROXINE; children 5-15 mg a day at first in divided doses.
Availability: NHS and private prescription.
Side effects: rash, headache, nausea, joint pain, bone marrow depression; inform the doctor of sore throat, mouth ulcer.
Caution: in pregnant women. Your doctor may advise regular blood tests.
Not to be used for: nursing mothers or patients with a blocked trachea.
Caution needed with:
Contains: CARBIMAZOLE.
Other preparations:

Neo-Naclex *see* bendrofluazide tablets
(Goldshield Healthcare)

Neo-Naclex-K
(Goldshield Healthcare)

A double-layered pink/white tablet used as a DIURETIC with potassium supplement to treat high blood pressure, chronic fluid retention.

Dose: adults high blood pressure 1-4 tablets a day, fluid retention 2 tablets a day increasing to 4 tablets a day if needed then 1-2 tablets from time to time.
Availability: NHS and private prescription.
Side effects: rash, sensitivity to light, blood changes, impotence, stomach upset, dizziness, loss of appetite, pancreatitis, electrolyte and other disturbances, bowel disorders.
Caution: in the elderly, pregnant women, nursing mothers, and in patients

suffering from diabetes, liver or kidney disease, gout, SLE.
Not to be used for: children, or for patients suffering from severe kidney or liver failure, raised calcium or potassium levels, Addison's disease, allergy to some antibiotics.
Caution needed with: DIGOXIN, LITHIUM, some diuretics, potassium supplements, some antidiabetic drugs, STEROIDS, CARBENOXOLONE, NON-STEROIDAL ANTI-INFLAMMATORY DRUGS, alcohol, BARBITURATES, opiate ANALGESICS.
Contains: BENDROFLUAZIDE, POTASSIUM CHLORIDE.
Other preparations:

Neocon 1/35
(Janssen-Cilag)

A peach-coloured tablet used as an oestrogen, progestogen contraceptive.

Dose: 1 tablet a day for 21 days starting on day 5 of the period.
Availability: NHS and private prescription.
Side effects: enlarged breasts, bloating and fluid retention, cramps, leg pains, mood change, reduction in sexual desire, headaches, nausea, vaginal erosion, discharge, and bleeding, weight gain, skin changes, rarely thrombosis, raised blood pressure, jaundice.
Caution: in patients suffering from high blood pressure, diabetes, vascular disorders, asthma, depression, kidney disease, multiple sclerosis, womb diseases. Your doctor may advise you not to smoke, to have regular examinations. You should stop treatment at the first sign of serious symptoms such as severe headache or jaundice. Treatment should be stopped before surgery.
Not to be used for: pregnant women, or for patients suffering from sickle-cell anaemia, history of heart disease or thrombosis, liver disorders, some cancers, undiagnosed vaginal bleeding, some ear, skin, and kidney disorders.
Caution needed with: RIFAMPICIN, TETRACYCLINE ANTIBIOTICS, GRISEOFULVIN, BARBITURATES, PHENYTOIN, PRIMIDONE, CARBAMAZEPINE, ETHOSUXIMIDE, CHLORAL HYDRATE.
Contains: ETHINYLOESTRADIOL, NORETHISTERONE.
Other preparations: NORIMIN.

Neogest
(Schering Healthcare)

A brown tablet used as a progesterone contraceptive.

Dose: 1 tablet at the same time every day starting on day 1 of the period.
Availability: NHS and private prescription.
Side effects: irregular bleeding, breast discomfort, acne, headache, rarely

thrombosis, raised blood pressure, jaundice, ovarian cysts.
Caution: in patients suffering from high blood pressure, tendency to thrombosis, migraine, some cancers, liver abnormalities, ovarian cysts. Your doctor may advise regular check-ups.
Not to be used for: pregnant women, or for patients suffering from severe heart or artery disease, benign liver tumours, undiagnosed vaginal bleeding, previous ectopic pregnancy.
Caution needed with: BARBITURATES, PHENYTOIN, PRIMIDONE, CARBAMAZEPINE, CHLORAL HYDRATE, ETHOSUXIMIDE, RIFAMPICIN, CHLORPROMAZINE, MEPROBAMATE, GRISEOFULVIN.
Contains: NORGESTREL.
Other preparations:

---

neomycin *see* **Almevax, Audicort, Betnovate (-N), Cicatrin, Cloburate (-N), Dermovate (-NN), Dexa-Rhinaspray, Ervevax, Eumovate (-N), FML (-Neo), Gregoderm, Graneodin, Maxitrol, Mycifradin, Naseptin, Neo-Cortef, Neo-Medrone Cream, neomycin cream BPC, neomycin eye drops, Neosporin, Nivemycin, Otomize, Otosporin, Predsol (-N), Synalar (-N), Tri-Adcortyl, Tri-Adcortyl Otic, Vistamethasone (-N)**

---

neomycin cream BPC

A cream used as an antibacterial preparation to treat skin infection.

Dose: apply up to 3 times a day. Do not repeat within 3 months. For short-term use only.
Availability: NHS and private private prescription.
Side effects: allergy.
Caution: with large open wounds, and in patients allergic to other similar antibiotics.
Not to be used for:
Caution needed with:
Contains: NEOMYCIN cream BPC.
Other preparations:

---

neomycin elixir *see* **Mycifradin**

---

neomycin eye drops

Drops used as an aminoglycoside antibiotic to treat bacterial infections of the eye.

Dose: adults 1 or more drops into the eye as needed; children 1 drop into the eye as needed.
Availability: NHS and private prescription.
Side effects:
Caution:
Not to be used for:
Caution needed with:
Contains: NEOMYCIN sulphate.
Other preparations: Neomycin Minims. MYCIGUENT.

Neoral *see* Sandimmun
(Sandoz)

Neosporin
(Cusi)

Drops used as an antibiotic to treat eye infections, prevention of eye infections before and after eye operations, removal of foreign bodies from the eye.

Dose: 1-2 drops 2-4 times a day or more often if needed.
Availability: NHS and private prescription.
Side effects:
Caution: in patients suffering from existing eye defect.
Not to be used for:
Caution needed with:
Contains: POLYMYXIN B SULPHATE, NEOMYCIN sulphate, GRAMICIDIN.
Other preparations:

---

neostigmine *see* Prostigmin

Neotigason
(Roche)

A brown/white capsule or brown/yellow capsule according to strengths of 10 mg, 25 mg, and used to treat severe extensive psoriasis and other related skin disorders.

Dose: initially 25-30 mg once a day, increasing to a maximum of 75 mg a day if needed, and then usually 25-50 mg a day for a maximum of 6 months.
Availability: NHS and private prescription.
Side effects: dryness, erosion of mucous membranes, hair loss, itching,

liver disorder, blood changes, nausea, headache, drowsiness, sweating, joint or muscle pain, thickening of bones, sensitivity to light, changes in blood lipids, reddened skin.

Caution: in patients suffering from diabetes. Women of child-bearing age must use effective contraception during treatment and for 2 years afterwards. Blood must not be donated during treatment or for 1 year afterwards. Your doctor may advise regular tests and examinations.

Not to be used for: children, pregnant women, nursing mothers, or for patients suffering from kidney or liver damage.

Caution needed with: alcohol, sedatives, high doses of VITAMIN A, METHOTREXATE, some antibiotics.

Contains: ACITRETIN.

Other preparations:

Nephril
(Pfizer)

A white, scored tablet supplied at a strength of 1 mg and used as a DIURETIC to treat fluid retention, high blood pressure.

Dose: ½–4 tablets a day.

Availability: NHS and private prescription.

Side effects: low potassium levels, rash, sensitivity to light, blood changes, gout, tiredness, loss of appetite, impotence, pancreatitis, dizziness, upset stomach.

Caution: in the elderly, pregnant women, nursing mothers, and in patients suffering from diabetes, liver or kidney disease, gout, SLE. Potassium supplements may be needed. Your doctor may advise regular blood and urine tests.

Not to be used for: children or patients suffering from kidney or liver failure, raised calcium levels, Addison's disease, allergy to some antibiotics.

Caution needed with: DIGOXIN, LITHIUM, blood-pressure lowering drugs, STEROIDS, CARBENOXOLONE, NON-STEROIDAL ANTI-INFLAMMATORY DRUGS, antidiabetics, BARBITURATES, alcohol, opiate ANALGESICS.

Contains: POLYTHIAZIDE.

Other preparations:

Nericur
(Schering Healthcare)

A gel, available in 2 strengths, and used as an anti-bacterial, skin softener to treat acne.

Dose: wash and dry the affected area, then apply the gel once a day. Start

with the weaker-strength product and go on to the stronger one if necessary.
Availability: NHS, private prescription, over the counter.
Side effects: irritation, peeling.
Caution: in patients with sensitive skin (reduce frequency of application). Keep out of the eyes, nose, mouth. May bleach fabrics.
Not to be used for: children.
Caution needed with:
Contains: BENZOYL PEROXIDE.
Other preparations: ACETOXYL, ACNECIDE, ACNEGEL, BENOXYL, PANOXYL, QUINODERM. (Other brands also available over the counter.)

Nerisone
(Schering Healthcare)

A cream used as a strong STEROID treatment for skin disorders.

Dose: apply to the affected area 2-3 times a day reducing to once a day as soon as possible.
Availability: NHS and private prescription.
Side effects: fluid retention, suppression of adrenal glands, thinning of the skin may occur.
Caution: do not use for longer than 3 weeks for children under 4 years; do not use for prolonged periods for other patients, especially on the face.
Not to be used for: patients suffering from acne or any other skin infections caused by tuberculosis, ringworm, viruses, or fungi, leg ulcers, scabies, or continuously especially in pregnant women.
Caution needed with:
Contains: DIFLUCORTOLONE VALERATE.
Other preparations: Nerisone Oily Cream, Nerisone Ointment, Nerisone Forte.

Neulactil
(Rhône-Poulenc Rorer)

A yellow, scored tablet supplied at strengths of 2.5 mg, 10 mg, and used as a sedative to treat behavioural and character problems, schizophrenia, anxiety, tension, agitation.

Dose: elderly 15-30 mg a day at first; adults 15-75 mg a day at first, then increased to a maximum of 300 mg a day if needed; children as advised by physician.
Availability: NHS and private prescription.
Side effects: muscle spasms, restlessness, hands shaking, constipation, blurred vision, dry mouth, stuffy nose, urine retention, palpitations, low

N

blood pressure, weight gain, changes in sexual function, low body temperature, breast swelling, menstrual changes, jaundice, blood and skin changes, drowsiness, tiredness, rarely fits, heart disorders.
Caution: in pregnant women, nursing mothers, and the elderly in very hot or cold weather.
Not to be used for: unconscious patients, or for patients suffering from heart failure, bone marrow depression, liver or kidney disorder, epilepsy, Parkinson's disease, underactive thyroid, glaucoma, enlarged prostate.
Caution needed with: alcohol, sedatives, tranquillizers, pain killers, blood-pressure lowering drugs, antidepressants, anticonvulsants, antidiabetic drugs, LEVODOPA.
Contains: PERICYAZINE.
Other preparations: Neulactil Forte Syrup.

Neurontin
(Parke-Davis)

A white capsule, yellow capsule, or orange capsule according to strengths of 100 mg, 300 mg, 400 mg, and used as an anticonvulsant as an additional treatment for epilepsy.

Dose: 300 mg once a day on day 1, 300 mg twice a day on day 2, then 300 mg 3 times a day on day 3, increasing if necessary to a maximum of 800 mg 3 times a day.
Availability: NHS, private prescription.
Side effects: sleepiness, weakness, dizziness, lack of co-ordination, headache, shaking, nausea, vomiting, rhinitis, poor eyesight, involuntary eye movements, double vision.
Caution: in pregnant women, nursing mothers, the elderly, and in patients suffering from kidney disorder, or who are on dialysis. Withdraw gradually.
Not to be used for: children.
Caution needed with: ANTACIDS, alcohol, sedatives.
Contains: GABAPENTIN.
Other preparations:

---

nicardipine *see* Cardene

---

niclosamide *see* Yomesan

Niconil
(Elan)

A skin patch supplied at strengths of 11 mg, 22 mg per 24 hours, and used as a nicotine replacement aid to giving up smoking.

Dose: 1 22 mg patch applied once a day for the first 4 weeks, then an 11 mg patch once a day for 2 weeks. (Maximum treatment period of 3 months.) Apply one patch at a time to a different area of of non-hairy skin on the trunk or upper arm. Stop smoking when starting treatment and dispose of used patches carefully. Replace patches at 24-hour intervals.
Availability: private prescription, over the counter.
Side effects: headache, nausea, dizziness; reactions at the site of the patch, sleeplessness (stop treatment if severe).
Caution: in patients suffering from raised blood pressure, stomach ulcer, underactive thyroid gland, diabetes, PHAEOCHROMOCYTOMA, or with a history of heart, brain, or hormonal disorders. Stop smoking completely when treatment starts.
Not to be used for: children, pregnant women, nursing mothers, or for patients suffering from skin diseases, recent heart attack, severe abnormal heart rhythm, angina, reduced blood flow to the brain.
Caution needed with: CAFFEINE, THEOPHYLLINE, IMIPRAMINE, PENTAZOCINE, GLUTETHAMIDE, DEXTROPROPOXYPHENE, FRUSEMIDE, HYDROCORTISONE, PROPANOLOL.
Contains: NICOTINE.
Other preparations: NICOTINELL.

---

nicorandil *see* Ikorel

Nicorette Gum
(Pharmacia)

Chewing gum supplied at strengths of 2 mg, and used as a nicotine-replacement aid to end smoking addiction.

Dose: chew 1 piece slowly for 30 minutes when required, up to a maximum of 15 pieces a day, and withdraw gradually after 3 months.
Availability: private prescription and over the counter.
Side effects: addiction, hiccups, indigestion, irritated throat, increased saliva, headache, dizziness, palpitations.
Caution: in patients with a history of stomach ulcer, gastric inflammation, angina, recent heart attack, or suffering from coronary disease, stroke, severe abnormal heart rhythm, high blood pressure, circulatory disorders, diabetes, PHAEOCHROMCYTOMA, severe kidney disorder, angina, gastritis, stomach ulcer.
Not to be used for: children, pregnant women, nursing mothers.
Caution needed with: WARFARIN, INSULIN, PARACETAMOL, CAFFEINE, IMIPRAMINE, PENTAZOCINE, OXAZEPAM, THEOPHYLLINE, AMINOPHYLLINE, some drugs used to treat high blood pressure.
Contains: NICOTINE.

Other preparations: Nicorette nasal spray (also available on NHS), Nicorette Plus 4 mg, Nicorette patches (left in place for 18 hours). NICONIL, NICOTINELL, (other brands also available over the counter).

nicotinamide *see* nicotinamide tablets, vitamin B₃

nicotinamide tablets

A tablet supplied at a strength of 50 mg and used to treat vitamin B_3 deficiency.

Dose: as advised by a doctor.
Availability: NHS and private prescription.
Side effects:
Caution:
Not to be used for:
Caution needed with:
Contains: VITAMIN B₃.
Other preparations: NICOTINIC ACID TABLETS.

nicotine *see* Niconil, Nicorette, Nicotinell

Nicotinell
(Zyma Healthcare)

A patch supplied at sizes 10 cm, 20 cm, 30 cm, and used to treat nicotine addiction as an aid to giving up smoking.

Dose: apply a patch to a clean, non-hairy dry area of skin on upper arm or trunk. Change daily. Patch size depends on number of cigarettes smoked. Reduce patch size at monthly intervals. Maximum daily dose 30 cm. Maximum treatment period 3 months.
Availability: private prescription and over the counter.
Side effects: skin reactions.
Caution: in patients suffering from high blood pressure, angina, blood vessel disease, heart failure, overactive thyroid, diabetes, kidney or liver disorder, stomach ulcer. Stop smoking completely when starting treatment. Dispose of patches carefully.
Not to be used for: pregnant women, nursing mothers, children under 18 years, or for patients suffering from heart attack, uncontrolled angina, severe heart rhythm disorder, recent stroke, skin disease. Also not suitable for occasional smokers.
Caution needed with: THEOPHYLLINE, WARFARIN, INSULIN.

Contains: NICOTINE.
Other preparations: Nicotinell chewing gum. NICONIL, NICORETTE.

nicotinic acid *see* nicotine acid tablets, vitamin B₃

nicotinic acid tablets

Tablets supplied at a strength of 50 mg and used as a lipid-lowering agent to treat high blood lipid levels.

Dose: adults, 2-4 tablets 3 times a day, increased if necessary to 20-40 tablets 3 times a day.
Availability: NHS, private prescription, over the counter.
Side effects: flushing, dizziness, headache, irregular heartbeat, itching, nausea, vomiting, liver disorder, rash.
Caution: in patients suffering from diabetes, gout, liver disease, stomach ulcer.
Not to be used for: pregnant women, nursing mothers.
Caution needed with:
Contains: NICOTINIC ACID (VITAMIN B₃)
Other preparations:

nicotinyl alcohol tartrate *see* Ronicol

nicoumalone *see* Sinthrome

nifedipine *see* Adalat, Adalat Retard, Angiopine, Beta Adalat, Calanif, Calcilat, Cardilate MR, Coracten, Hypolar Retard, nifedipine capsules, nifedipine modified release, Tenif

nifedipine capsules

An orange, liquid-filled capsule supplied at a strength of 5 mg and 10 mg, and used as a calcium antagonist treatment for angina, and to treat Raynaud's phenomenon.

Dose: for angina, 10 mg 3 times a day at first, then according to response up to 60 mg a day with or after food. (The capsule may be bitten for immediate effect.) For Raynaud's phenomenon, 10-20 mg 3 times a day with or after food.
Availability: NHS and private prescription.

Side effects: headache, flushes, fluid retention, dizziness, chest pain, gum swelling, rash, eye pain, depression, tiredness, abnormal heart rate, nausea, increased frequency of passing urine.
Caution: in nursing mothers and in patients with weak hearts, liver disease, low blood pressure, or diabetes.
Not to be used for: children, pregnant women, or for patients suffering from PORPHYRIA.
Caution needed with: blood-pressure lowering drugs, CIMETIDINE, QUINIDINE, RIFAMPICIN, DIGOXIN, CYCLOSPORIN, some anticonvulsants, SYMPATHOMIMETICS.
Contains: NIFEDIPINE.
Other preparations: ADALAT CAPSULES, BETA ADALAT, CALCILAT. (For longer-acting products *see* nifedipine modified release.)

---

nifedipine modified release

An long-acting tablet or capsule supplied at strengths of 10 mg, 20 mg, 30 mg, and used as a calcium-antagonist ANTIHYPERTENSIVE to treat high blood pressure and to prevent angina.

Dose: 20-40 mg a day adjusted according to response. (Usual maximum 80-100 mg a day.) Doses may be supplied once a day or divided into two 12-hourly doses depending on brand supplied.
Availability: NHS and private prescription.
Side effects: headache, flushes, fluid retention, dizziness, chest pain, gum swelling, rash, eye pain, depression, tiredness, abnormal heart rate, nausea, increased frequency of passing urine.
Caution: in nursing mothers and in patients with weak hearts, liver or kidney disease, low blood pressure, bowel disorder, or diabetes.
Not to be used for: children, pregnant women, or for patients suffering from PORPHYRIA.
Caution needed with: blood-pressure lowering drugs, CIMETIDINE, QUINIDINE, RIFAMPICIN, DIGOXIN, CYCLOSPORIN, some anticonvulsants, SYMPATHOMIMETICS.
Contains: NIFEDIPINE.
Other preparations: NIFEDIPINE CAPSULES. ADALAT LA, ADALAT RETARD, CARDILATE MR, CORACTEN, HYPOLAR RETARD, NIFELEASE, NIFENSAR XL.

Nifelease *see* nifedipine modified release
(Lennon)

Nifensar XL *see* nifedipine modified release
(Rhône-Poulenc Rorer)

Niferex
(Tillomed)

An elixir used as an iron supplement to treat iron-deficiency anaemia.

Dose: adults treatment 5 ml 1-2 times a day, prevention 2.5 ml a day; children 0-2 years 1 drop of paediatric elixir per 0.45 kg bodyweight a day, 2-6 years 2.5 ml a day, 6-12 years 5 ml a day.
Availability: NHS, private prescription, and over the counter.
Side effects:
Caution: in patients with a history of stomach ulcer.
Not to be used for:
Caution needed with: some antibiotics, ANTACIDS, LEVODOPA.
Contains: POLYSACCHARIDE-IRON COMPLEX.
Other preparations: Niferex-150 Capsules, Niferex Paediatric Elixir (available on NHS only for treating premature babies).

---

nimodipine *see* Nimotop

Nimotop
(Bayer)

A white tablet supplied at a strength of 30 mg and used to treat symptoms following stroke.

Dose: 2 tablets every 4 hours for 21 days.
Availability: NHS and private prescription.
Side effects: low blood pressure, flushing, headache, changes in heart rate, stomach upset.
Caution: in pregnant women and in patients suffering from fluid retention in the brain or high blood pressure in the brain, kidney damage, cirrhosis of the liver
Not to be used for: children.
Caution needed with: ß-BLOCKERS, other similar drugs, anticonvulsants, CIMETIDINE.
Contains: NIMODIPINE.
Other preparations: Nimotop Infusion.

Nindaxa see indapamide tablets
(Ashbourne)

Nitoman
(Lifehealth)

A yellow/buff, scored tablet supplied at a strength of 25 mg and used as a sedative to treat Huntington's chorea, hemiballismus, senile chorea (movement disorders).

Dose: 1 tablet 3 times a day at first increasing if needed by 1 tablet a day every 3-4 days to a maximum of 8 tablets a day.
Availability: NHS and private prescription.
Side effects: drowsiness, depression, low blood pressure on standing, tremor, rigidity.
Caution: in pregnant women.
Not to be used for: children or for nursing mothers.
Caution needed with: alcohol, sedatives, RESERPINE, LEVODOPA, MAOIS.
Contains: TETRABENAZINE.
Other preparations:

---

nitrate
a drug used to treat poor blood supply to the heart muscle (angina). Nitrates reduce the work which the heart has to do. Example GLYCERYL TRINITRATE *see* Suscard Buccal.

---

nitrazepam *see* Mogadon, nitrazepam tablets

---

nitrazepam tablets

A tablet supplied at a strength of 5 mg and used as a sleeping tablet for the short-term treatment of sleeplessness.

Dose: elderly ½-1 tablet before going to bed; adults 1-2 tablets before going to bed.
Availability: NHS and private prescription.
Side effects: drowsiness (which may persist the next day), confusion, forgetfulness, unsteadiness. Rarely low blood pressure, rash, headache, changes in vision, interference with sexual function, retention of urine, liver and blood changes. Risk of addiction increases with dose and length of treatment. May impair judgement.
Caution: in the elderly, pregnant women, nursing mothers, and in patients suffering from lung disorders, kidney or liver disorders, PORPHYRIA, personality problems, history of drug or alcohol abuse. Avoid long-term use and withdraw gradually.
Not to be used for: children, or for patients suffering from acute lung diseases, some chronic lung diseases, some obsessional and psychotic

diseases.
Caution needed with: alcohol, sedatives, other tranquillizers, anticonvulsants, opiate ANALGESICS, CIMETIDINE, RIFAMPICIN.
Contains: NITRAZEPAM.
Other preparations: nitrazepam oral suspension. MOGADON, REMNOS, SOMNITE, UNISOMNIA (none available on NHS).

Nitro-Dur see Transiderm-Nitro
(Schering-Plough)

Nitrocontin Continus see glyceryl trinitrate tablets
(ASTA Medica)

---

nitrofurantoin see Furadantin, Macrobid, Macrodantin, nitrofurantoin tablets

---

nitrofurantoin tablets

A tablet supplied at strengths of 50 mg, 100 mg and used as an antiseptic to treat infection of the urinary tract.

Dose: adults treatment 50-100 mg 4 times a day with food or milk for 7 days, prevention 50-100 mg a day; children over 3 months use suspension.
Availability: NHS and private prescription.
Side effects: stomach upset, anorexia, allergy, jaundice, nerve inflammation, blood changes, possible liver damage, hair loss, lung disorders, rash, itching, brown-coloured urine, joint disorders.
Caution: in patients suffering from anaemia, diabetes, electrolyte imbalance, VITAMIN B deficiency, lung disease, liver disorders.
Not to be used for: infants under 3 months, pregnant women, nursing mothers or for patients suffering from kidney problems resulting in reduced urine output, PORPHYRIA.
Caution needed with: MAGNESIUM TRISILICATE, PROBENECID.
Contains: NITROFURANTOIN.
Other preparations: FURADANTIN (also available as suspension), MACROBID, (long-acting capsule), MACRODANTIN.

Nitrolingual see Coro-Nitro
(Lipha)

Nivaquine
(Rhône-Poulenc Rorer)

A yellow tablet supplied at a strength of 150 mg and used as an antimalarial drug for the prevention and treatment of malaria, and to treat rheumatoid arthritis.

Dose: prevention of malaria adults 2 tablets on the same day once a week (start 1 week before entering endemic area and continue for 4 weeks after leaving); treatment as advised by the physician; Children use Nivaquine Syrup. Rheumatoid arthritis, adults 1 tablet a day.
Availability: NHS, private prescription, and over the counter if for prevention of malaria.
Side effects: headache, stomach upset, skin eruptions, hair loss, eye disorders, blood disorders, loss of pigment, allergy.
Caution: in pregnant women, nursing mothers, or in patients suffering from PORPHYRIA, kidney or liver disease, severe gastro-intestinal, nervous, or blood disorder, psoriasis or history of epilepsy. The eyes should be tested before and during prolonged treatment.
Not to be used for:
Caution needed with:
Contains: CHLOROQUINE sulphate.
Other preparations: Nivaquine Syrup, Nivaquine Injection. AVOCLOR.

Nivemycin
(Knoll)

A tablet supplied at a strength of 500 mg and used as an aminoglycoside antibiotic for preparation before bowel surgery, and as an additional treatment in liver disease coma.

Dose: adults 2 tablets every hour for 4 hours, then 2 tablets every 4 hours for 2-3 days; children 6-12 years ½-1 tablet every 4 hours for 2-3 days, over 12 years 2 tablets every 4 hours for 2-3 days.
Availability: NHS and private prescription.
Side effects: stomach disturbances.
Caution: in patients suffering from kidney or liver damage, Parkinson's disease, damaged hearing.
Not to be used for: children under 6 years, or for patients suffering from a blockage of the intestine.
Caution needed with:
Contains: NEOMYCIN sulphate.
Other preparations: MYCIFRADIN, NEOMYCIN ELIXIR.

---

nizatidine *see* **Axid**

Nizoral
(Janssen-Cilag)

A white scored tablet supplied at a strength of 200 mg and used as an anti-fungal treatment for severe fungus infections, including persistent vaginal thrush, and to prevent fungal infections in patients with a weak immune system.

Dose: adults 1-2 tablets a day with meals until at least 1 week after symptoms have gone; children use suspension.
Availability: NHS and private prescription
Side effects: liver disorders, allergy, stomach upset, rash, headache, blood changes, rarely breast enlargement.
Caution: liver should be checked regularly.
Not to be used for: pregnant women, patients with any form of liver disorder.
Caution needed with: ANTICHOLINERGICS, ANTACIDS, ASTEMIZOLE, CIMETIDINE, RANITIDINE, ANTICOAGULANTS, PHENYTOIN, RIFAMPICIN, CYCLOSPORIN, TERFENADINE, CISAPRIDE, CIMETIDINE, NIZATADINE, FAMOTIDINE.
Contains: KETOCONAZOLE.
Other preparations: NIZORAL CREAM, Nizoral Suspension.

Nizoral Cream
(Janssen)

A cream used as an antifungal treatment for fungus infections, skin thrush, seborrhoeic dermatitis.

Dose: apply to the affected area 1-2 times a day.
Availability: NHS and private prescription.
Side effects: irritation.
Caution:
Not to be used for:
Caution needed with:
Contains: KETOCONAZOLE.
Other preparations: Nizoral Shampoo (for scalp infections).

Noctec
(Squibb)

A liquid-filled, red capsule supplied at a strength of 500 mg and used as a sedative to treat sleeplessness.

N

Dose: usually 1-2 capsules taken with water 15-30 minutes before going to bed; maximum dose 4 capsules a day.
Availability: NHS and private prescription.
Side effects: stomach irritation, headache, excitement, delirium, skin allergies, ketones in the urine.
Caution: in patients suffering from PORPHYRIA. Patients should be warned of reduced judgement and abilities.
Not to be used for: children, pregnant women, nursing mothers, or for patients suffering from severe heart, liver, or kidney disease, or gastric inflammation.
Caution needed with: alcohol, sedatives, ANTICOAGULANTS.
Contains: CHLORAL HYDRATE.
Other preparations: WELLDORM.

NODS Tropicamide
(Chauvin)

Sterile ophthalmic applicator strips supplied at a strength of 125 micrograms and used as a short-acting ANTICHOLINERGIC preparation to dilate the pupil and paralyse the ciliary muscle of the eye in ophthalmic procedures.

Dose: 1 unit into the eye repeated after 30-45 minutes if necessary.
Availability: NHS, private prescription.
Side effects:
Caution: do not drive or operate machinery while affected.
Not to be used for: patients suffering from narrow-angle glaucoma.
Caution needed with:
Contains: TROPICAMIDE.
Other preparations: MYDRIACYL, TROPICAMIDE MINIMS.

Nolvadex-D *see* tamoxifen tablets
(Zeneca)

---

non-steroidal anti-inflammatory drug (NSAID)
an antirheumatic preparation which has pain-killing properties. An NSAID may cause stomach upsets. Example IBUPROFEN *see* ibuprofen tablets.

---

nonoxynol-9 *see* Delfen, Duragel, Gynol II, Ortho-Creme, Staycept

---

466

Nordox *see* **doxycycline capsules**
(Panpharma)

---

norethisterone *see* **BiNovum, Brevinor, Climagest, Estracombi, Estrapak, Evorel-Pak, Kliofem, Loestrin 20, Menophase, Menzol, Micronor, Micronor-HRT, Neocon 1/35, norethisterone tablets, Noriday, Norimin, Norinyl-1, Noristerat, Ortho-Novin 1/50, Ovysmen, Primolut N, Synphase, Trinovum, Trinovum-ED, Trisequens, Utovlan**

---

norethisterone tablets

A tablet supplied at a strength of 5 mg and used as a progestogen treatment for postponing menstruation, and for other menstrual and womb disorders (such as endometriosis, painful or heavy periods).

Dose: usually 1 tablet 2-3 times a day.
Availability: NHS and private prescription.
Side effects: liver disturbances, masculinization, may make epilepsy or migraine worse, acne, itch, fluid retention, weight change, stomach upset, breast discomfort, premenstrual symptoms, changes in sexual function, irregular periods, mood changes, sleeplessness, hair growth or loss, allergy.
Caution: in patients suffering from epilepsy or migraine, diabetes, high blood pressure, heart or kidney disease.
Not to be used for: children, pregnant women, or patients suffering from severe liver disease, undiagnosed vaginal bleeding, severe circulation problems, PORPHYRIA some cancers.
Caution needed with: CYCLOSPORIN.
Contains: NORETHISTERONE.
Other preparations: PRIMOLUT-N, UTOVLAN.

---

norfloxacin *see* **Utinor**

Norgalax *see* **Fletchers' Enemette**
(Norgine)

---

norgestimate *see* **Cilest**

Norgeston
(Schering Healthcare)

A white tablet used as a progesterone contraceptive.

Dose: 1 tablet at the same time every day starting on day 1 of the period.
Availability: NHS and over the counter.
Side effects: irregular bleeding, breast discomfort, acne, headache, rarely thrombosis, raised blood pressure, jaundice.
Caution: in patients suffering from high blood pressure, tendency to thrombosis, migraine, some cancers, liver abnormalities, ovarian cysts. Your doctor may advise regular check-ups.
Not to be used for: pregnant women, or for patients suffering from severe heart or artery disease, benign liver tumours, vaginal bleeding, previous ectopic pregnancy.
Caution needed with: BARBITURATES, PHENYTOIN, PRIMIDONE, CARBAMAZEPINE, CHLORAL HYDRATE, ETHOSUXIMIDE, RIFAMPICIN, CHLORPROMAZINE, MEPROBAMATE, GRISEOFULVIN.
Contains: LEVONORGESTREL.
Other preparations: MICROVAL.

---

norgestrel *see* **Cyclo-Progynova, Neogest, Ovran, Ovranette, Ovysmen, PC4, Prempak-C.** *See also* **levonorgestrel.**

Noriday
(Roche)

A white tablet used as a progesterone contraceptive.

Dose: 1 tablet at the same time every day starting on day 1 of the period.
Availability: NHS and private prescription.
Side effects: irregular bleeding, breast discomfort, acne, headache, rarely thrombosis, raised blood pressure, jaundice.
Caution: in patients suffering from high blood pressure, tendency to thrombosis, migraine, some cancers, liver abnormalities, ovarian cysts. Your doctor may advise regular check-ups.
Not to be used for: pregnant women, or for patients suffering from severe heart or artery disease, benign liver tumours, vaginal bleeding, previous ectopic pregnancy.
Caution needed with: BARBITURATES, PHENYTOIN, PRIMIDONE, CARBAMAZEPINE, CHLORAL HYDRATE, ETHOSUXIMIDE, RIFAMPICIN, CHLORPROMAZINE, MEPROBAMATE, GRISEOFULVIN.
Contains: NORETHISTERONE.
Other preparations: MICRONOR.

Norimin
(Roche)

A yellow tablet used as an oestrogen, progestogen contraceptive.

Dose: 1 tablet a day for 21 days starting on day 5 of the period.
Availability: NHS and private prescription.
Side effects: enlarged breasts, bloating and fluid retention, cramps, leg pains, mood change, reduction in sexual desire, headaches, nausea, vaginal erosion, discharge, and bleeding, weight gain, skin changes, rarely thrombosis, raised blood pressure, jaundice.
Caution: in patients suffering from high blood pressure, diabetes, vascular disorders, asthma, depression, kidney disease, multiple sclerosis, womb diseases. Your doctor may advise you not to smoke, to have regular examinations. You should stop treatment at the first sign of serious symptoms such as severe headache or jaundice. Treatment should be stopped before surgery.
Not to be used for: pregnant women, or for patients suffering from sickle-cell anaemia, history of heart disease or thrombosis, liver disorders, some cancers, undiagnosed vaginal bleeding, some ear, skin, and kidney disorders.
Caution needed with: RIFAMPICIN, TETRACYCLINE ANTIBIOTICS, GRISEOFULVIN, BARBITURATES, PHENYTOIN, PRIMIDONE, CARBAMAZEPINE, ETHOSUXIMIDE, CHLORAL HYDRATE.
Contains: ETHINYLOESTRADIOL, NORETHISTERONE.
Other preparations: NEOCON 1/35.

Norimode *see* loperamide capsules
(Tillomed)

Norinyl-1
(Syntex)

A white tablet used as an oestrogen, progestogen contraceptive.

Dose: 1 tablet a day for 21 days starting on day 5 of the period.
Availability: NHS and private prescription.
Side effects: enlarged breasts, bloating and fluid retention, cramps, leg pains, mood change, reduction in sexual desire, headaches, nausea, vaginal erosion, discharge, and bleeding, weight gain, skin changes, rarely thrombosis, raised blood pressure, jaundice.
Caution: in patients suffering from high blood pressure, diabetes, vascular disorders, asthma, depression, kidney disease, multiple sclerosis, womb diseases. Your doctor may advise you not to smoke, to have regular examinations. You should stop treatment at the first sign of serious

symptoms such as severe headache or jaundice. Treatment should be stopped before surgery.

Not to be used for: pregnant women, or for patients suffering from sickle-cell anaemia, history of heart disease or thrombosis, liver disorders, some cancers, undiagnosed vaginal bleeding, some ear, skin, and kidney disorders.

Caution needed with: RIFAMPICIN, TETRACYCLINE ANTIBIOTICS, GRISEOFULVIN, BARBITURATES, PHENYTOIN, PRIMIDONE, CARBAMAZEPINE, ETHOSUXIMIDE, CHLORAL HYDRATE.

Contains: MESTRANOL, NORETHISTERONE.

Other preparations: ORTHO NOVIN 1/50.

Normacol
(Norgine)

White granules in 7 g sachets or supplied as as 500 g and used as a bulking agent to treat constipation caused by lack of fibre in the diet.

Dose: adults 1-2 sachets or 1-2 heaped 5 ml spoonsful once or twice a day after meals swallowed with liquid; children half adult dose.

Availability: NHS, private prescription, over the counter.

Side effects:

Caution: do not take at bedtime

Not to be used for: patients suffering from blocked intestine, faecal impaction, inelastic colon.

Caution needed with:

Contains: STERCULIA.

Other preparations: Normacol Plus (also contains FRANGULA – used with caution in pregnancy).

Normasol
(Seton Healthcare)

A solution in a sachet used for washing out eyes, burns, wounds.

Dose: use as needed.

Availability: NHS, private prescription, over the counter.

Side effects:

Caution:

Not to be used for:

Caution needed with:

Contains: SODIUM CHLORIDE.

Other preparations: STERIPOD BLUE.

Normax
(Evans)

A brown capsule used as a stimulant and faecal softener to treat constipation in the elderly, in patients being treated with pain-killers, and those with heart failure or coronary thrombosis.

Dose: adults 1-3 capsules at night as required; children over 6 years 1 capsule at night.
Availability: NHS (when prescribed as a generic) and private prescription.
Side effects:
Caution: in pregnant women, nursing mothers.
Not to be used for: children under 6 years or for patients suffering from an obstruction of the intestine.
Caution needed with:
Contains: DANTHRON, DOCUSATE sodium.
Other preparations:

Normegon
(Organon)

An injection used as a hormone treatment for male and female infertility, and to induce ovulation for in-vitro fertilization treatment.

Dose: as advised by a doctor.
Availability: NHS and private prescription.
Side effects: rash, multiple pregnancy, miscarriage.
Caution: tests may be required before and throughout treatment.
Not to be used for: children, or for patients with some cancers.
Caution needed with:
Contains: HUMAN MENOPAUSAL GONADOTROPHINS.
Other preparations: HUMEGON.

Normison *see* tamazepam capsules
(Wyeth)

Norplant
(Hoechst Roussel)

An implant used as a long-term, reversible means of contraception for women.

Dose: six implants inserted beneath the skin (implants should be removed within 5 years).

Availability: NHS, private prescription.
Side effects: menstrual changes, spotting, vaginal bleeding, local reactions, ovarian cysts, headache, nausea, weight gain, hair loss or growth, enlargement of the sexual organs.
Caution: in patients suffering migraine, raised blood pressure,where there is a risk of arterial disease, raised blood pressure to the brain. Your doctor will advise regular check-ups.
Not to be used for: pregnant women or for patients suffering from liver disease, undiagnosed bleeding from the vagina, recent disease of the uterine wall, or with a history of severe arterial disease, blood clots, heart disease, some cancers.
Caution needed with: CARBAMAZEPINE, BARBITURATES, PHENYTOIN, PRIMIDONE, RIFAMPICIN, GRISEOFULVIN.
Contains: LEVONORGESTREL.
Other preparations:

Norprolac
(Sandoz)

A pink tablet, blue tablet, or white tablet according to strengths of 25 micrograms, 50 mcg, 75 mcg, 150 mcg and used as a hormone treatment for infertility.

Dose: 25 mcg once a day at bedtime for the first 3 days, increasing to 50 mcg once a day for the next 3 days, then 75 mcg a day up to 150 mcg a day if needed.
Availability: NHS, private prescription.
Side effects: mental disturbances, low blood pressure, blocked nose, flushing, fluid retention, sleeplessness, stomach upset, tiredness, dizziness, headache, nausea, loss of appetite.
Caution: in patients with a history of mental disorders. Your doctor will advise you to stop treatment if you become pregnant.
Not to be used for: children or for patients suffering from kidney or liver disorder.
Caution needed with: tranquillizers, alcohol.
Contains: QUINAGOLIDE hydrochloride.
Other preparations:

---

nortriptyline *see* Allegron, Motipress, Motival

NOVA-T
(Schering Health Care)

A copper wire with silver core on a plastic T-shaped carrier used as an intra-uterine device to prevent conception.

Dose: as advised. Replace after 5 years.
Availability: NHS, private prescription.
Side effects: pelvic infection, pain, abnormal bleeding, perforation of the uterus. On insertion, persistent low heart rate, asthma attack, epileptic attack.
Caution: in patients suffering from anaemia, heavy periods, diabetes, epilepsy, or who have had inflammatory heart conditions or pelvic inflammatory disease, or who are risk from sexually transmitted diseases. Patients should be checked 3 months after insertion and then annually.
Not to be used for: children, pregnant women, or for patients suffering from allergy to copper, abnormal uterus, severe infections, acute pelvic inflammatory disease, endometrial disease, abnormal vaginal bleeding, or some other urinogenital tract disorders, or with a history of ectopic pregnancies.
Caution needed with: ANTICOAGULANTS.
Contains: copper wire.
Other preparations: MULTILOAD, NOVAGARD, ORTHO-GYNE-T.

Novagard
(Pharmacia)

A copper wire with silver core on a plastic T-shaped carrier used as an intra-uterine device to prevent conception.

Dose: as advised. Replace after 5 years.
Availability: NHS, private prescription.
Side effects: pelvic infection, pain, abnormal bleeding, perforation of the uterus. On insertion, persistent low heart rate, asthma attack, epileptic attack.
Caution: in patients suffering from anaemia, heavy periods, diabetes, epilepsy or who have had inflammatory heart conditions or pelvic inflammatory disease, or who are at risk from sexually transmitted diseases. Patients should be checked 3 months after insertion and then annually.
Not to be used for: children, pregnant women, or for patients suffering from allergy to copper, abnormal uterus, severe infections, acute pelvic inflammatory disease, endometrial disease, abnormal vaginal bleeding, or some other urinogenital tract disorders, or with a history of ectopic pregnancies.
Caution needed with: ANTICOAGULANTS.
Contains: copper wire.
Other preparations: MULTILOAD, NOVA-T, ORTHO-GYNE-T.

Nozinan
(Link)

A white, scored tablet supplied at a strength of 25 mg, and used as a sedative to treat schizophrenia and other mental disorders, and to treat severe pain accompanied by restlessness, distress, or vomiting.

Dose: 25-200 mg a day.
Availability: NHS and private prescription.
Side effects: muscle spasms, restlessness, hands shaking, constipation, blurred vision, dry mouth, stuffy nose, urine retention, palpitations, low blood pressure, weight gain, changes in sexual function, low body temperature, breast swelling, menstrual changes, jaundice, blood and skin changes, drowsiness, tiredness, fits, heart disorder.
Caution: in pregnant women, nursing mothers, and in patients suffering from heart or circulation disease, liver damage, Parkinson's disease, or epilepsy.
Not to be used for: children, or for patients with bone marrow disorder, or who are in a coma.
Caution needed with: alcohol, sedatives, tranquillizers, pain killers, blood-pressure lowering drugs, antidepressants, anticonvulsants, antidiabetics, LEVODOPA.
Contains: METHOTRIMEPRAZINE.
Other preparations:

Nu-Seals Aspirin *see* aspirin 300 mg tablets
(Eli Lilly)

Nu-Seals 75 mg *see* aspirin 75 mg tablets
(Eli Lilly)

Nuelin
(3M Health Care)

A white tablet supplied at a strength of 125 mg, and used as a BRONCHODILATOR to treat bronchial spasm in bronchitis, asthma, and emphysema.

Dose: adults 1-2 tablets 3-4 times a day after food; children 2-6 years use liquid, 7-12 years half adult dose.
Availability: NHS, private prescription, over the counter.
Side effects: rapid heart rate, stomach upset and nausea, headache, abnormal heart rhythm, sleeplessness.
Caution: in pregnant women, nursing mothers, and in patients suffering

from heart or liver disease, stomach ulcer.
Not to be used for: children under 7 years (tablets) or under 2 years (liquid).
Caution needed with: CIMETIDINE, ERYTHROMYCIN, CIPROFLOXACIN, STEROIDS, DIURETICS, some other asthma treatments.
Contains: THEOPHYLLINE.
Other preparations: Nuelin SA, Nuelin SA-250 (both sustained release tablets), Nuelin Liquid. LASMA, SLO-PHYLLIN, THEO-DUR, UNIPHYLLIN (all long-acting products).

Nuelin SA *see* Nuelin
(3M Health Care)

Nupercainal
(Zyma Healthcare)

An ointment used as a local anaesthetic and a treatment for haemorrhoids.

Dose: apply sparingly up to 3 times a day.
Availability: NHS, private prescription, over the counter.
Side effects:
Caution:
Not to be used for:
Caution needed with:
Contains: CINCHOCAINE.
Other preparations:

Nutraplus *see* Aquadrate
(Novex)

Nutrizym GR
(Merck)

A green/orange capsule used as a source of pancreatic enzymes to treat cystic fibrosis, steatorrhoea, pancreatic disorders.

Dose: 1-2 capsules with meals, adjusted according to response.
Availability: NHS, private prescription, over the counter.
Side effects: irritation in the mouth and around the anus.
Caution:
Not to be used for:
Caution needed with:
Contains: PANCREATIN.

Other preparations: Nutrizym 10, Nutrizym 22. CREON, PANCREASE, PANCREX-V, PANZYTRAT 25000.

Nuvelle *see* **Cyclo-Progynova**
(Schering Health Care)

Nycopren *see* **naproxen tablets**
(Nycomed)

Nyspes *see* **Nystan Pessaries**
(DDSA)

Nystadermal
(Squibb)

A cream used as a strong STEROID and antibacterial treatment for thrush, itch, and eczema.

Dose: apply to the affected area 2-4 times a day.
Availability: NHS and private prescription.
Side effects: fluid retention, suppression of adrenal glands, thinning, spotting, or streaking of the skin may occur.
Caution: use for short periods of time only, especially in children or on the face.
Not to be used for: patients suffering from acne or any other skin infections caused by tuberculosis, ringworm, viruses, or fungi, leg ulcers, scabies, or continuously especially in pregnant women.
Caution needed with:
Contains: NYSTATIN, TRIAMCINOLONE ACETONIDE.
Other preparations:

Nystaform
(Bayer)

A cream used as an antifungal and antibacterial treatment for skin infections or skin conditions where infection may occur.

Dose: apply freely to the affected area 2-3 times a day until 7 days after the wounds have healed.
Availability: NHS and private prescription.
Side effects:
Caution:

476

Not to be used for:
Caution needed with:
Contains: NYSTATIN, CHLORHEXIDINE.
Other preparations:

Nystaform-HC
(Bayer)

A cream used as a STEROID and antifungal treatment for skin disorders where there is also infection.

Dose: apply to the affected area 2-3 times a day until 7 days after the condition has healed.
Availability: NHS and private prescription.
Side effects: fluid retention, suppression of adrenal glands, thinning, spotting, or streaking of the skin may occur.
Caution: use for short periods of time only, especially in children or on the face.
Not to be used for: patients suffering from acne or any other skin infections caused by tuberculosis, ringworm, viruses, or fungi, leg ulcers, scabies, or continuously especially in pregnant women.
Caution needed with:
Contains: NYSTATIN, CHLORHEXIDINE, HYDROCORTISONE.
Other preparations: Nystaform-HC Ointment. TIMODINE.

Nystamont *see* nystatin oral suspension
(Rosemont)

Nystan
(Squibb)

A yellow, diamond-shaped pessary or a brown tablet used as an antifungal treatment for vaginal, oral, or intestinal thrush.

Dose: vaginal thrush 1-2 pessaries into the vagina for at least 14 nights; children use cream. Other infections 1-2 tablets by mouth 4 times a day.
Availability: NHS and private prescription.
Side effects: irritation and burning from pessaries, nausea, vomiting, diarrhoea in high doses of tablets.
Caution: in pregnant women, nursing mothers.
Not to be used for:
Caution needed with:
Contains: NYSTATIN.
Other preparations: Nystan Vaginal Cream, Nystan Gel, Nystan Oral

477

Suspension, Nystan Oral Tablets, Nystan Pastilles (sucked to treat oral thrush).

Nystan Cream
(Squibb)

A cream used as an antifungal treatment for thrush of the skin and mucous membranes.

Dose: apply to the affected area 2-4 times a day.
Availability: NHS and private prescription.
Side effects: irritation and burning.
Caution:
Not to be used for:
Caution needed with:
Contains: NYSTATIN.
Other preparations: Nystan Ointment, Nystan Gel, Nystan Powder.

Nystan Oral Suspension *see* nystatin oral suspension
(Squibb)

nystatin *see* Dermovate (NN), Gregoderm, Nystadermal, Nystaform, Nystaform-HC, Nystamont, Nystan, Nystan Cream, Nystan Oral Suspension, nystatin oral suspension, Terra-Cortril (Nystatin), Timodine, Tinaderm-M, Tri-Adcortyl, Tri-Adcortyl Otic, Trimovate

Nystatin-Dome Oral Suspension *see* nystatin oral suspension
(Lagap)

nystatin oral suspension

A suspension used as an antifungal treatment for oral or intestinal thrush.

Dose: intestinal thrush, adults 5 ml every 6 hours; oral thrush, adults and children 1 ml 4 times a day (hold the dose in the mouth for as long as possible). Continue for 48 hours after healed.
Availability: NHS and private prescription.
Side effects: irritation and burning, rash, nausea, vomiting, diarrhoea in high doses.
Caution:
Not to be used for:

Caution needed with:
Contains: NYSTATIN.
Other preparations: NYSTAMONT, NYSTAN, NYSTATIN-DOME.

Nytol
(Stafford-Miller)

A white, scored tablet supplied at a strength of 25 mg, and used as an antihistamine treatment for relief of temporary sleep disturbance.

Dose: adults over 16 years 2 tablets 20 minutes before bedtime.
Availability: NHS, private prescription, over the counter.
Side effects: drowsiness, dizziness, dry mouth, nausea, nervousness, reduced effect with continuous use, and rarely blood disorders.
Caution: in patients suffering from MYASTHENIA GRAVIS. Causes drowsiness – your doctor should advise you not to drive or operate machinery if affected.
Not to be used for: children under 16 years, pregnant women, nursing mothers, or for patients suffering from asthma, narrow-angle glaucoma, enlarged prostate, some kinds of stomach ulcer, obstruction of the bladder or duodenum.
Caution needed with: other sedating drugs, MAOIS, alcohol.
Contains: DIPHENHYDRAMINE HYDROCHLORIDE.
Other preparations: Nytol One-a-Night. MEDINEX (a liquid form). Other brands are available for purchase without a prescription.

---

oatmeal *see* **Aveeno**

Occlusal
(Euroderma)

A liquid used as a skin softener to treat warts.

Dose: apply to wart, allow to dry, then apply a second coat; treat once a day, paring down wart before using solution.
Availability: NHS, private prescription, over the counter.
Side effects:
Caution: do not use on healthy skin.
Not to be used for: warts on the face or around the anus or genitals.
Caution needed with:
Contains: SALICYLIC ACID.
Other preparations: VERRUGON (ointment form).

Ocufen
(Allergan)

A solution supplied in unit dose vials, and used as a NON-STEROID ANTI-INFLAMMATORY DRUG to prevent closing of the pupil during eye surgery and to treat inflammation after glaucoma operations when CORTICOSTEROIDS can not be used.

Dose: as advised by your doctor.
Availability: NHS, private prescription.
Side effects:
Caution:
Not to be used for:
Caution needed with:
Contains: FLURBIPROFEN sodium.
Other preparations:

Ocusert Pilo
(Cusi)

An eye insert used as a cholinergic treatment for glaucoma.

Dose: 1 unit under the eyelid replaced every 7 days.
Availability: NHS and private prescription.
Side effects: irritation, reduced sharpness of vision.
Caution:
Not to be used for: children or for patients suffering from acute eye infection or inflammation.
Caution needed with:
Contains: PILOCARPINE.
Other preparations: ISOPTO-CARPINE, PILOCARPINE EYE DROPS, SNO PILO.

Odrik *see* Gopten
(Hoechst Roussel)

---

oestradiol *see* Climagest, Climaval, Cyclo-Progynova 1mg, Estracombi, Estraderm, Estrapak, Estring, Evorel, Evorel-Pak, Fematrix, Femoston 2/10, Hormonin, Kliofem, Menorest, Nuvelle, oestradiol implant, Oestrogel, Progynova, Tridestra, Trisequens, Vagifem, Zumenon

---

oestradiol implant

An implant used as a hormone replacement therapy to relieve menopausal symptoms, such as hot flushes, vaginal discomfort, and to prevent osteoporosis in women after the menopause.

Dose: 25-100 mg usually every 4-8 months by implantation under the skin.
Side effects: stomach upset, weight changes, enlargement of breasts, tender breasts, fluid retention, liver function changes, rash, depression, headache, skin pigmentation.
Caution: in patients suffering from migraine, history of lumps in the breasts, fibroids, endometriosis, gall bladder disease, PORPHYRIA, raised blood pressure, heart or kidney disease, diabetes, asthma, epilepsy, skin tumours, LUPUS, multiple sclerosis, PORPHYRIA, some ear disorders. Patients with an intact uterus may also be advised to take progestogen supplements.
Not to be used for: children, pregnant women, nursing mothers, or for patients suffering from some cancers, thrombophlebitis, liver disease, undiagnosed bleeding from the vagina.
Caution needed with: few interactions at low doses used for HRT.
Contains: OESTRADIOL.
Other preparations:

Oestrifen *see* tamoxifen tablets
(Ashbourne)

---

oestriol *see* Hormonin, Ortho-Gynest, Ovestin, Trisequens

Oestrogel
(Hoechst Roussel)

A gel supplied in a pressurized dispenser and used as a hormone replacement therapy to treat muscular disorder and inflammation of the vagina and urethra.

Dose: 2 measures applied once a day to arms, shoulders, or inner thighs, increasing if needed after a month to 4 measures. (Progestogen supplements may be needed if the uterus is intact.)
Availability: NHS, private prescription.
Side effects: enlarged breasts, fluid retention, nausea, vaginal bleeding, weight gain, headache, dizziness. Rarely jaundice, raised blood pressure, thrombosis.
Caution: in patients suffering from high blood pressure, diabetes, epilepsy, womb diseases, gall bladder disorder, migraine, multiple

sclerosis, PORPHYRIA, liver disorders, some ear disorders, or a history or increased risk of breast disorders (including cancer) and thrombosis. Your doctor may advise you to have regular examinations.

Not to be used for: children, pregnant women, nursing mothers, or for patients suffering from thombosis, severe liver, kidney, or heart disorders, some cancers, undiagnosed vaginal bleeding, endometriosis.

Caution needed with: ACE INHIBITORS, ANTICOAGULANTS, BARBITURATES, ß-BLOCKERS, CARBAMAZEPINE, PHENYTOIN, RIFAMPICIN.

Contains: OESTRADIOL.

Other preparations:

---

oestrogen *see* **Premique**

---

oestrone *see* **Hormonin**

---

ofloxacin *see* **Exocin, Tarivid**

Oilatum Cream
(Stiefel)

A cream used as an emollient to treat dermatitis and other dry itchy skin conditions.

Dose: apply after washing and as required.
Availability: NHS, private prescription, over the counter.
Side effects:
Caution:
Not to be used for:
Caution needed with:
Contains: ARACHIS OIL.
Other preparations: OILATUM EMOLLIENT, Oilatum Shower Gel, Oilatum Plus.

Oilatum Emollient
(Stifel)

A liquid used as a bath emollient to treat dermatitis and dry itchy skin conditions.

Dose: adults 1-3 capsful added to the bath and soak for 10-20 minutes, or rub a small amount on to wet skin, rinse and dry; children as for adults; infants ½-2 capsful added to a wash basin and apply over entire body.
Availability: NHS, private prescription, over the counter.

482

Side effects:
Caution: bath may become slippery
Not to be used for:
Caution needed with:
Contains: acetylated wool alcohols, LIQUID PARAFFIN.
Other preparations: OILATUM CREAM, Oilatum Shower Gel. Ashbourne.

Oilatum Plus
(Stiefel)

A liquid used as an antiseptic bath emollient to treat eczema, particularly if infection is likely or possible.

Dose: 2 capsful added to the bath and soak for 10-15 minutes; infants over 6 months 1 ml added to baby bath and soak for 10-15 minutes
Availability: NHS, private prescription, over the counter.
Side effects:
Caution: guard against slipping in the bath.
Not to be used for: infants under 6 months.
Caution needed with:
Contains: LIQUID PARAFFIN, BENZALKONIUM CHLORIDE, TRICLOSAN.
Other preparations: OILATUM EMOLLIENT, OILATUM CREAM, Oilatum Gel (all used only for dry skin conditions).

oily cream *see* hydrous ointment

Olbetam
(Pharmacia)

A red-brown/dark-pink capsule supplied at a strength of 250 mg and used as a lipid-lowering agent to treat elevated lipids.

Dose: 2-3 capsules a day with meals, no more than 1200 mg a day.
Availability: NHS and private prescription.
Side effects: flushes, rash, redness, stomach upset, headache, general feeling of being unwell.
Caution:
Not to be used for: children, pregnant women, nursing mothers, or for patients suffering from stomach ulcer.
Caution needed with:
Contains: ACIPIMOX.
Other preparations:

oleyl alcohol *see* **Polytar Liquid**

olive oil *see* **Rowachol, Rowatinex**

olsalazine sodium *see* **Dipentum**

omeprazole *see* **Losec**

ondansetron *see* **Zofran**

One-Alpha
(Leo)

A white capsule or a brown capsule according to strengths of 0.25 microgram, 1 microgram, and used as a source of VITAMIN D to treat bone disorders due to kidney disease, rickets, over- or underactive parathyroid glands, low calcium levels in newborn infants, other bone disorders.

Dose: adults and children over 20 kg body weight 1 microgram a day at first adjusting as needed; children under 20 kg 0.05 micrograms per kg a day at first.
Availability: NHS and private prescription.
Side effects:
Caution: in pregnant women, nursing mothers, and patients suffering from kidney failure. Your doctor may advise that calcium levels should be checked regularly.
Not to be used for:
Caution needed with: BARBITURATES, anticonvulsants, DIGOXIN, some DIURETICS, ANTACIDS, MINERAL OILS, CHOLESTYRAMINE, COLESTIPOL, SUCRALFATE.
Contains: ALFACALCIDOL (VITAMIN D).
Other preparations: One-Alpha Solution.

One Touch
(LifeScan)

A plastic reagent strip used in conjunction with either a One Touch Basic or a One Touch II meter to detect blood glucose levels. Blood-glucose monitoring enables individual patients suffering from diabetes accurately to control blood glucose and manage their condition.

Ophthaine
(Squibb)

Drops used as a local anaesthetic for eye procedures.

Dose: 1-2 drops into the eye before the procedure.
Availability: NHS and private prescription.
Side effects: Irritation, rarely severe allergy.
Caution: in patients with a history of allergy, heart disease, or overactive thyroid. Do not use over extended periods.
Not to be used for:
Caution needed with:
Contains: PROXYMETACAINE hydrochloride.
Other preparations:

Opilon
(Parke-Davis)

A yellow tablet supplied at a strength of 40 mg and used as a vasodilator to treat Raynaud's syndrome (a condition caused by spasms of arteries in the hand).

Dose: 1 tablet 4 times a day, increasing if necessary to 2 tablets 4 times a day.
Availability: NHS and private prescription.
Side effects: nausea, diarrhoea, vertigo, headache, liver disorder.
Caution: in patients suffering from diabetes, angina, recent heart attack.
Not to be used for: children, pregnant women, nursing mothers, or for patients who are allergic to thymoxamine.
Caution needed with: TRICYCLIC ANTIDEPRESSANTS, blood-pressure lowering drugs.
Contains: THYMOXAMINE HYDROCHLORIDE.
Other preparations:

Opticrom
(Fisons)

Drops used as a NON-STEROIDAL ANTI-INFLAMMATORY preparation to treat allergic conjunctivitis.

Dose: 1-2 drops into the eyes 4 times a day.
Availability: NHS and private prescription.
Side effects: temporary smarting.
Caution:
Not to be used for: patients who wear soft contact lenses.

O

Optimax
(Merck)

A tablet used as an antidepressant to treat severe depression (used only by hospital specialists).

Dose: 2 tablets 3 times a day, or up to a maximum of 12 tablets in 24 hours.
Availability: NHS and private prescription.
Side effects: muscle pain, blood changes, drowsiness, nausea, headache.
Caution: in pregnant women, nursing mothers, the elderly, and in patients suffering from kidney or liver disorders.
Not to be used for: patients with a history of eosinophilia myalgia (a muscle disorder).
Caution needed with: MAOIS, other antidepressants, sedatives, alcohol.
Contains: TRYPTOPHAN.
Other preparations:

Optimine
(Schering-Plough)

A syrup supplied at a strength of 0.5 mg/5 ml and used as an ANTIHISTAMINE and serotonin antagonist (hormone blocker) to treat bites and stings, itch, allergic rhinitis, urticaria.

Dose: adults 10-20 ml twice a day; children 1-6 years 2.5 ml twice a day, 6-12 years 5-10 ml twice a day.
Availability: NHS, private prescription, over the counter.
Side effects: drowsiness, reduced reactions, greater appetite, anorexia, nausea, headache, ANTICHOLINERGIC effects.
Caution:
Not to be used for: infants under 1 year or for patients suffering from prostate enlargement, retention of urine, glaucoma, stomach ulcer causing blockage, stomach obstruction.
Caution needed with: sedatives, MAOIS, alcohol.
Contains: AZATADINE MALEATE.
Other preparations: Optimine Tablets.

Opumide *see* indapamide tablets
(Opus)

Opustan *see* mefenamic acid tablets/capsules
(Opus)

Orabase
(Convatec)

An ointment used as a mucoprotectant to protect lesions in the mouth and on moist body surfaces.

Dose: apply to the affected area without rubbing in.
Availability: NHS, private prescription, over the counter.
Side effects:
Caution:
Not to be used for:
Caution needed with:
Contains: CARMELLOSE SODIUM, PECTIN, GELATIN.
Other preparations:

Orabet *see* metformin tablets
(Lagap)

Oral-B Fluoride Tablets *see* Fluor-a-day Tablets

Oraldene
(Warner Wellcome Consumer)

A solution used as an antiseptic rinse to treat thrush, ulcers, bad breath, inflammation of the mouth or gums, sore throat, and before and after dental surgery.

Dose: rinse out the mouth or gargle with 15 ml 2-3 times a day.
Availability: NHS, private prescription, over the counter.
Side effects: irritation.
Caution:
Not to be used for: children under 6 years.
Caution needed with:
Contains: HEXETIDINE.
Other preparations:

Oramorph SR
(Boehringer Ingelheim)

A buff tablet, violet tablet, orange tablet, or grey tablet (all long acting) according to strengths of 10 mg, 30 mg, 60 mg, 100 mg, and used as an opiate to control severe pain.

Dose: adults 10-20 mg every 12 hours, increased if necessary; children over 1 year use unit dose or concentrate.
Availability: controlled drug; NHS and private prescription.
Side effects: tolerance, addiction, constipation, nausea, vomiting, sedation.
Caution: in the elderly, nursing mothers, after surgery, and in patients suffering from underactive thyroid, liver or kidney disease, breathing difficulty, adrenal gland problems, enlarged prostate, shock.
Not to be used for: infants under 1 year, pregnant women, alcoholics, or for patients suffering from blocked airways, acute liver disease, head injury, coma, convulsions, or raised pressure in the brain.
Caution needed with: MAOIS, sedatives, alcohol.
Contains: MORPHINE sulphate
Other preparations: Oramorph Concentrated, Oramorph Unit Dose (liquid forms). MST CONTINUS, SEVREDOL.

Orap
(Janssen-Cilag)

A white, scored tablet or a green, scored tablet according to strengths of 2 mg, 4 mg, 10 mg and used as a sedative to treat schizophrenia.

Dose: 2-20 mg a day.
Availability: NHS and private prescription.
Side effects: muscle spasms, restlessness, weakness, hands shaking, blurred vision, constipation, dry mouth, stuffy nose, urine retention, palpitations, low blood pressure, weight gain, abnormal heart rhythm, changes in sexual function, low body temperature, breast swelling, menstrual changes, jaundice, blood and skin changes, drowsiness, tiredness, rarely fits.
Caution: in pregnant women and in patients suffering from depression, Parkinson's disease, epilepsy, kidney or liver damage, electrolyte disturbance.
Not to be used for: children or for patients suffering from some heart disorders.
Caution needed with: alcohol, sedatives, tranquillizers, pain killers, blood-pressure lowering drugs, TRICYCLIC ANTIDEPRESSANTS, anticonvulsants, antidiabetic drugs, antimalarials, LEVODOPA, some heart drugs, TERFENADINE, ASTEMIZOLE.

Contains: PIMOZIDE.
Other preparations:

Orbenin *see* **cloxacillin capsules**
(Forley)

---

orciprenaline sulphate *see* **Alupent**

Orelox
(Hoechst Roussel)

A white film-coated tablet supplied at a strength of 100 mg and used as an antibiotic to treat acute bronchitis and other respiratory infections, sinusitis, recurring or chronic tonsillitis, pharyngitis, acute inflammation of the middle ear.

Dose: 1-2 tablets twice a day with a meal depending on condition and severity. Children use paediatric suspension.
Availability: NHS, private prescription.
Side effects: stomach upset, headache, allergy, liver changes, colitis.
Caution: in pregnant women and in patients suffering from kidney disorder or who are allergic to certain antibiotics.
Not to be used for:
Caution needed with: ANTACIDS, H$_2$ ANTAGONISTS.
Contains: CEFPODOXIME.
Other preparations: Orelox Paediatric Suspension.

Orgafol *see* **Metrodin**
(Organon)

Orlept *see* **Epilim**
(CP Pharm)

---

orphenadrine *see* **Biorphen, Disipal**

Ortho-Creme
(Janssen-Cilag)

A cream with a separately available applicator used as a spermicidal contraceptive either on its own or in conjuction with a diaphragm.

Dose: 1 applicatorful inserted into the vagina or spread over the surface and rim of the diaphragm before intercourse.
Availability: NHS, private prescription, over the counter.
Side effects:
Caution:
Not to be used for:
Caution needed with:
Contains: NONOXYNOL-9.
Other preparations:

Ortho-Dienoestrol
(Janssen-Cilag)

A cream with applicator used as an oestrogen treatment for atrophic inflammation of the vagina, other disease of the vulva or painful intercourse.

Dose: 1-2 applications into the vagina once a day for 1-2 weeks reducing to half that dose for 1-2 weeks, then 1 application 1-3 times a week.
Availability: NHS and private prescription.
Side effects: enlarged breasts, fluid retention, nausea, vaginal bleeding, weight gain, headache, dizziness. Rarely jaundice, raised blood pressure, thrombosis.
Caution: in patients suffering from high blood pressure, diabetes, epilepsy, womb diseases, gall bladder disorder, migraine, multiple sclerosis, PORPHYRIA, liver disorders, some ear disorders, or a history or increased risk of breast disorders (including cancer) and thrombosis. Your doctor may advise you to have regular examinations.
Not to be used for: children, pregnant women, nursing mothers, or for patients suffering from thombosis, severe liver, kidney, or heart disorders, some cancers, undiagnosed vaginal bleeding, endometriosis.
Caution needed with: ACE INHIBITORS, ANTICOAGULANTS, BARBITURATES, ß-BLOCKERS, CARBAMAZEPINE, PHENYTOIN, RIFAMPICIN.
Contains: DIENOESTROL.
Other preparations:

Ortho-Gyne T 380 S
(Janssen-Cilag)

A copper-bearing coil used as an intra-uterine device to prevent conception.

Dose: as advised. Replace after 8 years.
Availability: NHS, private prescription.
Side effects: pelvic infection, pain, abnormal bleeding, perforation of the

uterus. On insertion, persistent low heart rate, asthma attack, epileptic attack.

Caution: in patients suffering from anaemia, heavy periods, diabetes, epilepsy or who have had inflammatory heart conditions or pelvic inflammatory disease, or who are at risk from sexually transmitted diseases. Patients should be checked 3 months after insertion and then annually.

Not to be used for: children, pregnant women, or for patients suffering from allergy to copper, abnormal uterus, severe infections, acute pelvic inflammatory disease, endometrial disease, abnormal vaginal bleeding, or some other urinogenital tract disorders, or with a history of ectopic pregnancies.

Caution needed with: ANTICOAGULANTS.

Contains: copper wire.

Other preparations: MULTILOAD, NOVA-T, ORTHO-GYNE-T.

Ortho-Gynest
(Janssen-Cilag)

A pessary supplied at a strength of 0.5 mg and used as an oestrogen treatment for atrophic inflammation of the vagina, other disease of the vulva or painful intercourse.

Dose: 1 pessary inserted into the vagina each evening at first, then 1 pessary twice a week.

Availability: NHS and private prescription.

Side effects: enlarged breasts, fluid retention, nausea, vaginal bleeding, weight gain, headache, dizziness. Rarely jaundice, raised blood pressure, thrombosis.

Caution: in patients suffering from high blood pressure, diabetes, epilepsy, womb diseases, gall bladder disorder, migraine, multiple sclerosis, PORPHYRIA, liver disorders, some ear disorders, or a history or increased risk of breast disorders (including cancer) and thrombosis. Your doctor may advise you to have regular examinations.

Not to be used for: children, pregnant women, nursing mothers, or for patients suffering from thombosis, severe liver, kidney, or heart disorders, some cancers, undiagnosed vaginal bleeding, endometriosis.

Caution needed with: ACE INHIBITORS, ANTICOAGULANTS, BARBITURATES, ß-BLOCKERS, CARBAMAZEPINE, PHENYTOIN, RIFAMPICIN.

Contains: OESTRIOL.

Other preparations: Ortho-Gynest Cream.

Ortho-Gynol
(Janssen-Cilag)

A jelly with a separately available applicator used as a spermicidal contraceptive either on its own or in conjuction with a diaphragm.

Dose: 1 applicatorful inserted into the vagina or spread over the surface and rim of the diaphragm before intercourse.
Availability: NHS, private prescription, over the counter.
Side effects:
Caution:
Not to be used for:
Caution needed with:
Contains: DI-ISOBUTYLPHENOXY-POLYETHOXYETHANOL.
Other preparations:

Ortho-Novin 1/50
(Janssen-Cilag)

A white tablet used as an oestrogen, progestogen contraceptive.

Dose: 1 tablet a day for 21 days starting on day 5 of the period.
Availability: NHS and private prescription.
Side effects: enlarged breasts, bloating and fluid retention, cramps, leg pains, mood change, reduction in sexual desire, headaches, nausea, vaginal erosion, discharge, and bleeding, weight gain, skin changes, rarely thrombosis, raised blood pressure, jaundice.
Caution: in patients suffering from high blood pressure, diabetes, vascular disorders, asthma, depression, kidney disease, multiple sclerosis, womb diseases. Your doctor may advise you not to smoke, to have regular examinations. You should stop treatment at the first sign of serious symptoms such as severe headache or jaundice. Treatment should be stopped before surgery.
Not to be used for: pregnant women, or for patients suffering from sickle-cell anaemia, history of heart disease or thrombosis, liver disorders, some cancers, undiagnosed vaginal bleeding, some ear, skin, and kidney disorders.
Caution needed with: RIFAMPICIN, TETRACYCLINE ANTIBIOTICS, GRISEOFULVIN, BARBITURATES, PHENYTOIN, PRIMIDONE, CARBAMAZEPINE, ETHOSUXIMIDE, CHLORAL HYDRATE.
Contains: MESTRANOL, NORETHISTERONE.
Other preparations: NORINYL-I.

Orudis *see* ketoprofen capsules
(Rhône-Poulenc Rorer)

Oruvail *see* ketoprofen capsules
(Rhône-Poulenc Rorer)

Ossopan 800
(Sanofi Winthrop)

A buff-coloured tablet supplied at a strength of 830 mg and used as a calcium-phosphorus supplement to treat osteoporosis, rickets, osteomalacia (bone disorders), and for nursing mothers.

Dose: adults 4-8 tablets a day in divided doses before food; children as advised by the physician.
Availability: NHS, private prescription, over the counter.
Side effects:
Caution: in patients suffering from kidney disease, severe immobility, or a history of kidney stones.
Not to be used for: patients suffering from elevated blood or urine calcium.
Caution needed with:
Contains: HYDROXYAPATITE compound.
Other preparations: Ossopan Powder.

Otomize
(Stafford-Miller)

A suspension supplied in a pump spray, and used as an antibiotic and STEROID to treat outer ear conditions.

Dose: 1 spray 3 times a day until 2 days after symptoms disappear.
Availability: NHS and private prescription.
Side effects: temporary stinging or burning.
Caution: in pregnant women, and in patients suffering from perforated ear drum.
Not to be used for:
Caution needed with:
Contains: NEOMYCIN, DEXAMETHASONE, ACETIC ACID.
Other preparations:

Otosporin
(Wellcome)

Drops used as an antibiotic, STEROID treatment for bacterial infections and inflammation of the outer ear.

Dose: 3 drops into the ear 3-4 times a day.

Availability: NHS and private prescription.
Side effects: additional infection.
Caution: with long-term use in infants.
Not to be used for: patients suffering from perforated ear drum, or untreated viral, fungal, or tubercular infections.
Caution needed with:
Contains: POLYMYXIN B SULPHATE, NEOMYCIN sulphate, HYDROCORTISONE.
Other preparations:

Otrivine
(Zyma Healthcare)

A spray and drops used as a SYMPATHOMIMETIC preparation to clear blocked nose.

Dose: adults 2-3 drops or 1 spray into each nostril 2-3 times a day; children use paediatric drops.
Availability: NHS (when prescribed as a generic), private prescription, over the counter.
Side effects: itching nose, headache, sleeplessness, rapid heart rate.
Caution: in pregnant women; do not use for extended periods.
Not to be used for: infants under 3 months.
Caution needed with: MAOIS.
Contains: XYLOMETAZOLINE hydrochloride.
Other preparations: Otrivine Paediatric.

Otrivine-Antistin Eye Drops
(Ciba Vision Ophthalmics)

Drops used as a SYMPATHOMIMETIC, ANTIHISTAMINE treatment for allergic conjunctivitis and other eye inflammations.

Dose: adults 1-2 drops into the eye 2-3 times a day; children over 5 years and elderly patients 1 drop 2-3 times a day.
Availability: NHS, private prescription, over the counter.
Side effects: temporary smarting, headache, drowsiness, blurred vision, additional congestion.
Caution: in patients suffering from high blood pressure, overactive thyroid, dry eyes, heart disease, diabetes.
Not to be used for: children under 5 years, or for patients suffering from glaucoma or who wear contact lenses.
Caution needed with: alcohol, sedatives, MAOIS, CLONIDINE.
Contains: XYLOMETAZOLINE HYDROCHLORIDE.
Other preparations:

Ovestin
(Organon)

A white tablet supplied at a strength of 1 mg, and used as an oestrogen for treating genital or urinary complaints caused by oestrogen deficiency.

Dose: genital/urinary complaints, 0.5-3 mg a day for 1 month then 0.5-1 mg a day.
Availability: NHS and private prescription.
Side effects: enlarged breasts, fluid retention, nausea, vaginal bleeding, weight gain, headache, dizziness. Rarely jaundice, raised blood pressure, thrombosis.
Caution: in patients suffering from high blood pressure, diabetes, epilepsy, womb diseases, gall bladder disorder, migraine, multiple sclerosis, PORPHYRIA, liver disorders, some ear disorders, or a history or increased risk of breast disorders (including cancer) and thrombosis. Your doctor may advise you to have regular examinations.
Not to be used for: children, pregnant women, nursing mothers, or for patients suffering from thrombosis, severe liver, kidney, or heart disorders, some cancers, undiagnosed vaginal bleeding, endometriosis.
Caution needed with: ACE INHIBITORS, ANTICOAGULANTS, BARBITURATES, ß-BLOCKERS, CARBAMAZEPINE, PHENYTOIN, RIFAMPICIN.
Contains: OESTRIOL.
Other preparations: OVESTIN CREAM (used to treat vaginal conditions requiring oestrogen therapy).

Ovestin Cream
(Organon)

A cream used as an oestrogen treatment for inflammation of the vagina, itch, as a treatment before vaginal surgery, other diseases of the vulva.

Dose: 1 application a day for 3 weeks, then 1 application twice a week.
Availability: NHS and private prescription.
Side effects: tender breasts, fluid retention, headaches, nausea, vaginal bleeding, weight gain, dizziness. Rarely, jaundice, raised blood pressure, thrombosis.
Caution: in patients suffering from high blood pressure, diabetes, womb diseases, epilepsy, gall bladder disease, liver disorders, some ear disorders, or a history of increase risk of breast disorders (including cancer and thrombosis), migraine, PORPHYRIA, multiple sclerosis. Your doctor may advise you to have regular examinations.
Not to be used for: children, pregnant women, nursing mothers, or for patients suffering from thrombosis, severe kidney, heart, or liver disorders, some cancers, undiagnosed vaginal bleeding, endometriosis.
Caution needed with: BARBITURATES, CARBAMAZEPINE, PHENYTOIN, ß-BLOCKERS,

ANTICOAGULANTS, ACE INHIBITORS.
Contains: OESTRIOL.
Other preparations: OVESTIN.

Ovran
(Wyeth)

A white tablet used as an oestrogen, progestogen contraceptive.

Dose: 1 tablet a day for 21 days starting on day 5 of the period.
Availability: NHS and private prescription.
Side effects: enlarged breasts, bloating and fluid retention, cramps, leg pains, mood change, reduction in sexual desire, headaches, nausea, vaginal erosion, discharge, and bleeding, weight gain, skin changes, rarely thrombosis, raised blood pressure, jaundice.
Caution: in patients suffering from high blood pressure, diabetes, vascular disorders, asthma, depression, kidney disease, multiple sclerosis, womb diseases. Your doctor may advise you not to smoke, to have regular examinations. You should stop treatment at the first sign of serious symptoms such as severe headache or jaundice. Treatment should be stopped before surgery.
Not to be used for: pregnant women, or for patients suffering from sickle-cell anaemia, history of heart disease or thrombosis, liver disorders, some cancers, undiagnosed vaginal bleeding, some ear, skin, and kidney disorders.
Caution needed with: RIFAMPICIN, TETRACYCLINE ANTIBIOTICS, GRISEOFULVIN, BARBITURATES, PHENYTOIN, PRIMIDONE, CARBAMAZEPINE, ETHOSUXIMIDE, CHLORAL HYDRATE.
Contains: ETHINYLOESTRADIOL, LEVONORGESTREL.
Other preparations: Ovran 30 (lower-strength preparation).

Ovranette
(Wyeth)

A yellow tablet used as an oestrogen, progestogen contraceptive.

Dose: 1 tablet a day for 21 days starting on day 5 of the period.
Availability: NHS and private prescription.
Side effects: enlarged breasts, bloating and fluid retention, cramps, leg pains, mood change, reduction in sexual desire, headaches, nausea, vaginal erosion, discharge, and bleeding, weight gain, skin changes, rarely thrombosis, raised blood pressure, jaundice.
Caution: in patients suffering from high blood pressure, diabetes, vascular disorders, asthma, depression, kidney disease, multiple sclerosis, womb diseases. Your doctor may advise you not to smoke, to have regular

examinations. You should stop treatment at the first sign of serious symptoms such as severe headache or jaundice. Treatment should be stopped before surgery.

Not to be used for: pregnant women, or for patients suffering from sickle-cell anaemia, history of heart disease or thrombosis, liver disorders, some cancers, undiagnosed vaginal bleeding, some ear, skin, and kidney disorders.

Caution needed with: RIFAMPICIN, TETRACYCLINE ANTIBIOTICS, GRISEOFULVIN, BARBITURATES, PHENYTOIN, PRIMIDONE, CARBAMAZEPINE, ETHOSUXIMIDE, CHLORAL HYDRATE.

Contains: ETHINYLOESTRADIOL, LEVONORGESTREL.

Other preparations: MICROGYNON-30.

Ovysmen
(Janssen-Cilag)

A white tablet used as an oestrogen, progestogen contraceptive.

Dose: 1 tablet a day for 21 days starting on day 5 of the period.
Availability: NHS and private prescription.
Side effects: enlarged breasts, bloating and fluid retention, cramps, leg pains, mood change, reduction in sexual desire, headaches, nausea, vaginal erosion, discharge, and bleeding, weight gain, skin changes, rarely thrombosis, raised blood pressure, jaundice.
Caution: in patients suffering from high blood pressure, diabetes, vascular disorders, asthma, depression, kidney disease, multiple sclerosis, womb diseases. Your doctor may advise you not to smoke, to have regular examinations. You should stop treatment at the first sign of serious symptoms such as severe headache or jaundice. Treatment should be stopped before surgery.
Not to be used for: pregnant women, or for patients suffering from sickle-cell anaemia, history of heart disease or thrombosis, liver disorders, some cancers, undiagnosed vaginal bleeding, some ear, skin, and kidney disorders.
Caution needed with: RIFAMPICIN, TETRACYCLINE ANTIBIOTICS, GRISEOFULVIN, BARBITURATES, PHENYTOIN, PRIMIDONE, CARBAMAZEPINE, ETHOSUXIMIDE, CHLORAL HYDRATE.
Contains: ETHINYLOESTRADIOL, NORGESTREL.
Other preparations: BREVINOR.

---

oxazepam

A tablet supplied at strengths of 10 mg, 15 mg, 30 mg and used as a sedative to treat anxiety.

Dose: elderly 10-20 mg 3-4 times a day; adults 15-30 mg 3-4 times a day

(with associated sleeplessness, one single dose of 15-50 mg at night).
Availability: NHS and private prescription.
Side effects: drowsiness, confusion, unsteadiness, low blood pressure, rash, changes in vision, changes in sexual function, retention of urine. Risk of addiction increases with dose and length of treatment. May impair judgement.
Caution: in the elderly, pregnant women, nursing mothers, in women during labour, and in patients suffering from lung disorders, kidney or liver disorders. Avoid long-term use and withdraw gradually.
Not to be used for: children, or for patients suffering from acute lung diseases, some chronic lung diseases, some obsessional and psychotic diseases.
Caution needed with: alcohol, sedatives, other tranquillizers, anticonvulsants, RIFAMPICIN.
Contains: oxazepam.
Other preparations: oxazepam capsules.

---

oxerutins *see* **Paroven**

---

oxethazaine *see* **Mucaine**

---

oxitropium bromide *see* **Oxivent**

Oxivent
(Boehringer Ingelheim)

An inhaler supplied at a strength of 100 micrograms per dose, and used as an ANTICHOLINERGIC treatment for asthma and other diseases associated with breathing obstruction.

Dose: 2 puffs 2-3 times a day.
Availability: NHS and private prescription.
Side effects: irritation, nausea, dry mouth, anticholinergic effects.
Caution: in patients suffering from glaucoma, enlarged prostate, wheezing, or coughing. Avoid the eyes.
Not to be used for: children, pregnant women, nursing mothers, or for patients allergic to ATROPINE or IPRATROPIUM bromide.
Caution needed with:
Contains: OXITROPIUM BROMIDE.
Other preparations: Oxivent Autohaler.

---

oxpentifylline *see* **Trental**

---

oxprenolol *see* **oxprenolol tablets, Slow-Trasicor, Trasicor, Trasidrex**

---

oxprenolol tablets

A tablet supplied at strengths of 20 mg, 40 mg, 80 mg, 160 mg and used as a ß-BLOCKER to treat angina, abnormal heart rhythm, high blood pressure, anxiety.

Dose: for abnormal rhythm adults 20-40 mg 3 times a day at first. For angina 40-160 mg 3 times a day. For high blood pressure 160-480 mg a day in divided doses. For anxiety (short term only) 80-160 mg a day in divided doses.
Availability: NHS and private prescription.
Side effects: cold hands and feet, sleep disturbance, slow heart rate, tiredness, wheezing, heart failure, stomach upset, dry eyes, skin rash.
Caution: in pregnant women, nursing mothers, and in patients suffering from diabetes, kidney or liver disorders, MYASTHENIA GRAVIS. May need to be withdrawn before surgery. Withdraw gradually. Your doctor may advise additional treatment with DIURETICS or DIGOXIN.
Not to be used for: patients suffering from asthma, heart block, or failure.
Caution needed with: VERAPAMIL, CLONIDINE withdrawal, some anti-arrhythmic drugs and anaesthetics, some blood-pressure lowering drugs, ERGOTAMINE, sedatives, antidiabetics, SYMPATHOMIMETICS, alcohol, NON-STEROIDAL ANTI-INFLAMMATORY DRUGS, MEFLOQUINE, DILTIAZEM, NIFEDIPINE.
Contains: OXPRENOLOL hydrochloride.
Other preparations: OXYPRENIX, TRASICOR. (Long-acting preparations available – SLOW-TRASICOR.)

---

oxybutynin *see* **Ditropan, Cystrin**

Oxymycin *see* **oxytetracycline tablets**
(DDSA)

Oxyprenix *see* **oxprenolol tablets**
(Ashbourne)

---

oxytetracycline dihydrate *see* **oxytetracycline tablets**

---

oxytetracycline hydrochloride *see* **Terra-Cortril Ear Suspension, Terra-Cortril Ointment, Trimovate**; *see also* **Tetracycline**

oxytetracycline tablets

A coated tablet supplied at a strength of 250 mg and used as a broad-spectrum antibiotic to treat infections, including bronchitis and acne.

Dose: 1-2 tablets every 6 hours.
Availability: NHS and private prescription.
Side effects: stomach upsets, headache, vision changes, raised blood pressure, pancreatitis, colitis, sensitivity to light, skin changes.
Caution: in patients suffering from liver or kidney failure.
Not to be used for: children under 12 years, pregnant women, nursing mothers, or for patients suffering from PORPHYRIA, LUPUS.
Caution needed with: ANTICOAGULANTS, BARBITURATES, anti-epileptic drugs, QUINAPRIL, ANTACIDS, calcium, iron, and zinc supplements, dairy products, the contraceptive pill, ISOTRETINOIN.
Contains: OXYTETRACYCLINE DIHYDRATE.
Other preparations: BERKMYCIN, OXYMYCIN, OXYTETRAMIX, TERRAMYCIN (capsule form available).

Oxytetramix-250 *see* oxytetracycline tablets
(Ashbourne)

Paldesic *see* paracetamol paediatric elixir
(Rosemont)

Palfium
(Boehringer Mannheim)

A white, scored tablet or a peach, scored tablet according to strengths of 5 mg, 10 mg and used as an opiate to control severe and prolonged pain.

Dose: adults up to 5 mg initially, and then as advised by physician; children up to 80 micrograms per kg body weight or as advised by the physician.
Availability: controlled drug; NHS and private prescription.
Side effects: tolerance, addiction, dizziness, sweating, nausea.
Caution: in the elderly, in pregnant women, and in patients suffering from liver disease, underactive thyroid gland.
Not to be used for: women in labour or for patients suffering from breathing disorder or blocked airways.

Caution needed with: MAOIS, sedatives.
Contains: DEXTROMORAMIDE TARTRATE.
Other preparations: Palfium Suppositories.

Paludrine
(Zeneca)

A white, scored tablet supplied at a strength of 100 mg and used as an antimalarial drug for the prevention of malaria.

Dose: adults and children over 14 years 2 tablets a day after meals; reduced doses for children under 14 years. Begin taking tablets at least 24 hours before entering infected area and continue for 4 weeks after leaving.
Availability: NHS, private prescription, over the counter.
Side effects: stomach upset, skin reactions, hair loss, mouth ulcers, and inflammation of the mouth.
Caution: in patients suffering from severe kidney failure.
Not to be used for: .
Caution needed with:
Contains: PROGUANIL HYDROCHLORIDE.
Other preparations:

Pameton
(SmithKline Beecham)

A white tablet used as an ANALGESIC (with antidote included) to relieve pain and reduce fever, especially where misuse of PARACETAMOL may occur.

Dose: adults 2 tablets up to 4 times a day; children 6-12 years ½-1 tablet every 4 hours to a maximum of 4 doses a day.
Availability: private prescription and over the counter.
Side effects:
Caution: in pregnant women and in patients suffering from liver disease.
Not to be used for: children under 6 years.
Caution needed with: LEVODOPA, other medicines containing paracetamol.
Contains: PARACETAMOL, METHIONINE.
Other preparations:

Pancrease
(Janssen-Cilag)

A white capsule used as a source of pancreatic enzymes to treat deficiency as in cystic fibrosis and chronic pancreatitis.

Dose: 1-3 capsules during meals or 1 capsule with a snack
Availability: NHS, private prescription, over the counter.
Side effects: irritation around the anus.
Caution:
Not to be used for: pregnant women, nursing mothers, or for anyone with allergy to pork.
Caution needed with:
Contains: PANCREATIN.
Other preparations: PANCREASE HL (higher-strength product). CREON, NUTRIZYM GR, PANCREX V, PANZYTRAT 25000.

P

Pancrease HL
(Janssen-Cilag)

A white/red capsule used to supply pancreatic enzymes in the treatment of pancreatic exocrine insufficiency such as in cystic fibrosis and chronic inflammation of the pancreas.

Dose: 1-2 capsules with each meal and 1 capsule with a snack; up to 3 capsules may be taken with meals.
Availability: NHS, private prescription, over the counter.
Side effects: irritation around the anus, intestinal obstruction (withdraw if this occurs).
Caution:
Not to be used for: pregnant women, nursing mothers, or for patients allergic to pork. (Patients suffering from cystic fibrosis should not be treated under the age of 15 years.)
Caution needed with:
Contains: PANCREATIN.
Other preparations: PANCREASE (weaker-strength product). PANCREX-V FORTE, PANZYTRAT 25000, CREON, NUTRIZYM GR.

pancreatin *see* **Creon, Nutrizym GR, Pancrease, Pancrease HL, Pancrex V Forte Tablets, Panzytrat 25000**

Pancrex V Forte Tablets
(Paines & Byrne)

A white tablet used as a source of pancreatic enzymes to treat cystic fibrosis, steatorrhoea, pancreatic enzyme deficiency states due to pancreatic disease.

Dose: 6-10 tablets before each meal.
Availability: NHS, private prescription, over the counter.

Side effects: blocked intestines (withdraw if this occurs).
Caution:
Not to be used for:
Caution needed with:
Contains: PANCREATIN.
Other preparations: Pancrex V Tablets, Pancrex V Capsules, Pancrex V Capsules '125', Pancrex V Powder, Pancrex Granules. CREON, NUTRIZYM GR, PANCREASE, PANZYTRAT 25000.

Pan-ex *see* paracetamol tablets
(Custom Pharmaceuticals)

Panoxyl
(Stiefel)

A gel, available in two strengths (5% and 10%), used as an antibacterial, skin softener to treat acne.

Dose: wash and dry the affected area, then apply once a day, starting with the lower-dose gel.
Availability: NHS, private prescription, over the counter.
Side effects: irritation, peeling.
Caution: keep out of the eyes, nose, mouth. May bleach fabrics.
Not to be used for:
Caution needed with:
Contains: BENZOYL PEROXIDE.
Other preparations: Panoxyl Aquagel, Panoxyl Wash. ACETOXYL, ACNECIDE, ACNEGEL, BENOXYL, NERICUR, QUINODERM.

panthenol *see* Lipoflavonoid, Lipotriad

pantothenic acid *see* vitamin B$_5$

Panzytrat 25000
(Knoll)

A capsule used to supply pancreatic enzymes in the treatment of pancreatic exocrine insufficiency such as in cystic fibrosis and chronic inflammation of the pancreas.

Dose: 1-2 capsules with meals at first adjusting according to response; children under 18 months 2 capsules a day with food, over 18 months 4

capsules a day with food, adjust as needed.
Availability: NHS, private prescription, over the counter.
Side effects: intestinal obstruction (withdraw if this occurs).
Caution:
Not to be used for: patients suffering from acute pancreatitis, or who are allergic to pork or pork products.
Caution needed with:
Contains: pancreatic enzymes.
Other preparations: CREON, NUTRIZYM GR, PANCREASE, PANCREASE HL, PANCREX-V FORTE.

---

papaveretum *see* Aspav

---

paracetamol *see* Alvedon, Calpol, Co-Codamol, co-dydramol, co-proxamol, Cosalgesic, Disprol, Distalgesic, Fortagesic, Galake, Midrid, Migraleve, Pameton, paracetamol paediatric elixir, paracetamol tablets, Parake, Paramax, Remedeine, Rimadol, Solpadol, Tylex

---

paracetamol paediatric elixir

An elixir supplied at a strength of 120 mg in 5 ml and used as an ANALGESIC and fever-reducing preparation to relieve pain and temperature in children.

Dose: at age 2 months 2.5 ml (for fever after immunization), age 3-12 months 2.5-5 ml, age 1-5 years 5-10 ml, age 6-12 years 10-20 ml (all 4 times a day). Lower doses used for children under 2 months.
Availability: NHS, private prescription, over the counter.
Side effects: rarely rash, blood disorders, inflamed pancreas.
Caution: in patients suffering from kidney or liver disorders.
Not to be used for:
Caution needed with: other medicines containing PARACETAMOL.
Contains: PARACETAMOL.
Other preparations: paracetamol soluble tablets, PARACETAMOL TABLETS, paracetamol oral suspension (two strengths). ALVEDON SUPPOSITORIES, CALPOL, DISPROL, PALDESIC (available on NHS only if prescribed as a generic). Many other brands available over the counter.

---

paracetamol tablets

A tablet supplied at a strength of 500 mg and used as an ANALGESIC to relieve pain and reduce fever.

Dose: adults 1-2 tablet 4 times a day; children 6-12 years ½-1 tablet 4 times a day.
Availability: NHS, private prescription, over the counter.
Side effects: rarely rash, blood disorders, pancreatitis, (liver damage after overdose).
Caution: in patients suffering from kidney or liver disease, and in alcoholics.
Not to be used for: children under 6 years.
Caution needed with: other medicines containing PARACETAMOL.
Contains: PARACETAMOL.
Other preparations: paracetamol soluble, PARACETAMOL PAEDIATRIC ELIXIR. RIMADOL. (Other brands available over the counter.)

---

paradichlorobenzene *see* **Cerumol**

Parake *see* **co-codamol tablets**

Paramax
(Lorex Synthélabo)

A white, scored tablet used as an ANALGESIC, anti-emetic treatment for migraine.

Dose: adults over 20 years 2 tablets at the beginning of the attack, then 2 tablets every 4 hours to a maximum of 6 tablets in 24 hours; 15-19 years and with a body weight over 60 kg, 2 tablets at the beginning of the attack to a maximum of 5 tablets in 24 hours; children 12-14 years and body weight over 30 kg 1 tablet at the beginning to a maximum of 3 tablets in 24 hours.
Availability: NHS and private prescription.
Side effects: extrapyramidal reactions (shaking and rigidity), drowsiness, diarrhoea, altered hormone levels (prolactin).
Caution: in pregnant women, nursing mothers, and in patients suffering from liver or kidney disease.
Not to be used for: children under 12 years, or for patients suffering from PHAEOCHROMOCYTOMA, some breast cancers, or who have recently undergone stomach surgery.
Caution needed with: ANTICHOLINERGICS, alcohol, sedatives, other medicines containing PARACETAMOL.
Contains: PARACETAMOL, METOCLOPRAMIDE hydrochloride.
Other preparations: Paramax Sachets.

Paratulle
(Seton Healthcare)

A sterile, impregnated gauze dressing, supplied at a size of 10 cm square, and used as a dressing for burns, wounds, and sensitive areas.

Availability: NHS, private prescription, over the counter. (Also available on a trial basis from nurses.)
Contains: yellow soft paraffin.

Parlodel *see* bromocriptine tablets
(Sandoz)

Parnate
(SmithKline Beecham)

A red tablet supplied at a strength of 10 mg, and used as an MAOI antidepressant to treat depression.

Dose: 1 tablet twice a day at first, increasing after 7 days if necessary to 1 tablet 3 times a day, then usually 1 tablet a day for maintenance.
Availability: NHS and private prescription.
Side effects: severe high blood pressure reactions with certain foods and medicines, sleeplessness, low blood pressure, dizziness, drowsiness, weakness, dry mouth, constipation, stomach upset, blurred vision, urinary difficulties, ankle swelling, rash, jaundice, weight gain, confusion, sexual desire changes, confusion.
Caution: in the elderly and in patients suffering from epilepsy.
Not to be used for: children, or for patients suffering from liver disease, blood disorders, heart disease, PHAEOCHROMOCYTOMA (a disease of the adrenal glands), overactive thyroid, brain artery disease.
Caution needed with: amphetamines or similar SYMPATHOMIMETIC drugs, ANTICHOLINERGICS, LEVODOPA, drugs that lower blood pressure, TRICYCLIC ANTIDEPRESSANTS, PETHIDINE and other opiate ANALGESICS, some cough/cold remedies, and appetite suppressants containing SYMPATHOMIMETICS. BARBITURATES, sedatives, alcohol, and antidiabetics may be enhanced. Cheese, Bovril, Oxo, meat extracts, broad beans, banana, Marmite, yeast extracts, wine, beer, other alcohol, pickled herrings, vegetable proteins. (Up to 14 days after cessation.)
Contains: TRANYLCYPROMINE SULPHATE.
Other preparations:

Paroven
(Zyma Healthcare)

A yellow capsule supplied at a strength of 250 mg and used as a vein constrictor to treat ankle swelling, varicose veins.

Dose: 2 capsules twice a day.
Availability: NHS, private prescription, over the counter.
Side effects: stomach disturbances, flushes, headache.
Caution:
Not to be used for: children.
Caution needed with:
Contains: OXERUTINS.
Other preparations:

---

paroxetine *see* Seroxat

Parstelin
(SmithKline Beecham)

A green tablet used as an MAOI to treat depression with anxiety.

Dose: 1 tablet twice a day at first, increasing to 1 tablet 3 times a day if needed after 7 days, then usually 1 tablet a day.
Availability: NHS and private prescription.
Side effects: severe high blood pressure reactions with certain foods and medicines, low blood pressure, sleeplessness, low blood pressure, dizziness, drowsiness, weakness, dry mouth, constipation, stomach upset, blurred vision, urinary difficulties, ankle swelling, rash, blood and skin changes, jaundice, weight gain, confusion, sexual desire changes.
Caution: in the elderly, and in patients suffering from epilepsy.
Not to be used for: children, or for patients suffering from liver disease, blood changes, heart disease, PHAEOCHROMOCYTOMA, overactive thyroid, brain artery disease.
Caution needed with: amphetamines or similar SYMPATHOMIMETIC drugs, anticholinergics, some drugs that lower blood pressure, TRICYCLIC ANTIDEPRESSANTS, tranquillizers, LEVODOPA, PETHIDINE and other opiate ANALGESICS, some cough/cold remedies, and appetite suppressants containing SYMPATHOMIMETICS. BARBITURATES, sedatives, alcohol, and antidiabetics may be enhanced. Cheese, Bovril, Oxo, meat extracts, broad beans, banana, Marmite, yeast extracts, wine, beer, other alcohol, pickled herrings, vegetable proteins. (Up to 14 days after cessation.)
Contains: TRANYLCYPROMINE SULPHATE, TRIFLUOPERAZINE.
Other preparations:

Pavacol-D
(Boehringer Ingelheim)

A mixture containing and opiate cough suppressant and demulcents used to treat cough.

Dose: adults 5-10 ml as needed; children 1-2 years 2.5 ml 3-4 times a day, 3-5 years 5 ml 3 times a day, 6-12 years 5 ml 4-5 times a day.
Availability: NHS, private prescription, over the counter.
Side effects: constipation.
Caution: patients suffering from asthma
Not to be used for: for infants under 1 year or for patients suffering from liver disease.
Caution needed with: MAOIS.
Contains: PHOLCODINE, with aromatic and volatile oils.
Other preparations: GALENPHOL, PHOLCODINE LINCTUS.

PC4
(Schering Healthcare)

A white tablet used as an oestrogen, progestogen contraceptive in an emergency within 72 hours of intercourse where no other precautions have been taken.

Dose: 2 tablets within 72 hours of intercourse, then a further 2 tablets exactly 12 hours later.
Availability: NHS and private prescription.
Side effects: vomiting, nausea, rarely thrombosis, raised blood pressure, jaundice, disturbed menstrual pattern, breast discomfort, headache (if vomiting occurs, consult your doctor).
Caution: in patients with a history of depression, diabetes, high blood pressure, epilepsy, PORPHYRIA, tetanus, liver and kidney disease, gallstones, cardiovascular disease.
Not to be used for: women whose menstrual bleeding is overdue.
Caution needed with: RIFAMPICIN, TETRACYCLINE ANTIBIOTICS, GRISEOFULVIN, BARBITURATES, PHENYTOIN, PRIMIDONE, CARBAMAZEPINE, MEPROBAMATE, CHLORAL HYDRATE, ETHOSUXIMIDE, CHLORPROMAZINE.
Contains: ETHINYLOESTRADIOL, NORGESTREL.
Other preparations:

Pecram *see* aminophylline tablets
(Zyma Healthcare)

---

pectin *see* **Orabase**

---

pemoline *see* **Volital**

Penbritin *see* **ampicillin capsules**
(Beecham)

Pendramine *see* **penicillamine tablets**
(ASTA Medica)

---

penicillamine *see* **Distamine, penicillamine tablets,
Pendramine**

---

penicillamine tablets

A tablet supplied at strengths of 125 mg, 250 mg and used as an anti-arthritic drug and binding agent to treat severe active rheumatoid arthritis, Wilson's disease (inherited disorders), heavy metal poisoning, liver disease, cystinuria (a rare kidney disease).

Dose: varies between 125 mg and 3 g a day, depending on condition. (Lower doses used for elderly patients and children.) Usually given only on expert advice.
Availability: NHS and private prescription.
Side effects: nausea, loss of apetite, fever, rash, loss of taste, blood changes, blood or protein in the urine, kidney changes, muscle disease, LUPUS-like symptoms.
Caution: in pregnant women, nursing mothers and in patients suffering from kidney disease, sensitivity to penicillin. Your doctor may advise that your blood and urine should be checked regularly. Tell your doctor if sore throat, rash, mouth ulcers, bruising, or other unidentified illness develop.
Not to be used for: very allergic patients, or for patients suffering from LUPUS erythematosus, blood disorders.
Caution needed with: ANTACIDS, iron or zinc supplements.
Contains: PENICILLAMINE
Other preparations: DISTAMINE, PENDRAMINE.

---

penicillin *see* **Apsin, phenoxymethylpenicillin**

---

penicillin V (phenoxymethylpenicillin) tablets

A tablet supplied at a strength of 250 mg and used as a penicillin treatment for ear, chest, and throat infections, some wound infections, and rheumatic fever.

Dose: adults 2-3 tablets 4 times a day; children 6-12 years 1 tablet 4 times a day, under 6 years use elixir. (Lower doses used for prevention of infection.)
Availability: NHS and private prescription.
Side effects: allergy including shock, skin rash and itch, fever, joint pains; diarrhoea, blood changes.
Caution: in patients with a history of allergy or kidney failure.
Not to be used for: patients allergic to penicillins.
Caution needed with: ANTICOAGULANTS, METHOTREXATE, the contraceptive pill, PROBENECID.
Contains: PHENOXYMETHYLPENICILLIN.
Other preparations: penicillin V elixir. APSIN.

---

pentaerythritol tetranitrate *see* Mycardol

Pentasa *see* Asacol
(Yamanouchi)

---

pentazocine *see* Fortagesic, Fortral, pentazocine capsules/tablets

---

pentazocine capsules/tablets

A capsule supplied at a strength of 50 mg (and tablet at 25 mg), and used as an opiate ANALGESIC to relieve pain.

Dose: adults 25-100 mg every 3-4 hours after food; children 1-6 years by injection; children 6-12 years 25 mg every 3-4 hours after food, 1-6 years use injection.
Availability: controlled drug; NHS and private prescription.
Side effects: sedation, dizziness, psychological effects, stomach upset, constipation, difficulty passing urine, dry mouth, sweating, headache, flushing, rash, itch, low body temperature, vertigo, altered heart rhythm, hallucinations.
Caution: in pregnant women, nursing mothers, the elderly, and in patients suffering from kidney, liver, or respiratory disease, PORPHYRIA, underactive thyroid, low blood pressure, asthma.

Not to be used for: children under 1 year or for patients suffering from respiratory disorder, raised pressure in the brain, high blood pressure, heart failure, head injury, certain brain conditions, or dependence on opiates.
Caution needed with: MAOIS, sedatives, alcohol, SELEGILINE, CIMETIDINE, other opiate analgesics.
Contains: PENTAZOCINE hydrochloride.
Other preparations: pentazocine suppositories, injection. FORTRAL.

Pentran see phenytoin tablets
(Berk)

Pentrax
(Euroderma)

A liquid used to treat psoriasis of the scalp, dandruff, seborrhoeic dermatitis.

Dose: shampoo using the liquid at least twice a week.
Availability: NHS, private prescription, over the counter.
Side effects: irritation.
Caution:
Not to be used for:
Caution needed with:
Contains: COAL TAR.
Other preparations: T-GEL, GELCOTAR LIQUID, CLINITAR SHAMPOO, BALTAR.

Pepcid
(Morson)

A biege, square tablet or a brown, square tablet supplied at strengths of 20 mg, 40 mg and used as a HISTAMINE H$_2$-BLOCKER in the prevention and treatment of duodenal and gastric ulcers, Zollinger-Ellison syndrome (high acid production).

Dose: adults prevention 20 mg at night, otherwise 40 mg at night and up to 800 mg a day in rare disorders.
Availability: NHS and private prescription.
Side effects: headache, dizziness, constipation, diarrhoea, dry mouth, nausea, rash, bowel discomfort, loss of appetite, fatigue. Rarely breast swelling, skin disorders.
Caution: in pregnant women, nursing mothers, and in patients suffering from impaired kidney function. Stomach cancer should be excluded as a diagnosis.

Not to be used for: children.
Caution needed with:
Contains: FAMOTIDINE.
Other preparations: Pepcid-AC (a 10 mg tablet available over the counter only to treat heartburn, indigestion, and excess acid).

---

peppermint oil *see* Colpermin, Mintec

Peptimax *see* cimetidine tablets
(Ashbourne)

Percutol
(Cusi)

An ointment used as a NITRATE for the prevention of angina.

Dose: apply every 3-4 hours or as advised.
Availability: NHS, private prescription, over the counter.
Side effects: headache.
Caution:
Not to be used for: children.
Caution needed with:
Contains: GLYCERYL TRINITRATE.
Other preparations: CORO-NITRO, DEPONIT, GLYCERYL TRINITRATE TABLETS, GLYTRIN, GTN, MINITRAN, NITRO-DUR, NITROCONTIN, NITROLINGUAL, SUSCARD BUCCAL, SUSTAC, TRANSIDERM-NITRO.

---

pergolide mesylate *see* Celance

Pergonal
(Serono)

An injection used as a sex hormone to treat underdeveloped sexual organs in males and to treat infertility through failure of ovulation in women.

Dose: to encourage male testicular descent: 1 ampoule by injection 3 times a week as an additional treatment; to treat infertility in women: as advised by the physician.
Availability: NHS, private prescription.
Side effects: in men: allergy; in women: allergy, multiple pregnancy, over-stimulation of the ovaries.

Caution: patients with hormonal disorders or brain disorders must be treated before using this drug.
Not to be used for: children, pregnant women.
Caution needed with:
Contains: MENOTROPHIN.
Other preparations:

Periactin
(M.S.D.)

A white, scored tablet supplied at a strength of 4 mg and used as an ANTIHISTAMINE, serotonin antagonist (hormone blocker) to improve appetite, and to treat allergies, itchy skin conditions, migraine.

Dose: adults 1 tablet 3-4 times a day; children reduced doses. (For migraine, adults 1 tablet repeated after 30 minutes if necessary, to a maximum of 2 tablets in 4-6 hours, then reduce to 1 every 4-6 hours; not suitable for treating migraine in children.)
Availability: NHS, private prescription, over the counter.
Side effects: ANTICHOLINERGIC effects, reduced reactions, drowsiness.
Caution: in pregnant women and in patients suffering from bronchial asthma, raised eye pressure, overactive thyroid, cardiovascular disease, high blood pressure.
Not to be used for: children under 2 years, nursing mothers, the elderly, or patients suffering from glaucoma, enlarged prostate, bladder obstruction, retention of urine, stomach blockage, stomach ulcer, or debilitation. Not to be used during asthma attack.
Caution needed with: MAOIS, alcohol, sedatives.
Contains: CYPROHEPTADINE HYDROCHLORIDE.
Other preparations: Periactin Syrup.

---

pericyazine *see* **Neulactil**

Perinal
(Dermal)

A metered-dose spray used as a local anaesthetic and STEROID treatment for pain and irritation in and around the anus.

Dose: spray the affected area with 2 applications up to 3 times a day.
Availability: NHS, private prescription.
Side effects: raised blood sugars, thinning of the skin, osteoporosis, euphoria, depression, stomach ulcer, weight gain, flushing, hair growth, raised blood pressure, mental disturbances.

Caution: in pregnant women. Do not use for extended periods.
Not to be used for: children, or for treating infected anal conditions.
Caution needed with:
Contains: HYDROCORTISONE, LIGNOCAINE hydrochloride.
Other preparations:

---

perindopril *see* **Coversyl**

---

permethrin *see* **Lyclear**

Permitabs *see* **potassium permanganate solution**
(Bioglan)

---

perphenazine *see* **Fentazin, Triptafen**

Persantin
(Boehringer Ingelheim)

An orange tablet or a white tablet according to strengths of 25 mg, 100 mg and used as an anti-platelet drug in addition to oral ANTICOAGULANTS to prevent blood clots after heart valve replacement.

Dose: adults 300-600 mg a day in 3-4 doses before meals; children 5 mg per kg body weight a day in divided doses.
Availability: NHS and private prescription.
Side effects: headache, dizziness, stomach upset, rash.
Caution: in patients suffering from rapidly worsening angina, and some other heart conditions.
Not to be used for:
Caution needed with: ANTACIDS.
Contains: DIPYRIDAMOLE.
Other preparations: CEREBROVASE.

Pertofran
(Ciba)

A pale-pink tablet supplied at a strength of 25 mg and used as a TRICYCLIC ANTIDEPRESSANT to treat depression.

Dose: adults 1 tablet 3 times a day for 3 days, increasing to 2 tablets 3-4 times a day; elderly 1 tablet a day at first. Maximum 12 tablets a day.

Availability: NHS and private prescription.
Side effects: dry mouth, constipation, urine retention, blurred vision, palpitations, rapid heart rate, tinnitus, drowsiness, sleeplessness, nervousness, dizziness, hands shaking, low blood presure, sweating, weakness, fits, weight change, skin reactions, jaundice or blood changes, loss of sexual function may occur.
Caution: in nursing mothers or in patients suffering from heart disease, liver disorders, thyroid disease, epilepsy, diabetes, glaucoma, adrenal tumour, urinary retention, kidney disorder, constipation, some other psychiatric conditions. Your doctor may advise regular blood tests.
Not to be used for: children, pregnant women, or for patients suffering from heart attacks, liver disease, heart block.
Caution needed with: alcohol, sedatives, ANTICHOLINERGICS, ADRENALINE, MAOIS, BARBITURATES, other antidepressants, blood-pressure lowering drugs, CIMETIDINE, oestrogens, CARBAMAZEPINE, PHENYTOIN, local anaesthetics.
Contains: DESIPRAMINE hydrochloride.
Other preparations:

P

---

pertussis vaccine

Pertussis (whooping cough) vaccine is usually given in combination with diphtheria and tetanus vaccines. See **diphtheria, tetanus, and pertussis (DTP) vaccine.** A single vaccination is available, however, for those children for whom the whooping cough vaccine was not given or not completed as part of the DTP vaccination.

Dose: 3 injections of 0.5 ml at monthly intervals.
Availability: NHS, private prescription.
Side effects: local redding, swelling, and hardening around the site of the injection, mild fever. Rarely, shock, breathing difficulties, swelling of the throat, collapse, unresponsiveness, screaming, convulsions.
Caution: in patients with a family history of feverish convulsions. For any patient with evolving brain disorder, vaccination should be delayed until the condition is stabilized.
Not to be used for: patients suffering from any acute illness, or for patients who have had severe local or more generalized reactions to previous vaccinations.
Caution needed with:
Contains: pertussin antigen.
Other preparations:

Peru balsam *see* **Anugesic-HC, Anusol, Anusol HC**

---

pethidine hydrochloride *see* **pethidine tablets**

---

pethidine tablets
(Roche)

Tablets supplied at strengths of 50 mg and used as an opiate ANALGESIC to treat moderate to severe pain.

Dose: 1-3 tablets every 4 hours; children 0.5-2 mg/kg body weight.
Availability: controlled drug; NHS and private prescription.
Side effects: nausea, vomiting, constipation, drowsiness, low blood pressure, breathing difficulties, difficulty passing urine, dry mouth, sweating, flushing, vertigo, slow or irregular heart beat, loss of body temperature, hallucinations, mood change, addiction, constricted pupils, rash, itching.
Caution: in pregnant women, nursing mothers, and in patients suffering from low blood pressure, underactive thyroid, asthma and breathing problems, liver and kidney damage. Withdraw slowly at end of treatment. Not suitable for treating severe prolonged pain.
Not to be used for: patients suffering from raised pressure in the head, severe kidney disorder, or head injury.
Caution needed with: MEXILETINE, MAOIS, alcohol, sedatives, tranquillizers, CISAPRIDE, DOMPERIDONE, METOCLOPRAMIDE, SELEGILINE, CIMETIDINE.
Contains: PETHIDINE HYDROCHLORIDE.
Other preparations:

Pevaryl
(Janssen-Cilag)

A cream used as an antifungal treatment for fungal skin infections, including those of the genital areas.

Dose: massage gently into the affected area 2-3 times a day.
Availability: NHS, private prescription, over the counter.
Side effects: irritation.
Caution:
Not to be used for:
Caution needed with:
Contains: ECONAZOLE nitrate.
Other preparations: Pevaryl Lotion. GYNO PEVARYL. Also Pevaryl TC (with strong STEROID for inflamed conditions).

---

phaeochromocytoma
a tumour of the adrenal gland which produces excess ADRENALINE-like

hormones.

---

phenelzine sulphate *see* Nardil

Phenergan
(Rhône-Poulenc Rorer)

A blue tablet supplied at strengths of 10 mg, 25 mg and used as an ANTIHISTAMINE treatment for allergies, nausea, vomiting, and for sedation (if recommended by a doctor).

Dose: adults 10-20 mg 2-3 times a day; children 2-5 years 5-15 mg a day, over 5 years 10-25 mg a day (using syrup).
Availability: NHS, private prescription, over the counter (for allergies and travel sickness only).
Side effects: drowsiness, reduced reactions, dizziness, disorientation, sensitivity to light, ANTICHOLINERGIC effects, extrapyramidal reactions (shaking and rigidity).
Caution:
Not to be used for: children under 2 years.
Caution needed with: sedatives, MAOIS, alcohol.
Contains: PROMETHAZINE hydrochloride.
Other preparations: Phenergan Elixir, Phenergan Injection. AVOMINE, SOMINEX.

---

phenindamine tartrate *see* Thephorin

---

phenindione *see* Dindevan

---

pheniramine *see* Daneral SA

---

phenobarbitone tablets

A white tablet supplied at strengths of 15 mg, 30 mg, 60 mg, 100 mg, and used as a BARBITURATE to treat epilepsy.

Dose: adults, 60-180 mg at night; children 5-8 mg/kg body weight a day.
Availability: controlled drug; NHS and private prescription.
Side effects: drowsiness, lethargy, depression, lack of co-ordination, skin rash, excitement, restlessness, confusion, anaemia.
Caution: in the elderly, pregnant women, nursing mothers, physically

weak patients, and in patients suffering from liver or kidney damage, or breathing difficulty. Withdrawal should be gradual.

Not to be used for: patients suffering from PORPHYRIA.

Caution needed with: DISOPYRAMIDE, QUINIDINE, CHLORAMPHENICOL, DOXYCYCLINE, METRONIDAZOLE, NICOUMALONE, WARFARIN, antidepressants, other anti-epileptics, sedatives, alcohol, FELODIPINE, israpidine, NICARDIPINE, NIFEDIPINE, DIGITOXIN, STEROIDS, GESTRINONE, TIBOLONE, the contraceptive pill, THEOPHYLLINE, THYROXINE, VITAMIN D, ISRADIPINE, VERAPAMIL, DILTIAZEM, CYCLOSPORIN, GRISEOFULVIN.

Contains: PHENOBARBITONE.

Other preparations:

---

phenol *see* **magnesium sulphate paste**

---

phenothrin *see* **Full Marks**

---

phenoxybenzamine *see* **Dibenyline**

---

phenoxymethylpenicillin *see* **Penicillin-V**

---

phentermine *see* **Duromine, Ionamin**

---

phenylephrine *see* **Betnovate Rectal, Dimotapp LA, Hayphryn, Isopto Frin, phenylephrine eye drops, Phenylephrine Minims**

---

phenylephrine eye drops

Drops supplied at a strength of 10% and used as a SYMPATHOMIMETIC pupil dilator.

Dose: 1 drop into the eye as needed.
Availability: NHS, private prescription, over the counter.
Side effects:
Caution: in the elderly, children, and in patients suffering from heart disease; do not drive for 1-2 hours after using these drops.
Not to be used for: patients suffering from narrow angle glaucoma, high blood pressure coronary disease, overactive thyroid, diabetes.
Caution needed with: MAOIS, TRICYCLIC ANTIDEPRESSANTS, ß-BLOCKERS.
Contains: PHENYLEPHRINE.
Other preparations: PHENYLEPHRINE MINIMS (single-use containers,

additionally available in a weaker strength).

Phenylephrine Minims *see* phenylephrine eye drops
(Chauvin)

phenylethyl alcohol *see* Ceanel Concentrate

phenylpropanolamine *see* Dimotapp LA

phenytoin *see* Epanutin, Pentran, phenytoin tablets/capsules

phenytoin tablets/capsules

A tablet or capsule supplied at strengths of 50 mg, 100 mg, and used as an anticonvulsant to treat epilepsy.

Dose: initially adults, 150-300 mg a day increasing as necessary to a maximum of 600 mg a day; children 5-8 mg per kilogram body weight a day. Take the dose with or after food.
Availability: NHS and private prescription.
Side effects: stomach upset, confusion, dizziness, headache, shaking, sleeplessness, nervousness, unstable movements, speech and vision disturbances, rash, acne, hair growth, LUPUS, skin and blood changes, gum disorders.
Caution: in pregnant women, nursing mothers, and in patients suffering from liver disorders. Withdraw slowly.
Not to be used for: patients suffering from PORPHYRIA.
Caution needed with: ASPIRIN, AZAPROPAZONE, ANTACIDS, drugs affecting heart rhythm, some antibiotics, ANTICOAGULANTS, some antidepressants, TOLBUTAMIDE, other anticonvulsants, antifungal drugs, sedatives, tranquillizers, drugs used to treat angina and high blood pressure, STEROIDS, CYCLOSPORIN, METHOTREXATE, DISULFIRAM, LITHIUM, OESTROGENS, the contraceptive pill, CIMETIDINE, OMEPRAZOLE, SULPHINPYRAZONE, FOLIC ACID, INFLUENZA VACCINE.
Contains: PHENYTOIN sodium.
Other preparations: EPANUTIN (also available as suspension, chewable tablets, and 25 mg capsules).

Phimetin *see* cimetidine tablets
(BHR Pharmaceuticals)

pHiso-Med
(Sanofi Winthrop)

A solution used as a disinfectant to treat acne, and for disinfecting infants' skin, cleansing and disinfecting skin before surgery.

Dose: use as a liquid soap.
Availability: NHS, private prescription, over the counter.
Side effects:
Caution: in newborn infants dilute 1 in 10. Avoid ears and eyes.
Not to be used for:
Caution needed with:
Contains: CHLORHEXIDINE gluconate.
Other preparations: HIBISCRUB, HIBISOL, HIBITANE, UNISEPT.

---

pholcodine *see* **Galenphol, Pavacol-D, pholcodine linctus BP**

---

pholcodine linctus BP

A linctus supplied at a strength of 5 mg in 5 ml and used as an opiate cough suppressant to treat dry or painful cough.

Dose: adults 5-10 ml 3-4 times a day; children 5-12 years 2.5-5 ml 3-4 times a day.
Availability: NHS, private prescription, over the counter.
Side effects: constipation, breathing difficulties.
Caution: in patients suffering from asthma, liver or kidney disorder, or with a history of drug abuse.
Not to be used for: children under 5 years, or for patients suffering from liver disease or breathing failure.
Caution needed with: MAOIS.
Contains: PHOLCODINE.
Other preparations: pholcodine linctus, strong BP; GALENPHOL, PAVACOL-D (other brands are available over the counter, but not on NHS prescription).

Phosphate-Sandoz
(Sandoz)

A white, effervescent tablet used as a phosphate supplement to treat elevated calcium levels and low phosphate levels.

Dose: adults and children over 5 years up to 6 tablets a day; children under 5 years half adult dose.
Availability: NHS, private prescription, over the counter.

Side effects: diarrhoea, nausea.
Caution: in patients suffering from kidney disease or those on a low sodium diet.
Not to be used for:
Caution needed with: ANTACIDS.
Contains: SODIUM ACID PHOSPHATE, SODIUM BICARBONATE, POTASSIUM BICARBONATE.
Other preparations:

Phyllocontin Continus *see* aminophylline tablets
(Napp)

Physeptone *see* methadone tablets
(Wellcome)

physostigmine *see* physostigmine eye drops

physostigmine eye drops

Eye drops supplied at strengths of 0.25%, 0.5%, and used to treat glaucoma.

Dose: adults apply 2-6 times a day
Availability: NHS and private prescription.
Side effects: blurred vision, sweating, slow heart beat, intestinal pain, excess saliva, breathing spasm.
Caution:
Not to be used for:
Caution needed with:
Contains: PHYSOSTIGMINE sulphate.
Other preparations: physostigmine and pilocarpine eye drops.

Phytex
(Pharmax)

A paint used as an antifungal treatment for skin and nail infections.

Dose: paint on to the affected area morning and evening and after bathing until 2-3 weeks after the symptoms have gone.
Availability: NHS, private prescription, over the counter.
Side effects:
Caution:

Not to be used for: children under 5 years or pregnant women.
Caution needed with:
Contains: TANNIC ACID, BORIC ACID, SALICYLIC ACID, METHYL SALICYLATE, ACETIC ACID.
Other preparations:

---

phytomenadione *see* vitamin K

Picolax
(Ferring)

Powder supplied in sachets and used as a stimulant and laxative for the evacuation of bowels prior to surgery etc.

Dose: adults 1 sachet dissolved in water before breakfast, repeated 6-8 hours later if required; children 2-4 years ½ sachet morning and afternoon, children 4-9 years 1 sachet in morning, ½ sachet in afternoon, children over 9 years adult dose.
Availability: NHS, private prescription, over the counter.
Side effects:
Caution: low-residue food should be eaten before treatment, and plenty of water drunk during treatment. Special care should be taken for patients suffering from inflammatory bowel disease.
Not to be used for: patients suffering from blocked intestine.
Caution needed with:
Contains: SODIUM PICOSULPHATE, MAGNESIUM CITRATE.
Other preparations: LAXOBERAL, SODIUM PICOSULPHATE.

---

pilocarpine *see* Isopto Carpine, Ocusert Pilo, pilocarpine eye drops, Pilocarpine Minims, Sno Pilo

---

pilocarpine eye drops

Drops, available in various strengths, used as a pupil constrictor to treat glaucoma.

Dose: 1 drop into the eye 3-6 times a day.
Availability: NHS and private prescription.
Side effects: blurred vision, and if significant amounts are absorbed, sweating, slow heart beat, intestinal colic, breathing difficulty.
Caution:
Not to be used for: patients with acute iritis.
Caution needed with:

Contains: PILOCARPINE nitrate.
Other preparations: PILOCARPINE MINIMS (packed in single-use containers).
ISOPTO CARPINE, SNO-PILO, OCUSERT (slow-release insert), physostigmine and pilocarpine eye drops.

Pilocarpine Minims see pilocarpine eye drops
(Chauvin)

---

pimozide *see* **Orap**

---

pindolol *see* **Viskaldix, Visken**

. **pinene** *see* **Rowachol, Rowatinex**

---

piperazine *see* **Pripsen Sachets**

---

piperazine oestrone sulphate *see* **Harmogen**

---

pirbuterol *see* **Exirel**

---

pirenzepine *see* **Gastrozepin**

---

piretanide *see* **Arelix**

Piriton *see* **chlorpheniramine tablets**
(A & H)

Piroflam *see* **piroxicam capsules**
(Opus)

---

piroxicam *see* **Feldene, Flamatrol, Piroflam, piroxicam capsules, Pirozip**

piroxicam capsules

A capsule supplied at strengths of 10 mg, 20 mg and used as a NON-STEROIDAL ANTI-INFLAMMATORY DRUG to treat rheumatoid arthritis, other muscle or bone problems, acute gout, juvenile chronic arthritis.

Dose: rheumatic disease, adults 20 mg a day at first then 10-30 mg a day in divided doses; for muscle or bone problems, adults 40 mg a day for 2 days at first then 20 mg a day for 7-14 days; for gout 40 mg a day for 4-6 days. Children over 6 years and under 15 kg body weight 5 mg, 16-25 kg 10 mg, 26-45 kg 15 mg, over 46 kg 20 mg (all daily).
Availability: NHS and private prescription.
Side effects: stomach upset, swelling, brain disturbances, feeling of being unwell, blood changes, tinnitus, skin reactions, fluid retention, severe allergy, headache, dizziness, ear disturbances, liver and kidney disorders.
Caution: in pregnant women, nursing mothers, the elderly, and in patients suffering from kidney, heart, or liver disease, asthma, PORPHYRIA, LUPUS, or with a history of stomach ulcer.
Not to be used for: children under 6 years or for patients suffering from anti-inflammatory- or ASPIRIN-induced allergy, stomach ulcer, history of recurring ulcers, recent anal inflammation (suppositories).
Caution needed with: ANTICOAGULANTS, other non-steroidal anti-inflammatory drugs, CYCLOSPORIN, some antidiabetics, LITHIUM, drugs that lower blood pressure, some antibiotics, DIGOXIN, STEROIDS, METHOTREXATE, DIURETICS.
Contains: PIROXICAM.
Other preparations: FELDENE, FLAMATROL, PIROFLAM, PIROZIP (suppository and soluble tablet forms available). Feldene P Gel (available over the counter only to relieve muscular and joint pain, including rheumatic and back pain).

Pirozip *see* piroxicam capsules
(Ashbourne)

---

pivampicillin *see* Pondocillin

Pixol
(Thames)

A liquid used as an antiseptic and skin softener to treat psoriasis, seborrhoea, eczema, dandruff, and other skin disorders.

Dose: add 20-30 ml to the bath and soak for 20-30 minutes, or use when showering or washing the hair.
Availability: NHS, private prescription, over the counter.

Side effects: irritation.
Caution: keep out of the eyes. Avoid bright sunlight.
Not to be used for: treating inflamed or broken skin.
Caution needed with:
Contains: TAR, COAL TAR solution, CADE OIL.
Other preparations: POLYTAR.

---

pizotifen hydrogen malate *see* **Sanomigran**

Plaquenil
(Sanofi Winthrop)

An orange tablet supplied at a strength of 200 mg and used as an anti-arthritic drug to treat rheumatoid arthritis, LUPUS erythomatosus (a multisystem disease), skin conditions sensitive to light.

Dose: adults 2 tablets a day with food at first, then 1-2 tablets a day or up to 6.5 mg per kg body weight per day; children as advised by the physician.
Availability: NHS and private prescription.
Side effects: eye disorders, skin reactions, bleached hair, hair loss, stomach intolerance.
Caution: in nursing mothers, and in patients suffering from PORPHYRIA, kidney or liver disease, psoriasis, history of stomach, nerve, or blood disorders. The eyes should be checked regularly.
Not to be used for: pregnant women, or for patients suffering from maculopathy (eye disease).
Caution needed with: ANTACIDS, some antibiotics, any drugs likely to cause eye damage.
Contains: HYDROXYCHLOROQUINE sulphate.
Other preparations:

Plendil
(Schwarz)

Tablets supplied at strengths of 5 mg, 10 mg, and used to treat high blood pressure.

Dose: initially 5 mg a day at first, increasing if needed to a maximum of 20 mg a day.
Availability: NHS and private prescription.
Side effects: fluid retention of the ankles, dizziness, tiredness, headache, flushing, palpitations, rash, mild gum swelling.
Caution: in patients suffering from severe liver disorder or recent coronary

heart disease.
Not to be used for: children, pregnant women, nursing mothers.
Caution needed with: CIMETIDINE, PHENYTOIN, CARBAMAZEPINE, PHENOBARBITONE.
Contains: FELODIPINE.
Other preparations:

Plesmet
(Napp)

A syrup used as an iron supplement to treat and prevent iron-deficiency anaemia.

Dose: adults 5-10 ml 3 times a day; children 2.5-5 ml 1-3 times a day.
Availability: NHS, private prescription, over the counter.
Side effects: stomach upset.
Caution:
Not to be used for:
Caution needed with: TETRACYCLINE ANTIBIOTICS, ANTACIDS, LEVODOPA, zinc salts.
Contains: FERROUS GLYCINE SULPHATE.
Other preparations: FERROCONTIN CONTINUS.

Pneumovax II
(Pasterur Merieux MSD)

A vaccination used to provide active immunization against pneumonia.

Dose: adults and children over 2 years old, 1 injection of 0.5 ml.
Availability: NHS, private prescription.
Side effects: mild fever, discomfort at the site of the injection, relapse in patients suffering from skin rash caused by low blood platelet levels.
Caution: in patients with severely weak heart or lungs, or who are suffering from feverish breathing illness or an active infection. Caution in revaccination.
Not to be used for: children under 2 years, pregnant women, nursing mothers, or in patients who have been given radio- or chemotherapy to treat Hodgkin's disease, or less than 10 days before or during any treatment that suppresses the immune system.
Caution needed with: drugs that suppress the immune system.
Contains: pneumococcal vaccine.
Other preparations:

podophyllotoxin *see* Condyline, Warticon

podophyllum resin *see* **Posalfilin**

---

poldine methylsulphate *see* **Nacton Forte**

---

poliomyelitis vaccine

Usually prescribed as a live vaccine taken by mouth to give active immunization against poliomyelitis, and given as a routine immunization at the same time as DTP vaccination.

Dose: for initial immunization 3 drops from a multidose container or total contents of single-dose container given as a course of 3 doses.
Availability: NHS, private prescription.
Side effects:
Caution:
Not to be used for: patients who are suffering from vomiting, diarrhoea, or altered immunity.
Caution needed with:
Contains: live poliomyelitis vaccine.
Other preparations: inactivated polio vaccine (an injectable form).

---

poloxamer 188 *see* **Codalax**

---

polyacrylic acid *see* **Viscotears**

---

polyethylene glycol *see* **Canesten, Dioctyl Ear Drops**

---

polyethylene granules *see* **Ionax**

Polyfax
(Cusi)

An ointment or eye ointment used as an antibiotic to treat styes, conjunctivitis, other eye inflammations, skin infections, impetigo, burns.

Dose: apply at least twice a day.
Availability: NHS and private prescription.
Side effects: kidney damage, allergy.
Caution: in patients suffering from large open wounds.
Not to be used for:

Caution needed with:
Contains: POLYMYXIN B SULPHATE, BACITRACIN.
Other preparations:

---

polymyxin B sulphate *see* **Gregoderm, Maxitrol, Neosporin, Otosporin, Polyfax, Polytrim**

P

polynoxylin *see* **Anaflex Cream**

---

polysaccharide-iron complex *see* **Niferex**

---

polysorbate *see* **coal tar and salicylic acid ointment, Unguentum Merck**

Polytar AF
(Stiefel)

A shampoo used to treat psoriasis of the scalp, dandruff, seborrhoeic scalp disorders.

Dose: shampoo 2-3 times a week for at least 3 weeks.
Availability: NHS, private prescription, over the counter.
Side effects:
Caution:
Not to be used for:
Caution needed with:
Contains: TAR, COAL TAR, CADE OIL, ARACHIS OIL EXTRACT OF COAL TAR, ZINC PYRITHIONE.
Other preparations: POLYTAR LIQUID, Polytar Plus, POLYTAR EMOLLIENT.

Polytar Emollient
(Stiefel)

A liquid bath emollient used to treat eczema, and other skin conditions.

Dose: 2-4 capsful added to a 20 cm deep bath. Soak for 15-20 minutes. Pat dry.
Availability: NHS, private prescription, over the counter.
Side effects:
Caution: guard against slipping in the bath.

Not to be used for:
Caution needed with:
Contains: TAR, CADE OIL, COAL TAR, ARACHIS OIL, light LIQUID PARAFFIN.
Other preparations: POLYTAR AF, POLYTAR LIQUID.

Polytar Liquid
(Stiefel)

A liquid used as an antipsoriatic treatment for psoriasis of the scalp, dandruff, seborrhoea, eczema.

Dose: shampoo once or twice a week.
Availability: NHS, private prescription, over the counter.
Side effects:
Caution:
Not to be used for:
Caution needed with:
Contains: TAR, CADE OIL, COAL TAR, ARACHIS OIL, COAL TAR EXTRACT, OLEYL ALCOHOL.
Other preparations: Polytar Plus, POLYTAR AF.

---

polythiazide *see* Nephril

Polytrim
(Cusi)

Drops used as an antibacterial treatment for eye infections.

Dose: 1 drop into the eye 4 times a day until 2 days after the symptoms have gone.
Availability: NHS and private prescription.
Side effects:
Caution:
Not to be used for:
Caution needed with:
Contains: TRIMETHOPRIM, POLYMYXIN B SULPHATE.
Other preparations: Polytrim Ointment.

---

polyvinyl alcohol *see* Hypotears, Liquifilm Tears, Ocufen, Sno Tears

---

Ponderax Pacaps
(Servier)

A blue/clear capsule supplied at a strength of 60 mg and used as an appetite suppressant to treat severe obesity.

Dose: 1 capsule a day 30 minutes before a meal; continue treatment for no more than 3 months.
Availability: NHS and private prescription.
Side effects: hallucinations, nervousness, sedation, diarrhoea, dry mouth, frequent urination, depression if the drug is withdrawn suddenly.
Caution:
Not to be used for: children, epileptics, or patients with a history of alcoholism, drug addiction, or depression.
Caution needed with: MAOIS, blood-pressure lowering drugs, antidepressants, antidiabetic drugs, sedatives, alcohol, other obesity drugs.
Contains: FENFLURAMINE hydrochloride.
Other preparations:

Pondocillin
(Leo)

A white, egg-shaped tablet supplied at a strength of 500 mg and used as a penicillin to treat bronchitis, pneumonia, ear, nose, and throat infections, skin, soft tissue infections, urine infections, gonorrhoea.

Dose: adults 1 tablet twice a day with food or drink; children use suspension.
Availability: NHS and private prescription.
Side effects: allergy, stomach disturbances.
Caution: in patients suffering from kidney disease.
Not to be used for: patients suffering from glandular fever.
Caution needed with:
Contains: PIVAMPICILLIN.
Other preparations: Pondocillin Suspension.

Ponstan *see* mefenamic acid capsules/tablets
(Parke-Davis)

Pork Insulatard *see* Insulin

Pork Mixtard *see* **Insulin**

---

porphyria
A rare inherited disorder that leads to abnormality in the red blood cells.

Posalfilin
(Norgine)

P

An ointment used as a skin softener to treat plantar warts (verrucae).

Dose: protect healthy skin, apply the ointment to the wart, and cover; repeat 2-3 times a week.
Availability: NHS, private prescription, over the counter.
Side effects: pain when the ointment is first applied.
Caution: do not use on healthy skin.
Not to be used for: pregnant women or on warts on the face or anal and genital areas.
Caution needed with:
Contains: SALICYLIC ACID, PODOPHYLLUM RESIN.
Other preparations:

PostMI *see* **aspirin 75 mg tablets**
(Ashbourne)

Potaba
(Glenwood)

A powder in a 3 g sachet used as a fibrous tissue dissolver to treat scleroderma (thickened skin), Peyronie's disease.

Dose: 1 sachet with food 4 times a day.
Availability: NHS, private prescription, over the counter.
Side effects: loss of appetite, nausea.
Caution: in patients suffering from kidney disease.
Not to be used for: for children.
Caution needed with: sulphonamide antibiotics.
Contains: POTASSIUM P-AMINOBENZOATE.
Other preparations: Potaba Tablets, Potaba Capsules.

---

potassium benzoate *see* **Kloref**

---

potassium bicarbonate *see* **Algicon, Kloref, Phosphate, Sando-K**

---

potassium citrate *see* **Effercitrate, potassium citrate mixture BP**

---

potassium citrate mixture BP

A solution used as an alkalinizing treatment for the relief of discomfort in mild infections of the urinary tract.

Dose: 10 ml diluted in water 3 times a day.
Availability: NHS, private prescription, over the counter.
Side effects: raised potassium levels on high doses, mild DIURETIC effects.
Caution: in the elderly and in patients suffering from kidney failure, heart disease.
Not to be used for:
Caution needed with: CYCLOSPORIN, potassium-sparing DIURETICS, ACE INHIBITORS.
Contains: POTASSIUM CITRATE.
Other preparations: various over-the-counter remedies containing the ingredient are available. EFFERCITRATE.

---

potassium chloride *see* **Burinex K, Diarrest, Dioralyte, Diumide-K Continus, Electrolade, Glandosane, Gluco-lyte, Kay-Cee-L, Kloref, Lasikal, Lasix + K, Neo-Naclex-K, Rehidrat, Salivace, Sando-K, Slow-K**

---

potassium clorazepate *see* **Tranxene**

---

potassium hydroxyquinolone sulphate *see* **Quinocort, Quinoderm Cream, Quinoped**

---

potassium p-aminobenzoate *see* **Potaba**

---

potassium permanganate solution

A solution used to cleanse and deodorize weeping eczema and wounds.

Dose: apply as a wet dressing, or soak the affected part.

Availability: NHS, private prescription, over the counter.
Side effects: irritation of mucous membrane.
Caution: stains skin and clothing.
Not to be used for:
Caution needed with:
Contains: potassium permanganate.
Other preparations: PERMITABS (tablets dissolved in water to make the solution).

---

povidone-iodine *see* **Betadine, Betadine Gargle and Mouthwash, Betadine Ointment, Betadine Scalp and Skin Cleanser, Betadine Spray**

Powergel *see* **Oruvail Gel**
(Searle)

Pragmatar
(Bioglan)

A cream used as an anti-itch, antiseptic, skin softener to treat scaly skin, scalp seborrhoea and similar disorders.

Dose: apply weekly, or daily in severe cases, to wet hair.
Availability: NHS, private prescription, over the counter.
Side effects: irritation.
Caution: dilute the cream first when using for infants. Avoid eyes, groin, or inflamed areas.
Not to be used for:
Caution needed with:
Contains: CETYL ALCOHOL/COAL TAR distillate, SULPHUR, SALICYLIC ACID.
Other preparations:

---

pramoxine *see* **Anugesic-HC, Epifoam, Proctofoam-HC**

---

pravastatin *see* **Lipostat**

Praxilene
(Lipha)

A pink capsule supplied at a strength of 100 mg and used as a blood vessel dilator to treat brain and blood vessel disorders.

Dose: 1-2 capsules 3 times a day.
Availability: NHS and private prescription.
Side effects: nausea, stomach pain, rash, rarely liver disorder.
Caution:
Not to be used for: children.
Caution needed with:
Contains: NAFTIDROFURYL OXALATE.
Other preparations: Praxilene Forte injection (restricted to hospitals).

P

prazosin *see* **Alphavase, Hypovase, prazosin tablets**

prazosin tablets

A tablet supplied at strengths of 500 micrograms, 1 mg, 2 mg, 5 mg and used as an alpha-blocker to treat congestive heart failure, high blood pressure, Raynaud's phenomenon, additional treatment in urinary obstruction caused by prostate enlargement.

Dose: for heart failure 500 micrograms 2-4 times a day at first, increasing to 1 mg 3-4 times a day, followed by 4-20 mg a day in divided doses to maintain treatment. For high blood pressure 500 micrograms on first evening, then 500 micrograms 2-3 times a day for 3-7 days increasing as needed to a maximum of 20 mg a day. For Raynaud's phenomenon or prostate enlargement 500 micrograms twice a day at first then 1-2 mg twice a day.
Availability: NHS and private prescription.
Side effects: low blood pressure on standing, dizziness, nausea, lassitude, headache, palpitations, increased urination, drowsiness.
Caution: in the elderly, pregnant women, nursing mothers, and in patients suffering from fainting when they urinate, kidney failure. Take the first dose when going to bed.
Not to be used for: children, or for patients suffering heart failure due to blockage.
Caution needed with: blood-pressure lowering drugs, anaesthetics, NON-STEROIDAL ANTI-INFLAMMATORY DRUGS, ß-BLOCKERS, STEROIDS, DIURETICS, sedatives, alcohol, some anti-angina treatments.
Contains: PRAZOSIN hydrochloride.
Other preparations: ALPHAVASE, HYPOVASE.

Preconceive
(Lane)

A tablet used as a FOLIC ACID supplement, taken before and during pregnancy to help prevent spina bifida and other neural tube defects in the developing foetus.

Dose: 1 tablet each day until the end of the third month of pregnancy.
Availability: NHS, private prescription, over the counter.
Side effects:
Caution: patients with epilepsy or anaemia should consul a doctor before using this medication.
Not to be used for:
Caution needed with: some anti-epileptic medications.
Contains: FOLIC ACID.
Other preparations:

Precortisyl *see* prednisolone tablets
(Hoechst Roussel)

Pred Forte
(Allergan)

Drops used as a STEROID treatment for inflammation of the eye where no infection is present.

Dose: 1-2 drops into the eye 2-4 times a day or 2 drops every hour for the first two days if needed.
Availability: NHS and private prescription.
Side effects: rise in eye pressure, secondary fungal or viral infections, thinning cornea, cataract.
Caution: in infants and pregnant women.
Not to be used for: patients suffering from glaucoma, viral, fungal, tubercular, or weeping eye infections, dendritic ulcer, or for patients who wear soft contact lenses.
Caution needed with:
Contains: PREDNISOLONE acetate.
Other preparations: PREDSOL EYE DROPS.

Predenema *see* Predsol Enema
(Pharmax)

Predfoam *see* Predsol Enema
(Pharmax)

Prednesol *see* **prednisolone tablets**
(Glaxo)

---

prednisolone *see* **Deltacortril, Deltastab, Precortisyl, Predenema, Pred Forte, Predfoam, Prednesol, Prednisolone Minims, prednisolone tablets, Predsol Enema, Predsol Drops, Scheriproct**

Prednisolone Minims
(Chauvin)

Drops used as a STEROID treatment for inflammation of the eye where no infection is present.

Dose: 1-2 drops as needed; children as advised by the physician.
Availability: NHS and private prescription.
Side effects: rise in eye pressure, fungal infection, cataract, thinning cornea.
Caution: in infants – do not use for extended periods.
Not to be used for: pregnant women or for patients suffering from glaucoma, viral, fungal, tubercular, or acute weeping infections.
Caution needed with:
Contains: PREDNISOLONE sodium phosphate.
Other preparations: PRED FORTE, PREDSOL EYE DROPS.

---

prednisolone tablets

A tablet supplied at strengths of 1 mg, 5 mg and used as a STEROID treatment for inflammatory and allergic conditions.

Dose: adults up to 60 mg a day, and then reduce to minimum effective dose. (Children used reduced doses.)
Availability: NHS and private prescription.
Side effects: high blood sugar, thin bones, mood changes, stomach ulcers, fluid retention, potassium loss, high blood pressure.
Caution: in pregnant women, in patients who have had recent bowel surgery, or who are suffering from inflamed veins, psychiatric disorders, virus infections, chickenpox, some cancers, some kidney diseases, thinning of the bones, stomach ulcers, tuberculosis, other infections, high blood pressure, glaucoma, epilepsy, diabetes, underactive thyroid, liver disease, stress. Withdraw gradually. Avoid contact with chicken pox and seek medical attention if exposed.
Not to be used for: infants under 1 year.
Caution needed with: RIFAMPICIN, DIURETICS, DIGOXIN, antidiabetic agents,

ANTICOAGULANTS, NON-STEROIDAL ANTI-INFLAMMATORY DRUGS, ASPIRIN, drugs that lower blood pressure, CYCLOSPORIN, some drugs used to treat asthma, anticonvulsants.

Contains: PREDNISOLONE.

Other preparations: prednisolone EC tablets (coated to protect the stomach – do not take with ANTACIDS). DELTACORTRIL (coated to protect the stomach – do not take with ANTACIDS), DELTASTAB, PRECORTISYL, PREDNESOL (soluble tablets).

---

prednisone *see* Decortisyl, prednisone tablets

---

prednisone tablets

A tablet supplied at a strength of 5 mg and used as a STEROID treatment for inflammatory conditions, allergies.

Dose: adults up to 60 mg a day, then reduce to minimum effective dose. (Children use reduced doses.)

Availability: NHS and private prescription.

Side effects: high blood sugar, thin bones, mood change, stomach ulcers, fluid retention, potassium loss, high blood pressure.

Caution: in pregnant women, in patients who have had recent bowel surgery, or who are suffering from inflamed veins, psychiatric disorders, virus infections, some cancers, some kidney diseases, thinning of the bones, stomach ulcers, tuberculosis, other infections, high blood pressure, glaucoma, epilepsy, diabetes, underactive thyroid, stress. Withdraw gradually. Avoid contact with chicken pox and seek medical attention if exposed.

Not to be used for: infants under 1 year, or for patients suffering from liver disease.

Caution needed with: RIFAMPICIN, DIURETICS, DIGOXIN, antidiabetic agents, ANTICOAGULANTS, NON-STEROIDAL ANTI-INFLAMMATORY DRUGS, ASPIRIN, drugs that lower blood pressure, CYCLOSPORIN, some drugs used to treat asthma, anticonvulsants.

Contains: PREDNISONE.

Other preparations: DECORTISYL.

Predsol Enema
(Evans)

An enema supplied at a strength of 20 mg and used as a STEROID treatment for ulcerative colitis.

Dose: 1 at night for 2-4 weeks.

Availability: NHS and private prescription.
Side effects: systemic CORTICOSTEROID effects (*see* prednisolone tablets).
Caution: in pregnant women. Do not use for prolonged periods.
Not to be used for: children, or for treating tuberculous, fungal, viral, or bacterial infections.
Caution needed with:
Contains: PREDNISOLONE.
Other preparations: Predsol Suppositories. PREDFOAM, PREDENEMA .

Predsol Drops
(Evans)

Drops used as a STEROID treatment for inflammation of the ear or eye where no infection is present.

Dose: 2-3 drops into the ear every 2-3 hours or 1-2 drops into the eye every 1-2 hours.
Availability: NHS and private prescription.
Side effects: allergy, resistance to NEOMYCIN (in Predsol-N), rise in eye pressure, thinning cornea, cataract.
Caution: do not use unless necessary, and avoid use over extended periods for infants or pregnant women.
Not to be used for: patients suffering from viral, fungal, tubercular, or weeping infections, dendritic ulcer, glaucoma or for patients who wear soft contact lenses; patients with perforated ear drum (Predsol-N).
Caution needed with:
Contains: PREDNISOLONE sodium phosphate.
Other preparations: Predsol-N (contains neomycin, for infected conditions). PRED FORTE, PREDNISOLONE MINIMS.

Preferid
(Yamanouchi)

A cream or ointment used as a strong STEROID to treat eczema, psoriasis, and dermatitis.

Dose: apply sparingly 2-3 times a day.
Availability: NHS and private prescription.
Side effects: fluid retention, suppression of adrenal glands, thinning, streaking, or spotting of the skin.
Caution: use for short periods of time only, especially in children or on the face.
Not to be used for: continuously, especially for pregnant women or for patients suffering from acne or any other tubercular, viral, fungal, or ringworm skin infections, scabies, leg ulcers.

Caution needed with:
Contains: BUDESONIDE.
Other preparations:

Prefil
(Norgine)

Brown granules used as a bulking agent to treat obesity.

Dose: 1 sachet swallowed with water ½-1 hour before eating.
Availability: NHS, private prescription, over the counter.
Side effects: stomach discomfort.
Caution: in patients suffering from ulcerative colitis.
Not to be used for: patients suffering from a blocked intestine, or lack of normal bowel motion.
Caution needed with:
Contains: STERCULIA.
Other preparations: NORMACOL.

Pregaday
(Evans)

A brownish-red tablet used as an iron and FOLIC ACID supplement for prevention of iron and folic acid deficiency in pregnancy.

Dose: 1 tablet a day.
Availability: NHS, private prescription, over the counter.
Side effects: stomach upset, allergy.
Caution: in patients with a history of stomach ulcer or who are in the first three months of pregnancy.
Not to be used for: patients suffering from VITAMIN B_{12} deficiency.
Caution needed with: PHENYTOIN, anticonvulsant drugs, CO-TRIMOXAZOLE, some antibiotics, ANTACIDS, LEVODOPA.
Contains: FERROUS FUMARATE, FOLIC ACID.
Other preparations: FOLEX-350, GALFER FA, METERFOLIC.

Pregnyl
(Organon)

An injection used as a sex hormone to treat low sperm count and underdeveloped sex organs in males, and as an additional treatment for infertility in women.

Dose: as prescribed by the physician.

Availability: NHS, private prescription.
Side effects: water and salt retention, rash.
Caution: in patients suffering from raised blood pressure, heart or kidney failure, epilepsy, migraine. Women will have hormone levels regularly checked.
Not to be used for: children, pregnant women, or patients who are suffering from certain types of cancer.
Caution needed with:
Contains: GONADOTROPHIN.
Other preparations: GONADOTROPHON LH, PROFASI.

Premarin
(Wyeth)

A maroon, oval tablet, yellow, oval tablet, or purple, oval tablet according to strengths of 0.625 mg, 1.25 mg, 2.5 mg and used as an oestrogen for hormone replacement during and after the menopause, and to prevent thinning of the bones.

Dose: menopause 0.625-1.25 mg a day for 21 days starting on the fifth day of the period if present, then 7 days without tablets. Other, as advised by the physician.
Availability: NHS and private prescription.
Side effects: enlarged breasts, fluid retention, nausea, vaginal bleeding, weight gain, headache, dizziness. Rarely jaundice, raised blood pressure, thrombosis.
Caution: in patients suffering from high blood pressure, diabetes, epilepsy, womb diseases, gall bladder disorder, migraine, multiple sclerosis, PORPHYRIA, liver disorders, some ear disorders, or a history or increased risk of breast disorders (including cancer) and thrombosis. Your doctor may advise you to have regular examinations.
Not to be used for: children, pregnant women, nursing mothers, or for patients suffering from thombosis, severe liver, kidney, or heart disorders, some cancers, undiagnosed vaginal bleeding, endometriosis.
Caution needed with: ACE INHIBITORS, ANTICOAGULANTS, BARBITURATES, ß-BLOCKERS, CARBAMAZEPINE, PHENYTOIN, RIFAMPICIN.
Contains: conjugated oestrogens.
Other preparations: Premarin Vaginal Cream.

Premique
(Wyeth)

A blue tablet used as an oestrogen, progestogen for hormone replacement in women over 54 years, who have not had a hysterectomy, and who are suffering from menopausal symptoms, or who are at risk from osteoporosis.

Dose: 1 tablet a day, taken continuously.
Availability: NHS and private prescription.
Side effects: enlarged breasts, fluid retention, nausea, vaginal bleeding, weight gain, headache, dizziness. Rarely jaundice, raised blood pressure, thrombosis.
Caution: in patients suffering from high blood pressure, diabetes, epilepsy, womb diseases, gall bladder disorder, migraine, multiple sclerosis, PORPHYRIA, liver disorders, some ear disorders, or a history or increased risk of breast disorders (including cancer) and thrombosis. Your doctor may advise you to have regular examinations.
Not to be used for: children, pregnant women, nursing mothers, or for patients suffering from thombosis, severe liver, kidney, or heart disorders, some cancers, undiagnosed vaginal bleeding, endometriosis.
Caution needed with: ACE INHIBITORS, ANTICOAGULANTS, BARBITURATES, ß-BLOCKERS, CARBAMAZEPINE, PHENYTOIN, RIFAMPICIN.
Contains: OESTROGEN, MEDROXYPROGESTERONE acetate.
Other preparations: Premique Cycle (where the two ingredients are contained in 2 separate tablets – used in postmenopausal women of any age, and taken so that a monthly withdrawal bleed occurs).

Prempak-C
(Wyeth)

A maroon, oval tablet or yellow, oval tablet according to strengths of 0.625 mg, 1.25 mg plus a brown tablet 0.15 mg and used as an oestrogen, progestogen for hormone replacement during and after the menopause, and treatment of post-menopausal osteoporosis.

Dose: beginning on the first day of the period if present,1 maroon or yellow tablet a day for 16 days then 1 maroon or yellow tablet plus 1 brown tablet a day for 12 days.
Availability: NHS and private prescription.
Side effects: enlarged breasts, fluid retention, nausea, vaginal bleeding, weight gain, headache, dizziness. Rarely jaundice, raised blood pressure, thrombosis.
Caution: in patients suffering from high blood pressure, diabetes, epilepsy, womb diseases, gall bladder disorder, migraine, multiple sclerosis, PORPHYRIA, liver disorders, some ear disorders, or a history or increased risk of breast disorders (including cancer) and thrombosis. Your doctor may advise you to have regular examinations.
Not to be used for: children, pregnant women, nursing mothers, or for patients suffering from thombosis, severe liver, kidney, or heart disorders, some cancers, undiagnosed vaginal bleeding, endometriosis.
Caution needed with: ACE INHIBITORS, ANTICOAGULANTS, BARBITURATES, ß-BLOCKERS, CARBAMAZEPINE, PHENYTOIN, RIFAMPICIN.
Contains: conjugated oestrogens plus NORGESTREL.

Other preparations:

Prepadine *see* **dothiepin capsules**
(Berk)

P

Prepulsid
(Janssen-Cilag)

A white, scored tablet supplied at a strength of 10 mg and used as a stomach-emptying drug to treat gastric reflux, inflamed oesophagus, indigestion, and to encourage emptying of the stomach in conditions where the nerve supply is impaired.

Dose: up to 40 mg a day in divided doses.
Availability: NHS and private prescription.
Side effects: abdominal cramps, stomach rumbling, diarrhoea, occasionally headaches and convulsions, shaking, rigidity.
Caution: in the elderly, nursing mothers, and in patients suffering from kidney or liver impairment.
Not to be used for: pregnant women or for patients suffering from blocked intestines, intestinal perforation or bleeding.
Caution needed with: sedatives, ANTICOAGULANTS, ANTICHOLINERGICS, KETOCONAZOLE, ITRACONAZOLE, MICONAZOLE, some antibiotics.
Contains: CISAPRIDE.
Other preparations: Prepulsid Suspension. ALIMIX.

Prescal
(Ciba)

A yellow scored tablet supplied at a strength of 2.5 mg and used as a calcium antagonist to treat high blood pressure.

Dose: adults 1 tablet morning and evening, increasing after 3-4 weeks to 2 tablets twice a day if needed, up to a maximum of 4 tablets twice a day; lower doses for the elderly.
Availability: NHS and private prescription.
Side effects: weight gain, palpitations, rapid heart rate, swelling, headache, flushing, dizziness, tiredness, abdominal pain, skin rash, liver enzyme changes, rise in liver enzymes, localized fluid retention.
Caution: pregnant women, nursing mothers, and in patients suffering from some rare heart conditions.
Not to be used for: children.
Caution needed with: anticonvulsants.
Contains: ISRADIPINE.

Prestim
(Leo)

A white, scored tablet used as a ß-BLOCKER/thiazide DIURETIC combination to treat high blood pressure.

Dose: 1-4 tablets a day.
Availability: NHS and private prescription.
Side effects: cold hands and feet, sleep disturbance, slow heart rate, tiredness, wheezing, heart failure, low blood pressure, stomach upset, sensitivity to light, weakness, blood changes, gout, dry eyes, rash.
Caution: in pregnant women, nursing mothers, and in patients suffering from diabetes, high blood lipids, kidney or liver disorders, gout. May need to be withdrawn before surgery. Withdraw gradually. Your doctor may advise additional treatment with diuretics or DIGOXIN.
Not to be used for: children, or for patients suffering from heart block or failure, severe kidney disease, low blood pressure, untreated PHAEOCHROMOCYTOMA, breathing difficulties, or a history of asthma.
Caution needed with: VERAPAMIL, CLONIDINE withdrawal, some anti-arrhythmic drugs and anaesthetics, RESERPINE, some blood-pressure lowering drugs, ERGOTAMINE, CIMETIDINE, sedatives, SYMPATHOMIMETICS, INDOMETHACIN, LITHIUM, DIGOXIN, AMANTADINE, ALLOPURINOL, antidiabetics.
Contains: TIMOLOL maleate, BENDROFLUAZIDE.
Other preparations: Prestim Forte.

Priadel
(Delandale)

A white, scored tablet supplied at strengths of 200 mg, 400 mg and used as a LITHIUM salt to treat mania, manic depression, recurring depression, aggression, and self-injuring behaviour.

Dose: to keep blood levels in a given range.
Availability: NHS and private prescription.
Side effects: nausea, diarrhoea, hand tremor, muscular weakness, brain and heart disturbances, weight gain, fluid retention, under- or overactive thyroid, thirst and excessive urination, skin reactions. Your doctor may advise blood tests to gauge dose.
Caution: treatment should start in hospital. Kidney, heart, and thyroid function should be checked regularly. Salt and fluid consumption should be maintained.
Not to be used for: children, pregnant women, nursing mothers, or for patients suffering from Addison's disease, weak kidneys or heart,

underactive thyroid, disturbed sodium balance.
Caution needed with: DIURETICS, NON-STEROIDAL ANTI-INFLAMMATORY DRUGS,
sedatives, other antidepressants, hypnotics, PHENYTOIN, CARBAMAZEPINE,
FLUPENTHIXOL, HALOPERIDOL, DIAZEPAM, METHYLDOPA, TETRACYCLINE ANTIBIOTICS,
METOCLOPRAMIDE.
Contains: LITHIUM CARBONATE.
Other preparations: CAMCOLIT, LISKONUM.

P

prilocaine *see* EMLA

Primalan
(Rhône-Poulenc Rorer)

A white tablet supplied at a strength of 5 mg and used as an ANTIHISTAMINE
treatment for allergy, itch, hay fever, rhinitis.

Dose: 1 tablet twice a day.
Availability: NHS and private prescription.
Side effects: drowsiness, reduced reactions, ANTICHOLINERGIC effects,
extrapyramidal reactions (shaking and rigidity).
Caution:
Not to be used for: children, pregnant women, or for patients suffering
from epilepsy, enlarged prostate, liver disease, glaucoma.
Caution needed with: sedatives, MAOIS, SYMPATHOMIMETICS, alcohol.
Contains: MEQUITAZINE.
Other preparations:

---

primidone *see* Mysoline

Primolut N *see* norethisterone tablets
(Schering Healthcare)

Primoteston Depot
(Schering Healthcare)

An injection containing male sex hormone to treat underdeveloped male
sexual organs.

Dose: 250 mg by inection every 2-3 weeks at first, then 250 mg every 3-6
weeks.
Availability: NHS, private prescription.
Side effects: persistent painful erection, fluid retention, weight gain,

decreased fertility, liver disorder, premature end to growth.
Caution: in patients suffering from heart, liver, or kidney disorders, raised blood pressure, epilepsy, migraine.
Not to be used for: children, or for patients suffering from some heart problems or kidney disorders, or some cancers.
Caution needed with: BARBITURATES, GRISEOFULVIN, anticonvulsants, RIFAMPICIN.
Contains: TESTOSTERONE.
Other preparations: VIRORMONE, SUSTANON-100, RESTANDOL (capsule form).

P

Primperan *see* metoclopramide tablets
(Berk)

Prioderm
(Seton Healthcare)

A lotion used as a pediculicide, scabicide to treat scabies, lice of the head and pubic areas.

Dose: rub in and shampoo hair after 2-12 hours; repeat after 7-9 days.
Availability: NHS, private prescription, over the counter.
Side effects:
Caution: in infants under 6 months, and in patients suffering from asthma, eczema. Keep out of the eyes.
Not to be used for:
Caution needed with:
Contains: MALATHION.
Other preparations: Prioderm Cream Shampoo. DERBAC-M, SULEO-M.

Pripsen Sachets
(Seton Healthcare)

A sachet used to treat worms.

Dose: adults and children over 6 years 1 sachet and then a second dose of 1 sachet after 14 days; infants 3 months-1 year ⅓ sachet then a second dose after 14 days; children 1-6 years ⅔ sachet then a second dose after 14 days.
Availability: NHS, private prescription, over the counter.
Side effects: rarely sight disorders, vertigo.
Caution: care in nursing mothers and in patients suffering from nervous disorders.
Not to be used for: patients suffering from epilepsy, liver or kidney disease.

Caution needed with:
Contains: PIPERAZINE phosphate, SENNOSIDES.
Other preparations:

Pripsen Tablets *see* **Vermox**
(Seton Healthcare)

P

Pro-Banthine
(Baker-Norton)

A peach-coloured tablet supplied at a strength of 15 mg and used as an anti-spasm, ANTICHOLINERGIC treatment for ulcers, irritable bowel syndrome, bed wetting.

Dose: adults up to 8 daily in divided doses.
Availability: NHS and private prescription.
Side effects: blurred vision, confusion, dry mouth.
Caution: in the elderly and in patients suffering from ulcerative colitis, heart disease, autonomic neuropathy, kidney and liver disease, overactive thyroid.
Not to be used for: children or for patients suffering from glaucoma, obstructive bowel disease, obstructive disease of the urinary tract.
Caution needed with: DIGOXIN.
Contains: PROPANTHELINE BROMIDE.
Other preparations:

Pro-Viron
(Schering Healthcare)

A white, scored tablet supplied at a strength of 25 mg and used as a male sex hormone to treat low hormone levels, infertility in men.

Dose: 1 tablet 3-4 times a day for several months, then 2-3 tablets a day.
Availability: NHS and private prescription.
Side effects: liver disorders, painful persistent erection.
Caution:
Not to be used for: children, or for patients suffering from liver or prostate cancer.
Caution needed with: liver-enzyme inducing drugs such as BARBITURATES, CARBAMAZEPINE, PHENYTOIN, PRIMIDONE, RIFAMPICIN.
Contains: MESTEROLONE.
Other preparations:

---

probenecid *see* **Benemid**

Probeta *see* **propanolol SR capsules**
(Trinity)

---

probucol *see* **Lurselle**

---

procainamide *see* **Pronestyl**

---

prochlorperazine *see* **Buccastem, prochlorperazine tablets, Prozière, Stemetil**

---

prochlorperazine tablets

A tablet supplied at a strength of 5 mg and used as a ANTIHISTAMINE anti-sickness medication to treat vertigo, severe nausea, vomiting, inner ear disturbances.

Dose: for nausea and vomiting, adults 20 mg at first then 10 mg after 2 hours; for prevention 5-10 mg 2-3 times a day; children use syrup. For ear disorders 5 mg 3 times a day increasing if necessary to 30 mg a day in divided doses, then reducing to 5-10 mg a day.
Availability: NHS and private prescription.
Side effects: brain disturbances, ANTICHOLINERGIC effects, heart and hormone changes, sensitivity to light, allergies, eye changes, rarely liver and skin changes, sleeplessness, depression, blocked nose, blood disorder, altered body temperature, drowsiness, heart rhythm disturbance, low blood pressure, muscle spasm, weight gain, blurred vision, changes in sexual function, breast swelling, menstrual changes, fits, shaking, rigidity.
Caution: in the elderly, pregnant women, nursing mothers, and in patients suffering from heart or circulatory disease, undiagnosed or prolonged vomiting, breathing disorders, epilepsy, Parkinson's disease, infections, kidney or liver disease, underactive thyroid, prostate disorders, glaucoma, MYASTHENIA GRAVIS, certain blood disorders.
Not to be used for: patients in an unconscious state, or patients suffering from bone marrow depression, PHAEOCHROMOCYTOMA.
Caution needed with: sedatives, alcohol, ANALGESICS, blood-pressure lowering drugs, antidepressants, ANTICHOLINERGICS, anticonvulsants, some antidiabetics, anaesthetics, ANTACIDS, anti-arrhythmic drugs, ASTEMIZOLE, TERFENADINE, LITHIUM, CIMETIDINE, LEVODOPA, ß-BLOCKERS, drugs affecting heart rhythm.
Contains: PROCHLORPERAZINE maleate.

Other preparations: STEMETIL, PROZIÈRE.

Proctofoam HC
(Stafford-Miller)

Foam supplied in an aerosol with an applicator and used as a STEROID, local anaesthetic treatment for haemorrhoids, bowel inflammation, fissures.

Dose: in the rectum 1 application 2-3 times a day and after passing motions; around the anus apply as required. Maximum treatment period 7 days.
Availability: NHS and private prescription.
Side effects: systemic CORTICOSTEROID effects (*see* prednisolone tablets).
Caution: in pregnant women; do not use for prolonged periods.
Not to be used for: children or for patients suffering from tuberculous, fungal and viral infections.
Caution needed with:
Contains: HYDROCORTISONE acetate, PROXAMINE hydrochloride.
Other preparations:

Proctosedyl
(Hoechst-Roussel)

Suppositories used as a STEROID, local anaesthetic treatment for haemorrhoids, anal fissure, inflammation, itch.

Dose: 1 suppository night and morning and after passing motions.
Availability: NHS and private prescription.
Side effects: systemic CORTICOSTEROID effects (*see* prednisolone tablets).
Caution: in pregnant women; do not use for prolonged periods.
Not to be used for: patients suffering from tuberculous, fungal or viral infections.
Caution needed with:
Contains: HYDROCORTISONE, CINCHOCAINE hydrochloride.
Other preparations: Proctosedyl Ointment.

---

procyclidine *see* Arpicolin, Kemadrin, procyclidine tablets

---

procyclidine tablets

A tablet supplied at a strength of 5 mg and used as an ANTICHOLINERGIC to treat Parkinson's disease.

Dose: ½ tablet 3 times a day after meals at first, increasing to a maximum of 12 tablets a day.
Availability: NHS and private prescription.
Side effects: dry mouth, stomach upsets, blurred vision, dizziness, retention of urine, rapid pulse, severe allergy, confusion at high doses.
Caution: in patients suffering from heart problems, enlarged prostate, liver or kidney disorders. Reduce dose slowly.
Not to be used for: children or patients suffering from untreated urinary retention, glaucoma, obstruction in stomach or intestines.
Caution needed with: some sedative drugs, ANTIHISTAMINES, antidepressants, some tranquillizers, other anticholinergic drugs, NITRATE drugs used to treat angina and heart failure.
Contains: PROCYCLIDINE hydrochloride
Other preparations: ARPICOLIN (available only as syrup), KEMADRIN (tablet and syrup form available).

Profasi
(Serono)

An injection used as a sex hormone to encourage testicles to descend in males, to treat infertility through failure of ovulation in women, and underdeveloped sexual organs in men.

Dose: as advised by the physician.
Availability: NHS, private prescription.
Side effects: in men: allergy, fluid retention; in women: allergy, fluid retention, over-stimulation of the ovaries.
Caution: patients with hormonal disorders must be treated before using this drug. Women should have their hormone levels checked regularly.
Not to be used for: children.
Caution needed with:
Contains: GONADOTROPHIN.
Other preparations: GONADOTROPHIN LH, PREGNYL.

---

proflavine cream BPC

A cream used to treat minor cuts and abrasions.

Dose: apply as necessary,
Availability: NHS, private prescription, over the counter.
Side effects:
Caution: stains clothing.
Not to be used for:
Caution needed with:
Contains: proflavine cream BPC.

Other preparations:

Proflex Cream
(Zyma Healthcare)

A cream used as a NON-STEROIDAL ANTI-INFLAMMATORY preparation to treat rheumatic and muscular pain, sprains, strains.

Dose: 4-10 cm cream applied to the affected area 3-4 times a day.
Availability: NHS, private prescription, over the counter.
Side effects: reddening of skin.
Caution: in nursing mothers. Avoid broken skin, lips, and eyes.
Not to be used for: children, pregnant women, or for patients suffering from allergy to ASPIRIN or anti-inflammatories.
Caution needed with:
Contains: IBUPROFEN.
Other preparations: Proflex Tablets, Proflex Capsules. IBUGEL, Ibuleve (both gel forms) IBUSPRAY (spray form).

Progesic *see* Fenopron
(Eli Lilly)

---

progesterone *see* Cyclogest, Gestone

---

proguanil hydrochloride *see* Paludrine

Progynova
(Schering Healthcare)

A beige tablet or a blue tablet according to strengths of 1 mg, 2 mg and used as a hormone replacement therapy for the treatment of menopausal symptoms in women who have had a hysterectomy.

Dose: initially 1 mg a day, increasing to 2 mg if necessary.
Availability: NHS and private prescription.
Side effects: enlarged breasts, fluid retention, nausea, vaginal bleeding, weight gain, headache, dizziness. Rarely jaundice, raised blood pressure, thrombosis.
Caution: in patients suffering from high blood pressure, diabetes, epilepsy, womb diseases, gall bladder disorder, migraine, multiple sclerosis, PORPHYRIA, liver disorders, some ear disorders, or a history or increased risk of breast disorders (including cancer) and thrombosis. Your

doctor may advise you to have regular examinations.

Not to be used for: children, pregnant women, nursing mothers, or for patients suffering from thombosis, severe liver, kidney, or heart disorders, some cancers, undiagnosed vaginal bleeding, endometriosis.

Caution needed with: ACE INHIBITORS, ANTICOAGULANTS, BARBITURATES, ß-BLOCKERS, CARBAMAZEPINE, PHENYTOIN, RIFAMPICIN.

Contains: OESTRADIOL valerate.

Other preparations: CLIMAVAL, ZUMENON.

Proluton Depot
(Schering Health Care)

An injection supplied at a strength of 250 mg/ml and used as a progestogen treatment to prevent abortion in pregnant women where this is habitual.

Dose: 1-2 injections a week during the first half of pregnancy.
Availability: NHS, private prescription.
Side effects:
Caution:
Not to be used for: children.
Caution needed with:
Contains: HYDROXY-PROGESTERONE HEXANOATE.
Other preparations:

promazine *see* promazine tablets, Sparine

promazine tablets

A coated tablet supplied at strengths of 50 mg, 100 mg, and used as a sedative to treat agitation or restlessness in the elderly, additional short-term treatment for other types of agitation.

Dose: adults 100-200 mg 4 times a day; elderly 25-50 mg 4 times a day for restlessness.
Availability: NHS and private prescription.
Side effects: muscle spasms, restlessness, hands shaking, low blood pressure, heart rhythm disturbance, weight gain, blurred vision, changes in sexual function, breast swelling, menstrual changes, jaundice, blood and skin changes, eye changes, apathy, nightmares, sleeplessness, depression, dry mouth, blocked nose, difficulty passing water, rarely fits, change in body temperature, drowsiness.
Caution: in pregnant women, nursing mothers, the elderly, and in patients suffering from liver or kidney disease, heart or circulatory disorder,

Parkinson's disease, epilepsy, infections, blood disorders, underactive thyroid, MYASTHENIA GRAVIS, glaucoma, enlarged prostate, respiratory disorders.

Not to be used for: unconscious patients, the elderly, or for patients suffering from bone marrow depression, PHAEOCHROMOCYTOMA.

Caution needed with: alcohol, sedatives, tranquillizers, blood-pressure lowering drugs, antidepressants, anticonvulsants, some antidiabetic drugs, LEVODOPA, anaesthetics, ANTACIDS, anti-arrhythmic drugs, ASTEMIZOLE, TERFENADINE, ANTICHOLINERGICS, SOTALOL, DIURETICS, LITHIUM, CIMETIDINE, pain killers.

Contains: PROMAZINE hydrochloride.

Other preparations: promazine syrup. SPARINE.

---

promethazine *see* **Avomine, Phenergan, Sominex**

Prominal
(Sanofi Winthrop)

A white tablet supplied at strengths of 30 mg, 60 mg, 200 mg and used as a BARBITURATE to treat epilepsy.

Dose: adults 100-600 mg a day; children 5-15 mg per kg body weight a day.

Availability: controlled drug; NHS and private prescription.

Side effects: tolerance, addiction, drowsiness, hangover, dizziness, allergies, headache, confusion, excitement, lack of co-ordination, breathing difficulties.

Caution: in patients suffering from kidney, liver, or lung disease. Dependence (addiction) may develop.

Not to be used for: children, young adults, pregnant women, nursing mothers, the elderly, the debilitated, patients with a history of drug or alcohol abuse, or suffering from PORPHYRIA, or in the management of pain.

Caution needed with: ANTICOAGULANTS, alcohol, sedatives, other tranquillizers, STEROIDS, the contraceptive pill, GRISEOFULVIN, RIFAMPICIN, PHENYTOIN, METRONIDAZOLE, CHLORAMPHENICOL.

Contains: METHYLPHENOBARBITONE.

Other preparations:

Pronestyl
(Squibb)

A white, scored tablet supplied at a strength of 250 mg and used as an anti-arrhythmic drug to treat abnormal heart rhythm.

Dose: up to 50 mg per kg body weight a day in divided doses every 3-6 hours.
Availability: NHS and private prescription.
Side effects: SLE (a multi-system disorder), stomach and brain disturbance, blood changes.
Caution: in the elderly, pregnant women, and in patients suffering from kidney, liver, or heart failure, MYASTHENIA GRAVIS. Your doctor may advise regular blood tests.
Not to be used for: for children, nursing mothers, or for patients suffering from heart block, SLE (a multi-system disorder).
Caution needed with: some antibiotics, blood-pressure lowering drugs, ANTICHOLINERGICS, CAPTOPRIL, other anti-arrhythmic drugs.
Contains: PROCAINAMIDE hydrochloride.
Other preparations: Pronestyl Injection.

Propaderm
(Glaxo)

A cream used as a strong STEROID treatment for skin disorders.

Dose: rub in a small quantity to the affected area twice a day.
Availability: NHS and private prescription.
Side effects: fluid retention, suppression of adrenal glands, thinning, spotting, or streaking of the skin may occur.
Caution: use for short periods of time only, especially in children or on the face.
Not to be used for: patients suffering from acne or any other skin infections caused by tuberculosis, ringworm, viruses, or fungi, leg ulcers, scabies, or continuously especially in pregnant women.
Caution needed with:
Contains: BECLOMETHASONE diprorionate.
Other preparations: Propaderm Ointment.

Propanix *see* propranolol tablets
(Ashbourne)

propantheline bromide *see* Pro-banthine

Propine
(Allergan)

Drops used as a SYMPATHOMIMETIC treatment for glaucoma, hypertension of the eye.

Dose: 1 drop into the eye every 12 hours.
Availability: NHS and private prescription.
Side effects: temporary smarting, redness, allergy, rarely raised blood pressure.
Caution: in patients suffering from narrow-angle glaucoma, absence of the lens.
Not to be used for: children or for patients suffering from closed angle glaucoma or who wear soft contact lenses.
Caution needed with:
Contains: DIPIVEFRIN hydrochloride.
Other preparations:

---

propranolol hydrochloride *see* **Angilol, Apsolol, Bedranol, Berkolol, Beta-Prograne, Cardinol, Half Beta-Prograne, Half-Inderal LA, Inderal, Inderal LA, Inderetic, Inderex, Probeta, Propanix, propranolol tablets**

---

propranolol tablets

A tablet supplied at strengths of 10 mg, 40 mg, 80 mg, 160 mg, and used as a ß-BLOCKER to treat high blood pressure, PHAEOCHROMCYTOMA, angina, heart rhythm disturbances, anxiety, and in the prevention of migraine and further attacks after a heart attack.

Dose: 80-320 mg a day depending on condition.
Availability: NHS and private prescription.
Side effects: cold hands and feet, sleep disturbance, slow heart rate, tiredness, wheezing, heart failure, stomach upset, bronchospasm, rash, blood changes, dry eyes.
Caution: in pregnant women, nursing mothers, and in patients suffering from diabetes, kidney or liver disorders, MYASTHENIA GRAVIS. May need to be withdrawn before surgery. Withdraw gradually. Your doctor may advise additional treatment with DIURETICS or DIGOXIN, blood tests.
Not to be used for: children or for patients suffering from heart block or failure, very slow heart rate, asthma, or history of blocked airways disease.
Caution needed with: VERAPAMIL, DILTIAZEM, DIGOXIN, STEROIDS, DIURETICS, CIMETIDINE, FLUVOXAMINE, MEFLOQUINE, CLONIDINE withdrawal, some anti-arrhythmic drugs, some blood-pressure lowering drugs, anaesthetics, sedatives, SYMPATHOMIMETICS, alcohol, antidiabetics, ERGOTAMINE, NON-STEROIDAL ANTI-INFLAMMATORY DRUGS, RIFAMPICIN, CHLORPROMAZINE.
Contains: PROPRANOLOL HYDROCHLORIDE.
Other preparations: propranolol SR capsules. ANGILOL, APSOLOL, BEDRANOL SR, BERKOLOL, BETA-PROGRANE, CARDINOL, HALF-INDERAL LA, HALF BETA-PROGRANE, INDERAL, LOPRANOL, PROBETA, PROPANIX.

---

propyl salicylate *see* **Monphytol**

propyl undecoanate *see* **Monphytol**

propylene glycol *see* **Aserbine, Unguentum Merck**

propylthiouracil tablets

A tablet supplied at a strength of 50 mg and used to treat overactive thyroid.

Dose: adults 6-12 tablets a day, reducing gradually to 1-3 tablets a day.
Availability: NHS and private prescription.
Side effects: nausea, headache, rash, itching, blood changes, bleeding tendency, LUPUS. Report any signs of infection, such as sore throat.
Caution: in pregnant women, nursing mothers, and in patients suffering from kidney damage.
Not to be used for:
Caution needed with:
Contains: propylthiouracil.
Other preparations:

Prosaid *see* **naproxen tablets**
(BHR)

Proscar
(M.S.D.)

A blue, apple-shaped tablet supplied at a strength of 5 mg and used to treat enlarged prostate gland.

Dose: 1 tablet a day for at least 6 months. If then found to be beneficial, treatment should be continued long-term.
Availability: NHS and private prescription.
Side effects: impotence, decreased sexual function, decreased volume of ejaculate, breast tenderness and swelling.
Caution: in patients suffering from urine outflow obstruction or prostate cancer. Your doctor may advise regular tests before and during treatment. Female partners of patients being treated who are or who may become pregnant should not handle the tablets and avoid exposure to semen by using a condom.
Not to be used for: children.

Caution needed with:
Contains: FINASTERIDE.
Other preparations:

---

prostaglandin

a substance that, when it occurs naturally in the body, influences such processes as fever, pain, contraction of smooth muscle, fever production, control of blood pressure, blood clotting, and secretion of stomach acid. NON-STEROIDAL ANTI-INFLAMMATORY DRUGS inhibit prostaglandins, and reduce their unwanted effects (such as pain and swelling in rheumatic conditions). Synthetic prostaglandins are used for such purposes as inducing labour, and thinning of blood (in hospital), producing an erection (when injected), and healing stomach ulcers. Examples MISOPROSTOL (*see* Cytotec) and ALPROSTADIL (*see* Caverject).

Prostap SR
(Lederle)

An injection supplied at a strength of 3.75 mg and used to treat endometriosis in women.

Dose: 1 injection a month for a maximum of 6 months beginning during the first 5 days of the period.
Availability: NHS, private prescription.
Side effects: hot flushes, headache, emotional upset, dryness of the vagina. Your doctor will advise you to use effective barrier contraceptive methods.
Caution: in patients who are at risk from osteoporosis.
Not to be used for: children, pregnant women, nursing mothers, or for patients suffering from undiagnosed bleeding from the vagina.
Caution needed with:
Contains: LEUPRORELIN acetate.
Other preparations:

Prostigmin
(Lifehealth)

A white, scored tablet supplied at a strength of 15 mg and used as an ANTICHOLINESTERASE to treat urinary retention following surgery, bowel paralysis, MYASTHENIA GRAVIS (a muscle disorder).

Dose: adults bowel paralysis 1-2 tablets as required; children ⅙-1 tablet as required. Adults myasthenia gravis 5-20 tablets a day in divided doses; infants 1-5 mg every 4 hours, children 1-6 tablets a day in divided doses; after surgery adults 1-2 tablets; children ⅙-1 tablet.

Availability: NHS and private prescription.
Side effects: nausea, diarrhoea, colic, salivation, vomiting.
Caution: in patients suffering from bronchial asthma, heart disease, epilepsy, Parkinson's disease, disorders of the vagus nerve.
Not to be used for: patients suffering from intestinal or urinary obstruction.
Caution needed with: some drugs used in anaesthesia.
Contains: NEOSTIGMINE bromide.
Other preparations: Prostigmin Injection.

Prothiaden *see* dothiepin capsules
(Knoll)

protriptyline *see* Concordin

Provera
(Upjohn)

A white, scored tablet supplied at strengths of 5 mg, 10 mg, 100 mg, 200 mg, 400 mg and used as a progestogen treatment for abnormal bleeding of the uterus, absence of periods, endometriosis, and other hormone-dependent disorders.

Dose: 2.5-10 mg a day or as advised by a doctor.
Availability: NHS and private prescription.
Side effects: stomach upset, disorders of the skin, nervous system, and mucous membranes; on high doses breast pain, lactation, abnormal menstrual bleeding, weight gain.
Caution: in patients suffering from diabetes, epilepsy, migraine, asthma, heart or kidney failure.
Not to be used for: children, pregnant women, or patients suffering from some cancers, liver disease.
Caution needed with:
Contains: MEDROXYPROGESTERONE.
Other preparations:

proxymetacaine hydrochloride *see* Ophthaine

Prozac
(Dista)

A green/white capsule supplied at a strength of 20 mg and used as an antidepressant to treat depression, bulimia nervosa (an eating disorder), obsessive-compulsive disorder.

Dose: adults 1 capsule a day up to a maximum of 3 capsules.
Availability: NHS and private prescription.
Side effects: nausea, vomiting, diarrhoea, headache, anxiety, sleeplessness, dizziness, drowsiness, rash, fever, weakness, reduced judgement and abilities; rarely convulsions, hypomania, mania.
Caution: in pregnant women and in patients suffering from epilepsy, liver failure, moderate kidney failure, heart disease, diabetes.
Not to be used for: children, nursing mothers, or for patients suffering from severe kidney failure, unstable epilepsy.
Caution needed with: MAOIS, TRYPTOPHAN (this is in many health foods), TRICYCLIC ANTIDEPRESSANTS, FLECAINIDE, vinblastine, CARBAMAZEPINE, PHENYTOIN, LITHIUM.
Contains: FLUOXETINE.
Other preparations:

Prozière 5 *see* **prochlorperazine tablets**
(Ashbourne)

---

pseudoephedrine *see* **Dimotane Expectorant, Dimotane Plus, Galpseud, Galpseud Plus, Sudafed, Sudafed Plus**

Psoradrate
(Procter & Gamble)

A cream used as an antipsoriatic, wetting agent to treat psoriasis.

Dose: wash and dry the area, then apply the cream twice a day.
Availability: NHS, private prescription, over the counter.
Side effects: irritation, allergy.
Caution:
Not to be used for: patients suffering from pustular psoriasis.
Caution needed with:
Contains: DITHRANOL, UREA.
Other preparations: DITHROCREAM.

Psoriderm
(Dermal)

An emulsion used as an antipsoriatic to treat psoriasis.

Dose: add 30 ml of the emulsion to the bath water, soak for 15 minutes, dry, then apply the cream to the affected area.
Availability: NHS, private prescription, over the counter.
Side effects: irritation, sensitivity to light.
Caution:
Not to be used for: patients suffering from acute psoriasis.
Caution needed with:
Contains: COAL TAR.
Other preparations: Psoriderm Cream, Psoriderm Scalp Lotion. CARBO-DOME, CLINITAR, GELCOTAR, PSORIGEL.

P

Psorigel
(Galderma)

A gel used as an antipsoriatic treatment for psoriasis, eczema, allergic and itching skin disorders.

Dose: rub into the affected area and allow to dry 1-2 times a day. Remove surplus cream.
Availability: NHS, private prescription, over the counter.
Side effects: irritation, sensitivity to light.
Caution:
Not to be used for: patients suffering from acute psoriasis.
Caution needed with:
Contains: COAL TAR solution.
Other preparations: CARBO-DOME, CLINITAR, GELCOTAR, PSORIDERM.

Psorin
(Thames)

An ointment used as an antipsoriatic, skin softener to treat psoriasis.

Dose: apply to the affected areas twice a day.
Availability: NHS, private prescription, over the counter.
Side effects:
Caution: keep out of the eyes, and avoid direct sunlight.
Not to be used for: patients suffering from unstable psoriasis. Do not use topical STEROID treatments as well.
Caution needed with:
Contains: COAL TAR, DITHRANOL, SALICYLIC ACID.
Other preparations: Psorin Scalp Gel.

Pulmadil
(3M Health Care)

An aerosol supplied at a strength of 0.2 mg and used as a BRONCHODILATOR to treat bronchial spasm brought on by chronic bronchitis, bronchial asthma.

Dose: 1-3 sprays and again after 30 minutes if needed, up to a maximum of 24 sprays in 24 hours.
Availability: NHS and private prescription.
Side effects: headache, widening of the blood vessels.
Caution: in pregnant women and in patients suffering from abnormal heart rhythms, high blood pressure, overactive thyroid, heart muscle disorders, angina.
Not to be used for:
Caution needed with: SYMPATHOMIMETICS.
Contains: RIMITEROL HYDROBROMIDE.
Other preparations:

Pulmicort
(Astra)

An aerosol supplied at a strength of 200 micrograms and used as a STEROID to treat bronchial asthma.

Dose: 1 spray twice a day up to a maximum of 8 sprays a day if needed; children reduced doses or use Pulmicort LS.
Availability: NHS and private prescription.
Side effects: hoarseness, thrush of the mouth and throat. Rarely skin disorder or breathing difficulty.
Caution: in pregnant women, in patients suffering from infections of the lungs, and in those transferring from steroids taken by mouth.
Not to be used for: patients suffering from tuberculosis.
Caution needed with:
Contains: BUDESONIDE.
Other preparations: Pulmicort LS, Pulmicort Respules, Pulmicort Turbohaler.

Pulmozyme
(Genentech/Roche)

A single-use ampoule supplied at a strength of 2.5 mg/2.5 ml and used through a jet nebulizer to control cystic fibrosis.

Dose: 1 inhalation a day, or 2 inhalations a day for patients over 21 years.

Availability: NHS, private prescription.
Side effects: pharyngitis, laryngitis, hoarseness, rash, temporary breathing difficulties.
Caution: in pregnant women, nursing mothers.
Not to be used for: children under 5 years.
Caution needed with: (do not mix with other drugs in the nebulizer.)
Contains: DORNASE ALFA.
Other preparations:

Pylorid
(Glaxo)

A pale-blue, film-coated, eight-sided, capsule-shaped tablet supplied at a strength of 400 mg and used as an anti-ulcer drug (including HISTAMINE H$_2$-ANTAGONIST) to treat stomach ulcer and, in combination, to prevent recurrence.

Dose: 1 tablet twice a day for up to 8 weeks depending on condition. No more than 16 weeks treatment to be given in any one year period.
Availability: NHS, private prescription.
Side effects: blackening of tongue and faeces, stomach upset, headache, mild anaemia, changed liver function, rarely inflammation of the pancreas or liver, blood changes, bone or muscle problems, male breast problems, confusion.
Caution: in the elderly, pregnant women, nursing mothers, and in patients suffering from kidney damage or with a history of acute PORPHYRIA.
Not to be used for: children, or for patients suffering from severe kidney damage, or for use as maintenance.
Caution needed with: antidiabetics.
Contains: RANITIDINE bismuth citrate.
Other preparations:

Pyralvex
(Norgine)

A liquid used as an anti-inflammatory treatment for mouth ulcers and soreness caused by dentures.

Dose: apply to the affected area 3-4 times a day.
Availability: NHS, private prescription, over the counter.
Side effects: irritation.
Caution:
Not to be used for: children.
Caution needed with:
Contains: ANTHRAQUINONE GLYCOSIDES, SALICYLIC ACID.

Other preparations:

pyrantel *see* **Combantrin**

pyrazinamide *see* **Rifater, Zinamide**

pyridostigmine *see* **Mestinon**

pyridoxine *see* **pyridoxine tablets, vitamin B₆**

pyridoxine tablets

A tablet supplied at strengths of 10 mg, 20 mg, 50 mg, and used to treat deficiency, nerve disorders due to ISONIAZID treatment, some forms of anaemia, and premenstrual syndrome.

Dose: deficiency 20-50 mg 3 times a day; nerve disorder 50 mg 3 times a day (treatment) or 10 mg a day (prevention); anaemia 100-400 mg a day in divided doses; premenstrual syndrome 50-100 mg a day.
Availability: NHS and private prescription.
Side effects: high dose may give toxic effects.
Caution:
Not to be used for:
Caution needed with: LEVODOPA.
Contains: VITAMIN B₆.
Other preparations: Benadon, Compliment (neither available on NHS).

pyrimethamine *see* **Daraprim, Fansidar, Maloprim**

Pyrogastrone
(Sanofi Withrop)

An off-white tablet used as an ANTACID and stomach-lining protection to treat inflammation of the gullet, acid reflux.

Dose: 1 tablet to be taken 3 times a day after meals and 2 at bedtime.
Availability: NHS and private prescription.
Side effects: sodium and water retention, low blood potassium levels, low blood pressure, heart failure.
Caution: in patients suffering from sodium or water retention.

Not to be used for: children, the elderly, pregnant women, or for patients suffering from heart disorders or kidney or liver failure.

Caution needed with: tablets coated to protect the stomach, some antibiotics, iron, DIGOXIN, DIURETICS, ANALGESICS, heart-rhythm drugs, antibacterials, drugs used to treat high blood pressure.

Contains: CARBENOXOLONE sodium, MAGNESIUM TRISILICATE, ALUMINIUM HYDROXIDE, SODIUM BICARBONATE, ALGINIC ACID.

Other preparations: Pyrogastrone Suspension.

Quellada
(Stafford-Miller)

A lotion used as a scabicide to treat scabies.

Dose: apply as directed (2 applications needed, 24 hours apart).
Availability: NHS, private prescription, over the counter.
Side effects:
Caution: in pregnant women, nursing mothers. Keep out of the eyes.
Not to be used for: infants under 1 month.
Caution needed with:
Contains: LINDANE.
Other preparations: Quellada Application PC (for treating lice).

Questran
(Bristol-Myers Squibb)

A powder in a sachet used as a lipid-lowering agent to treat raised cholesterol, and to relieve some cases of diarrhoea and itching.

Dose: adults usually 1-6 sachets a day in divided doses to a maximum of 9 sachets a day; children over 6 years in proportion to dose for 70 kg adult.
Availability: NHS and private prescription.
Side effects: constipation, VITAMIN K deficiency.
Caution: in pregnant women, nursing mothers, and patients on long-term treatment should take VITAMIN A, D, K supplements.
Not to be used for: children under 6 years or for patients suffering from complete bile duct blockage.
Caution needed with: DIGOXIN, antibiotics, DIURETICS. WARFARIN, THYROXINE; take **any** other medicines either 1 hour before or 4-6 hours after Questran.
Contains: CHOLESTYRAMINE.
Other preparations: Questran Light (low sugar with added sweetener – caution in patients suffering from phenylketonuria).

Quinaband
(Seton Healthcare)

A bandage supplied at a size of 7.5 cm x 6 m, and used, in conjunction with a compression bandage, to treat varicose and gravitational ulcers, and reduce the smell of leg ulcers.

Availability: NHS, private prescription, over the counter. (Also available on a trial basis from nurses.)
Contains: ZINC PASTE, CALAMINE, CLIOQUINOL.

---

quinagolide *see* **Norprolac**

---

quinalbarbitone *see* **Seconal Sodium, Tuinal**

---

quinapril *see* **Accupro, Accuretic**

---

quinidine *see* **Kinidin Durules**

---

quinine bisulphate tablets *see* **quinine sulphate tablets**

---

quinine sulphate tablets

Tablets supplied at strengths of 200 mg, 300 mg, and used to treat malaria and leg cramps at night.

Dose: for cramp, adults 200-300 mg at night. For malaria, as advised by a doctor.
Availability: NHS and private prescription.
Side effects: noise in the ears, headache, nausea, stomach pain, rash, disturbance of vision, confusion, allergy, blood disorders, kidney failure, low blood sugar, flushing.
Caution: in pregnant women, and in patients suffering from some heart conditions and blood enzyme deficiencies.
Not to be used for: patients suffering from some blood disorders or inflammation of the optic nerve.
Caution needed with: MEFLOQUINE, DIGOXIN, CIMETIDINE, FLECAINIDE.
Contains: quinine sulphate.
Other preparations: QUININE BISULPHATE TABLETS.

Quinocort
(Quinoderm)

A cream used as a STEROID, antifungal, antibacterial treatment for skin disorders where there is also infection.

Dose: massage into the affected area 2-3 times a day.
Availability: NHS and private prescription
Side effects: fluid retention, suppression of adrenal glands, thinning, streaking or spotting of the skin may occur.
Caution: use for short periods of time only, especially in children or on the face.
Not to be used for: patients suffering from acne or any other skin infections caused by tuberculosis, ringworm, viruses, or fungi, scabies, leg ulcers, or continuously especially in pregnant women.
Caution needed with:
Contains: POTASSIUM HYDROXYQUINOLONE SULPHATE, HYDROCORTISONE.
Other preparations:

Quinoderm Cream
(Quinoderm)

A cream used as an antibacterial, skin softener to treat acne, acne-like eruptions, inflammation of the follicles.

Dose: massage into the affected area 1-3 times a day.
Availability: NHS, private prescription, over the counter.
Side effects: irritation, peeling.
Caution: keep out of the eyes, nose, mouth. May bleach fabrics.
Not to be used for:
Caution needed with:
Contains: POTASSIUM HYDROXYQUINOLONE SULPHATE, BENZOYL PEROXIDE.
Other preparations: Quinoderm Cream 5, Quinoderm Lotio-Gel 5%.

Quinoped
(Quinoderm)

A cream used as an antifungal treatment for athlete's foot and similar infections.

Dose: rub lightly into the affected area night and morning.
Availability: NHS, private prescription, over the counter.
Side effects:
Caution: may bleach fabrics.
Not to be used for:

Caution needed with:
Contains: BENZOYL PEROXIDE, POTASSIUM HYDROXYQUINOLONE SULPHATE.
Other preparations:

Rabies Vaccine
(Pasteur Merieux MSD)

A vaccination used to prevent and treat rabies.

Dose: as advised by the physician.
Availability: NHS, private prescription.
Side effects: skin reaction at injection site, fever, general illness.
Caution:
Not to be used for:
Caution needed with:
Contains: inactivated rabies virus.
Other preparations:

---

ramipril *see* **Tritace**

Ramysis *see* **doxycycline capsules**
(ISIS)

---

ranitidine *see* **Pylorid, Zantac**

Rapitard *see* **insulin**
(Novo Nordisk)

Rapitil
(Fisons)

Drops used as an anti-inflammatory treatment for allergic and other types of conjunctivitis.

Dose: 1 drop into each eye 2-4 times a day.
Availability: NHS, private prescription.
Side effects: temporary irritation, taste in the mouth.
Caution: in pregnant women.
Not to be used for: children under 6 years or for patients wearing soft contact lenses.
Caution needed with:

Contains: NEDOCROMIL sodium.
Other preparations:

Rastinon *see* **tolbutamide tablets**
(Hoechst Roussel)

Recormon
(Boehringer Mannheim Pharmaceuticals)

An injection used as a hormone treatment for anaemia associated with kidney failure or dialysis.

Dose: as prescribed by the physician.
Availability: NHS, private prescription.
Side effects: raised blood pressure, allergic shock, blood clots in shunts.
Caution: in pregnant women, nursing mothers, and in patients suffering from raised blood pressure, epilepsy, chronic liver failure, blood disorders. Your doctor will recommend regular blood tests. Other forms of anaemia should be brought under control before using this therapy.
Not to be used for: children under 2 years or for patients suffering from uncontrolled raised blood pressure.
Caution needed with:
Contains: EPOETIN BETA.
Other preparations:

Rectubes *see* Diazepam Rectubes

Refolinon
(Pharmacia)

A light-yellow tablet supplied at a strength of 15 mg and used as a folinic acid treatment for megaloblastic anaemia. Also used in emergency treatment of METHOTREXATE poisoning.

Dose: for anaemia 1 tablet a day.
Availability: NHS and private prescription.
Side effects:
Caution:
Not to be used for: patients suffering from VITAMIN B_{12} deficiency anaemia.
Caution needed with:
Contains: CALCIUM FOLINATE.
Other preparations: Refolinon Injection.

Regaine
(Upjohn)

A liquid used as a hair restorer to treat hair loss in men and women.

Dose: 1 ml applied to the scalp twice a day for at least 4 months.
Treatment must be continued or hair loss will recur.
Availability: private prescription, over the counter.
Side effects: dermatitis.
Caution: in patients suffering from low blood pressure, and on broken
skin. Your doctor may recommend blood pressure checks.
Not to be used for: children.
Caution needed with:
Contains: MINOXIDIL.
Other preparations:

Regulan
(Procter & Gamble)

An effervescent powder supplied in sachets of 3.6 g and used as a gluten-
free bulking agent to treat constipation owing to lack of fibre in the diet.

Dose: adults 1 sachet in water 1-3 times a day; children over 6 years 2.5-5
ml in water 3 times a day.
Availability: NHS, private prescription, over the counter.
Side effects:
Caution:
Not to be used for: children under 6 years and patients suffering from
intestinal obstruction.
Caution needed with:
Contains: ISPAGHULA husk.
Other preparations: FYBOGEL, ISOGEL, METAMUCIL.

Regulose *see* lactulose solution
(Sandoz)

Rehidrat
(Searle)

A lemon and lime, orange-, or blackcurrant-flavoured powder which is
dissolved in water and used to provide electrolytes in fluid and electrolyte
loss, and diarrhoea.

Dose: adults and children drink until thirst is quenched; infants substitute for feeds or give after breast feeding. 1 sachet of powder should be dissolved in 250 ml of water.

Availability: NHS, private prescription, over the counter.

Side effects:

Caution:

Not to be used for: care in patients suffering from kidney disease, blocked intestine, bowel paralysis.

Caution needed with:

Contains: SODIUM CHLORIDE, POTASSIUM CHLORIDE, SODIUM BICARBONATE, CITRIC ACID, GLUCOSE, SUCROSE, LAEVULOSE.

Other preparations: DIORALYTE, ELECTROLADE, GLUCO-LYTE (formulas may vary between brands).

Relaxit
(Crawford)

A micro-enema used as a faecal softener to treat constipation.

Dose: 1 enema.

Availability: NHS and private prescription.

Side effects:

Caution:

Not to be used for:

Caution needed with:

Contains: SODIUM CITRATE, SODIUM LAURYL SULPHATE, SORBIC ACID, GLYCEROL, SORBITOL solution.

Other preparations:

Relaxyl *see* Spasmonal
(Whitehall)

Relifex
(Bencard)

A red tablet supplied at a strength of 500 mg and used as a NON-STEROIDAL ANTI-INFLAMMATORY DRUG to treat rheumatoid arthritis, osteoarthritis.

Dose: adults 2 tablets at bed time and, if needed, 1-2 tablets in the morning; elderly 1-2 tablets a day.

Availability: NHS and private prescription.

Side effects: diarrhoea, indigestion, nausea, constipation, stomach pain, wind, headache, dizziness, rash, drowsiness.

Caution: in the elderly and in patients suffering from kidney or liver disease or with a history of stomach ulcer, allergy to ASPIRIN or anti-

inflammatories.
Not to be used for: pregnant women, nursing mothers, children, or for patients suffering from stomach ulcer, severe liver disease.
Caution needed with: ANTICOAGULANTS taken by mouth, anticonvulsants, antidiabetics, alcohol, sedatives.
Contains: NABUMETONE.
Other preparations: Relifex Suspension.

Remedeine
(Napp)

A white tablet used as a pain killer to treat pain and fever.

Dose: 1-2 tablets every 4-6 hours to a maximum of 8 tablets a day.
Availability: NHS and private prescription.
Side effects: drowsiness, nausea, vomiting, headache, vertigo, retention of urine, constipation.
Caution: in patients suffering from underactive thyroid, chronic liver disease, severe kidney disease, allergic disorder.
Not to be used for: children, or for patients suffering from breathing difficulty, raised pressure in the brain.
Caution needed with: MAOIS, alcohol, sedatives, other medicines containing PARACETAMOL.
Contains: paracetamol, DIHYDROCODEINE tartrate.
Other preparations: Remedeine Forte. CO-DYDRAMOL.

Remnos *see* nitrazepam tablets
(DDSA)

---

reproterol *see* Bronchodil

Resonium-A
(Sanofi Winthrop)

A powder used for ion-exchange to lower potassium levels.

Dose: adults 15 g taken by mouth 3-4 times a day or 30 g a day taken rectally; children 1 g per kilogram bodyweight a day taken orally or rectally in divided doses reducing to 0.5 g/kg (newborn infants use rectal route only).
Availability: NHS, private prescription, over the counter.
Side effects: low potassium levels, high sodium levels, impaction of resin
Caution: in patients suffering from heart disease. Potassium and sodium

levels should be checked regularly.
Not to be used for: patients suffering from obstructive bowel disease or in newborn infants with reduced gut activity.
Caution needed with:
Contains: SODIUM POLYSTYRENE SULPHONATE.
Other preparations:

---

resorcinol *see* Eskamel

Respacal *see* Brelomax
(UCB Pharma)

Restandol
(Organon)

A brown, oval capsule supplied at a strength of 40 mg and used as a hormone to treat underdeveloped male sexual organs and osteoporosis in men caused by low hormone levels.

Dose: 3-4 tablets a day for 2-3 weeks, then 1-3 tablets a day as needed.
Availability: NHS and private prescription.
Side effects: fluid retention, weight gain, raised calcium levels, increased bone growth, erect penis, premature closure of epiphyses (bone ends), reduced fertility in males, masculinization of women, inflammation of the prostate in the elderly.
Caution: in patients suffering from heart, kidney, or liver impairment, high blood pressure, epilepsy, migraine.
Not to be used for: children, or for patients suffering from prostate or liver cancer, kidney damage, heart disease, untreated heart failure.
Caution needed with: liver-enzyme inducing drugs (such as CARBAMAZEPINE, PHENYTOIN, GRISEOFULVIN, BARBITURATES).
Contains: TESTOSTERONE undecanoate.
Other preparations: PRIMOTESTON DEPOT, SUSTANON, VIRORMINE (injectable forms).

Retcin *see* erythromycin tablets
(DDSA)

Retin-A
(Janssen-Cilag)

A lotion used as a VITAMIN A derivative to treat acne where there are comedones, papules, and pustules.

Dose: apply to the affected area 1-2 times a day for at least 8 weeks.
Availability: NHS and private prescription.
Side effects: redness, irritation, peeling, loss or gain of skin pigment.
Caution: in nursing mothers and in patients suffering from eczema or skin
irritation; avoid direct sunlight or ultra-violet lamps, and keep the lotion
away from the eyes, nose, and mouth etc.
Not to be used for: pregnant women, or for patients with a family history
of skin cancer, or suffering from cuts, abrasion.
Caution needed with: skin softener or any other skin preparations,
including cosmetics, likely to cause irritation.
Contains: TRETINOIN.
Other preparations: Retin-A Gel, Retin-A Cream. RETINOVA (a stronger
product used to treat sun-damaged skin).

R

retinol *see* **vitamin A**

Retinova
(Janssen-Cilag)

A cream used as a VITAMIN A treatment for skin damaged by over-exposure
to the sun.

Dose: massage lightly into the affected area once a day at night, reducing
to 1 application 1-3 times a week when improved.
Availability: NHS, private prescription.
Side effects: reddening, peeling, irritation, and change in pigmentation of
the skin.
Caution: in nursing mothers, and in patients suffering from eczema, skin
irritation. Keep away from the eyes, mouth, and mucous membranes, and
keep out of the sun.
Not to be used for: children, pregnant women, or for patients with a
history of skin cancer in the family.
Caution needed with: other skin treatments that cause skin irritation.
Contains: TRETINOIN.
Other preparations: RETIN-A (a weaker product used to treat acne).

Retrovir
(Wellcome)

A white capsule or blue/white capsule according to strengths of 100 mg,
250 mg and used as an anti-viral treatment for serious HIV infections in

patients suffering from AIDS, or to delay the onset of AIDS in HIV positive people.

Dose: 500-600 mg a day in divided doses; children and pregnant women as prescribed by physician.
Availability: NHS and private prescription.
Side effects: anaemia, blood changes, headache, nausea, rash, stomach pain, fever, pins and needles, loss of appetite, muscle pain, sleeplessness.
Caution: in the elderly, pregnant women, and in patients suffering from anaemia, kidney or liver disease. Regular blood tests should be carried out.
Not to be used for: children under 3 months, nursing mothers, young babies with excess bilirubin in the blood, or for patients suffering from low white cell counts in the blood.
Caution needed with: ANALGESICS, especially PARACETAMOL, drugs inhibiting liver enzymes (such as CIMETIDINE, BARBITURATES, GRISEOFULVIN, anticonvulsants), some cancer treatments, PROBENECID, PHENYTOIN, tribavirin.
Contains: ZIDOVUDINE.
Other preparations: Retrovir Syrup.

R

Revanil
(Roche)

A white, scored tablet supplied at a strength of 200 micrograms and used as a hormone blocker to treat Parkinson's disease.

Dose: 1 tablet at bedtime with food, gradually increasing to a maximum of 25 tablets a day.
Availability: NHS and private prescription.
Side effects: low blood pressure, nausea, vomiting, dizziness, headache, tiredness, general feeling of being unwell, drowsiness, skin eruptions, abdominal pain, constipation, mental disturbance, blood vessel disease in the hands and feet.
Caution: in pregnant women and in patients with tumour of the pituitary gland.
Not to be used for: children, or for patients suffering from severe disturbance of circulation, heart disease.
Caution needed with: antidepressants, tranquillizers, alcohol, sedatives, DOMPERIDONE, METOCLOPRAMIDE.
Contains: LYSURIDE maleate.
Other preparations:

Rheumacin LA *see* indomethacin capsules
(Hillcross)

Rheumox
(Wyeth)

A light/dark orange capsule supplied at a strength of 300 mg and used as a NON-STEROIDAL ANTI-INFLAMMATORY DRUG to treat rheumatoid arthritis, osteoarthritis, ankylosing spondylitis, acute gout.

Dose: adults 4 capsules a day in 2 or 4 divided doses; acute gout 6 capsules a day in divided doses for up to 4 days reducing to 4 capsules a day until symptoms are relieved. Elderly 1 capsule morning and night; acute gout 6 capsules in divided doses for 24 hours then 4 capsules a day for 4 days, reducing to 2 capsules until symptoms are relieved.
Availability: NHS and private prescription.
Side effects: sensitivity to light, fluid retention, stomach bleeding, inflammation of the lungs, interference with some blood tests.
Caution: in the elderly or ill patients, and in patients suffering from high blood pressure, heart failure, kidney disorder, asthma, allergy to ASPIRIN or anti-inflammatory drugs. Patients on long-term treatment should be checked regularly.
Not to be used for: children, pregnant women, nursing mothers, or for patients with a history of stomach ulcer, ulcerative colitis, or blood changes, or who are suffering from severe kidney or liver disease, PORPHYRIA.
Caution needed with: PHENYTOIN, ANTICOAGULANTS, antidiabetics, some antibiotics, LITHIUM, DIGOXIN, CIMETIDINE, METHOTREXATE.
Contains: AZAPROPAZONE.
Other preparations: Rheumox 600 Tablets.

Rhinocort
(Astra)

An aerosol supplied at a strength of 50 micrograms and used as a STEROID treatment for rhinitis (including hayfever).

Dose: 2 sprays into each nostril twice a day (or 4 sprays once a day) at first, reducing when controlled.
Availability: NHS and private prescription.
Side effects: sneezing.
Caution: in pregnant women and in patients suffering from fungal, viral, or tubercular infections of the nose.
Not to be used for: children for prolonged treatment.
Caution needed with:
Contains: BUDESONIDE.
Other preparations: Rhinocort Aqua.

Rhinolast
(ASTA Medica)

A pump-action nasal spray used as an ANTIHISTAMINE to treat hay fever and rhinitis.

Dose: 1 spray in each nostril twice a day.
Availability: NHS and private prescription.
Side effects: nasal irritation, taste change.
Caution: in pregnant women and nursing mothers.
Not to be used for: children.
Caution needed with:
Contains: AZELASTINE.
Other preparations:

Rhumalgan *see* diclofenac tablets
(Lagap)

---

riboflavine *see* vitamin B$_2$

Ridaura Tiltab
(Bencard)

A pale-yellow, square tablet supplied at a strength of 3 mg and used as an oral gold salt to treat progressive rheumatoid arthritis which cannot be controlled effectively by NON-STEROIDAL ANTI-INFLAMMATORY DRUGS.

Dose: 1 tablet in the morning and 1 tablet in the evening for the first 3-6 months, then increase to 3 tablets a day if needed.
Availability: NHS and private prescription.
Side effects: diarrhoea, nausea, stomach pain, ulcerative enterocolitis, rash, itch, mouth inflammation, hair loss, conjunctivitis, disturbance of taste, blood changes, kidney effects, lung fibrosis. Report any side effects to the doctor.
Caution: in patients suffering from kidney or liver disease, inflammatory bowel disease, rash, history of bone marrow depression. Your doctor may advise that blood counts should be checked regularly. Women should take contraceptive measures until 6 months after end of treatment.
Not to be used for: children, pregnant women, nursing mothers, or for patients suffering from severe kidney or liver disease, SLE (a multisystem disorder), history of intestinal disorder, lung fibrosis, exfoliative dermatitis, bone marrow disorders, severe blood changes.
Caution needed with:
Contains: AURANOFIN.

Other preparations:

---

rifabutin *see* **Mycobutin**

Rifadin
(Marion Merrell Dow)

A red/blue capsule or a red capsule according to strengths of 150 mg, 300 mg and used as an antibiotic in the additional treatment for tuberculosis, and other infections. Used to prevent meningitis in susceptible patients

Dose: as advised by doctor according to condition.
Availability: NHS and private prescription.
Side effects: symptoms similar to influenza, rash, stomach and liver disturbances, orange-coloured urine, faeces, and stained soft contact lenses.
Caution: in the elderly, pregnant women, nursing mothers, underfed or very young infants, and in patients suffering from liver disease, PORPHYRIA.
Not to be used for: patients suffering from jaundice.
Caution needed with: ANTICOAGULANTS, DIGOXIN, antidiabetics, contraceptive pill, STEROIDS, CYCLOSPORIN, DAPSONE, PHENYTOIN, QUINIDINE, some ANALGESICS.
Contains: RIFAMPICIN.
Other preparations: Rifadin Syrup, Rifadin Infusion. RIMACTANE.

---

rifampicin *see* **Rifadin, Rifinah, Rimactane**

Rifater
(Marion Merrell Dow)

A pink/beige tablet used as an antibiotic combination to treat tuberculosis of the lungs.

Dose: adults under 40 kg body weight 3 tablets a day, 40-49 kg 4 tablets a day, 50-64 kg 5 tablets a day, over 65 kg 6 tablets a day; all either before or 2 hours after a meal.
Availability: NHS and private prescription.
Side effects: flu-like symptoms, skin reactions, stomach and liver disturbances, orange-coloured urine and stools, insomnia, muscle twitch, mental disturbance, LUPUS-like symptoms, stained soft contact lenses.
Caution: in the elderly, pregnant women, nursing mothers, the undernourished, and in patients suffering from liver disease, gout, or coughing blood, PORPHYRIA, or with a history of epilepsy. Your doctor may advise regular liver tests.

Not to be used for: children, or for patients suffering from jaundice.
Caution needed with: ANTICOAGULANTS, DIGOXIN, QUINIDINE, STEROIDS, the contraceptive pill, DAPSONE, ANALGESICS, antidiabetics taken by mouth, CYCLOSPORIN, PHENYTOIN.
Contains: ISONIAZID, PYRAZINAMIDE, RIFAMPICIN.
Other preparations:

Rifinah
(Marion Merrell Dow)

A pink tablet or an orange, oblong tablet according to strength and used as an antibiotic combination to treat tuberculosis.

Dose: under 50 kg body weight 3 pink tablets once a day before breakfast; over 50 kg body weight 2 orange tablets once a day before breakfast.
Availability: NHS and private prescription.
Side effects: sleeplessness, muscle twitching, flu-like symptoms, skin reactions, stomach and liver disturbances, orange-coloured urine and faeces, stained soft contact lenses, LUPUS-like symptoms, mental disturbance.
Caution: in pregnant women, nursing mothers, the elderly, the undernourished, and in patients suffering from liver disease, PORPHYRIA, or with a history of epilepsy.
Not to be used for: children or for patients suffering from jaundice.
Caution needed with: ANTICOAGULANTS, DIGOXIN, STEROIDS, the contraceptive pill, antidiabetics, CYCLOSPORIN, DAPSONE, PHENYTOIN, QUINIDINE, some painkillers.
Contains: RIFAMPICIN, ISONIAZID.
Other preparations: RIMACTAZID.

Rimacid *see* indomethacin capsules
(Rima)

Rimacillin *see* ampicillin capsules
(Rima)

Rimactane
(Ciba)

A red capsule or a brown/red capsule according to strengths of 150 mg, 300 mg and used as an antibiotic in the additional treatment for tuberculosis and other similar infections. Used to prevent meningitis in susceptible patients.

Dose: as advised by doctor according to condition.
Availability: NHS and private prescription.
Side effects: flu-like symptoms, skin reactions, stomach and liver disturbances, orange urine and faeces.
Caution: in the elderly, pregnant women, nursing mothers, or in very young or undernourished patients, and in patients suffering from liver disease, PORPHYRIA.
Not to be used for: patients suffering from jaundice.
Caution needed with: ANTICOAGULANTS, contraceptive pill, STEROIDS, DIGOXIN, antidiabetics, CYCLOSPORIN, DAPSONE, PHENYTOIN, QUINIDINE, indigestion remedies, ANTICHOLINERGICS, some painkillers.
Contains: RIFAMPICIN.
Other preparations: Rimactane Syrup, Rimactane Infusion. RIFADIN.

Rimactazid *see* Rifinah
(Ciba)

Rimadol *see* paracetamol tablets
(Rima)

Rimafen *see* ibuprofen tablets
(Rima)

Rimapam *see* diazepam tablets
(Rima)

Rimapen *see* penicillin V tablets
(Rima)

Rimapurinol *see* allopurinol tablets
(Rima)

Rimarin *see* chlorpheniramine tablets
(Rima)

Rimasal *see* salbutamol tablets
(Rima)

---

rimiterol hydrobromide *see* **Pulmadil**

Rimoxallin *see* **amoxycillin capsules**
(Rima)

Rimoxyn *see* **naproxen tablets**
(Rima)

Rinatec
(Boehringer Ingelheim)

A nasal spray supplied at a strength of 20 micrograms per dose, and used as an ANTICHOLINERGIC to treat nasal discharge associated with rhinitis.

Dose: 1-2 sprays in the nostril(s) up to 4 times a day.
Availability: NHS and private prescription.
Side effects: dry nose, irritation.
Caution: in patients suffering from glaucoma or enlarged prostate.
Not to be used for: children.
Caution needed with:
Contains: IPRATROPIUM bromide.
Other preparations:

Risperdal
Janssen/Organon

A white, orange, yellow, or green oblong scored tablet according to strengths of 1 mg, 2 mg, 3 mg, or 4 mg, and used as an antipsychotic drug to treat schizophrenia and other mental disorders.

Dose: 1 mg twice a day on the first day, 2 mg twice a day on the second day, 3 mg twice a day on the third day, and then up to 8 mg twice a day; elderly 0.5 mg twice a day at first, increasing by 0.5 mg amounts to 1-2 mg a day.
Availability: NHS, private prescription.
Side effects: low blood pressure on standing, rapid heart rate, abnormal production of breast milk, disturbed menstrual periods, loss of sexual function, sleeplessness, anxiety, agitation, headache, tiredness, dizziness, lack of concentration, weight gain, stomach upset, rhinitis, blurred vision, rash, rarely fits, shaking, rigidity.
Caution: in the elderly, pregnant women, nursing mothers and in patients suffering from Parkinson's disease, heart kidney, or liver disease. You should not drive or operate machinery. Your doctor will monitor you for any

R

...ents.
...ren under 15 years.
...sedatives, tranquillizers, LEVODOPA, LYSURIDE,
..., SELEGILINE.

---

risperi... ...e **Risperdal**

Ritalin
(Ciba)

A white, scored tablet supplied at a strength of 10 mg, and used as a central nervous system stimulant to treat children with attention deficit disorder.

Dose: ½ tablet once or twice a day at first, increasing by ½-1 tablet at weekly intervals to a maximum of 6 tablets a day in divided doses.
Availability: NHS, private prescription. Controlled drug.
Side effects: stomach upset, poor appetite, headache, sleeplessness.
Caution: in pregnant girls, nursing mothers, or in patients suffering from mental disorder, raised blood pressure, emotional instability, epilepsy. Should be administered only under the supervision of a specialist; height, weight, blood pressure, and blood count should be checked regularly.
Not to be used for: adults or for patients suffering from severe angina, heart rhythm disturbances, glaucoma, overactive thyroid, severe anxiety, agitation, or stress, tics, or with a family history of Tourette's syndrome.
Caution needed with: ANTICOAGULANTS, anticonvulsants, MAOIS, GUANETHIDINE, alcohol, blood-pressure raising drugs, TRICYCLIC ANTIDEPRESSANTS, appetite suppressants.
Contains: METHYLPHENIDATE hydrochloride.
Other preparations:

---

ritodrine hydrochloride *see* **Yutopar**

Rivotril
(Roche)

A beige tablet or white tablet according to strengths of 0.5 mg, 2 mg and used as an anticonvulsant to treat epilepsy.

Dose: adults 1 mg a day at first, up to 4-8 mg a day; children and the elderly reduced doses.

Availability: NHS and private prescription.
Side effects: drowsiness, light-headedness, shaking, confusion, unsteadiness, vertigo, stomach upset, low blood pressure, rash, changes in vision, changes in sexual function, retention of urine. Rarely blood or liver disorders. Risk of addiction increases with dose and length of treatment. May impair judgement.
Caution: in children, the elderly, pregnant women, nursing mothers, in women during labour, and in patients suffering from lung disorders, kidney or liver disorders. Avoid long-term use and withdraw gradually.
Not to be used for: patients suffering from acute lung diseases, some chronic lung diseases, some obsessional and psychotic diseases.
Caution needed with: alcohol, sedatives, other tranquillizers, anticonvulsants.
Contains: CLONAZEPAM.
Other preparations: Rivotril Injection.

Roaccutane
(Roche)

A white/red capsule used as a VITAMIN A derivative to treat severe acne.

Dose: 0.5 mg per kg body weight a day with food for the first 4 weeks, then adjust according to response for another 8-12 weeks. Repeat courses not recommended.
Availability: NHS (hospitals only).
Side effects: dryness, erosion of mucous membranes, hair loss, rise in liver enzymes, fits, nausea, headache, sweating, moodiness, drowsiness, irregular periods, rarely blood changes, blood vessel inflammation, hair growth, eye and ear disorders.
Caution: women of child-bearing age must take contraceptive precautions before, during, and after treatment. Your doctor may advise that liver and blood should be checked regularly.
Not to be used for: children, pregnant women, nursing mothers, or for patients suffering from liver or kidney disease.
Caution needed with: vitamin A.
Contains: ISOTRETINOIN.
Other preparations: ISOTREX (a gel applied to the skin).

Robaxin
(Shire)

A white, oblong, scored tablet supplied at a strength of 750 mg and used as a muscle relaxant to treat skeletal muscle spasm.

Dose: adults 2 tablets 4 times a day; elderly 1 tablet 4 times a day.

Availability: NHS and private prescription.
Side effects: drowsiness, allergy.
Caution: in pregnant women, nursing mothers, and in patients suffering from kidney or liver disease.
Not to be used for: children or for patients in a coma or suffering from brain damage, epilepsy, MYASTHENIA GRAVIS.
Caution needed with: alcohol, sedatives, stimulants, ANTICHOLINERGICS.
Contains: METHOCARBAMOL.
Other preparations: Robaxin Injectable.

Robaxisal Forte
(Wyeth)

A pink/white, two-layered, scored tablet used as a muscle relaxant and ANALGESIC to treat skeletal muscle spasm.

Dose: adults 2 tablets 4 times a day; elderly 1 tablet 4 times a day.
Availability: private prescription only.
Side effects: drowsiness, allergy, stomach bleeding.
Caution: in pregnant women, nursing mothers, and in patients suffering from kidney or liver disease, allergy to anti-inflammatory drugs, or a history of asthma or breathing disorder.
Not to be used for: children or for patients suffering from coma, brain damage, epilepsy, MYASTHENIA GRAVIS, stomach ulcer, haemophilia.
Caution needed with: alcohol, sedatives, stimulants, ANTICHOLINERGICS, ANTICOAGULANTS, antidiabetics, some anticonvulsants.
Contains: METHOCARBAMOL, ASPIRIN.
Other preparations:

Rocaltrol
(Roche)

A white/red capsule or a red capsule according to strengths of 0.25 micrograms, 0.5 micrograms, and used as a source of VITAMIN D for correcting calcium and phosphate metabolism in patients suffering from bone disease due to kidney disorder, and to treat established osteoporosis.

Dose: in kidney disorder, 0.25-1 microgram a day increasing if needed by 0.25-0.5 microgram at a time to no more than 2-3 micrograms a day; in osteoporosis, 0.25 micrograms twice a day.
Availability: NHS and private prescription.
Side effects: increased blood and urine calcium levels.
Caution: in pregnant women. Do not take any other vitamin D preparations. Your doctor may advise that calcium levels should be checked regularly.

Not to be used for: children, or for patients suffering from calcification (laying down of calcium), raised calcium levels.
Caution needed with: other vitamin D preparations, some DIURETICS.
Contains: CALCITRIOL.
Other preparations:

Rohypnol
(Roche)

A purple, diamond-shaped, scored tablet supplied at a strength of 1 mg and used as a sedative for the short-term treatment of sleeplessness or to bring on sleep at other times.

Dose: elderly ½ tablet before going to bed; adults ½-1 tablet before going to bed.
Availability: private prescription only.
Side effects: drowsiness, confusion, light-headedness, unsteadiness, shaking, low blood pressure, vertigo, stomach upset, rash, changes in vision, changes in sexual function, retention of urine. Risk of addiction increases with dose and length of treatment. May impair judgement.
Caution: in the elderly, pregnant women, nursing mothers, in women during labour, and in patients suffering from lung disorders, kidney or liver disorders. Avoid long-term use and withdraw gradually.
Not to be used for: children, or for patients suffering from acute lung diseases, some chronic lung diseases, some obsessional and psychotic diseases.
Caution needed with: alcohol, sedatives, other tranquillizers, anticonvulsants.
Contains: FLUNITRAZEPAM.
Other preparations:

Rommix *see* **erythromycin tablets**
(Ashbourne)

Ronicol
(Tillomed)

A white, scored tablet supplied at a strength of 25 mg and used as a vasodilator to treat poor circulation.

Dose: 1-2 tablets 4 times a day.
Availability: NHS, private prescription, over the counter.
Side effects: flushes.
Caution: in long-term treatment of diabetics.

Not to be used for: children.
Caution needed with:
Contains: NICOTINYL ALCOHOL TARTRATE.
Other preparations: Ronicol Timespan (a long-acting preparation).

Rose Bengal Minims
(Chauvin)

Drops used as a dye to stain the eye for finding degenerated cells in dry eye syndrome.

Dose: 1-2 drops into the eye as needed.
Availability: NHS, private prescription, over the counter.
Side effects: severe smarting in dry eyes.
Caution:
Not to be used for: children.
Caution needed with:
Contains: rose Bengal.
Other preparations:

Rowachol
(Monmouth)

A capsule containing essential oils used to treat cholelithiasis (gall stones).

Dose: adults 1-2 capsules 3 times a day before meals.
Availability: NHS and private prescription.
Side effects:
Caution:
Not to be used for: children.
Caution needed with: ANTICOAGULANTS, contraceptive pill.
Contains: MENTHOL, MENTHONE, PINENE, CAMPHENE, CINEOLE, BORNEOL, OLIVE OIL.
Other preparations:

Rowatinex
(Monmouth)

A capsule containing volatile oils used to treat urinary stones, kidney disorders, prevention of urinary stones, and mild urine infections

Dose: 1 capsule 3-4 times a day before food.
Availability: NHS and private prescription.
Side effects:
Caution:

Not to be used for: children.
Caution needed with: ANTICOAGULANTS, contraceptive pill.
Contains: PINENE, CAMPHENE, BORNEOL, ANETHOL, FENCHONE, CINEOLE, OLIVE OIL.
Other preparations:

Rozex
(Stafford-Miller)

A gel used as an antibiotic to treat spots, pus-filled spots, and reddening of the skin associated with rosacea.

Dose: wash the affected area of skin and massage the gel into the area in a thin film; treat morning and evening.
Availability: NHS, private prescription.
Side effects: temporary irritation.
Caution: in pregnant women and in patients suffering from some blood disorders. Keep away from the eyes.
Not to be used for: children.
Caution needed with:
Contains: METRONIDAZOLE.
Other preparations: METROGEL.

Rubavax *see* rubella vaccine
(Pasteur Merieux MSD)

---

rubella vaccine

Rubella, or German measles, is an active virus which in childhood is usually quite mild but, if contracted by women in pregnancy, can lead to congenital defects in the baby. An attack of rubella usually gives the sufferer immunity for life. Formerly, the policy was to immunize only females of child-bearing age but this has now been extended to both sexes to eliminate rubella.

Dose: 1 injection of the live virus confers immunity.
Availability: NHS and private prescription.
Side effects: fever, rash, joint pain, swelling of lymph glands.
Caution: women should not become pregnant within 1 month of receiving the vaccine.
Not to be used for: women in early pregnancy, and patients suffering from changes to immunity system, acute feverish illness, cancer.
Caution needed with: some STEROIDS, some cancer treatments, radiation, some other live vaccines, transfusions, immunoglobulins.
Contains: rubella vaccine.

Other preparations: ALMEVAX, ERVEVAX, RUBAVAX (most brands also contain NEOMYCIN).

Rusyde *see* frusemide tablets
(CP Pharmaceuticals)

Rynacrom Spray
(Fisons)

A spray used as an anti-allergy treatment for allergic rhinitis.

Dose: 1-2 sprays into each nostril up to 4 times a day continuously.
Availability: NHS, private prescription, over the counter.
Side effects: temporary itching nose, rarely breathing difficulty.
Caution:
Not to be used for:
Caution needed with:
Contains: SODIUM CROMOGLYCATE.
Other preparations: Rynacrom Compound. Resiston-One (both have added decongestant).

Rythmodan
(Hoechst-Roussel)

A beige/green capsule or a white capsule according to strengths of 100 mg, 150 mg and used as an anti-arrhythmic treatment for abnormal heart rhythm

Dose: 300-800 mg a day in divided doses.
Availability: NHS and private prescription.
Side effects: ANTICHOLINERGIC effects, rarely jaundice, mood changes, low blood sugar.
Caution: in pregnant women, and in patients suffering from heart conduction block, heart, liver, and kidney failure, enlarged prostate, glaucoma, urine retention, low potassium levels.
Not to be used for: children, or for patients suffering from severe heart conduction block, heart failure.
Caution needed with: ß-BLOCKERS, DIURETICS, ANTICHOLINERGICS, other anti-arrhythmics, ERYTHROMYCIN.
Contains: DISOPYRAMIDE.
Other preparations: Rythmodan Retard, Rythmodan Injection. DIRYTHMIN, ISOMIDE.

Sabril
(Marion Merrell Dow)

A white, oval, scored tablet supplied at a strength of 500 mg and used to treat epilepsy.

Dose: adults, 4 tablets a day initially, adjusted to a maximum of 8 tablets a day; children reduced doses according to body weight.
Availability: NHS and private prescription.
Side effects: aggression, mental disturbance, confusion, drowsiness, tiredness, dizziness, nervousness, irritability, memory and visual disturbances, excitation, agitation, depression, increased frequency of seizures.
Caution: in the elderly, and in patients with a history of mental or behavioural problems, or suffering from kidney damage. Your doctor may recommend regular examinations.
Not to be used for: pregnant women, nursing mothers.
Caution needed with: PHENYTOIN.
Contains: VIGABATRIN.
Other preparations: Sabril Sachets.

S

Salactol
(Dermal)

A paint used as a skin softener to treat warts, corns, and calluses.

Dose: apply to the wart once a day and rub down with a pumice stone between treatments.
Availability: NHS, private prescription, over the counter.
Side effects:
Caution: do not apply to healthy skin.
Not to be used for: warts on the face or anal and genital areas.
Caution needed with:
Contains: SALICYLIC ACID, LACTIC ACID.
Other preparations: CUPLEX, DUOFILM, SALATAC (gel form).

Salamol *see* salbutamol inhaler
(Baker Norton)

Salatac *see* Salactol
(Dermal)

Salazopyrin *see* **sulphasalazine tablets**
(Pharmacia)

Salazopyrin-EN Tablets *see* **sulphasalazine tablets**
(Pharmacia)

Salbulin Inhaler *see* **salbutamol inhaler**
(3M Health Care)

---

salbutamol *see* **Aerocrom Inhaler, Aerolin, Airomir, Asmavan, Combivent, Maxivent, Rimasal, Salamol, Salbulin, salbutamol inhaler, salbutamol tablets, Steri-Neb Salamol, Ventide, Ventodisks, Ventolin, Volmax**

Salbutamol Cyclocaps *see* **salbutamol inhaler**
(Du Pont)

---

salbutamol inhaler

An aerosol used as a bronchodilator to treat bronchial spasm brought on by asthma, chronic bronchitis, and emphysema.

Dose: 1-2 puffs up to 4 times a day.
Availability: NHS and private prescription.
Side effects: altered heart rate, anxiety, hands shaking, nervous tension, dilation of the blood vessels, headache, allergy, low blood potassium levels.
Caution: in pregnant women, nursing mothers, and in patients suffering from overactive thyroid, heart or circulation disorder.
Not to be used for:
Caution needed with: SYMPATHOMIMETICS, STEROIDS, THEOPHYLLINE.
Contains: SALBUTAMOL sulphate.
Other preparations: SALBUTAMOL TABLETS. AIROMIR, AEROLIN, ASMAVEN, MAXIVENT, SALAMOL Inhaler, SALAMOL Easi-Breathe, SALBULIN, SALBUVENT, VENTIDE, VENTOLIN Inhaler. (Preparations with different inhalation devices include SALBUTAMOL CYCLOCAPS; SALAMOL, STERINEB, Ventolin Rotacaps, Ventolin Nebules, VENTODISKS.)

---

salbutamol tablets

A tablet supplied at strengths of 2 mg and 4 mg, and used as a bronchodilator to treat bronchial spasm brought on by asthma, chronic bronchitis, and emphysema. Also used to stop premature labour in pregnant women.

Dose: for bronchial spasm: adults 4 mg 3-4 times a day; children aged 6-12 years 2 mg 3-4 times a day, 2-6 years 1-2 mg 3-4 times a day, under 2 years smaller doses according to bodyweight. To prevent premature labour: 4 mg every 6-8 hours after initial treatment by injection .
Availability: NHS and private prescription.
Side effects: altered heart rate, anxiety, hands shaking, nervous tension, dilation of the blood vessels, headache, allergy, low blood potassium levels.
Caution: in pregnant women, nursing mothers, and in patients suffering from overactive thyroid, heart or circulation disorder. Heart rate of mother and foetus should be monitored to treat premature labour.
Not to be used for: women suffering from certain complications of pregnancy.
Caution needed with: SYMPATHOMIMETICS, STEROIDS, THEOPHYLLINE.
Contains: SALBUTAMOL sulphate.
Other preparations: SALBUTAMOL INHALER. ASMAVEN, RIMASAL, VENTOLIN Intravenous Infusion, VENTOLIN Syrup, VENTOLIN Tablets. (Long-acting tablet preparations include: VOLMAX.)

S

---

salicylamide *see* **Intralgin**

---

salicylic acid *see* **Acnisal, Aserbine, benzoic acid compound ointment, Capasal, coal tar and salicylic acid ointment, Cocois, Cuplex, Diprosalic, Dithrolan, Duofilm, Gelcosal, Ionil T, Meted, Monphytol, Movelat, Occlusal, Phytex, Posalfilin, Pragmatar, Psorin, Pyralvex, Salactol, Salatac, salicylic acid collodion, salicylic acid ointment BP, Verrugon**

---

salicylic acid collodion

A liquid used as a skin softener to treat warts and calluses.

Dose: apply to the wart or callus once a day or every other day.
Availability: NHS, private prescription, over the counter.
Side effects: irritation of the treated area.
Caution: protect surrounding skin and avoid broken skin.
Not to be used for: patients suffering from diabetes, poor circulation; or on the face or anal or genital areas.
Caution needed with:
Contains: SALICYLIC ACID, flexible collodion.

Other preparations: OCCLUSAL.

---

salicylic acid ointment BP

An ointment used as a skin softener to treat skin disorders such as psoriasis.

Dose: apply twice a day.
Availability: NHS, private prescription, over the counter.
Side effects: irritation of the treated area, allergy, drying of skin.
Caution: avoid broken skin and inflamed areas.
Not to be used for:
Caution needed with:
Contains: SALICYLIC ACID, WOOL ALCOHOLS OINTMENT.
Other preparations:

---

saline *see* sodium chloride, sterile saline

Saliva Orthana
(Nycomed)

A spray used as an artificial saliva to treat dry mouth.

Dose: as needed.
Availability: NHS, private prescription, over the counter.
Side effects:
Caution:
Not to be used for:
Caution needed with:
Contains: MUCIN, XYLITOL.
Other preparations: Saliva Orthana Lozenges.

Salivace
(Penn Pharmaceuticals)

A spray used as an artificial saliva to treat dry mouth.

Dose: 1-2 sprays as needed.
Availability: NHS, private prescription, over the counter.
Side effects:
Caution:
Not to be used for:
Caution needed with:

Contains: CALCIUM CHLORIDE, DIPOTASSIUM PHOSPHATE, SODIUM CHLORIDE, POTASSIUM CHLORIDE, CARBOXYMETHYLCELLULOSE, XYLITOL.
Other preparations:

Salivix
(Thames)

A brown pastille used as an artificial saliva to treat dry mouth.

Dose: as needed.
Availability: NHS, private prescription, over the counter.
Side effects:
Caution:
Not to be used for:
Caution needed with:
Contains: MALIC ACID.
Other preparations:

---

salmeterol *see* **Serevent**

Salofalk *see* Asacol
(Thames)

Salonair
(Salonpas)

An aerosol used as an ANALGESIC rub to relieve muscular and rheumatic pain, sprains, neuralgia, chilblains.

Dose: spray on to the affected area 1-2 times a day.
Availability: private prescription, over the counter.
Side effects: may be irritant.
Caution:
Not to be used for: areas such as near the eyes, on broken or inflamed skin, or on membranes (such as the mouth).
Caution needed with:
Contains: GLYCOL SALICYLATE, MENTHYL SALICYLATE, MENTHOL, CAMPHOR, SQUALANE, BENZYL NICOTINATE.
Other preparations:

Saluric
(M.S.D.)

A white, scored tablet supplied at a strength of 500 mg and used as a DIURETIC to treat fluid retention, high blood pressure.

Dose: adults fluid retention ½-2 tablets a day or from time to time up to 4 a day, high blood pressure ½-1 a day up to 2 a day if needed; children under 6 months up to 35 mg per kilogram bodyweight a day, 6 months-2 years 125-375 mg a day in two doses, 2-12 years 375-1 g a day in two doses.
Availability: NHS and private prescription.
Side effects: rash, stomach upset, sensitivity to light, blood changes, loss of appetite, impotence, dizziness, pancreatitis, electrolyte disturbances.
Caution: in pregnant women, nursing mothers, the elderly, and in patients suffering from diabetes, kidney or liver disease, gout, SLE. Potassium supplements may be needed.
Not to be used for: patients suffering from severe kidney or liver failure, Addison's disease, high calcium levels, allergy to some antibiotics.
Caution needed with: DIGOXIN, LITHIUM, alcohol, BARBITURATES, some ANALGESICS, blood-pressure lowering drugs, NON-STEROIDAL ANTI-INFLAMMATORY DRUGS, sedatives, antidiabetics, STEROIDS, CARBENOXOLONE.
Contains: CHLOROTHIAZIDE.
Other preparations:

Sandimmun
(Sandoz)

A pink, oval capsule, yellow, oblong capsule, or pink, oblong capsule according to strengths of 25 mg, 50 mg, 100 mg, and used to suppress the immune system and treat severe psoriasis and severe rheumatoid arthritis that has not responded to other treatments. Also used to prevent rejection following transplantation or grafts.

Dose: for psoriasis, initially 1.25 mg/kg body weight twice a day, increasing to 5 mg/kg a day. For rheumatoid arthritis, initially 2.5 mg/kg body weight a day in 2 doses, increasing to 4 mg/kg a day. After transplant/graft as advised by doctor.
Availability: NHS and private prescription.
Side effects: kidney or liver disorder, high blood pressure, shaking, stomach upset, swollen gums, hair growth, tiredness, muscle weakness or cramp, muscle disease, burning sensation; rarely high potassium, magnesium, and uric acid levels, gout, fluid retention, convulsions, headache, rash, anaemia, weight gain, colitis, menstrual changes, pancreatitis, pins and needles, brain disorders.
Caution: in pregnant women, nursing mothers, and in patients suffering from chicken pox or shingles, or with high potassium or uric acid levels.

Your doctor may advise regular tests during treatment. Avoid sunbathing. *Not to be used for:* children, or for patients suffering from malignant conditions, kidney damage, or uncontrolled high blood pressure or infection.

Caution needed with: antibiotics, some vaccines, PHENYTOIN, KETOCONAZOLE, FLUCONAZOLE, ITRACONAZOLE, ERYTHROMYCIN, RIFAMPICIN, CARBAMAZEPINE, BARBITURATES, COLCHICINE, drugs affecting the kidneys, the contraceptive pill, propafenone, PREDNISOLONE, METHYLPREDNISOLONE, potassium supplements, some DIURETICS, NON-STEROIDAL ANTI-INFLAMMATORY DRUGS, grapefruit juice, some drugs used to treat angina and high blood pressure.

Contains: CYCLOSPORIN.

Other preparations: Sandimmun Oral Solution, Sandimmun Infusion.

Sando-K
(Sandoz)

A white, effervescent tablet used as a potassium supplement to treat potassium deficiency.

Dose: 2-4 tablets a day dissolved in water.
Availability: NHS, private prescription, over the counter.
Side effects: stomach upset.
Caution: in patients suffering from Addison's disease.
Not to be used for: patients suffering from acute dehydration, crush injuries, raised potassium levels, reduced urine production, kidney disorder.
Caution needed with:
Contains: POTASSIUM BICARBONATE, POTASSIUM CHLORIDE.
Other preparations:

Sandocal
(Sandoz)

A white, effervescent tablet supplied at strengths of 400 mg, 1 g and used as a calcium supplement in additional treatment for osteoporosis, and where calcium is deficient in the diet or requirements are high.

Dose: adults 400 mg-2 g a day; children 400 mg-1 g a day.
Availability: NHS, private prescription, over the counter.
Side effects: diarrhoea.
Caution: in patients suffering from kidney disease, unbalanced electrolyte levels. Your doctor may advise that calcium levels should be checked regularly.
Not to be used for: patients suffering from raised calcium levels in the

blood or urine, kidney stones.

Caution needed with: TETRACYCLINE ANTIBIOTICS, VITAMIN D, SODIUM FLUORIDE, some DIURETICS.

Contains: CALCIUM LACTATE GLUCONATE, calcium carbonate, citric acid, SODIUM BICARBONATE, POTASSIUM BICARBONATE.

Other preparations: Calcium Sandoz Syrup, Calcium Sandoz Injection.

Sanomigran
(Sandoz)

An ivory, scored tablet supplied at strengths of 0.5 mg, 1.5 mg and used as a blood vessel stabilizer to prevent migraine or headache.

Dose: adults 1.5 mg a day as a single dose at night or in 3 divided doses to a maximum of 4.5 mg a day in divided doses; children up to 1.5 mg a day in divided doses, or 1 mg at night.
Availability: NHS and private prescription.
Side effects: drowsiness, weight gain, excitement.
Caution: in patients suffering from glaucoma or retention of urine.
Not to be used for:
Caution needed with: alcohol, sedatives.
Contains: PIZOTIFEN HYDROGEN MALATE.
Other preparations: Sanomigran Elixir.

Saventrine
(Pharmax)

A white, mottled tablet supplied at a strength of 30 mg and used to treat conduction defects in the heart.

Dose: as advised by physician.
Availability: NHS and private prescription.
Side effects: palpitations, shaking, sweating, headache, diarrhoea.
Caution: in patients suffering from high blood pressure and diabetes.
Not to be used for: patients suffering from some heart diseases and overactive thyroid.
Caution needed with:
Contains: ISOPRENALINE hydrochloride
Other preparations: Saventrine I.V. MEDIHALER-ISO.

Schering PC4 *see* PC4
(Schering Healthcare)

Scheriproct
(Schering Healthcare)

An ointment used as a STEROID, local anaesthetic treatment for haemorrhoids, anal fissure, itching around the anus or vulva.

Dose: apply 2-4 times a day for up to 7 days.
Availability: NHS and private prescription.
Side effects: systemic CORTICOSTEROID effects (*see* prednisolone tablets).
Caution: in pregnant women; do not use for prolonged periods.
Not to be used for: patients suffering from tuberculous, fungal, or viral infections.
Caution needed with:
Contains: PREDNISOLONE hexanoate, CINCHOCAINE hydrochloride
Other preparations: Scheriproct suppositories.

Secadrex
(Rhône-Poulenc Rorer)

A white tablet used as a ß-BLOCKER/DIURETIC combination to treat high blood pressure.

Dose: 1-2 tablets a day.
Availability: NHS and private prescription.
Side effects: cold hands and feet, sleep disturbance, slow heart rate, rash, gout, blood changes, tiredness, wheezing, heart failure, stomach upset, low blood pressure, sensitivity to light, dry eyes, rash, weakness.
Caution: in pregnant women, nursing mothers, and in patients suffering from diabetes, high blood lipids, gout, kidney or liver disorders, asthma. May need to be withdrawn before surgery. Withdraw gradually. Your doctor may advise additional treatment with diuretics or DIGOXIN.
Not to be used for: children, or for patients suffering from heart block or failure, kidney failure, low blood pressure, untreated PHAEOCHROMOCYTOMA, failure to produce urine.
Caution needed with: VERAPAMIL, CLONIDINE withdrawal, some anti-arrhythmic drugs and anaesthetics, RESERPINE, some blood-pressure lowering drugs, ERGOTAMINE, CIMETIDINE, sedatives, SYMPATHOMIMETICS, INDOMETHACIN, LITHIUM, digoxin, antidiabetics.
Contains: ACEBUTOLOL hydrochloride, HYDROCHLOROTHIAZIDE.
Other preparations:

Seconal Sodium
(Eli Lilly)

An orange capsule supplied at strengths of 50 mg, 100 mg and used as a BARBITURATE to treat severe sleeplessness.

Dose: 50-100 mg at night.
Availability: controlled drug; NHS and private prescription.
Side effects: drowsiness, hangover, dizziness, shaking, breathing difficulties, allergies, headache, confusion, excitement.
Caution: in patients suffering from kidney, liver, or lung disease. Dependence (addiction) may develop.
Not to be used for: children, young adults, pregnant women, nursing mothers, the elderly, the debilitated, patients with a history of drug or alcohol abuse, or suffering from PORPHYRIA, or in the management of pain.
Caution needed with: ANTICOAGULANTS, alcohol, sedatives, other tranquillizers, STEROIDS, the contraceptive pill, GRISEOFULVIN, RIFAMPICIN, PHENYTOIN, METRONIDAZOLE, CHLORAMPHENICOL.
Contains: QUINALBARBITONE SODIUM.
Other preparations:

Sectral
(Rhône-Poulenc Rorer.)

A buff/white capsule or a buff/pink capsule according to strengths of 100 mg, 200 mg, or a white tablet supplied at a strength of 400 mg and used as a ß-BLOCKER to treat angina, abnormal heart rhythm, or high blood pressure.

Dose: up to 1200 mg a day in divided doses; high blood pressure up to 800 mg a day.
Availability: NHS and private prescription.
Side effects: cold hands and feet, sleep disturbance, slow heart rate, tiredness, wheezing, heart failure, low blood pressure, stomach upset, dry eyes, rash.
Caution: in pregnant women, nursing mothers, and in patients suffering from diabetes, kidney or liver disorders, asthma. May need to be withdrawn before surgery. Withdraw gradually. Your doctor may advise additional treatment with DIURETICS or DIGOXIN.
Not to be used for: children or for patients suffering from heart block or failure, low blood pressure, untreated PHAEOCHROMCYTOMA.
Caution needed with: VERAPAMIL, CLONIDINE withdrawal, some anti-arrhythmic drugs and anaesthetics, RESERPINE, some blood-pressure lowering drugs, ERGOTAMINE, CIMETIDINE, sedatives, antidiabetics, SYMPATHOMIMETICS, INDOMETHACIN.
Contains: ACEBUTOLOL hydrochloride.
Other preparations:

Securon *see* verapamil tablets
(Knoll)

Securon SR *see* **verapamil tablets**
(Knoll)

---

selegiline *see* **Eldepryl, selegiline tablets**

---

selegiline tablets

A white, scored tablet supplied at strengths of 5 mg, 10 mg and used as an anti-parkinsonian treatment for Parkinson's disease.

Dose: usually 10 mg a day either as a single dose in the morning or 5 mg in the morning and 5 mg at midday.
Availability: NHS and private prescription.
Side effects: low blood pressure, nausea, vomiting, confusion, mental disorders.
Caution:
Not to be used for: children.
Caution needed with: PETHIDINE, FLUOXETINE, MAOIS.
Contains: SELEGILINE hydrochloride.
Other preparations: ELDEPRYL.

---

selenium sulphide *see* **Lenium, Selsun**

Selsun
(Abbott)

A suspension used as an antidandruff shampoo for dandruff, scaly scalp conditions.

Dose: shampoo twice a week for 2 weeks, then once a week for 2 weeks, and then as needed.
Availability: NHS, private prescription, over the counter.
Side effects:
Caution: keep away from the eyes or broken skin; do not use within 48 hours of using waving or colouring substances.
Not to be used for:
Caution needed with:
Contains: SELENIUM SULPHIDE.
Other preparations: LENIUM.

S

Semitard *see* **insulin**
(Novo Nordisk)

Semprex
(Wellcome)

A white capsule supplied at a strength of 8 mg and used as an
ANTIHISTAMINE treatment for allergic rhinitis, other allergies.

Dose: 1 capsule 3 times a day.
Availability: NHS and private prescription
Side effects: rarely drowsiness.
Caution: in pregnant women and nursing mothers.
Not to be used for: children, the elderly, or for patients suffering from
kidney failure.
Caution needed with: sedatives, alcohol.
Contains: ACRIVASTINE.
Other preparations:

---

senna tablets

A tablet supplied at a strength of 7.5 mg and used as a stimulant laxative
to treat constipation, and to evacuate the bowels before surgery or
examinations.

Dose: adults 2-4 tablets at bedtime; children 6-12 years half adult dose.
Availability: NHS, private prescription, over the counter.
Side effects: stomach cramps.
Caution: not for prolonged use.
Not to be used for: children under 6 years, or for patients suffering from
blocked intestine.
Caution needed with:
Contains: SENNOSIDES.
Other preparations: SENOKOT (also available as a liquid, suitable for
children over 2 years). Other brands available over the counter.

---

sennosides *see* **Manevac, Pripsen Sachets, senna tablets**

Senokot *see* **senna tablets**
(Reckitt & Colman)

Septrin *see* **co-trimoxazole tablets**
(Wellcome)

Serc *see* **betahistine tablets**
(Solvay Healthcare)

Serenace *see* **haloperidol tablets**
(Baker Norton)

Serevent
(Allen and Hanburys)

An aerosol supplied at a strength of 25 micrograms per dose, and used as a BRONCHODILATOR to treat asthma and chronic bronchitis (usually in addition to STEROID or other anti-inflammatory treatment).

Dose: adults 2-4 puffs twice a day; children over 4 years 2 puffs twice a day.
Availability: NHS and private prescription.
Side effects: low potassium levels, breathing difficulty; rarely headache, tremor, palpitations, skin reactions, cramps, chest pain, joint pain, shaking, local irritation.
Caution: in pregnant women, nursing mothers, and patients suffering from thyroid disorders.
Not to be used for: children under 4 years, or for emergency use.
Caution needed with: ß-BLOCKERS.
Contains: SALMETEROL.
Other preparations: Serevent Diskhaler.

Serophene
(Serono)

A white, scored tablet supplied at a strength of 50 mg and used as a anti-oestrogen treatment for infertility due to failure of ovulation and for impaired hypothalamic-pituitary gland function.

Dose: 1 tablet a day for 5 days beginning within 5 days of the start of the period, or 2 tablets a day (for up to 6 cycles) for ovulation problems.
Availability: NHS and private prescription.
Side effects: enlargement of the ovaries, hot flushes, uncomfortable abdomen, blurred vision.
Caution:
Not to be used for: children, pregnant women, or patients suffering from

liver disease, large ovarian cyst, endometrial cancer, undiagnosed
bleeding from the uterus.
Caution needed with:
Contains: CLOMIPHENE citrate.
Other preparations: CLOMID.

Serotulle
(Seton Healthcare)

A sterile, impregnated gauze dressing, supplied at sizes of 5 cm square
and 10 cm square, and used as a dressing for wounds where there may
be infection.

Availability: NHS, private prescription, over the counter. (Also available
on a trial basis from nurses.)
Contains: WHITE SOFT PARAFFIN, CHLORHEXIDINE ACETATE.
Other preparations: BACTIGRAS, CHLORHEXITULLE.

S

Seroxat
(SmithKline Beecham)

A white, oval, scored tablet or a blue, oval, scored tablet according to
strengths of 20 mg, 30 mg, and used as an antidepressant to treat
depression and anxiety, obsessive-compulsive disorders, and panic
disorders (including agoraphobia).

Dose: depression and anxiety, initially 20 mg once a day in the morning
with food, increased to a maximum of 50 mg a day; elderly, 20-40 mg a
day only. Obsessive-compulsive disorders, 20-60 mg once a day in the
morning with food. Panic disorders 10-50 mg a day.
Availability: NHS and private prescription.
Side effects: nausea, sleepiness, sweating, shaking, tingling, dry mouth,
insomnia, sexual disturbance.
Caution: in pregnant women, nursing mothers, and in patients suffering
from severe kidney or liver damage, heart or circulation disorder, epilepsy,
or a history of mental disturbance.
Not to be used for: children.
Caution needed with: MAOIS, TRYPTOPHAN, LITHIUM, PHENYTOIN,
anticonvulsants, drugs affecting liver enzymes (eg BARBITURATES,
CARBAMAZEPINE, PRIMIDONE, RIFAMPICIN, ALLOPURINOL, CIMETIDINE), alcohol,
sedatives.
Contains: PAROXETENE.
Other preparations:

---

sertraline *see* **Lustral**

Sevredol *see* **MST Continus**
(Napp)

---

silicic acid *see* **Unguentum Merck**

---

silver sulphadiazine *see* **Flamazine**

---

simple eye ointment

An eye ointment used to lubricate and protect the eye in various eye disorders.

Dose: apply as required.
Availability: NHS, private prescription, over the counter.
Side effects: vision may be blurred.
Caution:
Not to be used for: patients allergic to any of the ingredients.
Caution needed with:
Contains: WOOL FAT, YELLOW SOFT PARAFFIN, LIQUID PARAFFIN.
Other preparations:

---

simple linctus BP

A linctus used to soothe a dry, irritating cough.

Dose: 5 ml 3-4 times a day; children use paediatric simple linctus.
Availability: NHS, private prescription, over the counter.
Side effects:
Caution: in patients suffering from diabetes.
Not to be used for:
Caution needed with:
Contains: CITRIC ACID, anise flavouring.
Other preparations: paediatric simple linctus.

Simplene
(Chauvin)

Drops used as a SYMPATHOMIMETIC treatment for primary open angle or secondary glaucoma.

Dose: 1 drop into the eye 1-2 times a day.
Availability: NHS and private prescription.
Side effects: pain in the eye, headache, redness, skin reactions, melanosis, rarely general sympathomimetic effects (abnormal heart beat, dry mouth, brain stimulation).
Caution:
Not to be used for: patients suffering from narrow angle glaucoma, diabetes.
Caution needed with: MAOIS, TRICYCLIC ANTIDEPRESSANTS, ß-BLOCKERS.
Contains: ADRENALINE.
Other preparations: EPPY.

---

simvastatin *see* Zocor

Sinemet
(Du Pont)

A yellow, scored, oval tablet or a blue, scored, oval tablet according to strengths of LS 50/12.5 mg, 110 110/10 mg, Plus 100/25 mg, 275 250/25 mg and used as an anti-parkinsonian preparation to treat Parkinson's disease.

Dose: 1 'LS' or 1 'Plus' 3 times a day at first, increasing gradually to a maximum of the equivalent of 8 'Plus' a day, or as advised.
Availability: NHS and private prescription.
Side effects: nausea, vomiting, loss of appetite, low blood pressure on standing, involuntary movements, heart and brain disturbances, discoloration of urine.
Caution: in patients suffering from heart, circulation, liver, kidney, lung, or hormone disorders, stomach ulcer, or wide-angle glaucoma. Your doctor may advise that blood, liver, kidney, heart and circulation should be checked regularly.
Not to be used for: patients under 18 years, pregnant women, nursing mothers, or for patients suffering from severe mental disorders or narrow-angle glaucoma, or for patients with a history of skin cancer.
Caution needed with: MAOIS, blood-pressure lowering drugs, and SYMPATHOMIMETICS, VITAMIN B$_6$, iron supplements, sedatives.
Contains: LEVODOPA, CARBIDOPA monohydrate (CO-CARELDOPA).
Other preparations: Sinemet CR, Half Sinemet CR.

Sinequan
(Pfizer)

A red capsule, blue/red capsule, blue capsule, or blue/yellow capsule

according to strengths of 10 mg, 25 mg, 50 mg, 75 mg, and used as a
TRICYCLIC ANTIDEPRESSANT to treat depression.

Dose: 10-100 mg 3 times a day or once a day at bedtime.
Availability: NHS and private prescription.
Side effects: dry mouth, constipation, urine retention, blurred vision,
palpitations, rapid heart rate, tinnitus, nervousness, shaking, drowsiness,
sleeplessness, dizziness, hands shaking, low blood pressure, sweating,
weight change, skin reactions, jaundice or blood changes, breast
enlargement, stomach upset, weakness, unsteadiness, convulsions. Loss
of sexual desire may occur.
Caution: in the elderly, nursing mothers or in patients suffering from
adrenal tumour, urine retention, heart, liver, or kidney disease, thyroid
disease, epilepsy, diabetes, glaucoma, some other psychiatric conditions.
Your doctor may advise regular blood tests.
Not to be used for: children, pregnant women, or for patients suffering
from heart attacks, severe liver disease, heart block.
Caution needed with: alcohol, sedatives, ANTICHOLINERGICS, ADRENALINE,
MAOIS, BARBITURATES, other antidepressants, CIMETIDINE, oestrogens, blood-
pressure lowering drugs, CARBAMAZEPINE, PHENYTOIN, local anaesthetics.
Contains: DOXEPIN hydrochloride
Other preparations:

S

Sinthrome
(Ciba)

A white tablet supplied at a strength of 1 mg, and used as an
ANTICOAGULANT drug to treat blood clots.

Dose: 8-12 mg on the first day, 4-8 mg second day, and then adjust
according to blood test results.
Availability: NHS and private prescription.
Side effects: bleeding, allergies, liver damage, reversible hair loss, rarely
nausea, loss of appetite, headache, skin disorder.
Caution: in nursing mothers, the elderly, and in patients suffering from
high blood pressure, reduced ability of protein in blood to bind drugs,
severe heart failure, liver dysfunction, gastro-intestinal disorders.
Not to be used for: children, pregnant women, the unco-operative, and in
patients suffering from bleeding conditions, blood changes, damaged
kidney or liver function, inflammation of the heart or lungs, very high blood
pressure, or within 24 hours of surgery.
Caution needed with: NON-STEROIDAL ANTI-INFLAMMATORY DRUGS, VITAMIN K,
oral antidiabetics, QUINIDINE, antibiotics, PHENFORMIN, CIMETIDINE, STEROIDS,
drugs affecting liver enzymes (BARBITURATES, GRISEOFULVIN, anticonvulsants),
other drugs affecting blood clotting.
Contains: NICOUMALONE.

Other preparations:

Skinoren
(Schering Health Care)

A cream used to treat acne.

Dose: apply once or twice a day and rub in. (Maximum of 10 g a day.)
Continue for up to 6 months.
Availability: NHS and private prescription.
Side effects: irritation, sensitivity to light.
Caution: in pregnant women and nursing mothers. Avoid the eyes.
Not to be used for:
Caution needed with:
Contains: AZELAIC ACID.
Other preparations:

SLE *see* lupus

Slo-Phyllin *see* Lasma
(Lipha)

Slow Sodium
(Ciba)

A white tablet supplied at a strength of 600 mg and used as a salt
supplement to treat and prevent salt deficiency.

Dose: adults treatment 4-20 tablets a day, prevention 4-8 tablets a day;
children in proportion to dose for 70 kg adult.
Availability: NHS, private prescription, over the counter.
Side effects:
Caution:
Not to be used for: patients suffering from fluid retention, heart disease,
heart failure, adrenal tumour.
Caution needed with: DIURETICS, LITHIUM.
Contains: SODIUM CHLORIDE.
Other preparations:

Slow-Fe *see* ferrous sulphate tablets
(Ciba)

Slow-Fe Folic
(Ciba)

A cream-coloured long-acting tablet used as an iron and FOLIC ACID supplement for the prevention of iron and folic acid deficiencies in pregnancy.

Dose: 1-2 tablets a day.
Availability: NHS and private prescription.
Side effects: nausea, constipation.
Caution:
Not to be used for: children.
Caution needed with: PENICILLAMINE, PHENYTOIN, zinc, anticonvulsants, ANTACIDS, some antibiotics, LEVODOPA.
Contains: FERROUS SULPHATE, folic acid.
Other preparations: FERROGRAD FOLIC.

Slow-K
(Ciba)

An orange tablet supplied at a strength of 600 mg and used as a potassium supplement to treat potassium deficiency.

Dose: adults 2-12 tablets a day or every other day after food.
Availability: NHS, private prescription, over the counter.
Side effects: blocked or ulcerated small bowel.
Caution: in pregnant women, and in patients suffering from kidney disease, stomach ulcer, low magnesium levels.
Not to be used for: children, or for patients suffering from advanced kidney disease, Addison's disease, adrenal gland disorder, dehydration, acidic blood (may occur in diabetes).
Caution needed with: some DIURETICS, CYCLOSPORIN, ACE INHIBITORS, NON-STEROIDAL ANTI-INFLAMMATORY DRUGS.
Contains: POTASSIUM CHLORIDE.
Other preparations: KAY-CEE-L (liquid form).

Slow-Trasicor *see* oxprenolol tablets
(Ciba)

Slozem *see* diltiazem long-acting tablets
(Lipha)

Sno Phenicol *see* **chloramphenicol eye ointment**
(Chauvin)

Sno Pilo *see* **pilocarpine eye drops**
(Chauvin)

Sno Tears
(Chauvin)

Drops used to lubricate the eyes.

Dose: 1 or more drops into the eye as needed.
Availability: NHS, private prescription, over the counter.
Side effects: temporary stinging, blurred vision.
Caution:
Not to be used for: patients who wear soft contact lenses.
Caution needed with:
Contains: POLYVINYL ALCOHOL.
Other preparations: LIQUIFILM TEARS, HYPOTEARS.

---

soap spirit BP

A liquid used as a soap to remove crusts from the skin.

Dose: apply as needed.
Availability: NHS, private prescription, over the counter.
Side effects:
Caution:
Not to be used for:
Caution needed with:
Contains: soft soap, alcohol.
Other preparations:

---

sodium acid phosphate (anhydrous) *see* **Carbalax, Fletchers' Phosphate, Phosphate**

---

sodium alginate *see* **Algitec, Gaviscon, Pyrogastrone**

---

sodium alkylsulphoacetate *see* **Micralax**

Sodium Amytal
(Distriphar)

A blue capsule supplied at strengths of 60 mg, 200 mg and used as a BARBITURATE to treat sleeplessness.

Dose: 60-200 mg at night.
Availability: controlled drug; NHS and private prescription.
Side effects: drowsiness, hangover, dizziness, shaking, allergies, headache, confusion, excitement, unsteadiness, breathing difficulty.
Caution: in patients suffering from liver, kidney, or lung disease. Dependence (addiction) may develop.
Not to be used for: children, young adults, pregnant women, nursing mothers, the elderly, the debilitated, or for patients with a history of drug or alcohol abuse, or suffering from PORPHYRIA, or in the management of pain.
Caution needed with: ANTICOAGULANTS, alcohol, sedatives, other tranquillizers, STEROIDS, the contraceptive pill, GRISEOFULVIN, RIFAMPICIN, PHENYTOIN, METRONIDAZOLE, CHLORAMPHENICOL.
Contains: AMYLOBARBITONE sodium.
Other preparations: Sodium Amytal Injection (used for severe epilepsy). AMYTAL.

---

sodium aurothiomalate *see* Myocrisin

---

sodium bicarbonate *see* Carbalax, Caved-S, Dioralyte, Electrolade, Gastrocote, Gastron, Gaviscon, magnesium carbonate aromatic mixture, Mictral, Migravess, Phosphate, Pyrogastrone, Rehidrat, sodium bicarbonate ear drops BP

---

sodium bicarbonate ear drops BP

Ear drops used to remove ear wax.

Dose: use as needed. Lie down with treated ear uppermost for 5-10 minutes after inserting the drops.
Availability: NHS, private prescription, over the counter.
Side effects:
Caution:
Not to be used for:
Caution needed with:
Contains: SODIUM BICARBONATE, GLYCEROL.
Other preparations:

---

sodium cellulose *see* **Calcisorb**

---

sodium chloride *see* **Artificial Tears Minims, Diarrest, Dioralyte, Glandosane, Normasol, Rehidrat, Slow Sodium, Salivace, sodium chloride eye drops, Sodium Chloride Minims, Steri-Neb Saline, sterile saline**

---

sodium chloride eye drops

Drops used to irrigate the eyes.

Dose: use as needed.
Availability: NHS, private prescription, over the counter.
Side effects:
Caution:
Not to be used for:
Not to be used with:
Contains: SODIUM CHLORIDE.
Other preparations: SODIUM CHLORIDE MINIMS (packed in single-use containers).

Sodium Chloride Minims *see* **sodium chloride eye drops**
(Chauvin)

---

sodium citrate *see* **Diarrest, Micolette, Micralax, Mictral, Relaxit**

---

sodium cromoglycate *see* **Aerocrom Inhaler, Cromogen, Cusilyn, Hay-Crom, Intal, Nalcrom, Opticrom, Rynacrom Spray, sodium cromoglycate eye drops, Steri-Neb Cromogen, Vividrin**

---

sodium cromoglycate eye drops

Drops used as an anti-inflammatory preparation to treat allergic conjunctivitis.

Dose: 1-2 drops into the eyes 4 times a day.
Availability: NHS, private prescription, over the counter.
Side effects: temporary smarting, burning.
Caution:

Not to be used for: patients who wear contact lenses.
Caution needed with:
Contains: SODIUM CROMOGLYCATE.
Other preparations: sodium cromoglycate eye ointment. CUSILYN, HAY-CROM, OPTICROM, VIVIDRIN. (Various brands available without prescription only for the treatment of seasonal allergy such as hayfever – Brol-eze, Opticrom Allergy, Hay-crom Hayfever, Optrex Hayfever.)

---

sodium cromoglycate inhaler

An inhaler used as an anti-asthmatic drug for the prevention of bronchial asthma.

Dose: 2 puffs 4 times a day at regular intervals reducing to maintain effect. (May be required up to 8 times a day. Extra doses may be taken before exercise.) Treatment should be continuous.
Availability: NHS and private prescription.
Side effects: passing cough, irritated throat, rarely bronchial spasm.
Caution:
Not to be used for:
Caution needed with:
Contains: SODIUM CROMOGLYCATE.
Other preparations: Intal Fisonair, Intal Nebuliser Solution, Intal Spincaps, Intal Syncroner. CROMOGEN. Steri-Neb Cromogen. (Some have different inhalation devices, and some are for use with a nebulizer.) Intal Inhaler.

---

sodium docusate *see* Molcer

---

sodium fluorescein *see* Lignocaine and Fluorescein Minims

---

sodium fluoride *see* En-De-Kay, Fluor-a-day, Fluorigard Drops, Fluorigard Rinse, Fluorigard Tablets

---

sodium fusidate *see* Fucidin, Fucidin H

---

sodium hydrogen tartrate *see* Bocasan

---

sodium hypochlorite *see* Chlorasol

---

sodium iron edetate *see* **Sytron**

sodium lauryl sulphate *see* **Relaxit**

sodium lauryl sulphoacetate *see* **Micolette**

sodium nedocromil *see* **Tilade**

sodium perborate *see* **Bocasan**

sodium phosphate *see* **Fletchers' Phosphate**

sodium picosulphate *see* **Laxoberal, Picolax, sodium picosulphate elixir**

sodium picosulphate elixir

A stimulant laxative used to treat constipation, and to clear the bowels before medical procedures.

Dose: adults 5-15 ml at night; children 2-5 years 2.5 ml at night; children 5-10 years 5 ml at night.
Availability: NHS and private prescription.
Side effects: stomach cramp.
Caution: in patients suffering from inflammatory bowel disease. Not for prolonged use.
Not to be used for: children under 2 years, or for patients with blocked intestine.
Caution needed with:
Contains:
Other preparations: LAXOBERAL, PICOLAX.

sodium polystyrene sulphonate *see* **Resonium-A**

sodium pyrrolidone carboxylate *see* **Humiderm, Lacticare**

sodium sulphosuccinated undecylenic monoalkylolamide *see* **Genisol**

---

sodium valproate *see* **Epilim, Orlept, sodium valproate tablets**

---

sodium valproate tablets

A tablet supplied at strengths of 200 mg, 500 mg and used as an anticonvulsant to treat epilepsy.

Dose: adults 600 mg a day at first in 2 divided doses after food then increase by 200 mg every 3 days usually to 1-2 g a day and a maximum of 2.5 g a day; children under 20 kg body weight 20 mg per kg a day at first, over 20 kg 400 mg a day at first, increasing gradually to 35 mg per kg a day if needed.
Availability: NHS and private prescription.
Side effects: stomach irritation, nausea, drowsiness (withdraw immediately), rash, gain in weight, loss of hair, fluid retention, pancreatitis, liver failure, blood changes, neurological effects, liver disorder, disturbance of periods, unsteadiness, breast swelling.
Caution: in children, pregnant women, nursing mothers, and in patients suffering from LUPUS, PORPHYRIA, or who are undergoing major surgery, or who have a history of liver disorders.
Not to be used for: patients suffering from liver disease, or with a history in the family of severe liver failure.
Caution needed with: ASPIRIN, antidepressants, other anticonvulsants, antimalarial drugs, tranquillizers, sedatives.
Contains: SODIUM VALPROATE.
Other preparations: EPILIM, ORLEPT. (Liquid and long-acting forms available.)

Sofradex Drops
(Hoechst-Roussel)

Drops used as an aminoglycoside antibiotic, STEROID treatment for inflammation of the outer ear or eye.

Dose: 2-3 drops into the ear 3-4 times a day, or 1-2 drops into the eye up to 6 times a day.
Availability: NHS and private prescription.
Side effects: rise in eye pressure, fungal infection, thinning cornea, cataract.
Caution: in pregnant women and infants – do not use over extended periods.

Not to be used for: patients suffering from perforated ear drum, glaucoma, viral, fungal, tubercular, or weeping infections.
Caution needed with:
Contains: FRAMYCETIN sulphate, DEXAMETHASONE, GRAMICIDIN.
Other preparations: SOFRADEX OINTMENT.

Sofradex Ointment
(Roussel)

An ointment used as a STEROID, aminoglycoside antibiotic treatment for inflammation of the outer ear or eye.

Dose: apply to the eye 2-3 times a day or at night, apply to the ear once or twice a day.
Availability: NHS and private prescription.
Side effects: rise in eye pressure, additional infection in eye or ear, thinning cornea, cataract.
Caution: in pregnant women and infants – do not use for extended periods.
Not to be used for: patients suffering from glaucoma, viral, fungal, tubercular, or weeping infections, perforated ear drum.
Caution needed with:
Contains: DEXAMETHASONE, FRAMYCETIN sulphate, GRAMICIDIN.
Other preparations: Sofradex Drops.

Soframycin Drops
(Roussel)

Drops used as an aminoglycoside antibiotic treatment for conjunctivitis, styes, eyelid inflammation

Dose: 1-2 drops into the eye 3-4 times a day.
Availability: NHS and private prescription.
Side effects:
Caution:
Not to be used for:
Caution needed with:
Contains: FRAMYCETIN sulphate.
Other preparations: Soframycin Ointment.

Sofra-Tulle
(Hoechst-Roussel)

A sterile, impregnated gauze dressing, supplied at a size of 10 cm square, and used as a dressing for burns, wounds, ulcers, and other infected areas.

Availability: NHS, private prescription, over the counter. (Also available on a trial basis from nurses.)
Contains: FRAMYCETIN.

Solpadol
(Sanofi Winthrop)

A white, scored, effervescent tablet used as an ANALGESIC to treat severe pain.

Dose: 2 tablets dissolved in water every 4 hours to a maximum of 8 tablets in 24 hours.
Availability: NHS and private prescription.
Side effects: tolerance and addiction, constipation, dizziness, sedation, nausea, dry mouth, blurred vision.
Caution: in the elderly, pregnant women, during labour, nursing mothers, and in patients suffering from underactive thyroid, kidney or liver damage, inflammatory or obstructive bowel disease, enlarged prostate.
Not to be used for: children, or for patients suffering from breathing difficulty, acute alcoholism, head injury, raised brain pressure, or who have undergone biliary tract surgery.
Caution needed with: MAOIS, sedatives, other medicines containing PARACETAMOL.
Contains: paracetamol, CODEINE PHOSPHATE.
Other preparations: Solpadol Caplets.

S

Solvazinc
(Thames)

An off-white, effervescent tablet supplied at a strength of 200 mg and used as a zinc supplement to treat zinc deficiency.

Dose: adults and children over 30 kg body weight 1 tablet dissolved in water 1-3 times a day after food; children under 10 kg body weight ½ tablet in water once a day after food, 10-30 kg half adult dose.
Availability: NHS, private prescription, over the counter.
Side effects: stomach upset.
Caution: in patients suffering from kidney failure.
Not to be used for:
Caution needed with: TETRACYCLINE ANTIBIOTICS.
Contains: ZINC SULPHATE.
Other preparations: ZINCOMED, ZINCOSOL, Z-SPAN.

Sominex
(SmithKline Beecham)

A white, scored tablet supplied at a strength of 20 mg and used as an ANTIHISTAMINE treatment for occasional sleeplessness.

Dose: 1 tablet at bedtime.
Availability: NHS, private prescription, over the counter.
Side effects: ANTICHOLINERGENIC effects, brain and stomach upsets, allergies, blood disorders.
Caution: in patients suffering from glaucoma, enlarged prostate, epilepsy, liver disease. Patients should be warned of drowsiness and should not drive or carry out any functions requiring alertness.
Not to be used for: children under 16 years.
Caution needed with: alcohol, sedatives, ANTICHOLINERGICS.
Contains: PROMETHAZINE hydrochloride.
Other preparations:

Somnite *see* nitrazepam tablets
(Norgine)

Soneryl
(Rhone-Poulenc Rorer)

A pink, scored tablet supplied at a strength of 100 mg and used as a BARBITURATE to treat sleeplessness.

Dose: 1-2 tablets before going to bed.
Availability: controlled drug; NHS and private prescription.
Side effects: drowsiness, hangover, dizziness, shaking, allergies, headache, confusion, excitement, unsteadiness, breathing difficulty.
Caution: patients suffering from kidney or lung disease. Dependence (addiction) may develop.
Not to be used for: children, young adults, pregnant women, nursing mothers, the elderly, patients with a history of drug or alcohol abuse, or suffering from PORPHYRIA, or in the management of pain.
Caution needed with: ANTICOAGULANTS, alcohol, sedatives, other tranquillizers, STEROIDS, the contraceptive pill, GRISEOFULVIN, RIFAMPICIN, PHENYTOIN, METRONIDAZOLE, CHLORAMPHENICOL.
Contains: BUTOBARBITONE.
Other preparations:

Soni-Slo *see* **isosorbide dinitrate tablets**
(Lipha)

---

sorbic acid *see* **Micralax, Relaxit, Unguentum Merck**

Sorbichew *see* **isosorbide dinitrate tablets**
(Stuart)

Sorbid SA *see* **isosorbide dinitrate tablets**
(Stuart)

---

sorbitol *see* **Glandosane, Relaxit**

Sorbitrate *see* **isosorbide dinitrate tablets**
(Stuart)

Sorbsan
(Pharma Plast)

A sterile, alginate dressing, supplied at sizes of 5 cm square, 10 cm square, and used as a drying dressing for wet wounds, such as leg ulcers, bed sores, post-operative wounds.

Availability: NHS, private prescription, over the counter. (Also available on a trial basis from nurses.)
Contains: alginate.
Other preparations: TEGAGEL, KALTOSTAT, KALTOGEL.

Sotacor
(Bristol-Myers)

A white tablet supplied at strengths of 80 mg, 160 mg and used as a ß-BLOCKER to treat angina, abnormal heart rhythm, high blood pressure, and for the prevention of heart attacks.

Dose: angina 160 mg a day in single or divided doses; for other uses up to 320 mg a day depending on condition.
Availability: NHS and private prescription.
Side effects: cold hands and feet, sleep disturbance, slow heart rate, tiredness, wheezing, heart failure, stomach upset, low blood pressure, dry

eyes, skin rash.

Caution: in pregnant women, nursing mothers, and in patients suffering from diabetes, kidney or liver disorders, asthma. May need to be withdrawn before surgery. Withdraw gradually. Your doctor may advise additional treatment with DIURETICS or DIGOXIN.

Not to be used for: children, or for patients suffering from heart block or failure, low blood pressure, or untreated PHAEOCHROMOCYTOMA.

Caution needed with: VERAPAMIL, CLONIDINE withdrawal, some anti-arrhythmic drugs and anaesthetics, RESERPINE, some blood-pressure lowering drugs, ERGOTAMINE, CIMETIDINE, sedatives, antidiabetics, SYMPATHOMIMETICS, INDOMETHACIN.

Contains: SOTALOL hydrochloride.

Other preparations: Sotacor Injection. BETA-CARDONE.

---

sotalol *see* **Beta-Cardone, Sotacor, Sotazide, Tolerzide**

---

soya oil *see* **Balneum, Balneum Plus, Balneum with Tar**

Sparine *see* **promazine tablets**
(Wyeth)

Spasmonal
(Norgine)

A blue/grey capsule supplied at a strength of 60 mg and used as an anti-spasmodic treatment for irritable bowel syndrome and period pain.

Dose: adults 1-2 tablets 1-3 times a day; children over 8 years 1 tablet 3 times a day.

Availability: NHS, private prescription, over the counter.

Side effects:

Caution: in pregnant women.

Not to be used for: children under 8 years, or for patients without normal bowel movement.

Caution needed with:

Contains: ALVERINE CITRATE.

Other preparations: RELAXYL.

Spiretic *see* **spironolactone tablets**
(DDSA)

Spiro-Co *see* **Aldactide**
(Baker Norton)

Spiroctan *see* **spironolactone tablets**
(Boehringer Mannheim)

Spirolone *see* **spironolactone tablets**
(Berk)

---

spironolactone *see* **Aldactide, Aldactone, Lasilactone, Spiretic, Spiro-Co, Spiroctan, Spirolone, spironolactone tablets, Spirospare**

---

spironolactone tablets

A tablet supplied at strengths of 25 mg, 50 mg, 100 mg and used as a DIURETIC to treat fluid retention in congestive heart failure, liver cirrhosis, kidney disorder, and adrenal tumour.

Dose: adults 100-200 mg a day with food increasing to 400 mg a day if necessary; children 3 mg per kg bodyweight a day in divided doses.
Availability: NHS and private prescription.
Side effects: breast enlargement, impotence, lethargy, raised potassium levels, irregular periods, stomach upset, rash, headache, confusion, low sodium levels, liver and blood disorders, soft bones.
Caution: in the elderly, and in patients suffering from kidney or liver disease, PORPHYRIA. Your doctor may advise regular blood tests.
Not to be used for: pregnant women, nursing mothers, or for patients suffering from severe kidney disorder, raised potassium or low sodium levels, Addison's disease.
Caution needed with: potassium supplements, CARBENOXOLONE, ACE INHIBITORS, some blood-pressure lowering drugs, sedatives, alcohol, NON-STEROIDAL ANTI-INFLAMMATORY DRUGS, some heart drugs, TRICYCLIC ANTIDEPRESSANTS, CARBAMAZEPINE, DIGOXIN, CYCLOSPORIN.
Contains: SPIRONOLACTONE.
Other preparations: ALDACTONE, SPIRETIC, SPIROCTAN, SPIROLONE, SPIROSPARE.

Spirospare *see* **spironolactone tablets**
(Ashbourne)

Sporanox
(Janssen-Cilag)

A blue/pink capsule supplied at a strength of 100 mg and used as an antifungal treatment for skin, vaginal, or mouth infections.

Dose: 1-2 capsules a day for 1-30 days, or 2 capsules twice a day for 1 day, or as advised by a physician.
Availability: NHS and private prescription.
Side effects: headache, indigestion, nausea, stomach pain.
Caution: in patients suffering from liver disease, or with a history of liver disorder resulting from other treatments.
Not to be used for: children, the elderly, pregnant women, nursing mothers. Contraception must be used during and for 1 month after treatment.
Caution needed with: CYCLOSPORIN, ANTACIDS, HISTAMINE H_2-ANTAGONIST treatments for stomach ulcer, ASTEMIZOLE, TERFENADINE, CISAPRIDE, RIFAMPICIN.
Contains: ITRACONAZOLE.
Other preparations:

S

Sprilon
(Perstorp)

An aerosol spray used as a barrier to protect the skin from faeces and urine, and to treat eczema, leg ulcers, bedsores, cracked skin.

Dose: spray for 2-3 seconds from a distance of 20 cm.
Availability: NHS, private prescription, over the counter.
Side effects:
Caution:
Not to be used for:
Caution needed with:
Contains: DIMETHICONE, ZINC OXIDE.
Other preparations:

squalane *see* Dermalex, Salonair

Stafoxil *see* flucloxacillin tablets
(Yamanouchi)

stannous fluoride *see* Fluorigard Gelkam

stanozolol *see* **Stromba**

Staril
(Squibb)

A white, diamond-shaped tablet, and a white tablet according to strengths of 10 mg, 20 mg, and used as an ACE-INHIBITOR, to treat high blood pressure, and, in combination with a DIURETIC, heart failure.

Dose: for high blood pressure, 10-40 mg once a day; discontinue any diuretic several days before starting treatment; re-introduce later if needed. For heart failure, 10-40 mg once a day, starting treatment in hospital or under strict medical supervision.
Availability: NHS and private prescription.
Side effects: dizziness, cough, stomach upset, palpitations, chest pain, rash, muscle/bone pain, tiredness, taste disturbance, severe allergy.
Caution: in patients suffering from liver or kidney damage, congestive heart failure, salt or body fluid depletion, or who are undergoing dialysis.
Not to be used for: children, pregnant women, nursing mothers.
Caution needed with: some diuretics, potassium supplements, NON-STEROIDAL ANTI-INFLAMMATORY DRUGS, ANTACIDS, LITHIUM, blood-pressure lowering drugs.
Contains: FOSINOPRIL sodium.
Other preparations:

Staycept
(Roche)

A pessary used in conjunction with barrier contraceptives as a spermicidal preparation.

Dose: 1 pessary inserted into the vagina 10 minutes before intercourse, and 1 pessary placed inside the diaphragm or cap.
Availability: NHS, private prescription, over the counter.
Side effects:
Caution:
Not to be used for:
Caution needed with:
Contains: NONOXYNOL-9.
Other preparations: Staycept Jelly. ORTHO-FORMS, GYNOL II, DURAGEL, DOUBLE CHECK.

Stelazine
(SmithKline Beecham)

A blue tablet supplied at strengths of 1 mg, 5 mg and used as a sedative to treat anxiety, depression, agitation, schizophrenia, mental disorders, dangerous impulsive behaviour, nausea, vomiting, vertigo.

Dose: for anxiety, depression, nausea, vomiting adults 2-4 mg up to a maximum of 6 mg a day in divided doses; elderly 1 mg a day at first; children 3-5 years up to 1 mg a day, 6-12 up to 4 mg a day. For schizophrenia etc, adults 5 mg twice a day increasing after 7 days to 15 mg; elderly 1 mg a day at first; children up to 5 mg a day.
Availability: NHS and private prescription.
Side effects: brain disturbances, dry mouth, blurred vision, ECG and hormone changes, allergies, impaired judgement and ability, rarely extrapyramidal symptoms (shaking and rigidity).
Caution: in the elderly, pregnant women, nursing mothers, and in patients suffering from undiagnosed vomiting, epilepsy, cardiovascular disease or Parkinson's disease. Your doctor may advise you to watch for loss of dexterity.
Not to be used for: patients in an unconscious state or patients suffering from liver disease, bone marrow depression.
Caution needed with: sedatives, alcohol, ANALGESICS, blood-pressure lowering drugs.
Contains: TRIFLUOPERAZINE hydrochloride.
Other preparations: Stelazine Syrup, Stelazine Spansules (long-acting product), Stelazine Concentrate, Stelazine Injection.

Stemetil *see* prochlorperazine tablets
(Rhône-Poulenc Rorer)

Ster-Zac Bath Concentrate
(Hough, Hoseason)

A liquid used as an antibacterial treatment for skin infections.

Dose: add 28.5 ml to the bath water.
Availability: NHS, private prescription, over the counter.
Side effects:
Caution: keep out of the eyes.
Not to be used for:
Caution needed with:
Contains: TRICLOSAN.
Other preparations: AQUASEPT, MANUSEPT.

Ster-Zac Powder
(Hough, Hoseason.)

A powder used as a disinfectant for the prevention of infections in new-born infants, and to treat recurring skin infections.

Dose: adults apply to the affected area once a day; infants dust the affected area at each change of nappy.
Availability: NHS, private prescription, over the counter.
Side effects:
Caution: in patients where the skin is broken.
Not to be used for:
Caution needed with:
Contains: HEXACHLOROPHANE.
Other preparations:

---

sterculia *see* Alvercol, Normacol, Prefil

Sterexidine
(Galen)

A liquid used as a disinfectant to clean wounds and burns.

Dose: as needed.
Availability: NHS, private prescription, over the counter.
Side effects:
Caution:
Not to be used for:
Caution needed with:
Contains: CHLORHEXIDINE GLUCONATE.
Other preparations: UNISEPT, HIBISOL, HIBISCRUB.

Steri-Neb Cromogen *see* sodium cromoglycate inhaler
(Baker Norton)

Steri-Neb Ipratropium *see* Atrovent (Nebules)
(Baker Norton)

Steri-Neb Salamol *see* salbutamol inhaler
(Baker Norton)

S

Steri-Neb Saline
(Baker Norton)

A preservative-free solution used to dilute substances used in nebulizers (fine sprays).

Dose: as needed.
Availability: NHS, private prescription.
Side effects:
Caution:
Not to be used for:
Caution needed with:
Contains: SODIUM CHLORIDE.
Other preparations:

---

sterile saline

A solution used for washing out eyes, burns, wounds, and for general cleansing of the skin.

Dose: use as needed.
Availability: NHS, private prescription, over the counter.
Side effects:
Caution:
Not to be used for:
Caution needed with:
Contains: SODIUM CHLORIDE.
Other preparations: AMIDOSE SALINE, NORMASOL, STERIPOD BLUE.

Steripod Blue *see* sterile saline
(Seton)

Steripod Yellow *see* Unisept
(Seton)

---

steroid
A preparation which supplements the hormones naturally produced by the adrenal gland. Corticosteroids (example PREDNISOLONE *see* prednisolone tablets) are used to suppress inflammatory or allergic disorders, such as asthma, rheumatic conditions, or eczema. High doses may cause patients to develop a 'moon face' appearance. After long treatment periods, the drug should be withdrawn gradually. Anabolic STEROIDS (example

STANOZOLOL *see* Stromba) are used to treat vascular disorders, thinning of the bones, and some bone marrow disorders. They may be abused by some athletes because of their body-building properties.

Stesolid
(Dumex)

A solution supplied at strengths of 5 mg, 10 mg, in a unit dose rectal applicator and used as a sedative to treat acute anxiety, acute epilepsy or convulsions caused by fever, muscle spasm.

Dose: children 1-3 years 5 mg rectally, children over 3 years and adults 10 mg rectally; elderly half adult dose.
Availability: NHS, private prescription.
Side effects: drowsiness, light-headedness, unsteadiness, addiction, confusion, vertigo, stomach upset, low blood pressure, rash, disturbed eyesight, retention of urine, changes in sexual function; rarely blood disorders or jaundice.
Caution: in the elderly, pregnant women, women in labour, nursing mothers or for patients with chronic kidney, liver, or breathing disorders. Your doctor will warn you that your judgement or dexterity may be affected. Long-term therapy should be avoided and the treatment withdrawn gradually.
Not to be used for: children under 1 year, or for patients suffering from various mental disorders or acute breathing difficulties.
Caution needed with: alcohol, other sedatives, anticonvulsants.
Contains: DIAZEPAM.
Other preparations: DIAZEPAM RECTUBES.

Stiedex LP
(Stiefel)

An oily cream used as a STEROID treatment for skin disorders.

Dose: massage a small quantity into the affected area 2-3 times a day.
Availability: NHS and private prescription.
Side effects: fluid retention, suppression of adrenal glands, thinning, spotting, or streaking of the skin may occur.
Caution: use for short periods of time only, especially in children or on the face.
Not to be used for: patients suffering from acne or any other skin infections caused by tuberculosis, ringworm, viruses, or fungi, leg ulcers, scabies, or continuously especially in pregnant women.
Caution needed with:
Contains: DESOXYMETHASONE.

Other preparations: Stiedex Lotion (for psoriasis, eczema, and other skin disorders).

Stiemycin
(Stiefel)

A solution used as an antibiotic treatment for acne.

Dose: wash and dry the affected area and apply twice a day.
Availability: NHS and private prescription.
Side effects: irritation, dryness.
Caution:
Not to be used for:
Caution needed with:
Contains: ERYTHROMYCIN.
Other preparations:

---

stilboesterol *see* Tampovagan

Stilnoct
(Lorex)

A white, film-coated tablet used as a sedative for the short-term treatment of sleeplessness.

Dose: 2 tablets before going to bed; elderly, half adult dose.
Availability: NHS, private prescription
Side effects: stomach upset, drowsiness, headache, dizziness; very rarely, loss of memory, shaking, confusion, disturbed perception, depression.
Caution: in pregnant women, nursing mothers, and in patients suffering from liver or kidney disorders, depression, or with a history of alcohol or drug abuse. Your doctor will warn you not to drive or operate machinery if affected by drowsiness. Your doctor will also advise regular check-ups.
Not to be used for: children or for patients suffering from severe liver disorders, breathing difficulties, MYASTHENIA GRAVIS.
Caution needed with: alcohol, other sedatives.
Contains: ZOLPIDEM hemitartrate.
Other preparations:

Stimlor *see* Praxilene
(Berk)

Stromba
(Sanofi Winthrop)

A white, quarter-scored tablet supplied at a strength of 5 mg and used as an anabolic STEROID to treat blood vessel disorders.

Dose: adults ¼-2 tablets a day according to condition; children over 1 year use reduced doses.
Availability: NHS and private prescription.
Side effects: masculinization, liver poisoning, indigestion, cramp, headache, thyroid effects.
Caution: in children (avoid long-term use), women before the menopause, and in patients suffering from heart or kidney disease, or with a history of jaundice. Your doctor may advise blood tests for liver function.
Not to be used for: children under 1 year, or for pregnant women or for patients suffering from prostate cancer, liver disease, diabetes, PORPHYRIA.
Caution needed with: ANTICOAGULANTS taken by mouth, antidiabetics.
Contains: STANOZOLOL.
Other preparations:

S

Stugeron
(Janssen-Cilag)

A white, scored tablet supplied at a strength of 15 mg and used as an ANTIHISTAMINE treatment for vestibular disorders, travel sickness.

Dose: vestibular disorders adults, 2 tablets 3 times a day; travel sickness 2 tablets 2 hours before journey, then 1 every 8 hours during the journey. Children 5-12 years half adult dose.
Availability: NHS, private prescription, over the counter.
Side effects: brain and stomach disturbances, drowsiness, reduced reactions, rarely skin eruptions, allergy, blood disorders, ANTICHOLINERGIC effects.
Caution: in pregnant women, nursing mothers, and in patients suffering from liver or kidney disease, glaucoma, epilepsy, or enlarged prostate. Do not drive or operate machinery if affected by drowsiness.
Not to be used for: children under 5 years.
Caution needed with: alcohol, sedatives, some antidepressants (MAOIS), ANTICHOLINERGICS.
Contains: CINNARIZINE.
Other preparations:

Stugeron Forte
(Janssen-Cilag)

An orange/cream capsule supplied at a strength of 75 mg and used as an

ANTIHISTAMINE treatment for blood vessel disease including intermittent claudication (spasm of the arteries) and Raynaud's syndrome (a disease of the arteries of the hands).

Dose: 1 capsule 3 times a day.
Availability: NHS, private prescription, over the counter.
Side effects: drowsiness, rash.
Caution: in patients suffering from low blood pressure.
Not to be used for: children.
Caution needed with: alcohol, sedatives.
Contains: CINNARIZINE.
Other preparations:

---

sucralfate *see* **Antepsin**

---

sucrose *see* **Rehidrat**

S

Sudafed
(Warner Wellcome Consumer)

A brown tablet supplied at a strength of 60 mg and used as a SYMPATHOMIMETIC treatment to relieve congestion of the nose, sinuses, and upper respiratory tract.

Dose: adults 1 tablet 3 times a day; children over 2 years use elixir.
Availability: NHS, private prescription, over the counter.
Side effects: rapid or abnormal heart rate, dry mouth, brain stimulation.
Caution: in patients suffering from diabetes, overactive thyroid, raised blood pressure, heart disease, raised eye pressure, enlarged prostate.
Not to be used for: children under 2 years.
Caution needed with: MAOIS, TRICYCLIC ANTIDEPRESSANTS, other sympathomimetics, drugs to reduce appetite, FURAZOLIDONE.
Contains: PSEUDOEPHEDRINE.
Other preparations: Sudafed Elixir, Sudafed SA (not available over the counter), Sudafed-Co, Sudafed Expectorant (neither available on NHS). GALPSEUD.

Sudafed Plus
(Warner Wellcome Consumer)

A white, scored tablet used as an ANTIHISTAMINE, SYMPATHOMIMETIC treatment for allergic rhinitis.

Dose: adults 1 tablet 3 times a day; children over 2 years use syrup.
Availability: NHS, private prescription, over the counter.
Side effects: drowsiness, rash, disturbed sleep, rarely hallucinations.
Caution: in patients suffering from raised eye pressure, enlarged prostate, overactive thyroid, diabetes.
Not to be used for: infants under 2 years or for patients suffering from severe high blood pressure, heart disease.
Caution needed with: MAOIS, other sympathomimetics, alcohol, sedatives, FURAZOLIDONE.
Contains: TRIPROLIDINE HYDROCHLORIDE, PSEUDOEPHEDRINE hydrochloride.
Other preparations: Sudafed Plus Syrup. Actifed – not available on NHS.

Sudocrem
(Tosara)

A cream used as an antiseptic emollient to treat bedsores, burns, nappy rash, eczema.

Dose: apply a thin layer to the affected area as needed.
Availability: NHS, private prescription, over the counter.
Side effects:
Caution:
Not to be used for:
Caution needed with:
Contains: ZINC OXIDE, anhydrous WOOL FAT, BENZYL BENZOATE, BENZYL CINNAMATE, BENZYL ALCOHOL.
Other preparations:

---

sulconazole *see* Exelderm

Suleo-C
(Seton Healthcare)

A lotion used as a pediculicide to treat head lice.

Dose: rub into the scalp as directed. Shampoo off after 2-12 hours
Availability: NHS, private prescription.
Side effects:
Caution: in infants under 6 months, and in patients suffering from asthma, eczema. Keep out of the eyes.
Not to be used for:
Caution needed with:
Contains: CARBARYL.

Other preparations: Suleo-C Shampoo. CARYLDERM, CLINICIDE, DERBAC-C.

Suleo-M
(Seton Healthcare)

A lotion used as a pediculicide to treat head lice.

Dose: rub into the scalp as directed. Shampoo off after 2-12 hours.
Availability: NHS, private prescription, over the counter.
Side effects:
Caution: in infants under 6 months, and in patients suffering from asthma, eczema. Keep out of the eyes.
Not to be used for:
Caution needed with:
Contains: MALATHION.
Other preparations: DERBAC-M, PRIODERM.

---

sulfadoxine *see* Fansidar

---

sulfametopyrazine *see* Kelfizine W

---

sulindac *see* Clinoril

Sulparex
(Bristol-Myers Squibb)

A white, scored tablet supplied at a strength of 200 mg, and used to treat schizophrenia.

Dose: adults and young persons over 14 years, 2 tablets twice a day at first, increasing to up to 6 tablets twice a day if required.
Availability: NHS, private prescription.
Side effects: twitching, restlessness, rigidity, shaking, dry mouth, blocked nose, difficulty in urination, rapid heart rate, constipation, blurred vision, low blood pressure, weight gain, impotence, low body temperature, abnormal production of breast milk, absence of menstrual periods, breast enlargement in men, jaundice, blood changes, drowsiness, lethargy, tiredness, fits, abnormal heart rhythm, dermatitis.
Caution: in pregnant women, or in patients suffering from mood changes, epilepsy, kidney disorder.
Not to be used for: children under 14 years, or for patients suffering from PHAEOCHROMOCYTOMA, severe liver, kidney, or blood diseases.

Caution needed with: sedatives, alcohol, ANALGESICS, blood-pressure lowering drugs, antidepressants, anticonvulsants, antidiabetics, LEVODOPA.
Contains: SULPIRIDE.
Other preparations: SULPITIL.

---

sulphabenzamide *see* Sultrin

---

sulphacetamide *see* Sultrin

---

sulphadiazine tablets

Tablets supplied at a strength of 500 mg, and used as an antibiotic to treat meningococcal meningitis, and to prevent recurrence of rheumatic fever.

Dose: as directed by doctor.
Availability: NHS and private prescription.
Side effects: nausea, vomiting, tongue inflammation, rash, blood changes, diarrhoea, colitis, liver damage.
Caution: in the elderly, nursing mothers, and in patients suffering from kidney damage or sensitivity to light. A reasonable fluid intake must be maintained. Your doctor may advise regular blood tests.
Not to be used for: infants under 6 weeks, pregnant women, or for patients suffering from jaundice, blood disorders, or liver failure or severe kidney damage.
Caution needed with: ANTICOAGULANTS, antidiabetics, PYRIMETHAMINE, CYCLOSPORIN.
Contains: sulphadiazine.
Other preparations:

---

sulphadimidine tablets

Tablets supplied at a strength of 500 mg and used as an antibiotic to treat infections of the urinary system, and meningococcal meningitis.

Dose: initially 4 tablets, then 1-2 tablets every 6-8 hours; children use reduced doses.
Availability: NHS and private prescription.
Side effects: nausea, vomiting, tongue inflammation, rash, blood changes, diarrhoea, colitis, liver damage.
Caution: in the elderly, nursing mothers, and in patients suffering from kidney damage or sensitivity to light. A reasonable fluid intake must be maintained. Your doctor may advise regular blood tests.
Not to be used for: infants under 6 weeks, pregnant women, or for

S

patients suffering from jaundice, blood disorders, or kidney or liver failure.
Caution needed with: ANTICOAGULANTS, antidiabetics, PYRIMETHAMINE, CYCLOSPORIN.
Contains: sulphadimidine.
Other preparations:

---

sulphamethoxazole *see* **Bactrim, Chemotrim, co-trimoxazole tablets, Comixco, Fectrim, Laratrim, Septrin**

---

sulphasalazine *see* **Salazopyrin, Salazopyrin EN-tablets, sulphasalazine tablets**

---

sulphasalazine tablets

An tablet supplied at a strength of 500 mg and used as a salicylate-sulphonamide treatment for ulcerative colitis, Crohn's disease, rheumatoid arthritis that does not respond to NON-STEROIDAL ANTI-INFLAMMATORY DRUGS.

Dose: for colitis and Crohn's disease, adults 2-4 tablets 4 times a day at first, reducing to 4 a day; children over 2 years reduced doses. For rheumatoid arthritis, 1 tablet a day at first increasing every 7 days if needed to a maximum of 2-3 g a day in divided doses.
Availability: NHS and private prescription.
Side effects: headache, rash, high temperature, loss of appetite, stomach upset, brain, liver, pancreas, and kidney reactions, blood changes, diminished sperm production, sensitivity to light, orange-coloured urine, urine disorders, LUPUS-like symptoms; soft contact lenses may be stained.
Caution: in pregnant women, nursing mothers, and in patients with liver or kidney disease, with a history of allergy, PORPHYRIA. Your doctor may advise regular blood tests. Tell your doctor if sore throat, fever, or other unidentified illness develops.
Not to be used for: children under 2 years, or for patients who are allergic to sulphonamides or ASPIRIN.
Caution needed with: DIGOXIN, FOLIC ACID.
Contains: SULPHASALAZINE.
Other preparations: SALAZOPYRIN. (Liquid, and suppositories and enemas available; tablets coated to protect the stomach also available – do not take with ANTACIDS.)

---

sulphathiazole *see* **Sultrin**

---

sulphinpyrazone *see* **Anturan**

---

sulphur *see* **Actinac, Cocois, Eskamel, Meted, Pragmatar**

---

sulpiride *see* **Dolmatil, Sulparex, Sulpitil**

Sulpitil
(Pharmacia)

A white, scored tablet supplied at a strength of 200 mg and used as a sedative to treat schizophrenia.

Dose: elderly ¼-½ a tablet twice a day at first increasing to adult dose; adults over 14 years 1-2 tablets twice a day up to a maximum of 9 tablets a day.
Availability: NHS and private prescription.
Side effects: muscle spasms, restlessness, hands shaking, rigidity, constipation, blurred vision, dry mouth, stuffy nose, urine retention, palpitations, rapid heart rate, low blood pressure, weight gain, changes in sexual function, low body temperature, breast swelling, menstrual changes, jaundice, blood and skin changes, drowsiness, tiredness, rarely fits, heart disorder.
Caution: in pregnant women and in patients suffering from high blood pressure, kidney disease, hypomania, or epilepsy
Not to be used for: children under 14 years or for patients suffering from PHAEOCHROMOCYTOMA (a disease of the adrenal glands).
Caution needed with: alcohol, sedatives, tranquillizers, pain killers, blood-pressure lowering drugs, antidepressants, anticonvulsants, antidiabetic drugs, LEVODOPA.
Contains: SULPIRIDE.
Other preparations: DOLMATIL.

Sultrin
(Janssen-Cilag)

A cream used as a sulphonamide antibacterial treatment for bacterial inflammation of the vagina or cervix, and for care after surgery.

Dose: 1 applicatorful into the vagina twice a day for 10 days, reducing to once a day if needed.
Availability: NHS and private prescription.
Side effects: allergy.
Caution:

Not to be used for: children or patients suffering from kidney disease.
Caution needed with:
Contains: SULPHATHIAZOLE, SULPHACETAMIDE, SULPHABENZAMIDE.
Other preparations:

---

sumatriptan *see* Imigran

Suprax
(Lederle)

A white tablet supplied at a strength of 200 mg and used as a cephalosporin antibiotic to treat infections of the respiratory and urinary tract.

Dose: adults, 200-400 mg a day for 7-14 days; children use paediatric suspension.
Availability: NHS and private prescription.
Side effects: stomach upset, headache, dizziness, rash, rarely colitis.
Caution: in pregnant women, nursing mothers, and in patients suffering from severe kidney damage or allergy to this type of antibiotic.
Not to be used for: infants under 6 months.
Caution needed with: ANTICOAGULANTS.
Contains: CEFIXIME.
Other preparations: Suprax Paediatric Suspension.

Suprecur
(Hoechst Roussel)

A nasal spray with metered dose pump, used as a synthetic hormone to treat endometriosis and infertility.

Dose: for endometriosis,1 application in each nostril 3 times a day for up to 6 months. Start treatment on 1st or 2nd day of cycle. (Other conditions as advised by a doctor.)
Availability: NHS and private prescription.
Side effects: hot flushes, vaginal dryness, loss of sexual desire, emotional upset, headache, breast tenderness, alteration of breast size, ovarian cyst, nasal irritation.
Caution: in patients who may later develop thinning of the bones, and in depressed patients. A non-hormonal method of contraception must be used throughout treatment.
Not to be used for: children, pregnant women, nursing mothers, or patients suffering from undiagnosed vaginal bleeding or some cancers.
Caution needed with: decongestant sprays for the nose.

Contains: BUSERELIN.
Other preparations:

Surgam SA
(Hoechst Roussel)

A maroon/pink long-acting capsule supplied at a strength of 300 mg and used as a NON-STEROIDAL ANTI-INFLAMMATORY DRUG to treat rheumatoid arthritis, osteoarthritis, ankylosing spondylitis, lumbago, acute bone or muscular problems, soft tissue injuries.

Dose: 2 capsules once a day.
Availability: NHS and private prescription.
Side effects: stomach upset, headache, drowsiness, rash, bladder irritation, urinary disorders.
Caution: in the elderly, pregnant women, nursing mothers, and in patients suffering from kidney or liver disease, asthma, heart failure, allergy to ASPIRIN/non-steroidal anti-inflammatory drugs.
Not to be used for: children or for patients suffering from stomach ulcer or with a history of stomach ulcer, bladder or prostate disease, or with a history of urinary tract disorder.
Caution needed with: alcohol, sedatives, ANTICOAGULANTS, antidiabetics, some anticonvulsants, some antibiotics, DIURETICS.
Contains: TIAPROFENIC ACID.
Other preparations: Surgam Tablets (not long acting).

Surmontil
(Rhône-Poulenc Rorer)

A white tablet supplied at strengths of 10 mg, 25 mg and used as a TRICYCLIC ANTIDEPRESSANT to treat depression, anxiety, sleep disturbance, agitation.

Dose: 50-75 mg 2 hours before going to bed for at least 3 weeks, increasing to up to 300 mg a day; elderly start with 10-25 mg 3 times a day.
Availability: NHS and private prescription.
Side effects: dry mouth, constipation, urine retention, blurred vision, palpitations, rapid heart rate, drowsiness, tinnitus, nervousness, sweating, weakness, tiredness, sleeplessness, dizziness, hands shaking, low blood pressure, weight change, skin reactions, unsteadiness, convulsions, jaundice or blood changes. Loss of sexual desire may occur, breast enlargement.
Caution: in nursing mothers, the elderly, and in patients suffering from adrenal tumour, heart or liver disease, thyroid disease, epilepsy, diabetes,

urine retention, constipation, some other psychiatric conditions. Your
doctor may advise regular blood tests.
Not to be used for: children, pregnant women, or for patients suffering
from heart attacks, severe liver disease, heart block.
Caution needed with: alcohol, sedatives, ANTICHOLINERGICS, ADRENALINE,
MAOIS, BARBITURATES, other antidepressants, blood-pressure lowering drugs,
CIMETIDINE, CARBAMAZEPINE, PHENYTOIN, tranquillizers, some anaesthetics,
oestrogens, local anaesthetics.
Contains: TRIMIPRAMINE MALEATE.
Other preparations: Surmontil Capsules (stronger product).

Suscard Buccal *see* glyceryl trinitrate tablets
(Pharmax)

Sustac *see* glyceryl trinitrate tablets
(Pharmax)

Sustamycin *see* tetracycline tablets
(Boehringer Mannheim)

Sustanon 100
(Organon)

An injection containing male sex hormones, and used to treat male sex
hormone deficiencies including osteoporosis.

Dose: 1 injection every 2 weeks.
Availability: NHS, private prescription.
Side effects: fluid retention, weight gain, liver disorders, decreased
fertility, persistent painful erection, premature end to growth.
Caution: in patients suffering from epilepsy, migraine, raised blood
pressure, heart, liver, or kidney disorder.
Not to be used for: children, or for patients suffering from some kidney
disorders, some prostate or liver disorders, heart disease, heart failure.
Caution needed with: BARBITURATES, GRISEOFULVIN, anticonvulsants,
RIFAMPICIN.
Contains: TESTOSTERONE.
Other preparations: Sustanon 250.

Symmetrel
(Ciba)

A brownish-red capsule supplied at a strength of 100 mg and used as an anti-parkinsonian/antiviral drug to treat Parkinson's disease and shingles, and to treat or prevent influenza.

Dose: for Parkinson's disease1 tablet a day for 7 days then 1 tablet twice a day; shingles infections 1 tablet twice a day; influenza 1 tablet a day.
Availability: NHS and private prescription.
Side effects: skin changes, fluid retention, rash, sight, brain and stomach disturbances.
Caution: in pregnant women, confused patients, and in patients suffering from liver or kidney disease or congestive heart failure. Children over 10 years may be treated only for influenza.
Not to be used for: children under 10 years, or for patients suffering from severe kidney disease or with a history of convulsions or stomach ulcers.
Caution needed with: ANTICHOLINERGICS, LEVODOPA, stimulants, sedatives.
Contains: AMANTADINE hydrochloride.
Other preparations: Symmetrel Syrup.

---

sympathomimetic
A drug which functions like ADRENALINE and causes narrowing of the blood vessels but which may open other organs, such as the bronchial tubes. Example PSEUDOEPHEDRINE *see* Sudafed.

S

Synacthen Depot
(Ciba)

An injection used as a STEROID treatment for rheumatic and collagen disorders, ulcerative colitis, Crohn's disease.

Dose: as prescribed by the physician.
Availability: NHS, private prescription.
Side effects: raised blood sugars, osteoporosis, euphoria, depression, stomach ulcer, weight gain, flushing, hair growth, raised blood pressure, mental disturbances, allergy.
Caution: in pregnant women and in patients suffering from stress, underactive thyroid, cirrhosis of the liver, diabetes, epilepsy, glaucoma, raised blood pressure, chickenpox, tuberculosis, stomach ulcer, osteoporosis, kidney disorders, measle-like illnesses, mental disorders, thrombophlebitis, or who have undergone recent stomach surgery. Avoid contact with chicken pox.
Not to be used for: intravenous injection or where there is infection near the proposed injection site, or for patients suffering from asthma or allergic disorders.
Caution needed with: PHENYTOIN, PHENOBARBITONE, EPHEDRINE, RIFAMPICIN, DIURETICS, ANTICHOLINESTERASES, some antidiabetic drugs, ANTICOAGULANTS

taken by mouth, NON-STEROIDAL ANTI-INFLAMMATORY DRUGS, DIGOXIN.
Contains: TETRACOSACTRIN acetate, ZINC COMPLEX.
Other preparations:

Synalar
(Zeneca)

An ointment used as a strong STEROID treatment for skin disorders.

Dose: apply to the affected area twice a day, reducing to once or twice a week.
Availability: NHS and private prescription.
Side effects: fluid retention, suppression of adrenal glands, thinning, spotting, or streaking of the skin may occur.
Caution: use for short periods of time only, especially in children or on the face.
Not to be used for: patients suffering from acne or any other skin infections caused by tuberculosis, ringworm, viruses, or fungi, leg ulcers, scabies,or continuously especially in pregnant women.
Caution needed with:
Contains: FLUOCINOLONE acetonide.
Other preparations: Synalar Cream, Synalar 1:4, Synalar Cream 1:10 (diluted products), Synalar Gel (for scalp application); also Synalar C and Synalar N (for infected conditions).

Synarel
(Roche)

A metered-dose nasal spray supplied at a strength of 200 micrograms per dose, and used as a hormone treatment for endometriosis and for desensitizing the pituitary gland in in-vitro fertilization programmes.

Dose: for endometriosis: 1 spray to 1 nostril in the morning and 1 spray into the other nostril in the evening for up to 6 months, beginning the treatment between the second and fourth day of the cycle. For IVF programmes: 1 spray into each nostril morning and evening until ovarian down-regulation is achieved.
Availability: NHS, private prescription.
Side effects: hot flushes, dryness of the vagina, headache, migraine, emotional instability, depression, muscle problems, irritation of the nasal membranes, acne, hair loss, palpitations, blurred vision, ovarian cysts, allergy, changes in bone density, breast size, or sexual function.
Caution: in patients who are at risk of osteoporosis. Use barrier contraceptives.
Not to be used for: children, pregnant women, nursing mothers, or in

patients with undiagnosed bleeding from the vagina.
Caution needed with: nasal decongestants.
Contains: NAFARELIN.
Other preparations:

Synflex *see* naproxen tablets
(Roche)

Synphase
(Roche)

White tablets and yellow tablets used as an oestrogen, progestogen contraceptive.

Dose: 1 tablet a day for 21 days starting on day 5 of the period.
Availability: NHS and private prescription.
Side effects: enlarged breasts, bloating and fluid retention, cramps, leg pains, mood change, reduction in sexual desire, headaches, nausea, vaginal erosion, discharge, and bleeding, weight gain, skin changes, rarely thrombosis, raised blood pressure, jaundice.
Caution: in patients suffering from high blood pressure, diabetes, vascular disorders, asthma, depression, kidney disease, multiple sclerosis, womb diseases. Your doctor may advise you not to smoke, to have regular examinations. You should stop treatment at the first sign of serious symptoms such as severe headache or jaundice. Treatment should be stopped before surgery.
Not to be used for: pregnant women, or for patients suffering from sickle-cell anaemia, history of heart disease or thrombosis, liver disorders, some cancers, undiagnosed vaginal bleeding, some ear, skin, and kidney disorders.
Caution needed with: RIFAMPICIN, TETRACYCLINE ANTIBIOTICS, GRISEOFULVIN, BARBITURATES, PHENYTOIN, PRIMIDONE, CARBAMAZEPINE, ETHOSUXIMIDE, CHLORAL HYDRATE.
Contains: ETHINYLOESTRADIOL, NORETHISTERONE.
Other preparations:

Syntaris
(Roche)

A spray supplied at a strength of 25 micrograms and used as a STEROID treatment for rhinitis, hay fever.

Dose: adults 2 sprays into each nostril 2-3 times a day at first reducing according to response; children over 5 years 1 spray into each nostril 3

times a day.
Availability: NHS and private prescription.
Side effects: temporary itching.
Caution: in pregnant women, and in patients suffering from ulcerated nose, trauma, or who have undergone nasal surgery, or who are being transferred from steroids taken by mouth or injected.
Not to be used for: children under 5 years or for patients suffering from untreated nose or eye infections.
Caution needed with:
Contains: FLUNISOLIDE.
Other preparations: Syntaris Hayfever (available over the counter only to treat and to prevent hayfever).

Syntex Menophase *see* Menophase

Syntopressin
(Sandoz)

A nasal spray used as a hormone treatment for diabetes insipidus (a condition causing excess thirst and urination).

Dose: adults 1-2 sprays into one or both nostrils 3-4 times a day; children as advised by the physician.
Availability: NHS and private prescription.
Side effects: nausea, stomach pain, desire to defaecate, blocked nose and nasal ulceration.
Caution: in pregnant women and in patients suffering from epilepsy, or heart failure, high blood pressure, circulation disorders, bronchial asthma.
Not to be used for: patients suffering from heart disease, chronic inflammation of the kidneys.
Caution needed with: CARBAMAZEPINE, LITHIUM, CLOFIBRATE, CHLORPROPAMIDE, some anaesthetics.
Contains: LYPRESSIN.
Other preparations:

Synuretic *see* co-amilozide
(DDSA)

Sytron
(Link)

An elixir used as an iron supplement to treat iron-deficiency anaemia.

Dose: adults 5 ml 3 times a day at first increasing gradually to 10 ml 3 times a day; children 0-1 year 2.5 ml twice a day, 1-5 years 2.5 ml 3 times a day, 6-12 years 5 ml 3 times a day.
Availability: NHS, private prescription, over the counter.
Side effects: nausea, diarrhoea.
Caution:
Not to be used for:
Caution needed with: some antibiotics, ANTACIDS, LEVODOPA.
Contains: SODIUM IRON EDETATE.
Other preparations:

T Gel
(Neutrogena)

A shampoo used as an anti-psoriatic treatment for dandruff, scaly scalp disorders, and psoriasis of the scalp.

Dose: shampoo 1-2 times a week.
Availability: NHS, private prescription, over the counter.
Side effects: irritation.
Caution:
Not to be used for: patients suffering from acute psoriasis.
Caution needed with:
Contains: COAL TAR EXTRACT.
Other preparations: ALPHOSYL SHAMPOO, CLINITAR SHAMPOO, GELCOTAR LIQUID, POLYTAR LIQUID, PSORIDERM SCALP LOTION, PSORIGEL.

Tagamet *see* cimetidine tablets
(SmithKline Beecham)

Tambocor
(3M Health Care)

A white tablet and a white, scored tablet supplied at strengths of 50 mg, 100 mg and used as an anti-arrhythmic treatment for abnormal heart rhythm.

Dose: 50-100 mg twice a day at first up to 300-400 mg for 3-5 days, then reduce the dose to the minimum necessary to keep symptoms under control.
Availability: NHS and private prescription.
Side effects: dizziness, disturbed vision, sensitivity to light, nausea, vomiting, liver disturbance, tingling, weakness or numbness of hands and feet, unsteadiness.

Caution: in pregnant women, patients fitted with pacemakers, and in patients suffering from kidney or liver problems, some heart disorders. Your doctor may advise blood tests to check electrolytes and blood levels.
Not to be used for: children and for patients suffering from some heart disorders.
Caution needed with: DIGOXIN and some other heart drugs.
Contains: FLECAINIDE acetate.
Other preparations: Tambocor Injection.

Tamofen *see* tamoxifen tablets
(Pharmacia)

---

tamoxifen citrate *see* Emblon, Fentamox, Nolvadex-D, Oestrifen, Tamofen, tamoxifen tablets

---

tamoxifen tablets

A tablet supplied at strengths of 10 mg, 20 mg, 40 mg, and used as an anti-oestrogen treatment for infertility in women caused by failure of ovulation, and as a treatment and prophylactic for breast cancer.

Dose: 20 mg a day on the second, third, fourth, and fifth days of the period. If needed increase to 40 mg then 80 mg a day for further courses.
Availability: NHS and private prescription.
Side effects: hot flushes, bleeding from the vagina, stomach upset, dizziness, disturbed vision, vaginal itching, blood changes, fluid retention, hair loss, liver changes.
Caution: in patients suffering from PORPHYRIA.
Not to be used for: children, pregnant women, nursing mothers.
Caution needed with: WARFARIN, NICOUMALONE.
Contains: TAMOXIFEN CITRATE.
Other preparations: EMBLON, FENTAMOX, NOLVADEX-D, OESTRIFEN, TAMOFEN.

Tampovagan
(Norgine)

A pessary used as an oestrogen treatment for inflammation of the vagina after the menopause.

Dose: 2 pessaries in the vagina at night for 2-3 weeks.
Availability: NHS and private prescription.
Side effects: enlarged breasts, fluid retention, nausea, vaginal bleeding, weight gain, headache, dizziness. Rarely jaundice, raised blood pressure,

thrombosis.

Caution: in patients suffering from high blood pressure, diabetes, epilepsy, womb diseases, gall bladder disorder, migraine, multiple sclerosis, PORPHYRIA, liver disorders, some ear disorders, or a history or increased risk of breast disorders (including cancer) and thrombosis. Your doctor may advise you to have regular examinations.

Not to be used for: children, pregnant women, nursing mothers, or for patients suffering from thombosis, severe liver, kidney, or heart disorders, some cancers, undiagnosed vaginal bleeding, endometriosis.

Caution needed with: ACE INHIBITORS, ANTICOAGULANTS, BARBITURATES, ß-BLOCKERS, CARBAMAZEPINE, PHENYTOIN, RIFAMPICIN.

Contains: STILBOESTEROL, LACTIC ACID.

Other preparations:

---

tannic acid *see* **Phytex**

---

tar *see* **Gelcosal, Gelcotar, Polytar AF, Polytar Emollient, Pixol, Polytar Liquid**

Tarband
(Seton Healthcare)

A bandage supplied at a size of 7.5 cm x 6 m, and used, in conjunction with a compression bandage, to treat varicose and gravitational ulcers; chronic eczema, infantile eczema, and dermatitis.

Availability: NHS, private prescription, over the counter. (Also available on a trial basis from nurses.)

Contains: ZINC PASTE, COAL TAR.

Tarcortin
(Stafford-Miller)

A cream used as a STEROID, antipsoriatic treatment for eczema, psoriasis, other skin disorders.

Dose: apply to the affected area at least twice a day.

Availability: NHS and private prescription.

Side effects: fluid retention, suppression of adrenal glands, thinning, spotting, or streaking of the skin may occur.

Caution: use for short periods of time only, especially in children or on the face.

Not to be used for: patients suffering from acne or any other skin

infections caused by tuberculosis, ringworm, viruses, or fungi, leg ulcers, scabies, or continuously especially in pregnant women.
Caution needed with:
Contains: HYDROCORTISONE, COAL TAR EXTRACT.
Other preparations: ALPHOSYL HC.

Tarivid
(Hoechst Roussel)

A white, oblong, scored tablet or a yellow, oblong, scored tablet, according to strengths of 200 mg, 400 mg, and used as an antibiotic to treat urine or lung diseases, or sexually transmitted diseases.

Dose: 200-400 mg a day depending upon severity and type of condition.
Availability: NHS and private prescription.
Side effects: stomach upset, allergy, skin reactions, convulsions, nerve disorders, colitis, joint and muscle pain, changes in liver, kidneys, blood, or bone marrow, PORPHYRIA; rarely, weakness, joint or muscle pain, tendon disorders.
Caution: in patients suffering from psychiatric disorders or kidney or liver damage, or those exposed to strong sunlight, or who will be driving or operating machinery.
Not to be used for: children, pregnant women, nursing mothers, growing adolescents, or for patients with a history of epilepsy.
Caution needed with: magnesium or aluminium ANTACIDS, iron, NON-STEROIDAL ANTI-INFLAMMATORY DRUGS, ANTICOAGULANTS, SUCRALFATE, GLIBENCLAMIDE.
Contains: OFLOXACIN.
Other preparations: Tarivid Infusion.

Tavegil
(Sandoz)

A white, scored tablet supplied at a strength of 1 mg and used as an ANTIHISTAMINE treatment for allergic rhinitis, skin allergies, nettle rash, allergy to other drugs.

Dose: adults 1 tablet night and morning; children over 3 years ½-1 tablet night and morning according to age, under 3 years use elixir.
Availability: NHS, private prescription, over the counter.
Side effects: drowsiness, reduced reactions, rarely dizziness, dry mouth, palpitations, gastro-intestinal disturbances, excitement, rash, headache, tiredness, indigestion.
Caution: in pregnant women, nursing mothers, and in patients suffering from glaucoma, enlarged prostate, some stomach ulcers, urinary retention,

bladder and stomach blockage.
Not to be used for: children under 1 year.
Caution needed with: sedatives, MAOIS, alcohol.
Contains: CLEMASTINE.
Other preparations: Tavegil Elixir.

Tears Naturale
(Alcon)

Drops used to lubricate dry eyes.

Dose: 1-2 drops into the eye as needed.
Availability: NHS, private prescription, over the counter.
Side effects:
Caution:
Not to be used for: patients who wear soft contact lenses.
Caution needed with:
Contains: DEXTRAN, HYPROMELLOSE.
Other preparations: HYPROMELLOSE EYE DROPS, ISOPTO ALKALINE, ISOPTO PLAIN.

Tegagel
(3M Health Care)

A sterile, impregnated dressing, supplied at sizes of 5 cm square and 10 cm square, and used as an absorbent dressing for wet wounds such as leg ulcers and bed sores.

Availability: NHS, private prescription, over the counter. (Also available on a trial basis from nurses.)
Not to be used for: infected or very dry wounds.
Contains: calcium alginate.

Tegretol *see* carbamazepine tablets
(Ciba)

temazepam tablets

A tablet supplied at strengths of 10 mg, 20 mg, and used as a sleeping preparation to treat sleeplessness.

Dose: elderly 10-20 mg before going to bed; adults 10-40 mg before going to bed.
Availability: controlled drug; NHS and private prescription.

Side effects: drowsiness, confusion, unsteadiness, low blood pressure, rash, memory loss, changes in vision, changes in sexual function, retention of urine, headache, vertigo, low blood pressure. Risk of addiction increases with dose and length of treatment. May impair judgement.

Caution: in the elderly, pregnant women, nursing mothers, in women during labour, debilitated patients, and in patients suffering from lung disorders, kidney or liver disorders, PORPHYRIA. Avoid long-term use and withdraw gradually.

Not to be used for: children, or for patients suffering from acute lung diseases, some chronic lung diseases, some obsessional and psychotic diseases.

Caution needed with: alcohol, sedatives, anticonvulsants, other tranquillizers.

Contains: temazepam.

Other preparations: temazepam capsules, temazepam elixir. NORMISON (capsule forms not available on NHS).

Temgesic
(Reckitt & Colman)

A white tablet supplied at strength of 0.2 mg, 0.4 mg and used as a opiate to control pain.

Dose: 0.2-0.4 mg under the tongue every 6-8 hours or as needed; children use reduced doses.

Availability: controlled drug; NHS and private prescription.

Side effects: drowsiness, nausea, sweating, dizziness.

Caution: in pregnant women, women in labour, and in patients suffering from breathing or liver problems, or patients addicted to or with a history of addiction to opiate drugs.

Not to be used for: children under 16 kg body weight.

Caution needed with: MAOIS, alcohol, sedatives.

Contains: BUPRENORPHINE hydrochloride.

Other preparations: Temgesic Injection.

Tenchlor *see* co-tenidone tablets
(Berk)

Tenif
(Stuart)

A reddish-brown capsule used as a calcium blocker/ß-BLOCKER to treat high blood pressure, angina.

Dose: high blood pressure1 capsule a day at first increasing to 2 capsules

a day if needed; elderly a maximum of 1 capsule a day; angina 1 capsule twice a day.
Availability: NHS and private prescription.
Side effects: flushing, headache, dizziness, dry eyes, rash, fluid retention, jaundice, swollen gums.
Caution: in patients suffering from heart disease, kidney or liver disease, diabetes, or patients undergoing anaesthesia.
Not to be used for: children, pregnant women, nursing mothers, or for patients suffering from heart failure, block, or shock.
Caution needed with: CIMETIDINE, QUINIDINE, some heart drugs.
Contains: ATENOLOL, NIFEDIPINE.
Other preparations: BETA-ADALAT.

Tenoret 50 *see* co-tenidone tablets
(Stuart)

Tenoretic *see* co-tenidone tablets
(Stuart)

Tenormin *see* atenolol tablets
(Stuart)

---

tenoxicam *see* Mobiflex

Tensium *see* diazepam tablets
(DDSA)

Teoptic
(Ciba Vision Ophthalmics)

Drops available in 2 strengths used as a ß-BLOCKER to treat HYPERTENSION of the eye, open angle glaucoma, some secondary glaucomas.

Dose: 1 drop of the weaker strength into the eye twice a day at first. Go on to the stronger product if necessary.
Availability: NHS and private prescription.
Side effects: burning, stinging, and painful sensations of the eye, blurred vision, redness, corneal inflammation.
Caution: in patients suffering from heart conduction block, heart weakness, diabetes.
Not to be used for: children, pregnant women, or for patients suffering

from heart failure, asthma, chronic obstructive lung disease, or for those who wear contact lenses.
Caution needed with: ß-blockers taken by mouth or injection.
Contains: CARTEOLOL HYDROCHLORIDE.
Other preparations:

---

terazosin *see* Hytrin, Hytrin BPH

---

terbinafine *see* Lamisil

---

terbutaline *see* Bricanyl, Monovent

---

terfenadine *see* Histafen, terfenadine tablets, Terfenor, Terfinax, Triludan

---

terfenadine tablets

A tablet supplied at a strength of 60 mg, 120 mg, and used as an ANTIHISTAMINE treatment for allergies including hay fever, nettle rash, and rhinitis.

Dose: for hay fever and rhinitis, adults 60 mg a day, increasing to 120 mg if necessary; for allergy, use 120 mg a day; children 6-12 years 30 mg twice a day, 3-6 years 15 mg twice a day.
Availability: NHS, private prescription, over the counter.
Side effects: rash, sweating, headache, stomach disturbances, rapid heart beat, palpitations, hair loss, shock, dizziness, rash, visual disturbances, tiredness, breathing difficulty, pricking and itching, fits, muscle pain, blood changes, depression, low blood pressure, pins and needles, shaking hands. Rarely drowsiness, ANTICHOLINERGIC effects.
Caution: in pregnant women, nursing mothers, and in patients suffering from liver disease, some heart irregularities, epilepsy, prostate problems, glaucoma.
Not to be used for: children under 3 years or for patients suffering from severe liver damage, PORPHYRIA, or low blood potassium.
Caution needed with: KETOCONAZOLE, ERYTHROMYCIN, ITRACONAZOLE, DIURETICS, some antifungals, some antibiotics, anti-arrhythmic drugs, TRICYCLIC ANTIDEPRESSANTS, ASTEMIZOLE, some tranquillizers, MAOIS, CARBAMAZEPINE, other antihistamines, SOTALOL.
Contains: TERFENADINE.
Other preparations: HISTAFEN, TERFENOR, TERFINAX, TRILUDAN. (Liquid form

available on prescription.) Other brands available over the counter but not on NHS prescription.

Terfenor *see* **terfenadine tablets**
(Baker Norton)

Terfinax *see* **terfenadine tablets**
(Ashbourne)

Terra-Cortril Ointment
(Pfizer)

An ointment used as an antibiotic, STEROID treatment for weeping and infected eczema, insect bites, weeping intertrigo.

Dose: apply to the affected area 2-4 times a day.
Availability: NHS and private prescription.
Side effects: fluid retention, suppression of adrenal glands, thinning, spotting, or streaking of the skin may occur.
Caution: use for short periods of time only, especially in children or on the face.
Not to be used for: children or for patients suffering from acne or any other skin infections caused by tuberculosis, ringworm, viruses, or fungi, leg ulcers, scabies, or continuously especially in pregnant women.
Caution needed with:
Contains: OXYTETRACYCLINE HYDROCHLORIDE.
Other preparations: Terra-Cortril Nystatin (for infected conditions).

Terramycin *see* **oxytetracycline tablets**
(Pfizer)

Tertroxin
(Link)

A white, scored tablet supplied at a strength of 20 micrograms and used as a thyroid hormone to treat severe thyroid deficiency.

Dose: adults10-20 micrograms every 8 hours at first, increasing after 1 week to 60 micrograms a day in 2-3 divided doses; elderly and children 5 micrograms a day at first.
Availability: NHS and private prescription.

Side effects: abnormal heart rhythm, chest pain, rapid heart rate, muscle cramp or weakness, headache, restlessness, flushing, excitability, sweating, diarrhoea, rapid weight loss.
Caution: in nursing mothers, and in patients suffering from diabetes.
Not to be used for: patients suffering from heart or circulation problems or where effort causes anginal pain.
Caution needed with: ANTICOAGULANTS, TRICYCLIC ANTIDEPRESSANTS, PHENYTOIN, CHOLESTYRAMINE.
Contains: LIOTHYRONINE sodium.
Other preparations:

---

testosterone *see* **Primoteston Depot, Restandol, Sustanon 100, testosterone implant**

---

testosterone implant

An implant of male sex hormone used to maintain testosterone levels in men. Also used in the treatment of menopausal women.

Dose: 100-600 mg by implant under the skin.
Availability: NHS and private prescription.
Side effects: increase in weight, fluid retention, persistent erection, decreased fertility, liver disorders, high blood calcium levels.
Caution: in the elderly, and in patients suffering from high blood pressure, epilepsy, migraine, heart, liver, or kidney failure.
Not to be used for: children, pregnant women, nursing mothers, or for patients suffering from some prostate disorders, some kidney disorders, heart failure, high blood calcium levels.
Caution needed with:
Contains: TESTOSTERONE.
Other preparations:

---

tetanus vaccine

A vaccine that stimulates the body's production of antibodies to the tetanus bacillus thereby conferring active immunity.

Dose: in untreated subjects, an injection of 0.5 ml followed by second and third injections at 4-week intervals. A booster every 10 years maintains immunity.
Availability: NHS and private prescription.
Side effects: fever, general feeling of being unwell, local reactions.
Caution: in patients with a history of allergy to tetanus.
Not to be used for: patients suffering from acute infectious disease

except where there are wounds liable to tetanus infection.
Caution needed with:
Contains: tetanus vaccine.
Other preparations: CLOSTET, tetanus immunoglobulin injection (for passive immunity).

---

tetrabenazine *see* **Nitoman**

Tetrabid *see* **tetracycline tablets**
(Organon)

Tetrachel *see* **tetracycline tablets**
(Berk)

---

tetracosactrin *see* **Synacthen Depot**

---

tetracycline hydrochloride *see* **Achromycin, Berkmycen, Detecio, Economycin, Mysteclin, Sustamycin, Tetrabid, tetracycline tablets, Topicycline**

---

tetracycline tablets

An orange tablet supplied at a strength of 250 mg and used as an antibiotic treatment for infections, especially respiratory infections and acne.

Dose: 1-2 tablets 4 times a day. For acne, 2 tablets twice a day reducing to 1 tablet twice a day after 3 months
Availability: NHS and private prescription.
Side effects: stomach disturbances, headache, vision changes, pancreatitis, colitis, sensitivity to light, skin changes.
Caution: in patients suffering from liver or kidney disease.
Not to be used for: children, pregnant women, nursing mothers, or for patients suffering from systemic lupus erythematosus (SLE).
Caution needed with: ANTACIDS, iron and zinc supplements, the contraceptive pill, ANTICOAGULANTS, BARBITURATES, anti-epileptic drugs, QUINAPRIL, dairy products, ISOTRETINOIN.
Contains: TETRACYCLINE HYDROCHLORIDE.
Other preparations: ACHROMYCIN CAPSULES, BERKMYCEN, ECONOMYCIN,

T

SUSTAMYCIN, TETRABID (long-acting products), TOPICYCLINE (for application to the skin).

---

tetrahydrofurfuryl salicylate *see* **Transvasin**

Tetralysal
(Pharmacia)

A white capsule used as a TETRACYCLINE antibiotic to treat acne and other infections, such as bronchitis.

Dose: 1 capsule twice a day. (Use for 8 weeks for acne.)
Availability: NHS and private prescription.
Side effects: stomach upset, allergy, secondary infections, blood changes.
Caution: in patients suffering from liver or kidney disorders.
Not to be used for: children, pregnant women, nursing mothers.
Caution needed with: ANTACIDS, the contraceptive pill, some mineral supplements.
Contains: LYMECYCLINE.
Other preparations:

Theo-Dur *see* **Lasma**
(Astra)

---

theophylline *see* **Franol, Lasma, Nuelin, Slo-Phyllin, Theo-Dur, Uniphyllin**

Thephorin
(Sinclair)

A white tablet supplied at a strength of 25 mg and used as an ANTIHISTAMINE to treat allergies.

Dose: 1-2 tablets 1-3 times a day before 4.00 in the afternoon; children over 10 years 1 tablet 1-3 times a day.
Availability: NHS, private prescription, over the counter.
Side effects: dry mouth, stomach upset, rarely drowsiness, excitement in children.
Caution:
Not to be used for: children under 10 years.
Caution needed with: sedatives, MAOIS, ANTICHOLINERGICS, alcohol.

Contains: PHENINDAMINE TARTRATE.
Other preparations:

---

thiabendazole *see* Mintezol

---

thiamine *see* thiamine tabets, vitamin B₁

---

thiamine tablets

A tablet supplied at strengths of 25 mg, 50 mg, 100 mg, and used as a source of VITAMIN B₁ to treat deficiency.

Dose: 10-300 mg a day according to condition.
Availability: NHS and private prescription.
Side effects:
Caution:
Not to be used for:
Caution needed with:
Contains: VITAMIN B₁.
Other preparations: Benerva (not available on NHS).

---

thioridazine *see* Melleril

---

threonine *see* Cicatrin

---

thymoxamine hydrochloride *see* Opilon

---

thyroxine *see* Eltroxin, thyroxine tablets

---

thyroxine tablets

A tablet supplied at strengths of 25 micrograms, 50 micrograms, 100 micrograms and used as a thyroid hormone to treat underactive thyroid gland in adults or children.

Dose: adults 50-100 micrograms a day at first increasing as needed by 25-50 micrograms a day every 4 weeks to a maximum of 100-200 micrograms a day; infants 10 micrograms/kg a day up to 50 micrograms a

day, reaching 100 micrograms a day at age of 5 years and 100-200 mcg a day by 12 years. Dose is adjusted according to response.
Availability: NHS and private prescription.
Side effects: abnormal heart rhythms, chest pain, rapid heart rate, muscle cramp, headache, restlessness, excitability, flushing, sweating, diarrhoea, rapid weight loss.
Caution: in nursing mothers and in patients suffering from heart or circulatory disorders, adrenal gland weakness, or prolonged deficiency of thyroid hormones.
Not to be used for:
Caution needed with: ANTICOAGULANTS, TRICYCLIC ANTIDEPRESSANTS, antidiabetics, SYMPATHOMIMETICS, CHOLESTYRAMINE, RIFAMPICIN, anticonvulsants, PROPRANOLOL, SUCRALFATE, BARBITURATES.
Contains: SODIUM THYROXINE.
Other preparations: ELTROXIN.

---

tiaprofenic acid *see* **Surgam SA**

---

tibolone *see* **Livial**

Tiempe *see* **trimethoprim tablets**
(DDSA)

Tilade
(Fisons)

An aerosol supplied at a strength of 2 mg and used as a bronchial anti-inflammatory drug to treat bronchial asthma.

Dose: 2 puffs 4 times a day reducing to 2 puffs twice a day for maintenance.
Availability: NHS and private prescription.
Side effects: headache, stomach upset, cough, rarely wheezing.
Caution: in pregnant women.
Not to be used for: children under 6 years.
Caution needed with:
Contains: SODIUM NEDOCROMIL.
Other preparations: Tilade Syncroner (with spacer device).

Tilarin
(Fisons)

A nasal spray used as an anti-inflammatory treatment for hayfever.

Dose: 1 dose in each nostril 4 times a day.
Availability: NHS and private prescription.
Side effects: mild irritation, taste disturbance.
Caution: in pregnant women and nursing mothers.
Not to be used for: children.
Caution needed with:
Contains: SODIUM NEDOCROMIL.
Other preparations:

Tildiem *see* **diltiazem tablets**
(Lorex Synthélabo)

Tildiem Retard and LA *see* **diltiazem long-acting tablets**
(Lorex Synthélabo)

Tiloryth *see* **erythromycin tablets**
(Tillomed)

Timodine
(Reckitt & Colman)

A cream used as a STEROID, disinfectant, antifungal treatment for skin disorders, severe nappy rash with thrush.

Dose: apply a small quantity to the affected area 3 times a day or when the nappy is changed.
Availability: NHS and private prescription.
Side effects: fluid retention, suppression of adrenal glands, thinning, spotting, or streaking of the skin may occur.
Caution: use for short periods of time only, especially in children or on the face.
Not to be used for: patients suffering from acne or any other skin infections caused by tuberculosis, ringworm, viruses, or fungi, leg ulcers, scabies, or continuously especially in pregnant women.
Caution needed with:
Contains: NYSTATIN, HYDROCORTISONE, BENZALKONIUM CHLORIDE, DIMETHICONE.
Other preparations: NYSTAFORM-HC.

---

timolol *see* **Betim, Blocadren, Glavcol, Moducren, Prestim, Timoptol**

Timoptol
(M.S.D.)

Eye drops, available in 2 strengths, and used as a ß-BLOCKER to treat hypertension of the eye, glaucomas.

Dose: 1 drop of the weaker solution into the eye twice a day. Go on to the stronger solution if necessary.
Availability: NHS and private prescription.
Side effects: eye irritation, systemic ß-blocker effects (*see* propranolol tablets). MYASTHENIA GRAVIS may be made worse.
Caution: in pregnant women, nursing mothers. Treatment should be withdrawn gradually.
Not to be used for: children or patients suffering from asthma, heart conduction block, heart failure, a history of blocked lung disorder, or for patients who wear soft contact lenses.
Caution needed with: VERAPAMIL, blood-pressure lowering drugs, ADRENALINE.
Contains: TIMOLOL maleate.
Other preparations:

Timpron *see* naproxen tablets
(Berk)

Tinaderm-M
(Schering-Plough)

A cream used as an antifungal treatment for skin and nail infections

Dose: apply to the affected area 2-3 times a day.
Availability: NHS and private prescription.
Side effects:
Caution:
Not to be used for:
Caution needed with:
Contains: TOLNAFTATE, NYSTATIN.
Other preparations: Tinaderm Plus Aerosol, Tinaderm Cream (both containing tolnaftate only).

---

tinidazole *see* **Fasigyn**

---

tioconazole *see* **Trosyl**

Tisept
(Seton Healthcare)

A solution in a sachet used as a disinfectant for cleansing and disinfecting wounds and burns, changing dressings, obstetrics.

Dose: use neat as needed.
Availability: NHS, private prescription, over the counter.
Side effects:
Caution:
Not to be used for:
Caution needed with:
Contains: CHLORHEXIDINE gluconate, CETRIMIDE.
Other preparations: Tisept Concentrate.

Titralac
(3M Health Care)

A white tablet used as a calcium supplement, and to regulate blood phosphate levels in patients with kidney failure.

Dose: to be adjusted for individuals.
Availability: NHS, private prescription, over the counter.
Side effects:
Caution: your doctor may advise regular blood and urine tests.
Not to be used for: patients with low blood phosphate levels or high blood/urine calcium levels.
Caution needed with: TETRACYCLINE ANTIBIOTICS, STEROIDS, VITAMIN D, some DIURETICS, tablets coated to protect the stomach.
Contains: CALCIUM CARBONATE, GLYCINE.
Other preparations:

Tobralex
(Alcon)

Drops used as an aminoglycoside antibiotic treatment for eye infections.

Dose: 1-2 drops every 4 hours or up to 2 drops every hour in severe infections.

T

Availability: NHS and private prescription.
Side effects: temporary irritation.
Caution: reduce dose before stopping treatment.
Not to be used for:
Caution needed with:
Contains: TOBRAMYCIN.
Other preparations:

---

tobramycin *see* **Tobralex**

---

tocainide *see* **Tonocard**

---

tocopheryl acetate *see* **vitamin E**

Tofranil *see* **imipramine tablets**
(Ciba)

Tolanase
(Upjohn)

A white, scored tablet supplied at strengths of 100 mg, 250 mg and used as an antidiabetic treatment for diabetes

Dose: 100-250 mg a day in divided doses to a maximum of 1 g a day.
Availability: NHS and private prescription.
Side effects: allergy including skin rash.
Caution: in the elderly and in patients suffering from kidney failure.
Not to be used for: children, pregnant women, nursing mothers, during surgery, or for patients suffering from juvenile diabetes, liver or kidney disorders, raised ketone levels, stress, infections.
Caution needed with: ß-BLOCKERS, MAOIS, STEROIDS, DIURETICS, alcohol, ANTICOAGULANTS, lipid-lowering agents, ASPIRIN, some antibiotics (RIFAMPICIN, sulphonamides, CHLORAMPHENICOL), GLUCAGON, CYCLOPHOSPHAMIDE, the contraceptive pill.
Contains: TOLAZAMIDE.
Other preparations:

---

tolazamide *see* **Tolanase**

---

tolbutamide *see* **Glyconon, Rastinon, tolbutamide tablets**

tolbutamide tablets

A tablet supplied at a strength of 500 mg and used as an antidiabetic treatment for diabetes.

Dose: 1-4 tablets a day according to response.
Availability: NHS and private prescription.
Side effects: allergy including skin rash, stomach upset, headache. Rarely blood disorders.
Caution: in the elderly and in patients suffering from liver disorders.
Not to be used for: children, pregnant women, nursing mothers, during surgery, or for patients suffering from juvenile diabetes, liver disorders, stress, infections, ketosis (raised acid levels), PORPHYRIA.
Caution needed with: ß-BLOCKERS, ACE INHIBITORS, MAOIS, STEROIDS, DIURETICS, DIAZOXIDE, KETOTIFEN, NIFEDIPINE, LITHIUM, alcohol, ANTICOAGULANTS, lipid-lowering agents, ASPIRIN, some antibiotics, anti-epileptics, antifungals, tranquillizers, CIMETIDINE, RANITIDINE, GLUCAGON, cyclophosphamide, the contraceptive pill, SUPHINPYRAZONE, NON-STEROIDAL ANTI-INFLAMMATORY DRUGS.
Contains: TOLBUTAMIDE.
Other preparations: GLYCONON, RASTINON.

Tolectin
(Janssen-Cilag)

An orange/ivory capsule or orange capsule supplied at strengths of 200 mg, 400 mg and used as a NON-STEROIDAL ANTI-INFLAMMATORY DRUG to treat rheumatoid arthritis, osteoarthritis, ankylosing spondylitis, other joint disorders.

Dose: 600-1800 mg a day in divided doses; children 20-25 mg/kg a day in divided doses.
Availability: NHS and private prescription.
Side effects: stomach pain, fluid retention, rash.
Caution: in the elderly, pregnant women, nursing mothers, and in patients suffering from kidney, liver, or heart disease or a history of gastro-intestinal disease.
Not to be used for: patients suffering from stomach ulcer or allergy to ASPIRIN/anti-inflammatory drugs.
Caution needed with:
Contains: TOLMETIN.
Other preparations:

tolmetin *see* **Tolectin**

---

tolnaftate *see* **Tinaderm-M**

Tonocard
(Astra)

A yellow tablet supplied at a strength of 400 mg and used as an anti-arrhythmic drug to treat abnormal heart rhythms.

Dose: 1.2 g a day in 3 divided doses to a maximum of 2.4 g a day.
Availability: NHS and private prescription.
Side effects: shaking, dizziness, stomach upset, blood changes, SLE (a multisystem disorder).
Caution: in the elderly, pregnant women, and in patients suffering from severe liver or kidney disease or heart failure, low potassium levels.
Not to be used for: children or patients suffering from heart conduction block (unless pacemaker fitted).
Caution needed with: other anti-arrhythmics.
Contains: TOCAINIDE hydrochloride.
Other preparations:

Topal
(Novex)

A cream tablet used as an ANTACID to treat oesophagitis, heartburn, gastritis, acid indigestion, reflux oesophagitis, hiatus hernia.

Dose: adults 1-3 tablets 4 times a day after meals and at bedtime, children half adult dose.
Availability: NHS, private prescription, over the counter.
Side effects:
Caution:
Not to be used for: infants.
Caution needed with: tablets coated to protect the stomach, some antibiotics, iron.
Contains: ALUMINIUM HYDROXIDE, MAGNESIUM CARBONATE, ALGINIC ACID.
Other preparations:

Topamax
(Janssen-Cilag)

A pale-yellow, yellow, or pink tablet used as an additional anticonvulsant treatment for fits.

Dose: 100 mg a day at first, increasing to a maximum of 800 mg a day as needed.
Availability: NHS and private prescription.
Side effects: unsteadiness, inability to concentrate, confusion, dizziness, tiredness, pins and needles, drowsiness, emotional upset, depression, brain disturbance. Rarely kidney stones, weight loss.
Caution: in pregnant women, and in patients suffering from kidney disorders. Drink plenty of fluids. Withdraw treatment gradually.
Not to be used for: children, nursing mothers.
Caution needed with: PHENYTOIN, CARBAMAZEPINE, DIGOXIN, the contraceptive pill, other drugs affecting the kidneys.
Contains: TOPIRAMATE.
Other preparations:

Topicycline
(Monmouth)

A solution used as an antibiotic treatment for acne.

Dose: apply freely to the affected area twice a day.
Availability: NHS and private prescription.
Side effects: stinging or burning sensations.
Caution: in pregnant women, nursing mothers, and in patients suffering from kidney disease. Keep out of the eyes, nose, mouth, etc.
Not to be used for: children.
Caution needed with:
Contains: TETRACYCLINE HYDROCHLORIDE.
Other preparations:

---

topiramate *see* **Topamax**

Toradol
(Roche)

A white tablet supplied at a strength of 10 mg and used as a NON-STEROIDAL ANTI-INFLAMMATORY DRUG to treat pain after surgery.

Dose: 1 tablet every 4-6 hours for up to 7 days, to a maximum of 4 tablets a day or more if transferred from injectable form of the drug. Elderly patients 1 every 6-8 hours.
Availability: NHS and private prescription.
Side effects: stomach upset, ulcers, bleeding, liver abnormalities,

drowsiness, kidney failure, swelling, wheezing, severe allergy.
Caution: in the elderly, and in patients suffering from gastro-intestinal disease, heart, kidney, or liver disease, allergy, slow blood flow.
Not to be used for: children under 16 years, pregnant women, nursing mothers, or for patients suffering from stomach ulcer, allergy to ASPIRIN or anti-inflammatory drugs, blood-clotting disorders, asthma, severe kidney disease, decrease in blood volume, dehydration, polyps in the nose, fluid retention.
Caution needed with: alcohol, sedatives, LITHIUM, non-steroidal anti-inflammatory drugs, ANTICOAGULANTS, METHOTREXATE, PROBENECID, FRUSEMIDE OXYPENTIFYLLINE.
Contains: KETOROLAC TROMETAMOL.
Other preparations:

---

torasemide *see* Torem

Torem
(Boehringer Mannheim)

A white tablet supplied at strengths of 2.5 mg, 5 mg, 10 mg, and used as a DIURETIC to treat heart failure, fluid retention in the lungs or kidneys, and high blood pressure.

Dose: high blood pressure 2.5 mg a day at first, increasing to 5 mg a day if necessary; fluid retention 5 mg a day at first, increasing to a maximum of 40 mg a day if necessary.
Availability: NHS and private prescription.
Side effects: headache, stomach upset, blood changes, dry mouth, dizziness, cramps, pins and needles, electrolyte disturbances.
Caution: in patients suffering from gout, diabetes, low blood potassium or sodium, low blood volume, and urination disorders. Your doctor may advise regular checks on your electrolyte and lipid levels.
Not to be used for: children, pregnant women, nursing mothers, or for patients suffering from kidney or liver disorders, low blood pressure, allergy to some diabetic drugs, inability to produce urine.
Caution needed with: LITHIUM, DIGOXIN, STEROIDS, drugs that lower blood pressure, laxatives, some antibiotics, cisplatin, THEOPHYLLINE, NON-STEROIDAL ANTI-INFLAMMATORY DRUGS, PROBENICID, ACE-INHIBITORS, CHOLESTYRAMINE, antidiabetics.
Contains: TORASEMIDE.
Other preparations:

Totamol *see* **atenolol tablets**
(CP Pharm)

---

tramadol *see* **Zydol**

---

tramazoline *see* **Dexa-Rhinaspray**

Trandate *see* **labetolol tablets**
(Duncan, Flockhart)

---

trandolapril *see* **Gopten, Odrik**

---

tranexamic acid *see* **Cyklokapron**

Tranquax *see* **clomipramine capsules**
(Berk)

Transiderm-Nitro
(Ciba)

Patches supplied at strengths of 5 mg, 10 mg and used as a NITRATE for the prevention of angina and vein inflammation when a cannula (hollow tube) is inserted.

Dose: for angina apply a patch (begin with a 5 mg patch) to a hairless part of the chest every 24 hours on a different place each time (up to 2 patches may be needed). For other use as advised.
Availability: NHS, private prescription, over the counter.
Side effects: headache, rash, dizziness.
Caution: in patients suffering from heart failure or who have recently had a heart attack. The treatment should be reduced gradually and replaced with decreasing doses of an oral NITRATE.
Not to be used for: children, or for patients suffering from low blood pressure, raised pressure in the brain, or heart muscle weakness.
Caution needed with:
Contains: GLYCERYL TRINITRATE.
Other preparations: CORO-NITRO, DEPONIT, GLYCERYL TRINITRATE TABLETS, GLYTRIN, MINITRAN, NITRO-DUR, NITROCONTIN, NITROLINGUAL, PERCUTOL, SUSCARD BUCCAL, SUSTAC.

Transvasin
(Seton Healthcare)

A cream used as an ANALGESIC rub for the relief of rheumatic and muscular pain, strains and sprains.

Dose: massage into the affected area 2-3 times a day.
Availability: NHS, private prescription, over the counter.
Side effects:
Caution:
Not to be used for:
Caution needed with:
Contains: ETHYL NICOTINATE, HEXYL NICOTINATE, TETRAHYDROFURFURYL SALICYLATE.
Other preparations:

Tranxene
(Boehringer Ingelheim)

A maroon/grey capsule or a pink/grey capsule according to strengths of 7.5 mg, 15 mg, and used as a sedative to treat anxiety and depression.

Dose: elderly 7.5 mg a day; adults over 16 years 7.5-22.5 mg a day.
Availability: private prescription only.
Side effects: drowsiness, light-headedness, confusion, unsteadiness, shaking, vertigo, low blood pressure, rash, changes in vision, retention of urine, changes in sexual desire and blood, jaundice. Risk of addiction increases with dose and length of treatment. May impair judgement.
Caution: in the elderly, pregnant women, nursing mothers, in women during labour, and in patients suffering from lung disorders, kidney or liver disorders. Avoid long-term use and withdraw gradually.
Not to be used for: children under 16 years, or for patients suffering from acute lung diseases, some chronic lung diseases, some obsessional and psychotic diseases.
Caution needed with: alcohol, sedatives, other tranquillizers, anticonvulsants.
Contains: CLORAZEPATE POTASSIUM.
Other preparations:

---

tranylcypromine sulphate *see* **Parnate, Parstelin**

Trasicor *see* **oxprenolol tablets**
(Ciba)

Trasidrex
(Ciba)

A red, coated tablet used as a ß-BLOCKER/thiazide DIURETIC to treat high blood pressure.

Dose: 1 tablet every morning at first, increasing to 2 tablets a day if needed.
Availability: NHS and private prescription.
Side effects: cold hands and feet, sleep disturbance, slow heart rate, tiredness, wheezing, heart failure, stomach upset, low blood pressure, gout, breast enlargement, weakness, blood changes, sensitivity to light, dry eyes, skin rash.
Caution: in pregnant women, nursing mothers, and in patients suffering from diabetes, high blood lipid levels, kidney or liver disorders, gout. May need to be withdrawn before surgery. Withdraw gradually. Your doctor may advise additional treatment with DIURETICS or DIGOXIN.
Not to be used for: children or for patients suffering from heart block or failure, low blood pressure, untreated PHAEOCHROMOCYTOMA, severe liver or kidney disease, failure of the kidneys to produce urine.
Caution needed with: VERAPAMIL, CLONIDINE withdrawal, LITHIUM, DIGOXIN, some anti-arrhythmic drugs and anaesthetics, RESERPINE, some blood-pressure lowering drugs, ERGOTAMINE, CIMETIDINE, sedatives, antidiabetics, SYMPATHOMIMETICS, INDOMETHACIN, ALLOPURINOL, AMANTADINE.
Contains: OXPRENOLOL hydrochloride, CYCLOPENTHIAZIDE.
Other preparations:

T

Travogyn
(Schering Healthcare)

A white, almond-shaped vaginal tablet supplied at a strength of 300 mg and used as an antifungal treatment for thrush or other infections of the vagina. (This product may be purchased without prescription only for the treatment of vaginal thrush.)

Dose: 2 tablets inserted together into the vagina as a single dose.
Availability: NHS, private prescription, over the counter (*see* above).
Side effects: irritation and burning.
Caution:
Not to be used for: children.
Caution needed with:
Contains: ISOCONAZOLE nitrate.
Other preparations:

Traxam
(Lederle)

A clear gel used as a topical NON-STEROIDAL ANTI-INFLAMATORY rub to treat soft tissue injury such as strains, sprains.

Dose: massage gently into the affected area 2-4 times a day for up to 14 days up to a maximum of 25 g a day.
Availability: NHS and private prescription.
Side effects: mild local redness, dermatitis, itch.
Caution: in pregnant women and nursing mothers.
Not to be used for: children or for patients suffering from allergy to aspirin/anti-inflammatory drugs.
Caution needed with:
Contains: FELBINAC.
Other preparations: Traxam Foam.

---

trazodone *see* Molipaxin

Trental
(Hoechst Roussel)

A pink, oblong tablet supplied at a strength of 400 mg and used as a blood cell altering drug to treat peripheral vascular problems.

Dose: 1 tablet 2-3 times a day.
Availability: NHS and private prescription.
Side effects: stomach disturbances, vertigo, flushes.
Caution: in patients suffering from low blood pressure, severe heart artery disease, kidney disease.
Not to be used for: children.
Caution needed with: blood-pressure lowering drugs.
Contains: OXPENTIFYLLINE.
Other preparations:

---

tretinoin *see* Retin-A, Retinova

Tri-Adcortyl
(Princeton)

A cream used as an antifungal, antibacterial, strong STEROID treatment for inflammatory skin disorders where there is also infection.

Dose: apply to the affected area 2-4 times a day.
Availability: NHS and private prescription.
Side effects: fluid retention, suppression of adrenal glands, thinning, streaking, or spotting of the skin may occur.
Caution: use for short periods of time only, especially in children or on the face.
Not to be used for: patients suffering from acne or any other skin infections caused by tuberculosis, ringworm, viruses, or fungi, leg ulcers, scabies, or continuously especially in pregnant women.
Caution needed with:
Contains: TRIAMCINOLONE ACETONIDE, NYSTATIN, NEOMYCIN, GRAMICIDIN.
Other preparations: Tri-Adcortyl Ointment, TRI-ADCORTYL OTIC (for ear disorders).

Tri-Adcortyl Otic
(Squibb)

An ointment with an aural applicator used as an antibiotic, antifungal, STEROID treatment for inflammation of the external ear.

Dose: apply the ointment into the ear 2-4 times a day.
Availability: NHS and private prescription.
Side effects: additional infection, kidney disorder.
Caution: in infants, pregnant women, and in patients suffering from perforated ear drum, or established deafness – avoid using over extended periods.
Not to be used for: patients suffering from tubercular or viral wounds.
Caution needed with:
Contains: TRIAMCINOLONE ACETONIDE, NEOMYCIN sulphate, GRAMICIDIN, NYSTATIN.
Other preparations:

T

Tri-Minulet
(Wyeth)

Beige, brown, and white tablets used as an oestrogen, progestogen contraceptive.

Dose: 1 tablet a day, starting on day 1 of menstruation, for 21 days, then 7 days without tablets.
Availability: NHS and private prescription.
Side effects: enlarged breasts, bloating and fluid retention, cramps, leg pains, mood change, reduction in sexual desire, headaches, nausea, vaginal erosion, discharge and bleeding, weight gain, skin changes, rarely thrombosis, raised blood pressure, jaundice.
Caution: in patients suffering from high blood pressure, diabetes, vascular

disorders, asthma, depression, kidney disease, multiple sclerosis, womb diseases. Your doctor may advise you not to smoke, to have regular examinations. You should stop treatment at the first sign of serious symptoms such as severe headache or jaundice. Treatment should be stopped before surgery.

Not to be used for: pregnant women, or for patients suffering from sickle-cell anaemia, history of heart disease or thrombosis, liver disorders, some cancers, undiagnosed vaginal bleeding, some ear, skin and kidney disorders.

Caution needed with: RIFAMPICIN, TETRACYCLINE ANTIBIOTICS, GRISEOFULVIN, BARBITURATES, PHENYTOIN, PRIMIDONE, CARBAMAZEPINE, ETHOSUXIMIDE, CHLORAL HYDRATE.

Contains: ETHINYLOESTRADIOL, GESTODENE.
Other preparations: TRIADENE.

---

tri-potassium dicitrato bismuthate *see* **De-Nol**

Triadene *see* **Tri-minulet**
(Schering Healthcare)

Triamaxco *see* **co-triamterzide tablets**
(Ashbourne)

---

triamcinolone acetonide *see* **Adcortyl, Adcortyl in Orabase, Adcortyl intra-articular injection, Audicort, Aurecort, Kenalog, Ledercort, Lederspan 20 mg, Nystadermal, Pevaryl TC, Tri-Adcortyl, Tri-Adcortyl Otic**

Triamco *see* **co-triamterzide tablets**
(Baker Norton)

---

triamterene *see* **Dyazide, Dytac, Dytide, Frusene, Kalspare, Triamaxco, Triamco**

---

triclosan *see* **Aquasept, Manusept, Oilatum Plus, Ster-Zac Bath Concentrate**

---

tricyclic antidepressant

a drug used to treat depression but which may cause sedation and dryness of the mouth. Example AMITRIPTYLINE *see* amitriptyline tablets.

Tridestra
(Sanofi Winthrop)

White tablets, blue tablets, and yellow tablets used as an oestrogen/progestogen hormone replacement therapy to treat menopausal symptoms, and to prevent osteoporosis after the menopause.

Dose: 1 white tablet a day for 70 days starting on the fifth day of the cycle if present, then 1 blue tablet a day for 14 days, then 1 yellow tablet a day for 7 days.
Availability: NHS, private prescription.
Side effects: enlarged breasts, fluid retention, nausea, vaginal bleeding, weight gain, headache, dizziness. Rarely jaundice, raised blood pressure, thrombosis.
Caution: in patients suffering from high blood pressure, diabetes, epilepsy, womb diseases, gall bladder disorder, migraine, multiple sclerosis, PORPHYRIA, liver disorders, some ear disorders, or a history or increased risk of breast disorders (including cancer) and thrombosis. Your doctor may advise you to have regular examinations.
Not to be used for: children, pregnant women, nursing mothers, or for patients suffering from thombosis, severe liver, kidney, or heart disorders, some cancers, undiagnosed vaginal bleeding, endometriosis.
Caution needed with: ACE INHIBITORS, ANTICOAGULANTS, BARBITURATES, ß-BLOCKERS, CARBAMAZEPINE, PHENYTOIN, RIFAMPICIN.
Contains: OESTRADIOL, MEDROXYPROGESTERONE.
Other preparations:

---

trifluoperazine *see* **Parstelin, Stelazine, trifluoperazine tablets**

---

trifluoperazine tablets

A coated tablet supplied at strengths of 1 mg, 5 mg and used as a sedative to treat anxiety, depression, agitation, schizophrenia, mental disorders, severe agitation, dangerous impulsive behaviour, nausea, vomiting.

Dose: for anxiety adults 2-4 mg up to a maximum of 6 mg a day in divided doses; children 3-5 years up to 1 mg a day, 6-12 up to 4 mg a day. For schizophrenia and other mental disorders, adults 5 mg twice a day increasing after 7 days to 15 mg; children up to 5 mg a day. For nausea and vomiting adults 2-6 mg a day; children 3-5 years up to 1 mg a day, 6-

12 years up to 4 mg a day.
Availability: NHS and private prescription.
Side effects: muscle spasms, restlessness, hands shaking, dry mouth, palpitations, low blood pressure, weight gain, blurred vision, changes in sexual function, change in body temperature, breast swelling, menstrual changes, jaundice, blood and skin changes, drowsiness, apathy, nightmares, sleeplessness, depression, blocked nose, difficulty passing water, rarely fits.
Caution: in pregnant women, nursing mothers, and in patients suffering from heart or circulatory disorder, breathing disease, Parkinson's disease, epilepsy, infections, underactive thyroid, MYASTHENIA GRAVIS, enlarged prostate, glaucoma, some blood disorders.
Not to be used for: unconscious patients, the elderly, or for patients suffering from bone marrow depression, PHAEOCHROMOCYTOMA.
Caution needed with: alcohol, sedatives, tranquillizers, pain killers, blood-pressure lowering drugs, antidepressants, anticonvulsants, antidiabetic drugs, LEVODOPA, anaesthetics, ANTACIDS, ASTEMIZOLE, TERFENADINE, LITHIUM, CIMETIDINE, SOTOLOL.
Contains: TRIFLUOPERAZINE hydrochloride.
Other preparations: stelazine.

Trifyba
(Sanofi Winthrop)

A powder used as a bulking agent to treat constipation, diverticular disease, irritable colon, haemorrhoids, and fissures.

Dose: adults, 1 sachet 2-3 times a day; children ½-1 sachet once or twice a day. Mix powder with food.
Availability: NHS, private prescription, over the counter.
Side effects:
Caution: adequate fluids must be taken.
Not to be used for: patients suffering from blocked intestine.
Caution needed with:
Contains: concentrated extract of WHEAT HUSK.
Other preparations:

---

trilostane *see* Modrenal

Triludan *see* terfenadine tablets
(Merion Merrell Dow)

---

trimeprazine *see* **Vallergan**

---

trimethoprim *see* **Bactrim, Chemotrim, Comixco, Fectrim, Ipral, Laratrim, Monotrim, Polytrim, Septrin, Tiempe, trimethoprim tablets, Trimopan, Triprimix**

---

trimethoprim tablets

A tablet supplied at strengths of 100 mg, 200 mg and used as an antibiotic to treat infections such as bronchitis, urine infections.

Dose: adults 200 mg twice a day, children 6 weeks-5 months 25 mg twice a day, 6 months-5 years 50 mg twice a day, 6-12 years 100 mg twice a day. (Lower doses for prevention.)
Availability: NHS and private prescription.
Side effects: stomach upset, skin reactions, blood changes.
Caution: in nursing mothers, and in patients suffering from kidney disease from folate deficiency (vitamin deficiency), PORPHYRIA. Your doctor may advise regular blood tests.
Not to be used for: infants under 6 weeks, pregnant women, or for patients suffering from severe kidney disease, blood disorders.
Caution needed with: NICOUMALONE, WARFARIN, some antidiabetics, PHENYTOIN, PYRIMETHAMINE, CYCLOSPORIN, METHOTREXATE, PROCAINAMIDE.
Contains: TRIMETHOPRIM.
Other preparations: IPRAL, MONOTRIM, TIEMPE, TRIMOPAN (liquid forms available).

---

trimipramine maleate *see* **Surmontil**

Trimopan *see* **trimethoprim tablets**
(Berk)

Trimovate
(Glaxo)

A cream used as an antibiotic, antifungal, steroid treatment in skin disorders in moist or covered places where there is also infection.

Dose: apply to the affected area 1-4 times a day.
Availability: NHS and private prescription.
Side effects: fluid retention, suppression of adrenal glands, thinning, spotting, or streaking of the skin may occur.

T

Caution: use for short periods of time only, especially in children or on the face.

Not to be used for: patients suffering from acne or any other skin infections caused by tuberculosis, ringworm, viruses, or fungi, leg ulcers, scabies, or continuously especially in pregnant women.

Caution needed with:

Contains: CLOBETASONE BUTYRATE, NYSTATIN, CALCIUM OXYTETRACYCLINE.

Other preparations:

Trinordiol
(Wyeth)

Brown, white, and ochre tablets used as an oestrogen, progestogen contraceptive.

Dose: 1 tablet a day for 21 days starting on day 1 of the period.

Availability: NHS and private prescription.

Side effects: enlarged breasts, bloating and fluid retention, cramps, leg pains, mood change, reduction in sexual desire, headaches, nausea, vaginal erosion, discharge, and bleeding, weight gain, skin changes, rarely thrombosis, raised blood pressure, jaundice.

Caution: in patients suffering from high blood pressure, diabetes, vascular disorders, asthma, depression, kidney disease, multiple sclerosis, womb diseases. Your doctor may advise you not to smoke, to have regular examinations. You should stop treatment at the first sign of serious symptoms such as severe headache or jaundice. Treatment should be stopped before surgery.

Not to be used for: pregnant women, or for patients suffering from sickle-cell anaemia, history of heart disease or thrombosis, liver disorders, some cancers, undiagnosed vaginal bleeding, some ear, skin, and kidney disorders.

Caution needed with: RIFAMPICIN, TETRACYCLINE ANTIBIOTICS, GRISEOFULVIN, BARBITURATES, PHENYTOIN, PRIMIDONE, CARBAMAZEPINE, ETHOSUXIMIDE, CHLORAL HYDRATE.

Contains: ETHINYLOESTRADIOL, LEVONORGESTREL.

Other preparations: LOGYNON.

Trinovum
(Janssen-Cilag)

White tablets, pale peach tablets, and peach-coloured tablets used as an oestrogen, progestogen contraceptive.

Dose: 1 tablet a day for 21 days starting on day 1 of the period.

Availability: NHS and private prescription.

Side effects: enlarged breasts, bloating and fluid retention, cramps, leg pains, mood change, reduction in sexual desire, headaches, nausea, vaginal erosion, discharge, and bleeding, weight gain, skin changes, rarely thrombosis, raised blood pressure, jaundice.

Caution: in patients suffering from high blood pressure, diabetes, vascular disorders, asthma, depression, kidney disease, multiple sclerosis, womb diseases. Your doctor may advise you not to smoke, to have regular examinations. You should stop treatment at the first sign of serious symptoms such as severe headache or jaundice. Treatment should be stopped before surgery.

Not to be used for: pregnant women, or for patients suffering from sickle-cell anaemia, history of heart disease or thrombosis, liver disorders, some cancers, undiagnosed vaginal bleeding, some ear, skin, and kidney disorders.

Caution needed with: RIFAMPICIN, TETRACYCLINE ANTIBIOTICS, GRISEOFULVIN, BARBITURATES, PHENYTOIN, PRIMIDONE, CARBAMAZEPINE, ETHOSUXIMIDE, CHLORAL HYDRATE.

Contains: ETHINYLOESTRADIOL, LEVONORGESTREL.

Other preparations:

Trinovum-ED
(Janssen-Cilag)

White, light-peach, peach, and green tablets used as an oestrogen, progestogen contraceptive.

Dose: 1 tablet a day starting on day 1 of menstruation.

Availability: NHS and private prescription.

Side effects: enlarged breasts, bloating and fluid retention, cramps, leg pains, mood change, reduction in sexual desire, headaches, nausea, vaginal erosion, discharge and bleeding, weight gain, skin changes.

Caution: in patients suffering from high blood pressure, diabetes, vascular disorders, asthma, depression, kidney disease, multiple sclerosis, womb diseases. You should stop treatment at the first sign of serious symptoms such as severe headache or jaundice. Treatment should be stopped before surgery.

Not to be used for: pregnant women or for patients suffering from sickle-cell anaemia, history of heart disease or thrombosis, liver disorders, some cancers, undiagnosed vaginal bleeding, some ear, skin and kidney disorders.

Caution needed with: RIFAMPICIN, TETRACYCLINE ANTIBIOTICS, GRISEOFULVIN, BARBITURATES, PHENYTOIN, PRIMIDONE, CARBAMAZEPINE, ETHOSUXIMIDE, CHLORAL HYDRATE.

Contains: ETHINYLOESTRADIOL, NORETHISTERONE, LACTOSE.

Other preparations:

T

Triprimix-200 *see* **trimethoprim tablets**
(Ashbourne)

---

triprolidine hydrochloride *see* **Sudafed Plus**

Triptafen
(Forley)

A pink tablet used as a TRICYCLIC ANTIDEPRESSANT to treat depression with anxiety.

Dose: 1 tablet 3 times a day with 1 tablet at bed time if needed.
Availability: NHS and private prescription.
Side effects: dry mouth, constipation, urine retention, blurred vision, palpitations, rapid heart rate, tinnitus, nervousness, sweating, weakness, tiredness, drowsiness, heart disturbance, sleeplessness, dizziness, hands shaking, low blood pressure, weight change, skin reactions, fits, jaundice or blood changes, menstrual changes, breast enlargement. Loss of sexual desire may occur.
Caution: in pregnant women, nursing mothers or in patients suffering from Parkinson's disease, heart disease, liver disorder, kidney disease, constipation, thyroid disease, epilepsy, diabetes, glaucoma, adrenal tumour, urinary retention, some other psychiatric conditions. Your doctor may advise regular blood tests.
Not to be used for: children, or for patients suffering from heart attacks, severe liver disease, heart block, bone marrow depression, circulatory disorder.
Caution needed with: alcohol, sedatives, ANALGESICS, ANTICHOLINERGICS, ADRENALINE, MAOIS, BARBITURATES, other antidepressants, anticonvulsants, antidiabetics, CIMETIDINE, oestrogens, blood-pressure lowering drugs, CARBAMAZEPINE, PHENYTOIN.
Contains: AMITRYPTILINE hydrochloride, PERPHENAZINE.
Other preparations: Triptafen-M (a weaker-strength product).

Trisequens
(Novo-Nordisk)

Twelve blue tablets, 10 white tablets, and 6 red tablets used as a oestrogen, progestogen treatment for menopausal symptoms, and to prevent bone thinning after the menopause.

Dose: 1 tablet a day starting on the fifth day of the period if present, beginning with the blue tablets and continuing in sequence without a break.

Availability: NHS and private prescription.
Side effects: enlarged breasts, fluid retention, nausea, vaginal bleeding, weight gain, headache, dizziness. Rarely jaundice, raised blood pressure, thrombosis.
Caution: in patients suffering from high blood pressure, diabetes, epilepsy, womb diseases, gall bladder disorder, migraine, multiple sclerosis, PORPHYRIA, liver disorders, some ear disorders, or a history or increased risk of breast disorders (including cancer) and thrombosis. Your doctor may advise you to have regular examinations.
Not to be used for: children, pregnant women, nursing mothers, or for patients suffering from thombosis, severe liver, kidney, or heart disorders, some cancers, undiagnosed vaginal bleeding, endometriosis.
Caution needed with: ACE INHIBITORS, ANTICOAGULANTS, BARBITURATES, ß-BLOCKERS, CARBAMAZEPINE, PHENYTOIN, RIFAMPICIN.
Contains: OESTRADIOL, OESTRIOL, NORETHISTERONE acetate.
Other preparations: Trisequens Forte.

Tritace
(Hoechst Roussel)

A yellow/white capsule, orange/white capsule or crimson/white capsule according to strengths 1.25 mg, 2.5 mg and 5 mg, and used as an ACE INHIBITOR to treat high blood pressure, and as an extra treatment with DIURETICS in congestive heart failure.

Dose: initially 1.25 mg a day, increasing to a maximum of 10 mg a day.
Availability: NHS and private prescription.
Side effects: nausea, vomiting, tiredness, dizziness, headache, abdominal pain, low blood pressure, diarrhoea, cough, severe allergy, fainting, kidney damage, liver disorder, fluid retention, tiredness.
Caution: in patients suffering from congestive heart failure, liver or kidney damage, blood disorders, or for patients undergoing dialysis. Doses of diuretics may need to be reduced.
Not to be used for: children, pregnant women, nursing mothers, or for patients suffering from heart abnormalities, or with a history of severe allergy.
Caution needed with: blood-pressure lowering drugs, some DIURETICS, LITHIUM, potassium supplements, antidiabetics, NON-STEROIDAL ANTI-INFLAMMATORY DRUGS.
Contains: RAMIPRIL.
Other preparations:

Tropergen *see* Lomotil
(Norgine)

---

tropicamide *see* **Mydriacyl, NODS Tropicamide, Tropicamide Minims**

Tropicamide Minims
(Chauvin)

Drops used as an ANTICHOLINERGIC, short-acting pupil dilator.

Dose: 2 drops with 5 minutes between each drop, then 1-2 drops 30 minutes later if needed.
Availability: NHS and private prescription.
Side effects: temporary smarting.
Caution: care in infants.
Not to be used for: for patients suffering from narrow angle glaucoma.
Caution needed with:
Contains: TROPICAMIDE.
Other preparations: MYDRIACYL, NODS TROPICAMIDE.

Tropium *see* chlordiazepoxide tablets
(DDSA)

Trosyl
(Pfizer)

A solution used as an antifungal treatment for infections of the nails.

Dose: apply to the affected areas every 12 hours for 6-12 months.
Availability: NHS and private prescription.
Side effects: mild irritation.
Caution:
Not to be used for: pregnant women.
Caution needed with:
Contains: TIOCONAZOLE.
Other preparations: Trosyl Cream (also available over the counter).

Trusopt
(MSD)

Eye drops supplied at a strength of 2% and used as a treatment for high pressure in the eye, and some types of glaucoma.

Dose: 1 drop into the affected eye 3 times a day (or twice a day if ß-BLOCKERS are also being used).

Availability: NHS and private prescription.
Side effects: irritation, headache, bitter taste.
Caution: in patients with closed-angle glaucoma, allergy to some antibiotics, or impaired liver function.
Not to be used for: children, pregnant women, nursing mothers, or for patients suffering from impaired kidney function, or with abnormally high blood chlorides, or for people wearing soft contact lenses.
Caution needed with:
Contains: DORZOLAMIDE.
Other preparations:

Tryptizol *see* amitriptyline tablets
(Morson)

---

tryptophan *see* Optimax

---

tuberculosis vaccine (BCG)

An injection used to provide active immunity to tuberculosis. (Vaccination is carried out usually only after using a diagnostic test to determine suitability.)

Dose: one injection of 0.1 ml beneath the skin of the upper arm; children under 3 months, half dose.
Availability: NHS and private prescription.
Side effects: swollen glands, rash, fever, irritation, and reddening at the injection site. Within 2-6 weeks a small swelling appears at the injection site, and may progress to an ulcer that usually heals within 6-12 weeks.
Caution: in pregnant women, and in patients suffering from eczema.
Not to be used for: patients with acute illness, HIV infection, infected skin conditions, or who have altered immunity.
Caution needed with: live vaccines, CORTICOSTEROIDS, drugs that suppress immunity, treatments for tuberculosis.
Contains: live *Mycobacterium bovis.*
Other preparations:

Tuinal
(Distriphar)

An orange/blue capsule used as a BARBITURATE to treat sleeplessness in patients with barbiturate habit.

Dose: 1-2 tablets before going to bed.

Availability: controlled drug; NHS and private prescription.
Side effects: drowsiness, hangover, dizziness, shaking, allergies, headache, confusion, excitement, unsteadiness, breathing difficulty.
Caution: in patients suffering from kidney, liver, or lung disease. Dependence (addiction) may develop.
Not to be used for: children, young adults, pregnant women, nursing mothers, the elderly, patients with a history of drug or alcohol abuse, or suffering from PORPHYRIA, or in the management of pain.
Caution needed with: ANTICOAGULANTS, alcohol, sedatives, other tranquillizers, STEROIDS, the contraceptive pill, GRISEOFULVIN, RIFAMPICIN, PHENYTOIN, METRONIDAZOLE, CHLORAMPHENICOL.
Contains: QUINALBARBITONE sodium, AMYLOBARBITONE sodium.
Other preparations:

---

tulobuterol *see* Brelomax, Respacal

Tylex
(Janssen-Cilag)

A red/white capsule used as an ANALGESIC to relieve severe pain.

Dose: 1-2 tablets every 4 hours to a maximum of 8 tablets in 24 hours.
Availability: NHS and private prescription.
Side effects: tolerance, addiction, constipation, dizziness, sedation, nausea, dry mouth, blurred vision.
Caution: in the elderly, and in patients suffering from underactive thyroid, or kidney or liver disease, obstructive bowel disorders, Addison's disease, head injury, raised brain pressure, enlarged prostate.
Not to be used for: children, pregnant women, nursing mothers, or for patients suffering from breathing difficulty or blocked airways, chronic alcoholism.
Caution needed with: MAOIS, sedatives, other medicines containing PARACETAMOL.
Contains: paracetamol, CODEINE PHOSPHATE.
Other preparations:

Typhim VI *see* typhoid vaccine

---

typhoid vaccine

A killed vaccine used to provide active immunization against typhoid.

Dose: 2 injections, at 4-6 week intervals, of 0.5 ml; children 1-10 years

half adult dose.
Availability: NHS and private prescription.
Side effects: flu-like symptoms of headache, fever, and general feeling of being unwell, irritation and swelling at injection site.
Caution: in pregnant women, nursing mothers.
Not to be used for: children under 1 year, or for patients suffering from acute infections or altered immunity.
Caution needed with: drugs that affect immunity.
Contains: killed *Salmonella typhi* vaccine.
Other preparations: TYPHIM VI (single-dose product), VIVOTIF (oral form).

Ubretid Tablets
(Rhône-Poulenc Rorer)

A white, scored tablet supplied at a strength of 5 mg and used as an ANTICHOLINESTERASE to treat MYASTHENIA GRAVIS, post-operative bladder or intestine problems.

Dose: adults myasthenia gravis 1 tablet a day ½ hour before breakfast at first adjusting every 3-4 days up to 4 tablets a day; children up to 2 tablets a day. Otherwise 1 tablet a day or alternate days.
Availability: NHS and private prescription.
Side effects: nausea, vomiting, colic.
Caution: in patients suffering from bronchial asthma, heart disease, stomach ulcer, epilepsy, Parkinson's disease, vagus nerve disorder.
Not to be used for: pregnant women, or for patients suffering from bowel or urinary blockage, or with weak circulation or in shock after surgery.
Caution needed with: some medicines used during anaesthesia.
Contains: DISTIGMINE bromide.
Other preparations: Ubretid Injection.

U

Ucerax *see* Atarax
(UCB Pharma)

Ultec *see* cimetidine tablets
(Berk)

Ultrabase *see* Diprobase
(Schering Healthcare)

Ultralanum Plain Cream
(Schering Healthcare)

A cream used as a STEROID treatment for skin disorders.

Dose: apply to the affected area 2-3 times a day at first reducing to once a day as soon as possible.
Availability: NHS and private prescription.
Side effects: fluid retention, suppression of adrenal glands, thinning, spotting, or streaking of the skin may occur.
Caution: use for short periods of time only, especially in children or on the face.
Not to be used for: patients suffering from acne or any other skin infections caused by tuberculosis, ringworm, viruses, or fungi, leg ulcers, scabies, or continuously especially in pregnant women.
Caution needed with:
Contains: FLUOCORTOLONE PIVALATE, FLUOCORTOLONE HEXANOATE.
Other preparations: Ultralanum Plain Ointment.

Ultraproct
(Schering Healthcare)

A suppository supplied at a strength of 1 mg and used as a STEROID, local anaesthetic, ANTIHISTAMINE treatment for haemorrhoids, anal itch, vaginal itch. (Short-term use only.)

Dose: 1 suppository 1-3 times a day for 5-7 days.
Availability: NHS and private prescription.
Side effects: systemic CORTICOSTEROID effects (*see* prednisolone tablets).
Caution: do not use for prolonged periods; care in pregnant women.
Not to be used for: children, or for patients suffering from tuberculous, fungal, or viral infections.
Caution needed with:
Contains: FLUOCORTOLONE PIVALATE, FLUOCORTOLONE HEXANOATE, CINCHOCAINE hydrochloride,
Other preparations: Ultraproct ointment.

Ultratard *see* insulin
(Novo Nordisk)

---

undecenoic acid *see* Ceanel

Unguentum Merck
(Merck)

A cream used as an emollient to treat dermatitis, nappy rash, and dry, scaly skin.

Dose: apply thinly 3 times a day or as required.
Availability: NHS, private prescription, over the counter.
Side effects:
Caution:
Not to be used for:
Caution needed with:
Contains: SILICIC ACID, LIQUID PARAFFIN, WHITE SOFT PARAFFIN, CETOSTEARYL ALCOHOL, POLYSORBATE-40, GLYCEROL monostearate, saturated neutral oil, SORBIC ACID, PROPYLENE GLYCOL.
Other preparations:

Unilet Superlite
(Owen Mumford)

A device (lancet) for obtaining blood samples from the finger, compatible with Autolet, Autolet Lite, and Glucolet finger-pricking devices. Blood-glucose monitoring enables individual patients suffering from diabetes accurately to control blood glucose and manage their condition.

Unilet Superlite G
(Owen Mumford)

A device (lancet) for obtaining blood samples from the finger, compatible with Autoclix, Auto Lancet, Hypolet, Monojector, Penlet II, and Soft Touch finger-pricking devices. Blood-glucose monitoring enables individual patients suffering from diabetes accurately to control blood glucose and manage their condition.

Uniphyllin Continus *see* Lasma
(Napp)

Uniroid-HC
(Unigreg)

An ointment used as a STEROID and local anaesthetic treatment for pain, irritation, and itching associated with haemorrhoids and other itchy anal conditions.

Dose: apply a small amount 3 times a day and after each bowel movement, for a maximum of 7 days.
Availability: NHS and private prescription.
Side effects: allergy, systemic CORTICOSTEROID effects (*see* prednisolone tablets).
Caution: in pregnant women; do not use for prolonged periods.
Not to be used for: children, or for patients suffering from tuberculous, fungal, or viral infections, or allergy to any ingredient.
Caution needed with:
Contains: HYDROCORTISONE, CINCHOCAINE hydrochloride.
Other preparations: Uniroid-HC Suppositories.

Unisept
(Seton Healthcare)

A solution used as a disinfectant and general antiseptic.

Dose: use neat as needed.
Availability: NHS, private prescription, over the counter.
Side effects:
Caution:
Not to be used for:
Caution needed with:
Contains: CHLORHEXIDINE gluconate.
Other preparations: HIBISCRUB, HIBISOL, PHISOMED.

U

Unitulle *see* Jelonet
(Hoechst Roussel)

Univer *see* verapamil tablets
(Rhône-Poulenc Rorer)

Urantoin *see* nitrofurantoin tablets
(DDSA)

---

urea hydrogen peroxide *see* Exterol

---

urea *see* Alphaderm, Aquadrate, Calmurid, Calmurid HC, Psoradrate

---

Uriben *see* **nalidixic acid tablets**
(Rosemont)

Urispas
(Roche)

A white tablet supplied at a strength of 200 mg and used as an anti-spasmodic treatment for incontinence, abnormally frequent or urgent urination, bed wetting, painful urination.

Dose: 1 tablet 3 times a day.
Availability: NHS and private prescription.
Side effects: headache, nausea, tiredness, diarrhoea, blurred vision, dry mouth.
Caution: in pregnant women, and in patients suffering from glaucoma.
Not to be used for: children or for patients suffering from obstruction of the urinary or gastro-intestinal tracts.
Caution needed with:
Contains: FLAVOXATE HYDROCHLORIDE.
Other preparations:

---

urofollitrophin *see* **Metrodin High Purity, Orgafol**

---

ursodeoxycholic acid *see* **Combidol, Destolit, Ursofalk**

Ursofalk *see* **Destolit**
(Thames)

Utinor
(M.S.D.)

A white oval tablet supplied at a strength of 400 mg, and used as an antibiotic to treat infections of the urinary tract.

Dose: cystitis: 1 tablet twice a day for 3 days; complicated infections: 1 tablet twice a day for 7-10 days; chronic infections; 1 tablet twice a day for up to 12 weeks.
Availability: NHS, private prescription.
Side effects: nausea, headache, dizziness, rash, heartburn, stomach cramps, diarrhoea, loss of appetite, disturbed sleep, anxiety, mood changes, allergy, confusion, convulsions, pins and needles, blood changes, inflammation of the pancreas, liver disorder, sensitivity to light.

Caution: in patients with a history of epilepsy. Avoid excessive sunlight.
Not to be used for: children, adolescents, pregnant women, nursing
mothers.
Caution needed with: NITROFURANTOIN, THEOPHYLLINE, CYCLOSPORIN,
ANTICOAGULANTS taken by mouth, SULCRAFATE, iron, zinc, ANTACIDS, PROBENECID,
some other antibiotics, FENBUFEN, NON-STEROIDAL ANTI-INFLAMMATORY DRUGS.
Contains: NORFLOXACIN.
Other preparations:

Utovlan *see* norethisterone tablets
(Roche)

Vagifem
(Novo Nordisk)

Pessaries supplied with applicators, and used as an oestrogen treatment
for atrophic inflammation of the vagina.

Dose: 1 pessary inserted into the vagina daily for 2 weeks, then twice a
week.
Availability: NHS and private prescription.
Side effects: enlarged breasts, fluid retention, nausea, vaginal bleeding,
weight gain, headache, dizziness. Rarely jaundice, raised blood pressure,
thrombosis.
Caution: in patients suffering from high blood pressure, diabetes,
epilepsy, womb diseases, gall bladder disorder, migraine, multiple
sclerosis, PORPHYRIA, liver disorders, some ear disorders, or a history or
increased risk of breast disorders (including cancer) and thrombosis. Your
doctor may advise you to have regular examinations.
Not to be used for: children, pregnant women, nursing mothers, or for
patients suffering from thombosis, severe liver, kidney, or heart disorders,
some cancers, undiagnosed vaginal bleeding, endometriosis.
Caution needed with: ACE INHIBITORS, ANTICOAGULANTS, BARBITURATES,
ß-BLOCKERS, CARBAMAZEPINE, PHENYTOIN, RIFAMPICIN.
Contains: OESTRADIOL.
Other preparations:

Vaginyl *see* metronidazole tablets
(DDSA)

---

valciclovir *see* Valtrex

Valclair *see* **diazepam suppositories**
(Sinclair)

Valenac *see* **diclofenac tablets**
(Shire)

Valium *see* **diazepam tablets**
(Roche)

Vallergan
(Rhône-Poulenc Rorer)

A blue tablet supplied at a strength of 10 mg and used as an antihistamine treatment for itch, allergy.

Dose: adults 1 tablet 2-3 times a day or up to 10 a day if needed; elderly 1 tablet 1-2 times a day; children over 2 years use syrup.
Availability: NHS and private prescription.
Side effects: drowsiness, reduced reactions, rash, elation, depression, convulsions on high doses, extrapyramidal reactions (shaking and rigidity), stomach disturbances, ANTICHOLINERGIC effects, heart disturbances, low blood pressure, breathing difficulty, blood changes, jaundice, sensitivity to light.
Caution:
Not to be used for: pregnant women, nursing mothers, infants under 2 years, or for patients suffering from epilepsy, PHAEOCHROMOCYTOMA, glaucoma, parkinsonism, underactive thyroid, enlarged prostate, MYASTHENIA GRAVIS, kidney or liver disorder.
Caution needed with: sedatives, MAOIS, SYMPATHOMIMETICS, alcohol, antidiabetics, blood-pressure lowering drugs, ANTICHOLINERGICS.
Contains: TRIMEPRAZINE tartrate.
Other preparations: Vallergan Syrup, Vallergan Forte Syrup.

V

Valoid
(Wellcome)

A white, scored tablet supplied at a strength of 50 mg and used as an ANTIHISTAMINE treatment for vomiting, nausea, vertigo, inner ear disorders.

Dose: adults and children over 12 years 1 tablet 3 times a day; children 6-12 years ½ tablet 3 times a day.
Availability: NHS, private prescription, over the counter.
Side effects: drowsiness, reduced reactions, ANTICHOLINERGIC reactions,

allergy, blood disorders, rarely skin eruptions.
Caution: in nursing mothers, and in patients suffering from liver or kidney disease, glaucoma, epilepsy, enlarged prostate.
Not to be used for: children under 6 years, pregnant women.
Caution needed with: alcohol, sedatives, anticholinergics.
Contains: CYCLIZINE hydrochloride.
Other preparations: Valoid Injection (not available over the counter).

---

valproic acid *see* **Convulex**

Valtrex
(Wellcome)

A white tablet supplied at a strength of 500 mg, and used as an antiviral to treat shingles and herpes infections of the skin and genital areas.

Dose: for shingles 2 tablets 3 times a day for 7 days; for other herpes infections, 1 tablet twice a day for 5 days.
Availability: NHS, private prescription.
Side effects: headache, nausea.
Caution: in pregnant women, nursing mothers, and in patients with kidney disorders.
Not to be used for: children.
Caution needed with:
Contains: VALCICLOVIR.
Other preparations:

V

Vascace
(Roche)

A pink, white, yellow, red, or brown tablet supplied at strengths of 0.25 mg, 0.5 mg, 1.0 mg, 2.5 mg, 5 mg and used as an ACE-INHIBITOR to treat high blood pressure, including that associated with kidney disease.

Dose: initially 1 mg a day, adjusted as needed usually to 1-2.5 mg a day. Stop DIURETICS 2-3 days before starting treatment. Lower doses used for the elderly, and for patients with kidney involvement.
Availability: NHS and private prescription.
Side effects: headache, dizziness, tiredness, stomach discomfort, indigestion, rash, cough, severe allergy, blood changes, inflamed pancreas.
Caution: in patients suffering from kidney or liver damage, congestive heart failure, salt or body fluid depletion, or undergoing surgery, dialysis, or anaesthesia.

Not to be used for: children, pregnant women, nursing mothers, or for patients suffering from some heart defects or fluid in the abdomen.
Caution needed with: some DIURETICS, NON-STEROIDAL ANTI-INFLAMMATORY DRUGS.
Contains: CILAZAPRIL.
Other preparations:

Velosef
(Squibb)

A blue/orange capsule or a blue capsule according to strengths of 250 mg, 500 mg and used as a cephalosporin antibiotic to treat infections, and for the prevention of infections in surgery.

Dose: adults 1-2 g a day in 2-4 divided doses up to a maximum of 4 g a day; children 25-50 mg per kg body weight a day in 2-4 divided doses.
Availability: NHS and private prescription.
Side effects: allergy, stomach disturbances, thrush, blood changes, change in liver.
Caution: in pregnant women, nursing mothers, and in patients suffering from kidney disease or who are sensitive to penicillin.
Not to be used for:
Caution needed with: some antibiotics.
Contains: CEPHRADINE.
Other preparations: Velosef Syrup, Velosef Injection.

Velosulin *see* insulin
(Novo Nordisk)

---

venlafaxine *see* Efexor

Ventide
(A & H)

An aerosol used as a bronchodilator and steroid to treat asthma.

Dose: adults 2 sprays 3-4 times a day; children 1-2 sprays 2-4 times a day.
Availability: NHS and private prescription.
Side effects: hand shaking, nervous tension, headache, hoarseness, thrush, dilation of the blood vessels.
Caution: in pregnant women, and in patients suffering from overactive thyroid gland, heart muscle disease, abnormal heart rhythms, angina, high

V

blood pressure, tuberculosis of the lungs, or in those transferring from steroids taken by mouth.

Not to be used for:
Caution needed with: SYMPATHOMIMETICS.
Contains: SALBUTAMOL, BECLOMETHASONE diproprionate.
Other preparations: Ventide Rotacaps, Ventide Paediatric Rotacaps.

Ventodisks *see* salbutamol inhaler
(A & H)

Ventolin *see* salbutamol inhaler/tablets
(A & H)

Veracur
(Typharm)

A gel used as a skin softener to treat plantar warts (verrucae).

Dose: apply to the wart twice a day and cover, rubbing down with a pumice stone between treatments.
Availability: NHS, private prescription, over the counter.
Side effects:
Caution: do not apply to healthy skin.
Not to be used for: warts on the face or anal and genital areas.
Caution needed with:
Contains: FORMALDEHYDE.
Other preparations: formaldehyde lotion.

verapamil *see* Cordilox, Cordilox 160, Securon, Securon SR, verapamil tablets

verapamil tablets

A coated tablet supplied at strengths of 40 mg, 80 mg, 120 mg, 160 mg and used as a calcium antagonist to treat angina, high blood pressure, heart rhythm disturbances.

Dose: heart rhythm distrubance: adults 40-120 mg 3 times a day. For angina 80-120 mg 3 times a day. For high blood pressure 240-480 mg a day. Children as advised by a physician.
Availability: NHS and private prescription.
Side effects: constipation, flushes, nausea, vomiting, headache,

dizziness, tiredness, swollen ankles, liver damage, allergy, low blood pressure, slow heart rate, breast swelling, gum swelling.

Caution: in pregnant women, nursing mothers, and in patients suffering from some types of heart conduction block or failure, liver or kidney disease, slow heart rate, heart attack, or low blood pressure.

Not to be used for: patients suffering from severe heart conduction block, very slow heart rates, very low blood pressure, PORPHYRIA.

Caution needed with: ß-BLOCKERS, QUINIDINE, DIGOXIN, ACE INHIBITORS, anaesthetics, some anti-arrhythmics, TRICYCLIC ANTIDEPRESSANTS, some anti-epileptics, tranquillizers, MEFLOQUINE, CYCLOSPORIN, LITHIUM, THEOPHYLLINE some antibiotics, SYMPATHOMIMETICS, CIMETIDINE.

Contains: VERAPAMIL hydrochloride.

Other preparations: BERKATENS, CORDILOX, SECURON. (Long-acting preparations available.)

Vermox
(Janssen-Cilag)

A sugar-free suspension used as a vermicide to treat worms.

Dose: adults and children over 2 years 5 ml morning and evening for 3 days or 5 ml repeated after 2-3 weeks according to the type of infestation.
Availability: NHS and private prescription.
Side effects: stomach upset.
Caution:
Not to be used for: children under 2 years or pregnant women.
Caution needed with:
Contains: MEBENDAZOLE.
Other preparations: Vermox Tablets. (Various brands available over the counter only for the treatment of threadworm – Ovex, Pripsen.)

V

Verrugon
(Pickles)

An ointment with corn rings and plasters used as a skin softener to treat warts.

Dose: protect healthy skin, apply the ointment to the wart, and cover with a plaster, rubbing down with a pumice stone between treatments. Repeat once only.
Availability: NHS, private prescription, over the counter.
Side effects:
Caution: do not apply to healthy skin.
Not to be used for: warts on the face or anal and genital areas.
Caution needed with:

Contains: SALICYLIC ACID.
Other preparations:

Verucasep
(Galen)

A gel used as a virucidal, anhidrotic treatment for viral warts.

Dose: apply twice a day, cover, pare down any hard skin around the wart.
Availability: NHS, private prescription, over the counter.
Side effects: stains the skin.
Caution: do not apply to healthy skin.
Not to be used for: warts on the face or anal and genital areas.
Caution needed with:
Contains: GLUTARALDEHYDE.
Other preparations: GLUTAROL.

Vibramycin *see* doxycycline capsules
(Invicta)

Vibramycin 50 *see* doxycycline capsules
(Invicta)

Videx
(Bristol-Myers Squibb)

A white tablet supplied at strengths of 25 mg, 100 mg, and used as an antiviral drug to treat the symptoms of HIV infection where ZIDOVUDINE cannot be used.

Dose: under 60 kg bodyweight: 125 mg twice a day at first; over 60 kg: 200 mg twice a day at first. Dose must be given as 2 tablets to provide enough antacid, and should be chewed or dispersed in water, and taken at least ½ hour before food.
Availability: NHS, private prescription.
Side effects: inflammation of the pancreas, weakness and numbness of the hands and feet, stomach upset, brain disturbances, blood and urine changes; rarely liver failure, eyesight changes.
Caution: in pregnant women, nursing mothers, and in patients suffering from kidney or liver disorders, inflamed pancreas, or who are on diets with restricted sodium intake. Your doctor may advise regular blood and urine tests.
Not to be used for: children.

Caution needed with: TETRACYCLINE ANTIBIOTICS, GANCICLOVIR, drugs that affect or are affected by acidity of the stomach, drugs that cause pancreatitis, or weakness and numbness of hands and feet.
Contains: DIDANOSINE.
Other preparations:

Vidopen *see* ampicillin capsules
(Berk)

---

vigabatrin *see* Sabril

---

viloxazine hydrochloride *see* Vivalan

Vioform-Hydrocortisone
(Zyma Healthcare)

A cream used as a steroid, antibacterial, antifungal treatment for skin disorders, infected skin in the anal and genital areas.

Dose: apply to the affected area 1-3 times a day for up to 7 days.
Availability: NHS and private prescription.
Side effects: fluid retention, suppression of adrenal glands, thinning, streaking, or spotting of the skin may occur.
Caution: use for short periods of time only, especially in children or on the face.
Not to be used for: children under 2 years, or for patients suffering from acne or any other skin infections caused by tuberculosis, ringworm, viruses, or fungi, scabies, leg ulcers, or continuously especially in pregnant women.
Caution needed with:
Contains: CLIOQUINOL, HYDROCORTISONE.
Other preparations: Vioform-Hydrocortisone Ointment.

V

Virudox
(Bioglan)

A transparent, colourless solution used as an antiviral treatment for herpes, shingles.

Dose: apply 4 times a day for 4 days within 2-3 days of the appearance of the rash.
Availability: NHS and private prescription.

Side effects: local stinging, taste change.
Caution: keep away from eyes, mucous membranes, and clothing.
Not to be used for: children, pregnant women, nursing mothers.
Caution needed with:
Contains: IDOXURIDINE, DIMETHYL SULPHOXIDE.
Other preparations: HERPID, IDURIDIN.

Visclair
(Sinclair)

A yellow tablet supplied at a strength of 100 mg and used as a mucus softener to treat bronchitis, phlegm.

Dose: adults 2 tablets 3-4 times a day for 6 weeks then 2 tablets twice a day; children over 5 years 1 tablet 3 times a day.
Availability: private prescription and over the counter.
Side effects: stomach upset.
Caution:
Not to be used for: children under 5 years.
Caution needed with:
Contains: METHYLCYSTEINE HYDROCHLORIDE.
Other preparations:

Viscotears
(Ciba Vision)

A liquid gel used to treat tear deficiencies.

Dose: 1 drop into each eye 3-4 times a day.
Availability: NHS, private prescription, over the counter.
Side effects: temporary irritation and blurred vision.
Caution: in pregnant women, nursing mothers, and in patients who wear contact lenses.
Not to be used for: children.
Caution needed with:
Contains: POLYACRYLIC ACID.
Other preparations:

Viskaldix
(Sandoz)

A white, scored tablet used as a ß-BLOCKER and DIURETIC to treat high blood pressure.

Dose: 1 tablet in the morning at first, then increase to 2-3 tablets a day after 2-3 weeks.
Availability: NHS and private prescription.
Side effects: cold hands and feet, sleep disturbance, slow heart rate, rash, gout, blood changes, tiredness, wheezing, heart failure, stomach upset, low blood pressure, sensitivity to light, dry eyes, rash, weakness.
Caution: in pregnant women, nursing mothers, and in patients suffering from diabetes, high lipid levels, gout, kidney or liver disorders, asthma. May need to be withdrawn before surgery. Withdraw gradually. Your doctor may advise additional treatment with diuretics or DIGOXIN.
Not to be used for: children, or for patients suffering from heart block or failure, kidney failure, low blood pressure, untreated PHAEOCHROMOCYTOMA, failure to produce urine.
Caution needed with: VERAPAMIL, CLONIDINE withdrawal, some anti-arrhythmic drugs and anaesthetics, RESERPINE, some blood-pressure lowering drugs, ERGOTAMINE, CIMETIDINE, sedatives, SYMPATHOMIMETICS, INDOMETHACIN, LITHIUM, DIGOXIN, ALLOPURINOL, AMANTADINE, antidiabetics.
Contains: PINDOLOL, CLOPAMIDE.
Other preparations:

Visken
(Sandoz)

A white, scored tablet supplied at strengths of 5 mg, 15 mg and used as a ß-BLOCKER to treat angina, high blood pressure.

Dose: angina 2.5-5 mg up to 3 times a day. High blood pressure 10-15 mg a day at first increasing if needed at weekly intervals to 45 mg a day.
Availability: NHS and private prescription.
Side effects: cold hands and feet, sleep disturbance, slow heart rate, tiredness, wheezing, heart failure, low blood pressure, stomach upset, dry eyes, skin rash.
Caution: in pregnant women, nursing mothers, and in patients suffering from diabetes, kidney or liver disorders, asthma. May need to be withdrawn before surgery. Withdraw gradually. Your doctor may advise additional treatment with DIURETICS or DIGOXIN.
Not to be used for: children or for patients suffering from heart block or failure, low blood pressure, untreated PHAEOCHROMOCYTOMA.
Caution needed with: VERAPAMIL, CLONIDINE withdrawal, some anti-arrhythmic drugs and anaesthetics, RESERPINE, other blood-pressure lowering drugs, ERGOTAMINE, CIMETIDINE, sedatives, antidiabetics, SYMPATHOMIMETICS, INDOMETHACIN.
Contains: PINDOLOL.
Other preparations:

V

Vista-Methasone *see* **Betnesol Drops**
(Daniel)

---

vitamin A see **Abidec, Ketovite, Halycitrol, vitamins capsules BPC**. *See also* **retinol**.

---

vitamin B$_1$ *see* **Abidec, Dalivit Drops, Ketovite, Lipoflavonoid, Lipotriad, vitamins capsules BPC**. *See also* **thiamine**.

---

vitamin B$_2$ *see* **Abidec, Dalivit Drops, Ketovite, Lipoflavonoid, vitamins capsules BPC**. *See also* **riboflavine**.

---

vitamin B$_3$ *see* **Abidec, Dalivit Drops, Ketovite, Lipoflavonoid, Lipotriad, nicotinamide tablets, nicotinic acid tablets, vitamins capsules BPC**. *See also* **nicotinamide, nicotinic acid**.

---

vitamin B$_5$ *see* **Ketovite**. *See also* **pantothenic acid**.

---

vitamin B$_6$ *see* **Abidec, Dalivit Drops, Ketovite, Lipoflavonoid, Lipotriad**. *See also* **pyridoxine**.

---

vitamin B$_{12}$ *see* **Cytacon, Cytamen, Ketovite, Lipoflavonoid, Lipotriad**. *See also* **cyanocobalamin**.

V

vitamin B compound tablets

A tablet used as a source of B vitamins to prevent VITAMIN B deficiency.

Dose: adults 1-2 tablets a day.
Availability: NHS, private prescription, over the counter.
Side effects:
Caution:
Not to be used for: children.
Not to be used with:
Contains: vitamins B$_1$, B$_2$, B$_3$.
Other preparations: Benerva Compound (not available on NHS).

---

vitamin B compound strong tablets

A tablet used as a source of B vitamins to treat VITAMIN B deficiency.

Dose: adults 1-2 tablets 3 times a day.
Availability: NHS, private prescription, over the counter.
Side effects:
Caution:
Not to be used for: children.
Not to be used with: some anti-parkinson drugs.
Contains: vitamins B_1, B_2, B_3, B_6.

---

vitamin C *see* Abidec, ascorbic acid tablets, Dalivit Drops, Ketovite, Lipoflavonoid, vitamins capsules BPC. *See also* ascorbic acid.

---

vitamin D *see* Abidec, AT 10, calciferol tablets, calcium and ergocalciferol tablets, Dalivit Drops, Halycitrol, Ketovite, One-Alpha, Rocaltrol, vitamins capsules BPC. *See also* calciferol, cholecalciferol, ergocalciferol.

---

vitamin E *see* Ketovite, vitamin E suspension. *See also* tocopheryl acetate.

---

vitamin E suspension

A suspension used as a vitamin E supplement to treat deficiency (e.g. in cystic fibrosis).

Dose: as advised by a doctor.
Availability: NHS and private prescription.
Side effects: diarrhoea and stomach pain with high doses.
Caution: in patients with a tendency to blood clots, a form of enterocolitis in infants.
Not to be used for:
Caution needed with:
Contains: VITAMIN E (ALPHA TOCOPHERYL ACETATE).
Other preparations: Ephynal, Vita-E.

---

vitamin H *see* Ketovite. *See also* biotin.

V

vitamin K *see* **Konakion.** *See also* **phytomenadione.**

---

vitamins capsules BPC

Capsules used as a multivitamin supplement.

Dose: as advised by the doctor or manufacturer.
Availability: NHS, private prescription, over the counter.
Side effects:
Caution: in pregnant women.
Not to be used for:
Caution needed with: some DIURETICS.
Contains: VITAMIN C, VITAMIN B$_3$, VITAMIN B$_2$, VITAMIN B$_1$, VITAMIN A, VITAMIN D.
Other preparations:

Vivalan
(Zeneca)

A yellow tablet supplied at a strength of 50 mg and used as an antidepressant to treat depression, especially in patients for whom sedation is not required.

Dose: adults usually 6 tablets a day in divided doses up to a maximum of 8 tablets a day; elderly 2 tablets a day at first.
Availability: NHS and private prescription.
Side effects: vomiting, headache, impaired reactions, ANTICHOLINERGIC effects, jaundice, convulsions.
Caution: in pregnant women and in patients with suicidal tendencies, or suffering from heart disease including congestive heart failure, heart block, epilepsy.
Not to be used for: children, nursing mothers, or patients suffering from mania, severe liver disease, history of stomach ulcer, recent heart attack.
Caution needed with: MAOIS, CLONIDINE, PHENYTOIN, LEVODOPA, sedatives, CARBAMAZEPINE, THEOPHYLLINE some drugs used to treat heart failure, high blood pressure, Raynaud's disease (a circulation disorder), or enlarged prostate.
Contains: VILOXAZINE HYDROCHLORIDE.
Other preparations:

Vivapril *see* selegiline tablets

Vividrin
(Novex)

Eye drops or a nasal spray used as an anti-inflammatory preparation to treat allergic conjunctivitis or allergic rhinitis.

Dose: 1-2 drops into the eye up to 4 times a day; or 1 spray into each nostril 4-6 times a day; in both cases treatment should be continuous.
Availability: NHS, private prescription, (nasal spray available over the counter).
Side effects: temporary irritation; nasal spray may rarely cause bronchial spasm.
Caution:
Not to be used for: eye drops not to be used for patients who wear soft contact lenses.
Caution needed with:
Contains: SODIUM CROMOGLYCATE.
Other preparations: SODIUM CROMOGLYCATE EYE DROPS, CUSYLIN, HAY-CROM, OPTICROM, RYNACROM. (Other brands also available over the counter.)

Vivotif
(Evans)

A white/pink, coated capsule used as a vaccine to provide active immunization against typhoid fever.

Dose: 1 capsule swallowed whole with a cold drink an hour before a meal on days 1, 3, and 5. Regular travellers to infected areas take 3 capsules as a booster dose every year.
Availability: NHS, private prescription.
Side effects: temporary stomach upset, rarely nettle rash.
Caution: in pregnant women, nursing mothers.
Not to be used for: children under 6 years, or for patients suffering from acute feverish illness or stomach upsets, or whose immune systems are changed (including patients suffering from HIV).
Caution needed with: antibiotics, drugs that suppress the immune system, MEFLOQUINE.
Contains: live typhoid vaccine.
Other preparations: TYPHOID VACCINE, TYPHIM VI (injectable vaccines).

Viz-on *see* **sodium cromoglycate eye drops**
(Opus)

Volital
(L.A.B.)

A white, scored tablet supplied at a strength of 20 mg and used as a brain stimulant to treat movement disorders in children.

Dose: children 6-12 years 1 tablet a day in the morning, increasing if necessary to 6 a day.
Availability: NHS and private prescription.
Side effects: dizziness, sweating, palpitations, headache, irritability, dry mouth, loss of appetite and weight.
Caution:
Not to be used for: children under 6 years or for adults.
Caution needed with: MAOIS.
Contains: PEMOLINE.
Other preparations:

Volmax *see* salbutamol tablets
(A & H)

Volraman *see* diclofenac tablets
(Eastern)

Voltarol *see* diclofenac tablets
(Ciba)

---

warfarin *see* Marevan, warfarin tablets

---

warfarin tablets

A tablet supplied at strengths of 1 mg, 3 mg, 5 mg and used as an ANTICOAGULANT to thin the blood in the treatment of blood clots (thrombosis), and to prevent blood clotting in susceptible patients (e.g. after heart valve surgery).

Dose: 10 mg a day initially, then as directed (according to blood test results).
Availability: NHS and private prescription.
Side effects: rash, diarrhoea, blood changes, hair loss, nausea, vomiting, liver disorder, inflamed pancreas, skin problems, allergy.
Caution: in the elderly or very ill patients, and for patients suffering from high blood pressure, weight changes, kidney or liver disease, VITAMIN K deficiency, or who have had recent surgery.
Not to be used for: children, pregnant women, within 24 hours of surgery or labour, or for patients suffering from haemorrhagic conditions, stomach ulcer, very high blood pressure, heart valve infection.

Caution needed with: NON-STEROIDAL ANTI-INFLAMMATORY DRUGS, oral antidiabetics, anti-arrhythmic drugs, QUINIDINE, antibiotics, CIMETIDINE, OMEPRAZOLE, INFLUENZA VACCINE, VITAMIN K, THYROXINE, drugs affecting liver chemistry, alcohol, OXYMETHOLONE, STANOZOLOL, ASPIRIN, some antidepressants, some anticoagulants, some antifungals, PROGUANIL, DIPYRIMADOLE, CHLORAL, CLOFIBRATE, DISULFIRAM, SUCRALFATE, AMINOGLUTETHIMIDE, DANAZOL, FLUTAMIDE, TAMOXIFEN, the contraceptive pill, ACITRETIN, SIMVASTATIN.
Contains: WARFARIN sodium.
Other preparations: MAREVAN.

Warticon
(Perstorp)

A solution with applicators used as a cell softener and remover to treat genital warts.

Dose: apply twice a day for 3 days and repeat after 7 days if needed. (Maximum of 4 weeks total treatment.)
Availability: NHS and private prescription.
Side effects: irritation.
Caution:
Not to be used for: children, pregnant women, nursing mothers.
Caution needed with:
Contains: PODOPHYLLOTOXIN.
Other preparations: Warticon Fem, Warticon Cream. CONDYLINE.

Waxsol
(Norgine)

Drops used as a wax softener to remove ear wax.

Dose: fill the ear with the solution for 2 nights before they are to be syringed.
Availability: NHS, private prescription, over the counter.
Side effects: temporary irritation.
Caution:
Not to be used for: patients suffering from inflammation of the ear or perforated ear drum.
Caution needed with:
Contains: sodium DOCUSATE.
Other preparations: DIOCTYL.

Welldorm
(Smith & Nephew Healthcare)

A purple, oval tablet supplied at a strength of 707 mg and used as a sedative-hypnotic to treat sleeplessness.

Dose: 1-2 tablets before going to bed.
Availability: NHS and private prescription.
Side effects: nausea, vomiting, headache, rash, rarely blood changes, excitement, abdominal enlargement, wind.
Caution:
Not to be used for: pregnant women, nursing mothers, or for patients suffering from acute intermittent PORPHYRIA, severe kidney, liver, or heart disease, stomach inflammation.
Caution needed with: alcohol, sedatives, ANTICHOLINERGICS, ANTICOAGULANTS.
Contains: CHLORAL HYDRATE.
Other preparations: NOCTEC.

Wellvone
(Wellcome)

A yellow, film-coated tablet supplied at a strength of 250 mg, and used as an antibiotic to treat some forms of pneumonia in patients unable to take CO-TRIMOXAZOLE.

Dose: 3 tablets 3 times a day with food, continued for 21 days.
Availability: NHS, private prescription.
Side effects: rash, nausea, diarrhoea, headache, vomiting, fever, sleeplessness, liver changes.
Caution: in the elderly, pregnant women, nursing mothers, and in patients suffering from diarrhoea, kidney or liver disorders, or who have difficulty taking the drug with food.
Not to be used for: children.
Caution needed with: METOCLOPRAMIDE, RIFAMPICIN, ZIDOVUDINE, some other drugs.
Contains: ATOVAQUONE.
Other preparations:

---

wheat husk *see* **Trifyba**

---

white soft paraffin *see* **Bactigras, calamine and coal tar ointment, Chlorhexitulle, coal tar and salicyic acid ointment,**

Dermamist, Diprobase, Jelonet, Lipobase, Serotulle, Unguentum Merck

---

Whitfields Ointment *see* **benzoic acid compound ointment**

---

wool fat *see* **calamine and coal tar ointment, Lubrifilm, Sudocrem**

---

xamoterol *see* **Corwin**

Xanax
(Upjohn)

A white, oval, scored tablet or a pink, oval, scored tablet according to strengths of 0.25 mg, 0.5 mg and used as a sedative for the short-term treatment of anxiety and depression.

Dose: elderly 0.25 mg 2-3 times a day; adults 0.25-0.5 mg 3 times a day to a maximum of 3 mg a day.
Availability: private prescription only.
Side effects: drowsiness, light-headedness, confusion, vertigo, stomach disturbances, unsteadiness, low blood pressure, rash, changes in vision, changes in sexual function, retention of urine, jaundice. Risk of addiction increases with dose and length of treatment. May impair judgement.
Caution: in the elderly, pregnant women, nursing mothers, in women during labour, and in patients suffering from lung disorders, kidney or liver disorders. Avoid long-term use and withdraw gradually.
Not to be used for: children, or for patients suffering from acute lung diseases, some chronic lung diseases, some obsessional and psychotic diseases.
Caution needed with: alcohol, sedatives, other tranquillizers, anticonvulsants.
Contains: ALPRAZOLAM.
Other preparations:

X

Xanthomax *see* **allopurinol tablets**
(Ashbourne)

Xatral
(Lorex)

A white, film-coated tablet supplied at a strength of 2.5 mg, and used as an ALPHA-BLOCKER to treat enlarged prostate.

Dose: 1 tablet 3 times a day, up to a maximum of 4 tablets a day; elderly 1 tablet night and morning at first, up to 4 tablets a day.
Availability: NHS, private prescription.
Side effects: dizziness, vertigo, stomach upset, low blood pressure on standing, fainting, rapid heart rate, palpitations, fluid retention, chest pain, tiredness, drowsiness, rash, itching, flushing, headache.
Caution: in patients suffering from raised blood pressure, weak heart, or liver or kidney disorders. Your doctor may advise regular blood pressure tests. Withdraw treatment if chest pain worsens. Withdraw 24 hours before anaesthesia.
Not to be used for: children, or for patients suffering from severe liver disorder, or with a history of low blood pressure on standing.
Caution needed with: other similar drugs, blood-pressure lowering drugs, some drugs used to treat heart or circulation disorders.
Contains: ALFUZOSIN hydrochloride.
Other preparations: Xatral SR.

---

xipamide *see* **Diurexan**

Xuret *see* **Metenix**
(Galen)

---

xylitol *see* **Saliva Orthana, Salivace**

Xylocaine
(Astra)

An ointment used to anaesthetize the skin or mucous membranes.

Dose: as advised by your doctor.
Availability: NHS, private prescription, over the counter.
Side effects:
Caution: in patients suffering from epilepsy.
Not to be used for:
Caution needed with:
Contains: LIGNOCAINE.
Other preparations: Xylocaine Gel, Xylocaine Antiseptic Gel, Xylocaine

Topical, Xylocaine Pump Spray, Xylocaine Injection.

---

xylometazoline hydrochloride *see* **Otrivine, Rynacrom (compound)**

Xyloproct
(Astra)

A suppository used as a local anaesthetic and STEROID treatment for haemorrhoids, anal itch, anal fissure and fistula.

Dose: 1 at night and after passing motions.
Availability: NHS and private prescription.
Side effects: systemic CORTICOSTEROID effects (*see* prednisolone tablets).
Caution: in pregnant women, and in patients suffering from tuberculous, fungal, or viral infections, dermatitis. Do not use for prolonged periods.
Not to be used for:
Caution needed with:
Contains: LIGNOCAINE, ALUMINIUM ACETATE, ZINC OXIDE, HYDROCORTISONE acetate.
Other preparations: Xyloproct ointment.

---

yellow soft paraffin *see* **Lubrifilm**

Yomesan
(Bayer)

A yellow tablet supplied at a strength of 500 mg, and used as a vermicide to treat tapeworm.

Dose: as advised by your doctor.
Availability: NHS, private prescription.
Side effects: stomach upset, itching, light-headedness.
Caution:
Not to be used for:
Caution needed with: alcohol.
Contains: NICLOSAMIDE.
Other preparations:

Yutopar
(Solvay Healthcare)

A yellow, scored tablet supplied at a strength of 10 mg and used as a ß-agonist to treat premature labour.

Dose: 1 tablet about 30 minutes before ending intravenous treatment, 1 tablet every 2 hours for 24 hours, and then 1-2 tablets every 4-6 hours.
Availability: NHS and private prescription.
Side effects: rapid heart rate, flushing, sweating, nausea, chest pain, abnormal heart rhythm, anxiety, rise in blood sugar level, shaking, blood changes, liver changes.
Caution: in patients suffering from diabetes, or overactive thyroid. The heart rate of mother and foetus should be checked carefully.
Not to be used for: children or for patients suffering from heart disease or certain complications of pregnancy.
Caution needed with: MAOIS, ß-BLOCKERS, TRICYCLIC ANTIDEPRESSANTS, STEROIDS, SYMPATHOMIMETICS, ANAESTHETICS, some DIURETICS.
Contains: RITODRINE HYDROCHLORIDE.
Other preparations: Yutopar Injection.

Z Span Spansule
(Goldshield Healthcare)

A blue/clear capsule used as a zinc supplement for the prevention and treatment of zinc deficiency.

Dose: treatment, 1 capsule 1-3 times a day; prevention 1 capsule once a day.
Availability: NHS, private prescription, over the counter.
Side effects: stomach upset.
Caution: in patients suffering from kidney failure. Do not use high (treatment) doses for long periods.
Not to be used for: children.
Caution needed with: TETRACYCLINE ANTIBIOTICS.
Contains: ZINC SULPHATE monohydrate.
Other preparations: SOLVAZINC, ZINCOMED, ZINCOSOL.

Zaditen
(Sandoz)

A white, scored tablet supplied at a strength of 1 mg and used as an ANTIHISTAMINE preparation for the prevention of bronchial asthma, and the treatment of allergic rhinitis, conjunctivitis.

Dose: adults 1-2 tablets twice a day with food; children over 2 years 1 tablet twice a day with food.
Availability: NHS and private prescription.
Side effects: drowsiness, reduced reactions, dizziness, dry mouth,

Z

excitement, weight gain.
Caution: withdraw gradually.
Not to be used for: children under 2 years, pregnant women, nursing mothers.
Caution needed with: alcohol, sedatives, antidiabetics taken by mouth, other ANTIHISTAMINES.
Contains: KETOTIFEN.
Other preparations: Zaditen Capsules, Zaditen Elixir.

Zadstat *see* metronidazole tablets (and suppositories)
(Lederle)

---

zalcitabine *see* Hivid

Zantac
(Glaxo)

A white, five-sided tablet or white tablet supplied at strengths of 150 mg, 300 mg and used as a HISTAMINE H$_2$-ANTAGONIST to treat duodenal and gastric ulcers, oesophagitis, indigestion, oesophageal reflux, reduction of gastric acid.

Dose: children over 2 years for peptic ulcer only 2-4 mg per kilogram bodyweight twice a day up to 300 mg a day; adults 150 mg twice a day or 300 mg at bedtime for 28 days, 150 mg at bedtime thereafter; or as advised by a physician.
Availability: NHS and private prescription.
Side effects: headache, dizziness, occasionally hepatitis, low platelet counts, low white blood cell counts, allergy, confusion, breast symptoms.
Caution: exclude malignant disease. Care in pregnant women, nursing mothers, and in patients suffering from impaired kidney function.
Not to be used for: children under 2 years.
Caution needed with:
Contains: RANITIDINE.
Other preparations: Zantac effervescent, Zantac syrup, Zantac injection, Zantac-75 (a 75 mg tablet available over the counter only to treat heartburn and indigestion).

Zarontin
(Parke-Davis)

An amber-coloured capsule supplied at a strength of 250 mg and used as an anticonvulsant to treat epilepsy.

Z

Dose: adults and children over 6 years 2 tablets a day increasing as needed by 1 tablet a day every 4-7 days up to 8 tablets a day; children under 6 years 1 tablet a day at first increasing according to response.
Availability: NHS and private prescription.
Side effects: stomach and brain disturbances, rash, blood changes, SLE (a multisystem disorder).
Caution: in pregnant women, nursing mothers, and in patients suffering from kidney or liver disease. Dose should be decreased gradually.
Not to be used for:
Caution needed with:
Contains: ETHOSUXIMIDE.
Other preparations: Zarontin Syrup. EMESIDE.

Zeasorb
(Stiefel)

A dusting powder used to treat skin inflammation in areas such as between the thighs or beneath the breasts, excessive sweating, sweating brought on by using certain drugs.

Dose: as needed.
Availability: NHS, private prescription, over the counter.
Side effects:
Caution:
Not to be used for:
Caution needed with:
Contains: CHLOROXYLENOL, ALUMINIUM DIHYDROXYALLANTOINATE.
Other preparations:

Zestoretic *see* Carace Plus
(Zeneca)

Zestril
(Zeneca)

A white, pink, or red tablet according to strengths of 2.5 mg, 5 mg, 10 mg, 20 mg and used as an ACE INHIBITOR to treat congestive heart failure in addition to DIURETICS and DIGOXIN, high blood pressure.

Dose: 2.5 mg once a day at first increasing over 2-4 weeks to 5-20 mg once a day, or up to 40 mg a day for high blood pressure.
Availability: NHS and private prescription.
Side effects: low blood pressure, kidney failure, rash, dizziness, diarrhoea, cough, tiredness, palpitations, chest pain, fluid retention,

Z

weakness, headache, nausea, severe allergy.
Caution: in nursing mothers and in patients suffering from kidney disease, severe congestive heart failure, or who are undergoing anaesthesia or dialysis.
Not to be used for: children, pregnant women, or for patients suffering from some heart diseases or previous allergy to ACE inhibitors, kidney disorder following heart attack.
Caution needed with: some diuretics, potassium supplements, INDOMETHACIN, LITHIUM, blood-pressure lowering drugs.
Contains: LISINOPRIL.
Other preparations: CARACE.

---

zidovudine *see* Retrovir

Zimovane
(Rhône-Poulenc Rorer)

A white, scored tablet supplied at a strength of 7.5 mg and used as a sedative to treat sleeplessness.

Dose: 1 at bedtime; elderly ½ tablet only at first.
Availability: NHS and private prescription.
Side effects: metallic aftertaste, stomach upset, minor mental disturbance, allergy, drowsiness, impaired judgement and ability.
Caution: in patients suffering from liver disorder or during withdrawal.
Not to be used for: children, pregnant women, nursing mothers, or for patients suffering from severe breathing difficulties, MYASTHENIA GRAVIS.
Caution needed with: alcohol, other sedatives, TRIMIPRAMINE.
Contains: ZOPICLONE.
Other preparations:

Zinamide
(MSD)

A white, scored tablet supplied at a strength of 500 mg and used as an anti-tubercular drug in the additional treatment for tuberculosis.

Dose: 20-35 mg per kg body weight to a maximum of 3 g a day in divided doses.
Availability: NHS and private prescription.
Side effects: hepatitis.
Caution: in patients with a history of gout or diabetes. Your doctor may advise that liver function and blood should be checked regularly.
Not to be used for: children or for patients suffering from liver disease.

Z

Caution needed with:
Contains: PYRAZINAMIDE.
Other preparations:

---

zinc acetate *see* **Zineryt**

---

zinc and castor oil ointment BP *see* **zinc cream**

---

zinc and coal tar paste *see* **coal tar paste**

---

zinc cream BP

A cream used as an emollient to treat nappy and urine rashes, and eczema.

Dose: apply as needed.
Availability: NHS, private prescription, over the counter.
Side effects:
Caution:
Not to be used for:
Caution needed with:
Contains: ZINC OXIDE.
Other preparations: ZINC OINTMENT BP, ZINC AND CASTOR OIL OINTMENT BP.

---

zinc ointment BP *see* **zinc cream BP**

---

zinc oxide *see* **Anugesic-HC, Anusol, Anusol HC, Caladryl, calamine and coal tar ointment, coal tar paste, Sprilon, Sudocrem, Xyloproct, zinc cream BP**

---

zinc paste *see* **Ichthopaste, Icthaband, Quinaband, Tarband, Zincaband**

---

zinc pyrithione *see* **Polytar AF**

---

zinc sulphate eye drops

Eye drops supplied at a strength of 0.25% and used as an astringent to treat excessive tear production.

Dose: as advised by doctor.
Availability: NHS, private prescription, over the counter.
Side effects:
Caution:
Not to be used for:
Caution needed with:
Contains: ZINC SULPHATE.
Other preparations:

---

zinc sulphate *see* **Efalith, Solvazinc, Z Span Spansule, zinc sulphate eye drops, Zincomed, Zincosol**

Zincaband
(Seton Healthcare)

A zinc paste bandage used, in conjunction with a compression bandage, to treat varicose and gravitational ulcers, and chronic skin eczema or dermatitis.

Availability: NHS, private prescription, over the counter. (Also available on a trial basis from nurses.)
Contains: ZINC PASTE.

Zincomed *see* **Z Span Spansule**
(Medo)

Zincosol *see* **Z Span Spansule**
(Bioceuticals)

Zineryt
(Yamanouchi)

A solution used as an antibiotic to treat acne.

Dose: apply twice a day.
Availability: NHS and private prescription.
Side effects: irritation.
Caution: avoid eyes and mucous membranes.
Not to be used for:
Caution needed with:

Z

Contains: ERYTHROMYCIN, ZINC ACETATE.
Other preparations:

Zinga *see* Axid Capsules
(Ashbourne)

Zinnat
(Glaxo)

A white tablet supplied at strengths of 125 mg, 250 mg and used as a cephalosporin antibiotic to treat respiratory, ear, nose, and throat, skin, soft tissue, and urinary infections.

Dose: adults usually 250-500 mg twice a day, urinary infections 125 mg twice a day, gonorrhoea 1 g as one dose; children 3 months-2 years 125 mg twice a day, over 2 years 250 mg twice a day.
Availability: NHS and private prescription.
Side effects: stomach disturbances, allergy, colitis, blood changes, thrush, change in liver chemistry, headache, interference with some blood tests.
Caution: in pregnant women, nursing mothers, and in patients who are allergic to penicillin.
Not to be used for:
Caution needed with:
Contains: CEFUROXIME AXETIL.
Other preparations:

Zirtek
(UCB Pharma)

A white, oblong, scored tablet supplied at a strength of 10 mg and used as an ANTIHISTAMINE treatment for rhinitis, allergy.

Dose: adults and children over 6 years 1 tablet a day in the morning.
Availability: NHS private prescription.
Side effects: drowsiness, dizziness, headache, agitation, stomach disturbances, dry mouth.
Caution: in pregnant women and in patients suffering from kidney disease.
Not to be used for: children under 6 years, nursing mothers.
Caution needed with: sedatives, alcohol.
Contains: CETIRIZINE DIHYDROCHLORIDE.
Other preparations:

Z

Zita *see* **cimetidine tablets**
(Eastern)

Zithromax
(Richborough)

A white capsule supplied at a strength of 250 mg, and used as an antibiotic to treat respiratory, soft tissue, skin, ear, and genital infections.

Dose: adults, 2 capsules a day for 3 days. For genital infection 4 capsules as a single dose. Children use suspension.
Availability: NHS and private prescription.
Side effects: stomach upset, liver changes, allergy, rash, fluid retention, shock.
Caution: in pregnant women, nursing mothers, and in patients with kidney or liver damage.
Not to be used for: patients suffering from liver disease.
Caution needed with: ERGOTAMINE, ANTACIDS, CYCLOSPORIN, DIGOXIN, WARFARIN.
Contains: AZITHROMYCIN.
Other preparations: Zithromax Suspension.

Zocor
(M.S.D.)

A peach-coloured, oval tablet or a tan, oval tablet according to strengths of 10 mg, 20 mg and used as a lipid-lowering agent to treat raised cholesterol to reduce risk of heart attack, and slow progression of coronary heart disease.

Dose: 10-40 mg taken at night.
Availability: NHS and private prescription.
Side effects: headache, indigestion, diarrhoea, tiredness, rash, constipation, wind, nausea, stomach pain, cramps, dizziness, hair loss, muscle weakness, liver disorder, anaemia, pins and needles, inflamed pancreas, sensitivity to light.
Caution: in patients suffering from or with a history of liver disease. Your doctor may advise liver and eye checks. Use non-hormonal contraceptive methods.
Not to be used for: children, pregnant women, nursing mothers, or for patients suffering from liver disease.
Caution needed with: DIGOXIN, some ANTICOAGULANTS, CYCLOSPORIN, GEMIFIBROZIL, ERYTHROMYCIN, some antifungals, VITAMIN B_3, drugs affecting the immune system.
Contains: SIMVASTATIN.
Other preparations:

Z

Zofran
(Glaxo)

Yellow, oval tablets supplied at strengths of 4 mg, 8 mg, and used to treat nausea and vomiting associated with cancer treatment or surgical operation.

Dose: as advised by doctor.
Availability: NHS and private prescription.
Side effects: constipation, headache, flushing, liver changes, allergy.
Caution: in pregnant women.
Not to be used for: nursing mothers.
Caution needed with:
Contains: ONDANSETRON.
Other preparations: Zofran Injection.

Zoladex
(Zeneca)

An implant supplied at a strength of 3.6 mg, and used as a hormone treatment for endometriosis or prethinning of the endometrium before surgical procedures.

Dose: endometriosis: 1 implant inserted beneath the skin into the front wall of the abdomen every 28 days for up to 6 months; prethinning: use same dosage for 4-8 weeks.
Availability: NHS, private prescription.
Side effects: hot flushes, emotional upsets, changes in size of breasts or in sexual function, rash, headaches, dryness of the vagina. Your doctor will advise you to use non-hormonal methods of contraception.
Caution: in patients at risk of osteoporosis.
Not to be used for: children, pregnant women, nursing mothers.
Caution needed with:
Contains: GOSERELIN.
Other preparations:

---

zolpidem *see* **Stilnoct**

---

zopiclone *see* **Zimovane**

Zoton
(Lederle)

A lilac and purple capsule supplied at a strength of 30 mg and used as a
710

drug to treat stomach ulcers and acid reflux.

Dose: 1 capsule a day taken in the morning before eating for 4-8 weeks depending on the condition.
Availability: NHS, private prescription.
Side effects: headache, stomach upset, changed liver function, skin irritation; rarely blood changes, swelling of the hands and feet, depression, joint pain.
Caution: in pregnant women and nursing mothers.
Not to be used for: children.
Caution needed with: the contraceptive pill, PHENYTOIN, THEOPHYLLINE, WARFARIN, ANTACIDS, SUCRALFATE.
Contains: LANSOPRAZOLE.
Other preparations:

Zovirax Tablets *see* aciclovir tablets
(Wellcome)

Zovirax Cream
(Wellcome)

A cream used as an antiviral treatment for cold sores on the skin.

Dose: apply 5 times a day (every 4 hours) for up to 10 days (5 days are usually enough).
Availability: NHS, private prescription.
Side effects: reddening and flaking of the skin.
Caution: in patients with kidney disorders.
Not to be used for: eye conditions.
Caution needed with: PROBENECID.
Contains: ACICLOVIR.
Other preparations: Zovirax tablets and suspension, Zovirax Cold Sore Cream (available over the counter only to treat cold sores on the mouth and face).

Zovirax Eye Ointment
(Wellcome)

An ointment used as an antiviral treatment for herpes simplex infection of the cornea.

Dose: insert 1 cm length of ointment into the corner of the eye 5 times a day every 4 hours for at least 3 days after healing.
Availability: NHS and private prescription.

Z

Side effects: mild smarting, superficial punctate inflammation of the cornea.
Caution:
Not to be used for:
Caution needed with:
Contains: ACICLOVIR.
Other preparations:

---

zuclopenthixol *see* **Clopixol**

Zumenon *see* **Climaval**
(Solvay Healthcare)

Zyda-Co *see* **co-amilozide tablets**
(Opus)

Zydol
(Searle Pharmaceuticals)

A green/yellow capsule supplied at a strength of 50 mg and used as an opiate analgesic to treat moderate to severe pain.

Dose: 1-2 capsules at first, then 1-2 no more often than every 4 hours up to a maximum of 8 capsules a day.
Availability: NHS, private prescription.
Side effects: nausea, vomiting, dry mouth, drowsiness, tiredness, dizziness, rash, sweating, confusion, hallucinations, headache; rarely heart or circulation changes, breathing difficulties, convulsions, dependence, blood changes, anxiety and restlessness.
Caution: in the elderly, and in patients suffering from severe liver or kidney disorders, raised pressure on the brain, or a history of breathing difficulties or convulsions.
Not to be used for: children, pregnant women, nursing mothers.
Caution needed with: alcohol, sedatives, MAOIS, CARBAMAZEPINE.
Contains: TRAMADOL hydrochloride.
Other preparations: Zydol SR (long-acting preparation), Zydol injection.

Zyloric *see* **allopurinol tablets**
(Wellcome)

Z

For each of the medicines described in detail in this book, there is a paragraph headed 'Not to be used with'. This paragraph includes other medicines, groups of medicines, substances such as alcohol, or even foods which should not be taken at the same time as the drug described. This is because the medicine may interact with one or more of the substances mentioned in an unpleasant, harmful, or potentially dangerous way. On the other hand, for an individual patient, there may be no serious interaction at all.

The purpose of the chart set out below is to depict, using a simple and familiar technique, whether or not major 'families' of medicines have been found to interact with one another in any way. It does not attempt to show the degree of interaction. To work out whether or not a medicine you have been prescribed is likely to interact with any other substance, just pick out the family to which it belongs in the vertical column, and trace it horizontally across the chart. Where a '●' occurs, trace down the chart and you will find the name of the substance with which it may interact.

For detailed information concerning interactions, you should, of course, refer to the 'Not to be used with' paragraph for the particular medicine you have been prescribed.

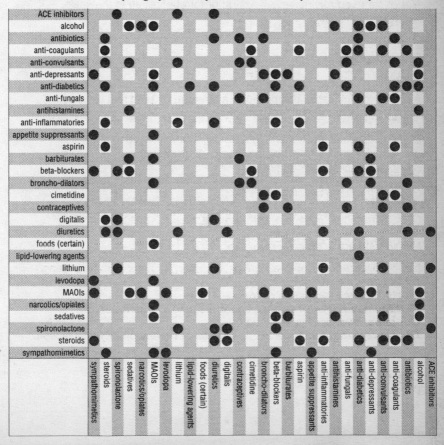

STOP PRESS

Curatoderm
(Merck)

An ointment used as a vitamin D treatment for some forms of psoriasis.

Dose: apply sparingly once daily at bedtime. (Maximum of 5 g per day.)
Up to 2 courses of 8 weeks treatment per year may be used.
Availability: NHS, private prescription.
Side effects: itching, reddening, burning and tingling of skin.
Caution: in pregnant women, and in patients suffering from kidney
disorders or certain forms of psoriasis. Avoid contact with eyes. Wash
hands after use. Avoid exposure to ultraviolet light immediately after
treatment.
Not to be used for: nursing mothers, or for application to the scalp.
Contains: tacalcitol.

Entocort CR
(Astra)

A grey and pink capsule supplied at a strength of 3 mg and used as a
CORTICOSTEROID treatment for Crohn's disease.

Dose: 3 capsules each morning before breakfast for up to 8 weeks.
(Reduce the dose for the last 2-4 weeks of treatment.)
Availability: NHS, private prescription.
Cautions, warnings, and side effects: as for other oral STEROID therapy
(*see* prednisolone tablets). In addition:
Side effects: indigestion, muscle cramps, heart rhythm disturbances,
blurred vision and menstrual disturbances have also been reported.
Not to be used for: pregnant women, nursing mothers.
Not to be used with: CHOLESTYRAMINE.
Contains: BUDESONIDE.

Notes

Notes

Notes

Notes

Notes

Notes